Hutchison's
Clinical Methods

The Educational Low-Priced Books Scheme is funded
by the Overseas Development Administration as part
of the British Government overseas aid programme.
It makes available low-priced, unabridged editions of
British publishers' textbooks to students in developing countries. Below is a list of some other medical
books published under the ELBS imprint.

Edwards *et al.* (editors)
Davidson's Principles and Practice of Medicine
Churchill Livingstone

Kumar and Clark (editors)
Clinical Medicine
Baillière Tindall

Munro and Edwards (editors)
Macleod's Clinical Examination
Churchill Livingstone

McMinn and Hutchings
A Colour Atlas of Human Anatomy
Wolfe Publishing

Ogilvie and Evans
**Chamberlain's Symptoms and Signs in Clinical
Medicine**
Butterworth-Heinemann

Romanes
**Cunningham's Manual of Practical Anatomy
Vols 1–3**
Oxford University Press

Hutchison's
Clinical Methods

Twentieth Edition

MICHAEL SWASH MD FRCP FRCPath
Consultant Physician, The Royal London Hospital, UK
Professor of Neurology, The London Medical College, London, UK

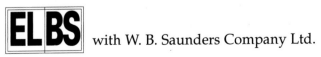 with W. B. Saunders Company Ltd.

Educational Low-Priced Books Scheme
funded by the British Government

W. B. Saunders Company Ltd
24–28 Oval Road, London NW1 7DX

First published 1897
Seventeenth edition 1980
Eighteenth edition 1984
Reprinted 1985
Nineteenth edition 1989
Reprinted 1990, 1992, 1993
Twentieth edition 1995

ELBS edition first published 1975
Reprinted 1975, 1976
ELBS edition of seventeenth edition 1980
Reprinted 1981 (twice), 1982
ELBS edition of eighteenth edition 1984
Reprinted 1985, 1986
ELBS edition of nineteenth edition 1989
Reprinted 1990, 1992, 1993
ELBS edition of twentieth edition 1995

ISBN 0 7020 1676 4

Typeset by Wyvern Typesetting, Bristol
Printed and bound in Great Britain by
BPC Paulton, Bristol

Contents

Sir Robert Hutchison MD FRCP (1871–1960)

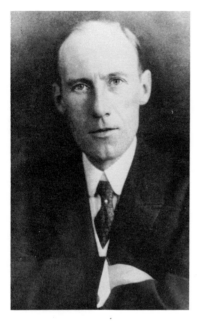

Clinical Methods began in 1897, three years after Robert Hutchison was appointed Assistant Physician to The London Hospital. He was appointed full physician to The London and to the Hospital for Sick Children, Great Ormond Street, in 1900. He steered *Clinical Methods* through no less than 13 editions, at first with the assistance of Dr H. Rainy and then, from the 9th edition, published in 1929, with the help of Dr Donald Hunter. Although Hutchison retired from hospital practice in 1934 he continued to direct new editions of the book wth Donald Hunter, and from 1949 with the assistance also of Dr Richard Bomford. The 13th edition, the first produced without Hutchison's guiding hand, was published in 1956 under the direction of Donald Hunter and Richard Bomford. Dr A. Stuart Mason and the present author joined Richard Bomford on Donald Hunter's retirement to produce the 16th edition, published in 1975, and following Richard Bomford's retirement prepared the 17th, 18th and 19th editions. Each of these editions was revised with the help of colleagues at The Royal London Hospital, in keeping with the tradition that lies behind the book.

During the many years of its continuous publication *Clinical Methods* has been translated into many languages. Indeed it is one of the great pleasures of association with the book to receive letters from far parts of the world, offering friendly advice, criticism and correction. Students have often noted errors that have escaped the eye of the editors.

Sir Robert Hutchison died in 1960 in his 90th year. It is evident from the memoirs of his contemporaries that he had a remarkable personality. Many of his clinical sayings became, in their day, aphorisms to be remembered and passed on to future generations of students. Of these the best known is his petition, written in his 82nd year:

'From inability to let well alone;
from too much zeal for the new and contempt for what is old;
from putting knowledge before wisdom, science before art, and
cleverness before common sense;
from treating patients as cases;
and from making the cure of the disease more grievous than the
endurance of the same, Good Lord, deliver us.'

Michael Swash
The Royal London Hospital

Preface to the twentieth edition

Clinical Methods is a book for students of all ages and all degrees of experience. We all have gaps in our knowledge and this book should help fill them. It is intended to provide insight into the acquisition of the traditional clinical skills of history-taking and physical examination, and of the increasingly complex and accurate methods available to the modern clinician from the biochemist, physicist, physiologist or computer engineer. If modern investigative methods are to be applied to patient care intelligently, with economy and with compassion, they must be integrated with traditional methods. The latter remain invaluable and irreplaceable clinical skills. Extended investigations and more complex managements must be both useful and humane. The art of the clinician, mentioned by Robert Hutchison in his petition, is essentially the art of understanding, communication and explanation.

In his own day Hutchison was concerned to explain those tests that were important in his clinical practice, particularly bacteriology, urine testing, radiology, and the beginnings of electrical tests of muscular function. In continuing this integrated approach to clinical practice, brief accounts of modern methods of investigation are given throughout the 20th edition of the book. These are intended to give some idea both of the principles underlying them, and of the indications for their use.

In this 20th edition of *Clinical Methods*, there are new chapters on the examination of elderly people, on endocrinology and on ethics. All the other chapters have been substantially revised and rearranged.

This comprehensive revision has included the development of a new colour format, designed to facilitate use of the book as a source of information and learning. None the less, faithful, older readers will continue to recognize in *Clinical Methods* an old friend; a friend offering some new information, together with much that is well-tried, and that ought to be as well-known to new generations of students as it was to their teachers when they were students. Good clinical method, Robert Hutchison said, is still the root of the matter.

Once again several new contributors have joined the book. Some have contributed entirely new chapters and others have modified the work of their predecessors. Thus *Hutchison's Clinical Methods* is not the work of any individual but is the result of close collaboration between clinical colleagues in their practice at The Royal London Hospital. The editor carefully moulds and modifies the individual contributions so as to integrate them into a single text. Throughout the book an attempt has been made to indicate particularly important matters, and to suggest the diagnostic relevance of certain findings. The book may therefore be used not only as a text of clinical methods but as a supplement to textbooks of medicine, surgery and the specialties. It may be read from cover to cover or approached piecemeal, as seems appropriate. Constructive criticisms are, as always, welcomed.

Michael Swash
The Royal London Hospital

Acknowledgements

This book represents the efforts of many colleagues. For many years, through many editions, the book has been formed from contributions by the staff of The Royal London Hospital. The final text, however, is a product of the editor's pen, since much work is required to avoid repetitions and omissions, and to make sure that the various parts of the clinical assessment and examination are described in the most relevant part of the book. Any errors, therefore, are the responsibility of the editor.

In this 20th edition there have been extensive revisions, with much new writing, reflecting the rapid pace of change in clinical practice that has occurred in recent years. The traditional reliance on colleagues at The Royal London Hospital has continued. I am most grateful for the hard work of my many colleagues in joining me in producing this new edition, and especially for their forebearance in allowing their ideas to be changed so as to be subservient to the whole endeavour. I record their contributions below. The list represents the major contributors to each chapter, upon whose work the final product is based.

I would also like to thank our patients, and our students, without whom the experience from which this book is ultimately derived would not have been gained.

Principal contributors to chapters:

1 Doctor and patient
   Professor Michael Swash
2 The psychiatric assessment
   Dr Jeremy Pfeffer
3 The skin, nails and hair
   Dr Rino Cerio
4 The endocrine system and metabolic disorders
   Dr John Monson
5 The gastrointestinal tract and abdomen
   Dr Paul Swain
6 The kidneys and the urinary system
   Dr Frank Marsh
7 The respiratory system
   Dr Duncan Empey
8 The cardiovascular system
   Dr Peter Mills
9 The ear, nose and throat
   Mr Guy Kenyon and Mr Duncan McRae
10 The eye
   Mr Ivor Levy
11 The locomotor system
   Dr David Perry
12 The nervous system
   Professor Michael Swash
13 The unconscious patient
   Professor Michael Swash
14 The examination of women
   Mr Trevor Beedham
15 The examination of children
   Dr Roger Harris
16 The examination of elderly people
   Dr Gerry Bennett
17 The genitalia and sexually transmitted diseases
   Dr Beng Goh
18 The blood
   Dr Brian Colvin and Professor Adrian Newland
19 Parasites in the blood and faeces
   Dr Christine Facer and Dr Gordon Cook
20 Using the laboratory
   Dr Elizabeth Shaw
21 Ethical issues in medicine
   Professor Michael Swash

CHAPTER 1

Doctor and patient

Introduction

The principles of medicine are difficult to define. They represent the interaction of clinical experience with knowledge acquired by study and are revealed gradually during a clinical lifetime; there is always something new to learn. *Clinical methods* is the term used to describe a properly organized approach to the patient and to his or her disease. It is a truism that 'diagnosis should precede treatment whenever possible', but the wise doctor should always strive not simply to be a diagnostician but rather someone who elucidates human problems, so as to help the patient and family manage the problems caused by a disease and, where possible, offer treatment, cure or prevention. Patients present with problems, i.e.

symptoms, that require definition and resolution. The underlying diagnosis is often of more interest to the doctor than it is to the patient, although the diagnosis is of fundamental importance in deciding how best to relieve the patient's presenting symptoms. In many instances it is possible to relieve these symptoms even though the underlying disease may be unresponsive to treatment. Labelling a disease process is but one step in the management of a clinical problem.

There are two main steps in making a diagnosis:
• The first is to establish the clinical features by history-taking, physical examination and investigation. This represents the clinical database.
• The second step is the interpretation of these data, if possible, in terms of disordered function and structure, that is pathology. Remember that pathology can mean disease or social pathology.

This book is about these two steps—the clinical database and its functional interpretation.

Communication: the art of history-taking

The aim of history-taking is to elicit an accurate account of the symptoms that represent the clinical problem and to set this against the background of the patient's life. The findings should be recorded under the headings listed in Box 1.1.

> **BOX 1.1 Headings to be used in history-taking.**
>
> - Age and address
> - Marital status
> - Social and occupational history
> - History of previous illness
> - Family history
> - Presenting complaint
> - History of present illness
> - Treatment history

Many experienced doctors prefer to obtain details of a patient's social, occupational, past medical and family history before discussing the presenting complaint, since this provides a context within which the presenting illness can be viewed. Further, it is often wise to find out about the patient's life, at least to some degree, before tackling the presenting illness itself. However, in taking the history it is neither possible nor desirable to tie a patient down to any particular sequence; the patient should always be encouraged to tell their story in their own way. The experienced doctor begins the consultation from the moment the patient walks into the room—the general appearance, dress, attitude, gait, vocabulary and personality—and only finishes when the patient has left. Occasionally, the physical examination may suggest new aspects of the history, or a vital piece of information may come out just as the patient is leaving.

The list of headings may appear formidable and it does take some experience to know in a given case which part of the history is particularly worth pursuing. Indeed, understanding the subtle variation of personal experience in a given syndrome, is both a skill and a joy in medical practice. If, for instance, the patient's complaint is bleeding, a careful *family*

history may suggest the diagnosis. If there are chest symptoms, a history of *occupational* exposure to asbestos even 20 years earlier may be the vital clue. If the symptoms are those of a severe anaemia, previous *treatment* with chloramphenicol may be all-important. If a businessman presents with fever and sweats, the fact that his plane put down in West Africa (*social history*) may be the clue. These are rare examples; more commonly it may be the *social circumstances*, e.g. interpersonal relations with spouse or employer, that are at fault. At least some enquiry should be made under all the headings listed. If given the opportunity the patient will usually provide the clue.

In a simple problem, provided one can be sure that the problem really is simple, a few direct questions may elicit all the necessary information. As a rule it is best just to let the patient talk, even if the process seems time-consuming.

Communicating with the patient

History-taking is a special form of communication. It is necessarily a two-way business, involving two people studying each other. This is the beginning of the doctor–patient relationship on which depends both the relevance of the patient's history and their confidence in the doctor. For many patients, consulting a doctor is an ordeal as daunting as a *viva voce* examination for students, and however anxious the patient is to seek medical advice, there is often a subconscious fear that the doctor is a threatening, formidable figure. The doctor must put the patient at ease and encourage him or her to talk freely.

Common courtesy goes a long way in establishing good communication, so greet the patient by name, if possible. Whenever meeting a patient for the first time, be friendly, say who you are and what your role is. It is usually possible to start the interview with some non-committal remarks. The discovery of a common town of origin or a mutual interest in a hobby or a pet may work wonders. Watch the patient's gestural language; the eyes, for example, may tell you more than what is actually said, and the hands can give valuable clues as to the underlying mood. Observe the patient's face from time to time and try to establish eye contact. Do they appear at ease, anxious, shifty or embarrassed? Consider whether something is being hidden or whether you have understood all the implications of the symptoms.

Make it clear from your stance, gestures and expression that the patient has your whole attention and that you will not be shocked or angered by anything said. If you *are* embarrassed try not to show it. Gazing out of the window or continually writing notes will put off the patient. Never underestimate the power of communication inherent in touching your patient. Try holding the hand of a frightened old lady and see how it gives her more comfort than your words of reassurance. When it comes to physical examination does the patient feel your touch as an attack or caress? Gentleness is all-important; abdominal palpation, for example, must be both firm and gentle to be successful. Patients are often greatly reassured by a thorough and gentle examination. It is all part of gaining the patient's confidence. Always tell the patient what you are doing, and try never to cause pain.

In telling the history the patient may appear to be evasive; this is seldom, if ever, deliberate. It may be due to dementia, aphasia or subnormal intelligence, but more commonly it is due to anxiety or even fright. Evasiveness is, of course, particularly common if the real problem is a sexual one or involves feelings of guilt. Sometimes the symptoms cannot be put easily into words. 'I feel rotten' or 'I just don't feel myself' may be the presenting complaint of many different disorders. Psychological symptoms are often difficult to express. Many people feel that such symptoms are not respectable and substitute complaints of vaguely described physical discomfort, often implying multiple, unrelated symptoms. Later, such a patient may say that everything is hopeless and there is nothing left to live for; in other words, he or she is depressed. An anxious patient may present with symptoms of indigestion, headache or palpitations; later an ever-present feeling that something awful is about to happen may be voiced. Indeed this feeling may have become so much a part of everyday life that the patient is almost unaware of it.

It is important for the doctor to recognize that there is always a reason for difficult behaviour. Anger and exasperation are natural reactions if the doctor does not make a determined attempt to tolerate a patient and discover why an interview is arousing mutual antipathy, and should be recognized as warning signs of misunderstanding. We all have our own strengths and weaknesses in personal relationships. The doctor must know his or her own personality, recognize weaknesses, and develop strengths and abilities. This is an essential part of acquiring excellence in clinical methods.

If you find yourself feeling angry with your patient, or confused about the history, recognize that this is a problem in communication that may reflect an abnormality in the patient's ability to remember or to describe their problem, or consider the possibility of a cultural barrier between you. Do not allow your feelings to surface into confrontation; try starting the interview afresh by saying: 'I have not quite got this clear yet; let's go over it again so that I get it right'. Communication with the patient, to establish the patient's personal, social and medical background in relation to the details of the development of the current illness, together with the process of physical examination, are the means of developing the all-important relationship between patient and doctor.

There is no one technique of history-taking applicable to all patients in all situations. The approach will vary according to whether the history is being taken in the wards, the out-patient clinic, the surgery or the home, and also according to the state of the patient and the time available. Having introduced oneself by name and established the patient's identity, age and address, and made the patient feel at ease, it is wise to open any consultation with some general question such as 'What can I do for you?' or 'How can I help you?' or 'What's the trouble?' This gives the patient an opportunity to begin the consultation, and encourages relevance.

Patients must be allowed as far as possible to tell their story in their own words and in their own way. Only when they have done this should they be asked to enlarge on what appear to be the more important aspects of the story and only after that should specific questions be asked. History-taking must never become a stereotyped routine of asking standard questions and recording the answers, though questionnaires may be useful for special purposes. None the less, a structured approach to details of the past medical history, family history, personal and social background and drug history is a valuable means of avoiding omissions, and early enquiry about these matters will establish this information independently of the current problem.

In spite of the proliferation of modern diagnostic tests, history-taking and physical examination remain essential skills. Those who work in large modern hospitals are apt to forget that most of the world's population are treated with restricted facilities. Even where modern scientific and imaging technologies are freely available, they are in varying degrees costly and are not always without discomfort or risk to the patient. It was Hutchison, the original author of this book, who wrote: 'From making the cure of the disease more grievous than the endurance of the same, good Lord deliver us.'

The presenting complaint

Try to define the main complaint and its duration. The presenting complaint is simply the problem which made the patient seek medical help. Patients are rarely deliberately evasive, but many find considerable difficulty putting their symptoms into words, particularly when their symptoms are outside ordinary experience, as in many neurological problems. In these instances it may be helpful to supply a list of alternatives, e.g. does a pain feel hot, sharp, dull, throbbing, inside, etc?

Some patients have more than one main complaint and a few, particularly the anxious or neurotic, have so many that it is impossible to identify a single presenting complaint. For these patients, the presenting complaints themselves represent the problem, rather than the underlying diagnosis. Of course, if the latter proves to be a serious matter, for example a malignant tumour or other progressive disorder, then the underlying disease assumes overwhelming priority for both the patient and the doctor.

The timing and duration of symptomatic events is especially important since the chronology of the illness will provide valuable clues to the pathological process underlying it. The question of duration may be difficult. Many people, particularly the elderly, often find it difficult to remember the duration of their symptoms. One could, indeed, regard this as the normal state of affairs and suspect the patient who can remember every detail of his or her illness as being unduly introspective and hypochondriacal.

Most patients with long-standing symptoms tend to date them by events rather than by years, even though there is no causal relationship. The symptoms started 'after my husband died' or 'at the time of the last general election'. Sometimes it is possible to date symptoms only by referring them to the seasons of the year or to national or religious holidays, such as Christmas. With patience it is possible to ascertain the likely duration. After that it is wise to ask questions such as: 'Did you ever have anything wrong before that?' or even: 'When were you last perfectly well?' In this way earlier symptoms, which the patient regards as unimportant, may be revealed. Remember that some people use the word 'chronic' to mean 'severe', rather than of prolonged duration.

The history of the present illness

Ask the patient to tell you the story of the illness from the beginning. Ideally you should allow this to continue virtually without interruption, but this may be a counsel of perfection. It may require some tactful encouragement to make a dour or nervous patient tell you their story at all, while some talkative ones cannot keep anywhere near the point. A particular difficulty is the patient who will use pseudomedical terms without really knowing the medical meaning. Patients who insist on talking about rheumatism, migraine, acidity, catarrh or discs should be gently discouraged and asked to describe what they actually feel to be wrong. Others will insist on talking about 'what my other doctor said'. Remember that these attitudes are almost always the consequence of the patient having rehearsed the problem before coming to the consultation, and imply an interpreted, often thoughtful view of what the patient *expects* the doctor wants to know. Well-meaning though it is, this is not always appropriate.

The patient may be accompanied by a friend or relative, or even by several people. Always begin by talking with the patient, excluding others, however well-meaning, from the conversation. Later, you may find it helpful to seek clarification, or even an alternative or objective view of the history, for example of epileptic attack, from the relative or friend. The history must represent an exchange between the physician and the patient, however, and not a semi-public discussion about an illness, involving several people.

When the patient has given you an initial description of their symptoms, suggest that you would like to find out more about certain aspects. Choose one or two points that you think are important or that you may have misunderstood. Try to clear up doubts about the time of onset and the duration of the main symptoms. Some patients have symptoms which come and go, and it is then important to try to find out whether the relapses and remissions are related in any way to times, seasons or events in the patient's life.

When you think you have understood the patient's story clearly, you should take each main symptom in turn and examine it in detail. The first step is to make sure that you and the patient are talking about the same thing. Ask the patient to rephrase any part of the story if their original description was unclear to you. Sometimes the history has to be elaborated before it can be understood. A patient may, for instance, complain of wind or flatulence. Since flatus is considered in Western culture to be an indelicate subject, it may be assumed that this means bringing up wind, whereas the patient may well mean passing wind by the back passage; or it may mean a feeling of wanting to get rid of wind but being unable to do so. Therefore enquire directly: 'Do you mean that you bring the wind up or that you pass it down or that you feel that you want to get rid of it but can't?' Although one should avoid, as far as possible, leading questions which themselves suggest an answer, other direct questions, such as 'Have you ever coughed blood?' may be essential. With experience, certain suggestions lend themselves to a rather stereotyped pattern of analysis. Remember that symptom analysis can be achieved only when the database is complete. Completion of the database is itself a function of the success of communication between doctor and patient.

ANALYSIS OF PAIN

Perhaps the commonest complaint which brings a patient to a doctor is a pain of some sort and this will serve to illustrate aspects of the way in which the nature of a symptom can be further explored (see Box 1.2). Ask about the following points:

Site. Where is it? Note whether the patient points with a finger to one spot or with the hands to an area on the affected part of the body.

Radiation. Does it stay in one place, or does it move or spread? It may gradually extend, or shoot along the distribution of a peripheral nerve or nerve root.

Severity. Does it interfere with daily activities or keep you awake at night? If the answers to these questions are 'Never', the pain is unlikely to be severe; however, some people are quite stoic in enduring severe pain. Patients who use exaggerated terms such as 'continual agony' are usually seeking sympathy and one should try to discover the real reason for their distress, which is more often social or psychological than the result of serious physical illness. Headache that never lets up, day or night, and that apparently prevents sleep—'I can't sleep at all with it, doctor'—is strongly suggestive of anxiety and depressive symptoms.

Timing and duration. When did it start? When does it come and when does it go? Has it changed since it began?

Character. What is it like? Descriptions of the character of a pain, e.g. stabbing, burning, pricking or gnawing, may be helpful, although it is very difficult for anyone to describe a pain in words. The distinction between an abdominal colic, which waxes and wanes and may cause a patient to roll about, and a steady pain like that of peritonitis, which causes the patient to try to avoid all movement, is very important in diagnosis.

Occurrence or aggravation. What brings it on? And what makes it worse? A pain in the centre of the chest which always comes on after a certain amount of exertion, or is made worse by exertion, is almost certainly due to ischaemia of the heart (angina). A very similar pain which comes on a short time after eating is probably oesophageal.

Relief. What makes it better? Pains may be relieved by simple measures. Pain arising in the musculoskeletal system, for instance, may be relieved by a change of position. Upper gastrointestinal pains, e.g. duodenal ulcers, are usually promptly relieved by eating. Lower gastrointestinal pains may be relieved by defaecation or the passage of wind. Cardiac pain, brought on by exertion, is relieved by rest. The discomfort of oesophageal reflux is often relieved by belching. Any definite relief by simple responses or maneouvres may be a valuable clue to the disturbance of function or structure involved.

The effect of drugs may also be of diagnostic value. Ischaemic cardiac pain is usually promptly relieved by trinitrites. Musculoskeletal pains are usually relieved by simple analgesics like aspirin, while discomforts associated with stress and tension are not.

BOX 1.2 Analysis of pain as a symptom.

- Site
- Radiation
- Severity
- Timing and duration
- Character
- Occurrence or aggravation
- Relief

SYMPTOM ANALYSIS

Pain is a symptom which can be explored in *clinical terms* in order to direct physical examination, and then clinical investigation, toward delineation of the cause of the pain, and its treatment. Other symptoms may have a *physiological* basis and thus can be considered more specifically. As an example, let us look at thirst.

Thirst must first be distinguished from the dry mouth of oral infections or of defective salivary secretion. Compulsive water drinkers complain of severe thirst but are seldom woken up by it. Thirst, however, is most commonly the prime symptom of loss of body water (with or without loss of salt). The principal causes of loss of body water are diminished intake, vomiting, diarrhoea, increased sweating (with fever or exposure to heat), increased output of urine and severe haemorrhage. Observation or simple questions will therefore uncover the immediate disorder of function or functions that are responsible for the symptom, but further questions and investigations may be necessary to explain it in terms of pathology.

Thirst associated with loss of body water due to increased urinary output should suggest diabetes mellitus. In this disorder the urine contains glucose and is of high specific gravity. In diabetes insipidus, on the other hand, the urine is of low specific gravity (<1.010). The passage of large amounts of urine with a specific gravity of 1.010 (isotonic with plasma) in renal failure may be sufficient to cause a thirst that persists both by day and night. Hypercalcaemia, by diminishing the action of antidiuretic hormone and so increasing water loss, may produce thirst. Finally, the administration of diuretics (including excessive tea or coffee drinking and alcohol) may promote salt and water loss with increased urine volume and so thirst.

These two examples, pain and thirst, thus serve to illustrate different ways in which all-important symptoms should be explored, with the object of identifying, if possible, the disturbance of function and/or structure responsible for them.

Course of the illness

In analysing symptoms it is important to consider the course or shape of the illness. Did it begin insidiously and gradually worsen or is it intermittent? Is it of acute onset, slowly getting better, but not yet gone? Does it relate to some past illness or to a chronic disorder already diagnosed? Sometimes the shape of the illness may be more significant than individual symptoms. Sudden events are often due to trauma or to vascular disease; progressive painful disorders suggest infection or neoplasm, and inexorably progressive or chronic conditions suggest degenerative disease.

Reason for presentation

Another valuable question in patients with long-standing symptoms (particularly psychological ones) is: 'What made you decide to come and see me at this particular time?' The answer is sometimes illuminating. It may well be: 'I wouldn't have dreamt of coming, but my wife made me', or it may be because a friend died recently with rather similar symptoms.

Review of systems

Later in this chapter (pages 9–14) there is a scheme of the kinds of questions doctors often ask their patients. This scheme is arranged under anatomical systems (see Box 1.4), the main purpose being to ensure that no symptom or disorder is neglected. It is not intended that every patient should be asked all these questions, but some enquiry must be made by direct questioning in order to exclude, as far as possible, other disease processes, even if there is no immediate reason to suspect them. When the patient has told their story and the stage of examining individual symptoms is reached, the doctor should be thinking: 'Are we both talking about the same thing?' and then: 'What does this symptom mean in terms of disturbance of function and/or structure?' A list of standard questions is not an example of good communication.

The history of previous illness

The previous history should include all important illnesses, operations and injuries from infancy onwards. Beware of accepting ready-made diagnoses, particularly such ill-defined diagnostic labels as influenza, arthritis, rheumatism and so on. Even if more precise diagnostic terms are used, it is wise to ask a few questions about the nature of the illness to check whether the diagnosis seems likely. Questions about common infections should include a tactful enquiry about sexually transmitted disease and its treatment, when this is considered of possible relevance. When relevant either to diagnosis or management, sexual orientation should be discussed. Any risk of exposure to HIV infection may need to be assessed (Chapter 17).

In some cases, it may be necessary to communicate with doctors or hospitals that have treated the patient in the past. The name and, if possible, the address of any doctor or hospital should be recorded, together with the name and address of the patient at the time of the previous illness, if this has changed, and, in the case of a married woman, her maiden name.

The menstrual history

Women should be asked about menstruation. In the majority of women menstruation occurs about every 28 days. Ask at what age menstruation began and, if menstruation has ceased, ask when this occurred. The menopause usually occurs toward the end of the fifth decade. Enquire whether the patient is losing more or less menstrual blood than usual. The menstrual flow is probably abnormal if it lasts for fewer than 2 or more than 8 days. Ask about premenstrual tension and about the presence or absence of pain with periods; and ask whether the patient is or has been taking oral contraceptives.

The obstetric history

Data on a woman's experience of childbirth, including miscarriages and therapeutic abortions may also be important in assessing the medical and social background to illness (see Chapter 14). In women presenting with stress incontinence it is important to know whether childbirth was traumatic, requiring sutures to vaginal or sphincter tears. Excessive bleeding may occur in childbirth in haematological disorders. Endocrine disease may be accompanied by abnormalities of pregnancy, labour and lactation. Cardiac failure may be triggered by the circulatory demands of pregnancy and labour even when cardiac disease was unsuspected.

The treatment history

The treatment history, which should include medical and surgical treatments, is important, not only because of the possibility of clinically important drug interactions or unwanted effects but also because it gives a clue to unsuspected previous or background illness, e.g. recognition of antihypertensive treatment in a patient presenting with dizziness, or transient stroke. In addition, the dosage of self-medicated analgesic drugs is useful in assessing severity of pain. Details of drugs taken, including analgesics, oral contraceptives and psychotropic drugs, and of surgery, radiotherapy and psychotherapy are all important. Adverse reactions to drugs, including hypersensitivities, are common. It is essential to find out whether the patient has had previous adverse effects from a drug so that its prescription can be avoided. Knowledge of current therapy is also necessary to avoid adverse drug interaction when new drugs are prescribed. A major difficulty is that patients may not be able to remember past treatments, nor may any record about them exist. Many of these remedies may in any case have been bought across the counter. In this case, when relevant, it helps to ask about remedies taken for particular complaints, e.g. 'What do you take when you have a headache?'; 'What do you take for the bowels?'. Relatives often remember more than the patient.

It is often important to discover not only whether someone was given a drug, but whether they took it and for the appropriate time. Reasons for non-compliance may be relevant in future management. Terminology is important; the word 'medicine' is often taken to mean something liquid or something sold in a pharmacy; 'drugs' may mean doctors' prescriptions or illicit narcotics to a patient; and 'tablets' may not be distinguished from 'capsules'. It is often better to ask a patient what remedies were taken for particular complaints and whether these ever caused discomfort, than to use technical terms. Hospital pharmacists can help with the names of unusual drugs imported from overseas and with listing the adverse effects of any drug. Abuse of narcotics, psychotropic or neuroleptic drugs is common but usually concealed, and if this is suspected, direct enquiry should be made of the patient as well as of family or friends. Surgical operations and anaesthetics should be noted, and any untoward events carefully documented: they may be relevant to future management. Patients frequently ignore past serious illness, believing it to be cured or irrelevant to the current problem.

The family history

Note the patient's position in the family and the ages of children, if any. Usually it is only necessary to record the state of health, important illnesses and the cause of death of immediate relatives. If, however, there is a question of a hereditary disorder one should enquire about all known relatives and attempt to construct a family tree showing those affected and those not affected. The family tree is especially important in the modern era of developments in genetics.

The social history

The patient's physical and emotional environment, including their surroundings both at home and work, and their habits and mental attitude to life and to work are essential components of the history that are important in assessing the effect of the illness on the patient and on their family. Try to visualize the patient's family life, to understand their emotions and to view, step-by-step, the home, family, daily habits, diet and work. It may help to ask for an account of a typical day. Other areas to ask about include the following:

Domestic and marital relationships. Ascertain feelings about other members of the family; interests, hobbies, hopes, fears; holidays taken and whether they are enjoyed; the amount of exercise taken; games and sports, and, in general, the sort of lifestyle and the sort of person the patient is. In men, particularly if unmarried, consider the possibility of homosexuality. Both male and female homosexuality may be associated with personal and social stresses that may culminate in mental illness.

Home surroundings. Look at the possibility of overcrowding or of loneliness. What pets are kept? Where did they come from and were they recently imported?

Diet and use of alcohol and tobacco. It is important to ask about past habits in these respects. A patient who claims to neither drink nor smoke may have been a heavy drinker or smoker, even in the recent past. Remember too that many alcoholics will convincingly deny their dependence. Almost every drinker grossly underestimates the extent of their alcohol consumption. Cigarette smoking is a prominent cause of carcinoma of the lung, emphysema and vascular disease; therefore a detailed history of smoking is essential. Other drug usage may also be admitted in response to an expectant enquiry.

Travel abroad. Find out whether or not the patient has lived abroad and if so whether they were ill there. Recent travel may be important; a patient may, for instance, suffer from malaria in the UK if they have recently travelled from or even through a malarious area.

The occupational history

The occupational history is always valuable, and there are few surer and quicker means of gaining a patient's confidence than an intelligent knowledge of their job. If there is any suspicion that the patient's symptoms are occupational in origin a full occupational history should be taken from the time the patient left school. Record the dates of all subsequent jobs. The patient may be exposed to a noxious substance responsible for ill-health in their present occupation, but this should not be assumed. For example, an ice-cream vendor may have a mesothelioma due to exposure to asbestos many years before. Cancer of the genitourinary tract may be the result of exposure in the past to certain aromatic amines used as intermediates in the dyestuffs industry or as an antioxidant in rubber and cable-making. Ask the patient the name of their trade, the processes employed, the tools used and the substances handled, bearing in mind that the name of an occupation may be misleading, as different names are used for the same job in different places. The patient may be ignorant of the nature of a substance used and may know it only by its trade name. In such cases it is best to communicate with their works manager and ask about the substance in question. In addition, find out about the general conditions at work (Box 1.3).

BOX 1.3 Questions to ask about occupational history and conditions at work.

- Is the job dusty, and if so what tools make the dust?
- Are there fumes or vapours, and if so what are the chemical substances involved? Most of the toxic substances encountered in dangerous trades enter the body by inhalation, although some solvents penetrate the skin.
- Is a hood installed over the bench, and is it connected to a suction system?
- Is protective clothing provided?
- Is a special suit and goggles required, and why?
- Has any similar illness affected a fellow employee? Certain occupational hazards are associated with office work, e.g. repetitive strain injury, and migraine induced by stress or inappropriate lighting.

Other aspects of the occupational history are no less important. An illness may render someone temporarily or permanently unfit to work. The doctor should know that conditions peculiar to certain trades may cause disease which predisposes to infection. For example, silicosis, which is an occupational hazard for mine and quarry workers, leads to an excessive mortality from pulmonary tuberculosis and also from pneumonia. On the other hand, diseases other than infections may be involved. For example, among publicans, barmen and others who have ready access to alcohol, a heavy mortality from cirrhosis of the liver as well as from tuberculosis exists.

The doctor should have regard for a patient's work even when the patient is suffering from a disease which is non-occupational. One must know whether a patient has a job with responsibility for the safety of others. A shop assistant or nursery nurse with open tuberculosis can infect others, and those who handle food can initiate outbreaks of typhoid fever, dysentery and *Salmonella* infection by acting as carriers. Those who drive heavy goods or public transport vehicles come under stringent medical regulations, particularly regarding epilepsy and heart disease. The possible effect of any drug on the patient's occupation must always be considered. Antihistamines may cure hay fever but may make the patient so sleepy that they cannot work without danger to themselves or others.

Negative data

There are two more points about history-taking which should be mentioned. First, it is sometimes as important to record that a symptom was *not* present as to record that it was present. Under each system, therefore, the absence of the most important symptoms, e.g. breathlessness and cough in the case of the respiratory system, breathlessness on exertion or cardiac pain in the case of the cardiovascular system, and paralysis, headaches or fits in the case of the nervous system, should be recorded.

Second, the history does not end when the patient is first seen. Continuation notes should record the disappearance of symptoms or the appearance of new ones, or any other relevant fact which becomes apparent while the patient is under observation. In inpatients a daily progress note, recording the progress of symptoms and signs, the investigations and treatments arranged, and the outcome, is essential.

Review of systems

The following is intended as an outline of the questions (see Box 1.4) that most doctors ask, or note from the patient's story, when taking a history. The degree of detail varies according to the state of the patient, the context of the illness and the relevance of the information sought to the problem under consideration.

General

Weight
- Is it increasing, decreasing, or stationary?

Sleep
- Has the sleeping pattern changed?
- Is there difficulty in getting to sleep or unusually early waking?

BOX 1.4 Review of systems.

General
- Weight
- Sleep
- Energy

Gastrointestinal system, abdomen and pelvis

Upper alimentary tract
- Pain
- Appetite
- Vomiting
- General characteristics of vomited matter
- Flatulence
- Water brash
- Heartburn
- Dysphagia

Lower alimentary tract
- Diarrhoea
- Constipation
- Pain

Liver and gallbladder
- Jaundice
- Pain

Genital system

Cardiovascular system
- Dyspnoea
- Pain or tightness
- Palpitation
- Cough
- Oedema
- Other symptoms

The blood
- Lassitude, dyspnoea and awareness
- Infections
- Blood loss
- Skin problems
- Diet
- Past history
- Drug history
- Occupational history
- Glandular enlargement

Respiratory system
- Cough
- Sputum
- Breathing
- Wheeze
- Chest pain

Urinary system
- Symptoms suggestive of renal failure
- Urine

Skin diseases

Nervous system
- Stroke
- Epilepsy
- Common neurological symptoms

Locomotor system

Infants and children
- Special questions where relevant

- Is the patient sleepy during the day?
- Are 'sleeping pills' taken?

Energy
- Tiredness is a universal complaint.
- Is it loss of energy or boredom?
- Is it part of a general malaise?
- Is there unusual fatiguability?

The gastrointestinal system, abdomen and pelvis

UPPER ALIMENTARY TRACT

If the symptoms suggest disease of the upper alimentary tract, enquire about the following.

Pain
- What is its severity and site?
- Is it localized or diffuse?
- Does it radiate in any particular direction?
- For how long has the patient had it?
- Are there intervals of freedom? If so, for how long?
- What is its relation to meals (if any)?
- Does it wake the patient at night?
- What things aggravate it? What affords relief (e.g. food, antacid powders, vomiting)? Distinguish especially between 'pain', 'sense of discomfort' or 'fullness'.

Appetite
- Is it increased or reduced?
- If reduced, is the appetite poor, or is the patient afraid to eat on account of pain?

Vomiting
- What is the frequency, and the relation of vomiting to pain?
- Does it relieve the pain or not? Sometimes people deliberately induce vomiting.
- Vomiting in the morning is a rare feature of raised intracranial pressure, or of posterior fossa tumour.

General characteristics of vomited matter
- How much and what colour?
- Does it ever contain blood?
- Does it ever look like 'coffee grounds'?
- Is it ever sour and frothy?
- Does it contain residues of food taken the day before?

Flatulence
- Does the wind tend to escape downwards or upwards?
- Does either relieve the symptoms?

Water brash
- Does the patient ever experience excessive secretion of saliva into the mouth, with regurgitation of mouthfuls of clear, tasteless fluid?

Heartburn
- Does the patient suffer from pain behind the sternum?
- Does it come on especially when lying down?

Dysphagia
- Is there any difficulty in swallowing?
- If so, where does the food appear to stick?
- Is it worse with liquids or with solids?
- Is swallowing painful?

LOWER ALIMENTARY TRACT

If the symptoms point to a disorder of the lower alimentary tract, enquire about the following.

Diarrhoea
- How frequent and at what times are the motions during the day and what is their relation to meals or to special articles of food?
- What colour are the motions?
- Are they formed, unformed, porridge-like, frothy, or watery?
- Do they float in the lavatory pan or are they difficult to flush away?
- Has the patient ever passed any blood or slime?
- Is there pain during defaecation?
- Does the patient use purgatives or anything else, e.g. beer, which is likely to produce loose motions?
- Is there incontinence of formed stools?

Constipation
- What is the patient's usual bowel habit?
- Has there been any recent change in habit?
- If so, can this be explained by change in diet, medicines, etc.?
- Does the constipation alternate with diarrhoea? If so, can this be explained by the taking of purgatives?
- Is there any colicky pain?
- Is there blood in the stools?
- Does the patient take codeine in any form?

Pain
- What is the site, radiation and character?
- Is it persistent or intermittent?
- Where is it felt worst?
- Is it relieved by defaecation or by the passage of flatus?

Liver and gallbladder

If the symptoms point to disease of the liver or gallbladder, e.g. if the patient is jaundiced or has pain in the right upper abdomen, enquire about the following.

Jaundice
● Has the patient noticed any yellowing of conjunctival or skin, or any change of colour of the urine?
● Are the motions pale or dark?
● Does the skin itch?
● Have there been any other cases of jaundice among family, friends or workmates?
● Has any kind of injection been given in the last 3 or 4 months?
● Has the patient travelled abroad recently?
● How much alcohol does the patient consume?

Pain
● Where is it?
● Has the patient ever had attacks of very severe pain, coming on suddenly and lasting for a few hours?
● If so, did the pain radiate and in what direction?
● Was there any jaundice after the pain subsided?
● Did the pain radiate to the tip of the shoulder or the middle of the back?

The genital system

Patients will usually talk spontaneously about obvious structural abnormalities, such as a urethral discharge, swelling of the testicles or ulceration of the penis or scrotum in the male; and gynaecological abnormalities in the case of the female. Often, however, the real complaint is of a disorder of function which is intensely personal. Tact and sympathetic listening may enable such patients to discuss disorders of coital function, such as impotence, premature ejaculation or frigidity, problems of infertility and anxieties about masturbation or homosexuality. (see Chapter 2).

The cardiovascular system

If the symptoms point to disease of the circulatory system, enquire about the following.

Dyspnoea
● How short of breath is the patient?
● When does this come on? Is it present at rest or only on exertion?
● What degree of exertion is necessary to produce it?
● Are there attacks of breathlessness at night (*paroxysmal nocturnal dyspnoea*)?
● Does the patient have to sleep sitting up (*orthopnoea*)?

Pain or tightness
● What is its exact site and character?
● If the patient has chest pain or tightness, does it radiate to the left arm, neck, shoulder or interscapular region? If so, in what direction?
● What precipitates it, and what, if anything, relieves it? (Angina pectoris and cardiac pain are discussed on p. 186.) A cramp-like pain and tiredness in the legs on exercise may be due to intermittent claudication; this is felt in the muscles of the legs, especially in the calves.
● Is it present only on exertion, or also at rest?
● Is it relieved by rest?

Palpitation
● What brings on palpitation and how long does it last?
● Is it induced or relieved by exercise?
● Does the heart give an occasional thump now and then?
● Is the pulse rate increased during an attack and is the pulse regular or irregular?

Cough
● Enquire also about cough, sputum and haemoptysis, as detailed in the section on the respiratory system, below.

Oedema
● Do the feet or ankles swell?

Other symptoms
● Are there cramp-like pains in the calves when walking relieved by rest?
● Or is there undue coldness, redness or blueness of the extremities?
● Is there a past history of rheumatic fever or chorea?

The blood (see also Chapter 18)

If the clinical features suggest a blood disorder enquire about the following.

Lassitude, dyspnoea and awareness of the heart beat.
Infections involving the mouth, skin, lungs, urinary tract and perianal area.
Blood loss including gum bleeding, epistaxis, bruising, rectal bleeding, malaena (black stools), and menstrual disturbances. It is important to establish whether bleeding or bruising is spontaneous or is out of proportion to the degree of trauma.
Skin problems including red skin spots (*purpura*) and changes in skin colour.

Diet including meat and green vegetable consumption.

Past history including excessive bleeding after dental extraction and tonsillectomy.

Drug history including aspirin consumption and drugs known to cause bone marrow (aplasia) or haemolytic anaemia.

Family history of blood disorders and the country of origin of the patient and family.

Occupational history including exposure to dangerous chemicals.

Glandular enlargement.

The respiratory system

If the symptoms point to disease of the respiratory system, ask about any family history of tuberculosis, allergies or asthma, whether induced by pollens, dusts or exercise; occupation (including past occupations) and possible exposure to animal, mineral or vegetable dusts. Ask particularly about smoking habits, both past and present.

Cough
- Is it dry or productive?
- At what time of the day is it worst?
- Is it worsened by any particular conditions, such as cold, dust or pollen?
- Is it painful or not?

Sputum
- How much?
- Most produced at what time of day?
- What is the consistency, colour, and odour?
- Is it purulent or not?
- Is it ever blood-stained, and if so whether with streaks or clots, and on how many occasions?

Breathing
- Is the patient dyspnoeic?
- Does dyspnoea occur at rest, or after varying degrees of exertion? Various 'grades' of dyspnoea have been described, but, in talking with patients it is best to enquire what sort of activity, e.g. walking upstairs or running for a bus, produces dyspnoea. Patients with severe pulmonary disease may be dyspnoeic at rest.

Wheeze
- When does wheezing occur?
- Is it constant or intermittent?
- Does anything provoke it?
- Is it worse at any particular time of day or night?

Chest pain
- Where is it?
- Is it aggravated by deep breathing or coughing?
- Is it associated with an increase in cough, sputum or dyspnoea?
- Is the onset sudden, as in spontaneous pneumothorax?

The urinary system

If the symptoms point to disease of the kidneys, e.g. oedema, or of the urinary system, e.g. pain on micturition, ask about a history of tonsillitis, previous renal disease or of rheumatic fever or chorea, and ascertain any family history of renal disease or high blood pressure. What analgesics has the patient taken?

Symptoms suggestive of renal failure
- Has any pain been noted in the lumbar region or any attacks of acute pain shooting down into the groin or testicles?
- Have any of the following remote symptoms been noted: headache, vomiting, drowsiness, fits, dimness of vision, dyspnoea?
- Does the face ever look puffy in the morning? Are the ankles swollen?
- What is the state of the bowels?

Urine
- Is the urine altered in amount?
- Does the patient have to get up at night to pass water?
- Is the patient continent?
- Is the stream of urine normal or reduced in flow?
- Is it altered in colour?
- Is it clear or turbid when passed?
- Is there any blood in it? If so, at what period of micturition is it present?
- Is the urine frothy?
- Is there any increased frequency of micturition?
- Is the increase by day or by night?
- Is there an increase in volume passed?
- Is frequency associated with undue thirst?
- Distinguish between *polyuria*, as in diabetes mellitus and chronic renal failure and *frequency*, as in cystitis.
- Is there any pain during micturition? Is it before, during or after the act? What is its character, and where is it felt?

Skin diseases

- Enquire carefully into the patient's habits regarding diet, clothing and washing.

- Is there any occupational or other exposure to chemical substances or other irritants? Ask about recent drug therapy.
- Does the eruption itch? If so, when is the itching worst?
- Did the eruption appear all at once or in crops?
- Is there a history of asthma, hay fever or any other allergic disorder?
- Is there contact with animals, insects, or plants?
- What skin lotions have been used?
- What cosmetics are used?
- Is there a family history of skin disease, asthma, hay fever, urticaria?
- Is there a family history of loss of hair or of excessive hair?

The nervous system

Neurological symptoms may be of sudden or gradual onset.

Stroke, due to cerebrovascular disease, typically presents with the sudden onset of a neurological deficit, i.e. weakness, sensory loss or visual disturbance, usually on one side of the body. This may recover in a few minutes, or in less than 24 hours (*transient ischaemic attack*: *TIA*) or may resolve in a few days (*reversible ischaemic neurological deficit*: *RIND*) or may recover incompletely (*stroke*). These features should be established.

- Was headache associated with the onset? This suggests haemorrhage or migraine.
- Is there a history suggestive of generalized vascular disease, e.g. angina pectoris, intermittent claudication, past history of hypertension or heavy smoking, diabetes mellitus or a family history of vascular disease?
- Is there a history of heart disease, especially vascular disease.

Epilepsy, causing seizures consists of repetitive, even stereotyped convulsive events.

- What was the age at the first attack? Describe the first attack.
- What have been the shortest and longest intervals between attacks?
- Do they occur during sleep?
- Is there any warning or *aura*?
- What is the character of the aura?
- Does the patient lose consciousness in the attack (generalized epilepsy) or not (partial epilepsy)?
- Did the patient convulse; was there incontinence; was the tongue bitten?
- Were there any post-ictal symptoms, e.g. sleep, headache, automatism or paralysis?
- Was the mental state affected?
- What is the treatment history?
- Is a witnessed account of the attack available?

The words 'fit' and 'epilepsy' are often thought undesirable, or as carrying an unacceptable stigma, and 'seizure' is usually preferred nowadays. Enquire about antecendent events, especially serious head injury, ear infection, brain operation, brain injury and family history.

Other common neurological symptoms include dizziness, headache, loss of balance, visual failure, pain, tremor, speech disturbance, impairment of memory and intellect, proximal weakness (*myopathy*) and distal weakness and sensory loss (*peripheral neuropathy*). In each instance, enquire in detail about the mode and circumstances of onset of the symptom, its progression, and specific precipitating and relieving features.

- Is dizziness induced by moving the head in a particular way or into a particular posture?
- Did it follow an injury or a presumed viral infection?
- Regarding headache, is the symptom intermittent or continuous, associated with visual disturbance (migraine) or not, a family disorder (migraine), unilateral, frontal or generalized, induced by stress (migraine or tension headache) and what relieves it?
- Could the neurological symptom result from a complication of a systemic disorder, e.g. cerebral or spinal metastasis from primary cancer of another organ; or vasculitis; or infection?
- Is there evidence of an inherited disease, e.g. myotonic dystrophy, Huntington's chorea or Friedreich's ataxia?
- Is there a congenital malformation?
- Are there features of an underlying genetic disorder predisposing to a neurological problem, e.g. von Recklinghausen's neurofibromatosis (NF1).
- Could the neurological disorder be due to an infection, whether acquired in temperate climes, e.g. Lyme disease or HIV infection, or in the tropics?
- Has there been an exposure to toxic substances, e.g. in a case of subacute peripheral neuropathy?

The locomotor system

If the symptoms suggest a disorder of the bones or joints, enquire about previous manifestations of rheumatoid arthritis, rheumatic fever or gout. Ask about possible associated conditions in the skin (e.g. dermatomyositis, psoriasis, systemic lupus erythematosus, scleroderma and erythema nodosum), the bowels (ulcerative colitis) and the eyes (e.g. conjunctivitis, uveitis and Sjögren's disease). Ask about the presence of a urethral discharge in men or of vaginal discharge in women with arthritis (Reiter's syndrome).

● Has the patient been exposed to rubella?
● Is there a family history of gout or other rheumatic disorder?
● If there is pain referred to a bone, ask whether it is worse in the day or at night. Bone pains are often described as being deep or boring in character.
● If the pain is in a joint, ask whether it is present constantly or only when the joint is moved.
● Has the joint been visibly swollen?
● Does the pain move from one joint to another, as is characteristic of acute or subacute rheumatism?
● Describe the patient's gait and other disabilities.

Infants and children

If the patient is an infant or a very young child, the following special questions, where relevant, should be put to the mother or other responsible person (see also Chapter 15):

● How many other children are there in the family?
● What are their sexes and ages?
● Have there been any miscarriages or stillbirths? If so, when?
● Is there a history of illness in the parents or siblings, or in the parents' near relatives?
● Was the mother well during pregnancy and did she take any drugs?
● Was this a full-term infant?
● What was the birth weight?
● Was the child born at home or in hospital, and was the labour normal?
● Were there any unusual symptoms, such as jaundice, cyanosis or fits, in the newborn period?
● Was the baby breast-fed, and for how long?
● If bottle-fed, what type of milk was used?
● Were vitamin supplements given?
● When was mixed feeding introduced?
● Was there a satisfactory weight-gain in infancy?
● What immunizations were given, and when?

It is particularly important to enquire about the 'milestones of development' (see page 377 and Table 15.1).

● When did the baby first smile, sit up, walk and talk?
● Or acquire control of bowels and bladder?
● What are the child's present habits with regard to eating, sleeping, bowels and micturition?
● What is the general behaviour like in comparison with siblings or other children of the same age?
● If the child is of school age, does he or she attend school regularly, get on well with his lessons, and like school?

Social factors may be important:

● Has the child ever been separated from his mother? If so, when and for how long?
● What is the social background?
● Are the living conditions satisfactory? Does the mother go out to work?
● If she does, who looks after the child while she is away?
● Is this an immigrant family? If so, where do they come from, and how long have they been in this country?
● Did they suffer illness, injury or malnutrition in their home country?

Finally, enquire about previous illnesses, their nature and severity, and the ages at which they occurred—infectious diseases, fits, bowel disturbances, upper respiratory infections, or discharging ears.

● If there is a history of cough, was it spasmodic, associated with vomiting, particularly bad at night? And was there a whoop?
● What drugs has the child received?
● Has the child ever been in hospital?
● Have there ever been any accidents involving physical injury, burns or poisoning?

In taking the history try to discover what is really worrying the parents. It may be something deeper than is suggested by the child's symptoms, for example leukaemia or some other serious disease which affected another child in the family.

The physical examination

The general assessment of the patient and the techniques for examination of the different systems are described in Chapters 2 to 12. In general, it is important to develop a routine of physical examination which combines speed with thoroughness, sensitivity and alertness, but which disturbs the patient no more than necessary. It need hardly be said that the examination must be carried out as gently as possible, without tiring or exposing the patient more than necessary. In severely ill patients it may be necessary to postpone a routine examination and to perform only the examination necessary for a provisional diagnosis and treatment. Ill patients must obviously be treated with special care and consideration.

Different doctors have different routines for examining patients in different circumstances. Always plan the examination. Does the information obtained from the history suggest that particular abnormal features will be found on examination? What else should be looked for? If the patient has vomited blood, and has a history of heavy alcohol ingestion, the liver may be found to be enlarged, there may be signs of hepatic failure and there could be also be neurological abnormalities (see Chapter 2).

Start the examination in a manner that will appear relevant to the patient. For example, if the presenting symptom is sciatica, start with the legs and the spine. However, a systematic approach to each functional system is essential until considerable experience has been acquired, in order to gain information that is both complete and relevant. This routine serves to remind the clinician of any omissions. Always try to be thorough.

Remember that the examination can only reveal abnormalities present at the time of the examination. The history, on the other hand, can reveal aspects of the temporal development of the illness. The history and examination are thus complementary, but often the history is more important.

General approach

A good physical examination requires a co-operative patient and a quiet, warm and well-lit room. Daylight is better than artificial light, which may mask changes in skin colour, for example the faint yellow tinge of slight jaundice. Although in practice a physical examination may have to be made under all sorts of circumstances, every attempt should be made to reassure and relax the patient. For a complete examination the patient should be asked to undress completely and should then be covered by a blanket or dressing-gown. Patients are often examined while wearing underpants, but it is essential to remember to examine the buttocks and genitalia. Ideally a

chaperone should be present when a male doctor is examining a female patient and during rectal and vaginal examinations, both to reassure the patient and to protect the doctor from subsequent accusations of improper conduct.

Considering the general appearance, the most important step is to make a rapid assessment of the degree of illness. This is not making a diagnosis. One has simply to answer the question: 'Does this patient look well, mildly ill, or severely ill and, therefore, in need of urgent attention?' Experienced nurses are often highly skilled in this kind of assessment and their opinion should never be ignored. Some severely ill patients complain little; and occasionally one meets a patient whose appearance of excellent health belies his protestations of unbearable agony.

It has already been said that a good doctor begins the examination on meeting the patient, and continues taking the history until the consultation ends. An abnormal finding on examination may indicate the need for further questioning. Although the examination may provide information about organs and functions, in physical examination as well as in history-taking it is important to try to view the patient as a whole person, recognizing the patient's reaction to their illness as an important aspect of the approach to understanding the symptoms and presentation (see Box 1.5).

BOX 1.5 The physical examination.

- Mental and emotional state
- Physical attitude
- Gait
- Physique
- Face
- Skin
- Hands
- Feet
- Neck
  —lymphatic and salivary glands
  —thyroid gland
  —pulsation
- Breasts
- Axillae
- Temperature
- Pulse
- Respiration
  — odours

The mental and emotional state

Try to make some initial assessment of the patient's intelligence and mental and emotional state but recognize that this initial impression may be inaccurate. Vocabulary and command of language are generally a good guide. Sometimes a book or magazine carried by the patient may provide a reliable clue. Observation, as well as the history, assist in the assessment of the emotional state. Thus an anxious person may be restless, with wide palpebral fissures and sweating palms. Is the anxiety reasonable in the circumstances or is the patient overanxious? In depression, the lowered mood, inability to concentrate or make decisions, mental retardation, apathy or even obvious misery may be clearly evident; but so-called 'masked depression', in which these features are less obvious, is an important cause of physical symptoms. Apparently severe disability, without appropriate concern or anxiety, should suggest malingering or hysteria (*la belle indifférence*). The examination of the mental state is discussed in detail in Chapter 2.

The physical attitude

The posture of a patient may give valuable information. Severely ill patients slip down into the most uncomfortable attitudes and are unable to correct their position for themselves. Patients with congestive heart failure sit up because they may become dyspnoeic if they lie flat (*orthopnoea*). Patients with abdominal pain due to peritonitis lie still, while patients with colic are restless or even roll about in futile attempts to find relief. Patients with painful joint diseases often have an attitude of helplessness. Various neurological disorders produce characteristic postures (Chapter 12). In the severest cases of meningitis the neck may be bent backwards so that the head appears to bore into the pillow (*neck retraction*).

The gait

The gait should always be observed in patients able to walk. Important abnormalities of the gait are described in Chapters 12 and 16, but note that simple things like a painful corn, an ill-fitting shoe or a strained muscle may produce a temporary limp. The gait is best observed as the patient walks into the consulting room, or to the couch prior to the formal examination, since this represents the patient's natural gait. Under formal examination the gait may appear more abnormal as the patient may then try to demonstrate certain subjective abnormalities to the physician. Much can be learned by observing the unconscious signals of confidence, distress, anxiety, depression and other moods and emotions. An attempt should always be made to encourage a patient examined in bed to try to sit up, stand and walk. It may even be helpful to ask the patient to jump, hop or walk an imaginary narrow line.

Physique

Much can be learned from a general inspection of the patient's physique. Is the appearance consistent with the patient's chronological age? Is he or she tall, short, fat, thin, muscular or asthenic? Are there any obvious deformities and is the body proportionate? Height should be roughly equal to the fingertip-to-fingertip measurement of outstretched arms and twice the leg length from pubis to heel. Dwarfism, with a stocky body and very short legs, is characteristic of achondroplasia. Hypopituitarism arising in

Height			Small frame		Medium frame		Large frame	
ft	in	cm	lb	kg	lb	kg	lb	kg
5	2	157.5	112–120	50.8–54.4	118–129	53.8–58.5	126–141	57.2–64.0
5	3	160.0	115–123	52.2–55.8	121–133	54.9–60.3	129–144	58.5–65.3
5	4	162.6	118–126	53.5–57.2	124–136	56.2–61.7	132–148	59.9–67.1
5	5	165.1	121–129	54.9–58.5	127–139	57.6–63.0	135–152	61.2–68.9
5	6	167.6	124–133	56.2–60.3	130–143	59.0–64.9	138–156	62.6–70.8
5	7	170.2	128–137	58.1–62.1	134–147	60.8–66.7	142–161	64.4–73.0
5	8	172.7	132–141	59.9–64.0	138–152	62.6–68.9	147–166	66.7–75.3
5	9	175.3	136–145	61.7–65.8	142–156	64.4–70.8	151–170	68.5–77.1
5	10	177.8	140–150	63.5–68.0	146–160	66.2–72.6	155–174	70.3–78.9
5	11	180.3	144–154	65.3–69.9	150–165	68.0–74.8	159–179	72.1–81.2
6	0	182.9	148–158	67.1–71.7	154–170	69.9–77.1	164–184	74.4–83.5
6	1	185.4	152–162	68.9–73.5	158–175	71.7–79.4	168–189	76.2–85.7
6	2	188.0	156–167	70.8–75.7	162–180	73.5–81.6	173–194	78.5–88.0
6	3	190.5	160–171	72.6–77.6	167–185	75.7–83.5	178–199	80.7–90.3
6	4	193.0	164–175	74.4–79.4	172–190	78.1–86.2	182–204	82.7–92.5

Heights are measured wearing ordinary shoes and weights in ordinary indoor clothing. Notice that tables of this kind make no allowance for 'middle-aged spread'.

Table 1.1   Ideal weights for men aged 25 and over.

| Height | | | Small frame | | Medium frame | | Large frame | |
ft	in	cm	lb	kg	lb	kg	lb	kg
4	10	147.3	92– 98	41.7–44.5	96–107	43.5–48.5	104–119	47.2–54.0
4	11	149.9	94–101	42.6–45.8	98–110	44.5–49.9	106–122	48.1–55.3
5	0	152.4	96–104	43.5–47.2	101–113	45.8–51.3	109–125	49.4–56.7
5	1	154.9	99–107	44.9–48.5	104–116	47.2–52.6	112–128	50.8–58.1
5	2	157.5	102–110	46.3–49.9	107–119	48.5–54.9	115–131	52.2–59.4
5	3	160.0	105–113	47.6–51.3	110–122	49.9–55.3	118–134	53.5–60.8
5	4	162.6	108–116	49.0–52.6	113–126	51.3–57.2	121–138	54.9–62.6
5	5	165.1	111–119	50.3–54.0	116–130	52.6–59.0	125–142	56.7–64.0
5	6	167.6	114–123	51.7–55.8	120–135	54.4–61.2	129–146	59.5–66.2
5	7	170.2	118–127	53.5–57.6	124–139	56.2–63.0	133–150	60.3–68.0
5	8	172.7	122–131	55.3–59.4	128–143	58.1–64.9	137–154	62.1–69.9
5	9	175.3	126–135	57.2–61.2	132–147	59.9–66.7	141–158	64.0–71.7
5	10	177.8	130–140	59.0–63.5	136–151	61.7–68.5	145–163	65.8–73.9
5	11	180.3	134–144	60.8–65.3	140–155	63.5–70.3	149–168	67.6–76.2
6	0	182.9	138–148	62.6–67.1	144–159	65.3–72.1	153–173	69.4–78.5

Heights are measured wearing ordinary shoes and weights in ordinary indoor clothing.
Notice that tables of this kind make no allowance for 'middle-aged spread'.

Table 1.2   Ideal weights for women aged 25 and over.

childhood produces a proportionate but dwarfed adult with an unusually youthful appearance. In acromegaly the features are coarsened and the jaw, hands and feet are large.

'Ideal' weights, as used in life insurance assessment, are listed in Tables 1.1 and 1.2. Obesity is mostly a problem of developed countries. In some parts of the world signs of malnutrition such as wasting, apathy, anaemia and skin changes may be encountered; they should also be looked for in neglected elderly patients in developed countries such as Britain. A history of weight gain or loss can be checked by observation, remembering that fluid retention (*oedema*) will increase weight. Obvious weight loss, even when food intake has increased is seen in thyrotoxicosis and diabetes mellitus. Psychogenic loss of appetite in girls (anorexia nervosa) causes extreme emaciation while physical activity remains unimpaired. Vegetarians may be unusually thin.

The face

Observe the patient's face. The expression, and particularly the eyes, indicate real feelings better than words. Some diseases, e.g. Parkinson's disease, depression, hypothyroidism, thyrotoxicosis, acromegaly, third and seventh cranial nerve palsies and paralysis of the cervical sympathetic nerve (Horner's syndrome, Fig. 10.16), produce characteristic facial appearances.

Parotid swellings are obvious on inspection of the face. The tender bilateral parotid swelling of mumps or the unilateral swelling with reddening of the skin from acute parotitis can be contrasted with the non-bilateral persistent enlargement, accompanied by dry, tearless eyes of Sjögren's syndrome, or the more irregular unilateral painless lump of a mixed parotid tumour.

The cheeks give information regarding the patient's health: in anaemia and hypopituitarism they are pale; in the nephrotic syndrome they are pale and puffy; in cases of mitral stenosis there is sometimes a bright circumscribed flush over the malar bones; in many persons who lead an open-air life they are red and high-coloured; in congestive heart failure they may also be high-coloured, but the colour is of a bluish tint which cannot be mistaken for the red cheeks of weather-beaten people. In some cases of systemic lupus erythematosus there is a red raised eruption on the bridge of the nose extending on to the cheeks in a 'butterfly' distribution. *Telangiectases*, minute capillary tortuosities, or *naevi*, may be seen on the face in liver disease and, rarely, as a hereditary disorder (Fig. 1.1).

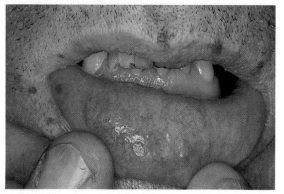

Fig. 1.1   Hereditary telangiectasia. The telangiectasia can be seen at the margin of the lips and on the lower lip.

The skin

The detailed examination of the skin is described in Chapter 3.

The most important abnormalities relevant to general examination are pallor, yellowness, pigmentation, cyanosis and cutaneous eruptions. In dehydration the skin is dry and inelastic so that it can be pinched up into a ridge. The skin is atrophied by age and sometimes after treatment with glucocorticoids. It is thickened, greasy and loose in acromegaly.

Pallor depends on the thickness and quality of the skin, and the amount and quality of the blood in the capillaries. Pallor occurs in persons with thick or opaque skins, who are always pale; in hypopituitarism; in states where the blood flow in the capillaries is diminished, such as shock, syncope or left heart failure; locally in a limb deprived of its blood supply; or in the fingers or toes when arterial spasm occurs on exposure to cold, as in Raynaud's disease. Generalized pallor may also occur in severe anaemia. Anaemia, however, is a feature of 'the colour of the blood rather than that of the patient' and the colour of the skin may be misleading. The colour of the mucous membranes of the mouth and conjunctivae gives a better indication, as does the colour of the creases of the palm of the hand.

Yellowness is usually due to jaundice. A pale lemon-yellow tint is characteristic of haemolytic jaundice; in obstructive jaundice, there is a dark yellow or orange tint. In obstructive jaundice there may be scratch marks from itching evoked by bile salts. In rare cases yellowness may be due to carotenaemia. Are there tobacco stains on the fingers, face or hair?

Pigmentation (see Chapter 3) is most commonly racial or actinic. The pigmentation of Addison's disease affects the buccal mucous membranes as well as exposed skin and parts subject to friction. In Von Recklinghausen's disease (neurofibromatosis type 1) patches of café au lait (milky coffee) pigment patches, ranging from freckling of the axillae to large (greater than 5 cm in length) areas on the limbs, trunk or face are a characteristic feature.

Cyanosis is a bluish colour of the skin and mucous membranes due to the presence of reduced haemoglobin in the blood. There are two physiological types; central and peripheral cyanosis. *Central cyanosis* results from imperfect oxygenation of blood, as in heart failure and some lung diseases, or from admixture of desaturated venous blood with arterial oxygenated blood due to right-to-left (venous-arterial) shunts in the heart. In this case the cyanosis is general and the cyanosed extremities are warm. It characteristically affects the tongue as well as the limbs. *Peripheral cyanosis* is due to excessive reduction of oxyhaemoglobin in the capillaries when the flow of blood is slowed. This may happen on exposure to cold, when there is venous obstruction, or in heart failure. The cyanosed extremity or extremities are cold, and the tongue is unaffected. The cyanosis of heart failure is often due to both central and peripheral causes. A similar bluish or leaden colour rarely may be produced by methaemoglobinaemia or sulphaemoglobinaemia, usually due to the taking of drugs such as phenacetin. This should be considered in any patient who is cyanosed but not breathless. Carbon monoxide poisoning produces a generalized cherry-red discoloration, due to the presence of carboxyhaemoglobin.

Cutaneous eruptions are described in Chapter 3.

An excess of fluid in the subcutaneous tissue causing swelling of the tissues is known as *oedema*. Thus in acute nephritis an early symptom is oedema of the face, which is most marked when the patient rises in the morning. In *dependent oedema*, however, which is typically present in congestive heart failure, and in conditions associated with a low plasma protein level, the swelling first appears at the ankles and over the dorsum of the foot, and only gradually involves the legs, thighs and trunk. In local *venous obstruction* the oedema is confined to the parts from which the return of blood is impeded. Thus, oedema of an arm occurs when malignant glands constrict the axillary vein; and oedema of a leg occurs in thrombosis of the popliteal or femoral vein. Oedema of the whole upper part of the body may result from intrathoracic tumours. Oedema can be recognized by the pallid and glossy appearance of the skin over the swollen part, by its doughy feel, and by the fact that it pits on finger pressure. In recumbent patients oedema often appears first over the sacrum. In recognizing pitting oedema it is important to press firmly and for a sustained period, or slight oedema may be missed. The oedema of lymphatic obstruction does *not* pit on pressure.

Localized oedema may be due to local changes in capillary permeability, as in angioneurotic oedema and giant urticaria. Oedema is also a feature of cutaneous or subcutaneous inflammation.

Subcutaneous emphysema is uncommon, but if present can be recognized by the crackling sensation produced by lightly compressing the part affected.

The hands

The hands of the patient should be examined carefully. Notice the strength of grip as you shake hands; this is a rough indicator of abnormality. Note the general shape of the hands, the state of the joints, the character of the nails, the presence or absence of finger-clubbing, the presence of nailbed infarcts, and of staining with nicotine.

In osteoarthrosis the finger joints are often implicated, and bony nodules, known as *Heberden's nodes* (Fig. 1.2), are formed at the bases of the terminal phalanges. In rheumatoid arthritis there is a spindle-shaped swelling of the interphalangeal joints and, later, ulnar deviation of the fingers. *Trophic changes* in the skin may be present in neurological disease and in disorders of the peripheral circulation (e.g. Raynaud's disease). Characteristic movements or attitudes of the hand may also be seen in athetosis, tetany and lead palsy. *Tremor* of the hands may occasionally be familial (essential tremor). In other cases it is due to nervousness, senility, Parkinsonism, thyrotoxicosis, alcoholism, multiple sclerosis, uraemia or hepatic failure (see Chapter 6). In ulnar paralysis the hand becomes deformed by overextension of the wrist, combined with excessive flexion of the ulnar two digits, so that a claw-like attitude is produced. Wasting of the small muscles of the hand, due for example to median or ulnar nerve lesions, cervical root (T1) disease or loss of anterior horn cells at the same level, gives the hand a flattened appearance. The characteristic posture of the hand in tetany is shown in Fig. 1.3(a) and (b). In *Dupuytren's contracture* there is a thickening of the palmar fascia, which may lead to flexion contracture of the ring and other fingers. In acromegaly the hands are massive, the fingers spatulate with square tips and the skin thickened.

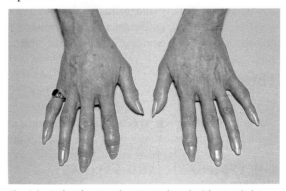

Fig. 1.2 Heberden's nodes. Reproduced with permission from M. A. Mir (1995) *Atlas of Clinical Diagnosis*, London, W. B. Saunders.

(a)

(b)

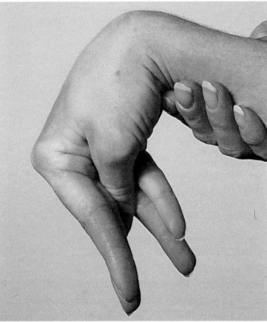

Fig. 1.3 Tetany. Reproduced with permission from M. A. Mir (1995) *Atlas of Clinical Diagnosis*, London, W. B. Saunders.

In *clubbing of the fingers* (Fig. 1.4(a) and (b)), the tissues at the base of the nail are thickened, and the angle between the nail base and the adjacent skin of the finger is obliterated. The nail itself loses its longitudinal ridges and becomes convex from above downwards as well as from side to side. In extreme cases the terminal segment of the finger is bulbous, like the end of a drumstick. The toes may also be affected. Clubbing is found in association with a number of cardiopulmonary and abdominal disorders (Box 1.6). Clubbing is an important sign of subacute bacterial endocarditis, when it may be associated with Osler's nodes. The latter consists of tender transient swellings about the size of a pea in the pulp of the fingers and

(a)

(b)

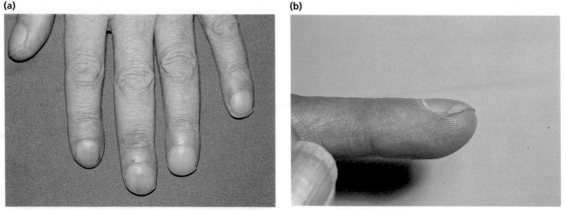

Fig. 1.4   Clubbing. Reproduced with permission from M. A. Mir (1995) *Atlas of Clinical Diagnosis*, London, W. B. Saunders.

BOX 1.6 Causes of clubbing of the fingers.

Acquired disorders
• Severe chronic cyanosis
• Congenital heart disease, e.g. Fallot's tetralogy
• Chronic fibrosing alveolitis
• Emphysema

Other pulmonary disorders
• Chronic suppuration in the lungs
  —bronchiectasis
  —empyema
• Carcinoma of the bronchus
• Pulmonary tuberculosis

Chronic abdominal disorders
• Crohn's disease
• Polyposis of the colon
• Ulcerative colitis
• Subacute bacterial endocarditis

---

toes. 'Splinter' haemorrhages occur beneath the nails in this condition. In hypertrophic pulmonary osteoarthropathy, besides clubbing of the fingers,

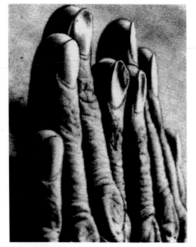

Fig. 1.5   Koilonychia.

there is thickening of the periosteum of radius, ulna, tibia and fibula. This gives rise to swelling above the wrist and ankle. Congenital clubbing is rare.

Koilonychia (Fig. 1.5) occurs in iron-deficiency anaemia. The nails are soft, thin, brittle and spoon-shaped. The normal convexity is lost and replaced by a concavity. *Nailbed infarcts* occur in vasculitis, especially in systemic lupus erythematosus and in polyarteritis.

The feet

The feet must not remain obscured under bedclothes or socks during the examination. Pitting oedema may be recognized only in the ankles and dorsal surfaces of the feet. The condition of the skin of the feet is especially important in diabetics and the elderly. Peripheral vascular disease will make the skin shiny, and hair does not grow on ischaemic legs or feet. The dorsalis pedis and posterior tibial pulses may be reduced or absent. If the toes of an ischaemic foot are compressed their dull purple colour will blanch and only slowly return. Passive elevation of an ischaemic leg will cause marked pallor of the foot as perfusion against gravity falls. Painless trophic lesions, often with deep ulceration, on the soles are seen frequently in diabetic peripheral neuropathy (*the diabetic foot*).

The neck

The neck should be inspected and palpated. Swellings in the neck are usually felt best from behind. Note the following:

THE LYMPHATIC AND SALIVARY GLANDS
In infection of the tonsils the lymph glands at the angles of the jaws are enlarged; those below the jaw

are enlarged in patients with metastases from cancer in the mouth. Glands draining an inflammatory focus are usually tender. Enlarged tuberculous glands may occur in groups or in long chains behind the sternomastoid, and scars may mark the sites of past suppuration in severe untreated cases. In human immunodeficiency virus (HIV) infection, Hodgkin's disease, other reticuloses and secondary neoplasms the glands are enlarged and discrete. In lymphatic leukaemia there may be great enlargement of the glands on both sides. In secondary syphilis the glands under the upper part of the trapezius are often palpable. If enlarged glands are found either in the neck or elsewhere, it is important to observe whether they are firm and distinct, or fused together; whether fluctuation can be elicited, and whether they are adherent to adjacent structures. The submandibular salivary glands should also be palpated when the neck is being examined from behind. If they are swollen and tender, the opening of their ducts into the mouth should be inspected with the tip of the patient's tongue rolled upwards; this may reveal a salivary calculus.

THE THYROID GLAND

Inspect the neck for any general or local enlargement of the gland, and observe its movement with the larynx during swallowing. Patients find this easier if they are given a glass of water. Next, stand behind the seated patient and palpate the gland with one hand on each side of the neck. Determine if any swelling exists and, if so, whether it is uniform or nodular, hard or soft. Sometimes such an enlargement presses on the trachea and, occasionally, it may extend into the thorax behind the sternum. At other times, particularly if the disease is malignant, the recurrent laryngeal nerves may become implicated. If it is difficult to determine whether a tumour is connected with the thyroid, remember that the gland and any tumour connected with it moves up and down on swallowing. Minor degrees of enlargement of the thyroid are often better seen than felt. A bruit heard over the thyroid is a sign that the gland is hyperactive.

PULSATION

Pulsations in the vessels must be noted. Any arterial pulsation is both seen and felt as a distinct thrust, whereas venous pulsation can be seen but not felt as a thrust, if it is felt at all. In aortic incompetence the carotid arteries are seen to pulsate forcibly. In aortic stenosis a systolic thrill is felt. In hypertensive patients carotid pulsation may be prominent. The jugular veins may be distended and pulsatile in congestive heart failure (p. 171). In superior mediastinal obstruction due to retrosternal goitre or malignant neoplasm in the mediastinum, non-pulsatile distended veins may be seen over the neck and upper part of the body; cyanosis and oedema of the upper part of the body may accompany this sign. Distended neck veins may also be seen in large pericardial effusions (see page 175).

The breasts

The chance of finding a treatable cancer should make a full examination of the breasts a necessary feature of every general examination of a woman older than 35 years. With the patient reclining, arms to the sides, inspect the development and symmetry of breasts and nipples. Look for any reddening of the skin, ulceration or dimpling (*peau d'orange*). Retraction (rather than inversion) of the nipple is a sign that suggests carcinoma of the breast. Gently squeeze deeply beneath the nipple to express any milk or discharge. Determine whether it is blood, serous or milky; the patient may well have noticed this herself.

Palpate each breast with the flat part of the fingers, working over the whole breast as if it were mapped out in quadrants. Repeat this when the patient has her hands placed behind her head. If a lump is found, the characteristics to describe it are the same as those for any lump felt anywhere in the body. Determine its situation, size, shape, surface and edge; feel its consistency and mobility in relation to deep and superficial structures.

Any swelling of the male breast is likely to be seen at a glance. The swelling can be distinguished as breast tissue rather than pectoral fat by palpation when the patient's hands are behind his head. At some stage of puberty the majority of normal boys will have a palpable disc of breast tissue beneath the areola.

AXILLAE

Examine the axillae. It is difficult to feel enlarged lymph glands unless the patient's arm is raised to allow the examining fingers to be pushed high into the axilla. The arm is then lowered in the flexed position to rest across the examiner's arm and palpation is continued downwards along the chest wall.

Temperature

When taking the temperature, the following points must be remembered:

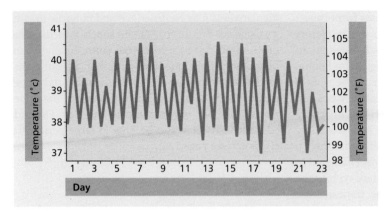

Fig. 1.6   Remittent fever. Patient died on day 23.

- The thermometer must be accurate.
- It must be kept in position long enough to allow the mercury to reach body temperature. It is advisable to exceed the period which the instrument professes to require. The ordinary 'half-minute' thermometer should be left in position for a full minute. Collapsed, comatose and elderly patients should have their rectal temperature taken with a special 'low-reading' thermometer. Accidental hypothermia is common in the elderly.
- In conscious adults the temperature is taken in the mouth or in the axilla. In young children the thermometer should be placed in the fold of the groin, and the thigh flexed on the abdomen; or it may be inserted into the rectum. The temperature of the mouth and rectum is generally at least half a degree higher than that of the groin or axilla. When the temperature is taken in the mouth, the patient must breathe through the nose and keep the lips firmly closed during the observation.
- Before inserting the thermometer, make it an invariable rule to wash it in antiseptic or in cold water, and see that the mercury is well shaken down. Wash it again before replacing it in its case. The centigrade (Celsius) scale is in general use in the UK, but many people are still more familiar with the Fahrenheit scale (Table 1.3).

	Centigrade	Fahrenheit
Normal	36.6–37.2	98–99
Subnormal	<36.6	<98
Febrile	>37.2	>99
Hyperpyrexia	>41.6	>107
Hypothermia	<35	<95

Table 1.3   Temperature ranges in centigrade and Fahrenheit.

In febrile disorders, there is a disturbance of heat regulation, so that the 'thermostatic' mechanism controlling heat gain and loss is set at a level higher than normal. While the temperature is rising to this new level, heat is conserved, the skin vessels are constricted so that the body feels cold, and the patient may even shiver violently. This shivering is called a *rigor*. When the higher temperature is reached, heat loss again becomes apparent; the skin vessels dilate and the body feels warm.

FEVER

There are three classical types of fever or pyrexia: continued, remittent and intermittent. When fever does not fluctuate more than about 1°C (1.5°F) during 24 hours, but at no time touches the normal, it is described as *continued*. When the daily fluctuations exceed 2°C, it is called *remittent* (Fig. 1.6), and when fever is present only for several hours during the day it is called *intermittent*. When a paroxysm of intermittent fever occurs daily, the fever is described as *quotidian*; when on alternate days, it is *tertian*; when two days intervene between consecutive attacks, it is *quartan* (Fig. 1.7). However, with the use of antibiotics and other specific drugs, these classical types of fever are less often encountered.

Pulse

Count the pulse for a full half minute when the patient is at rest and composed. Abnormalities due to cardiovascular causes, such as disturbances of the normal rhythm (*arrhythmia*) are described in Chapter 8. The rate in health during the stress of a medical examination varies from about 60 to 80 beats/minute. The common causes of a rapid pulse are recent exercise, excitement or anxiety, shock (e.g. bleeding), fever and thyrotoxicosis. A slow pulse is characteristic of severe hypothyroidism and of complete heart block.

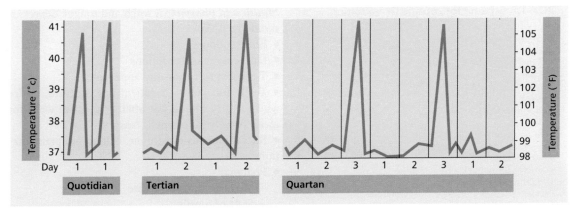

Fig. 1.7 Intermittent fever.

Respiration

Count the patient's respirations for a full half minute starting when the patient's attention is directed elsewhere. It is convenient to do this when the patient thinks you are still counting the pulse. The normal rate in an adult is about 14–18 respirations/minute, but wide variations occur in health. The main causes of fast breathing (*tachypnoea*) are recent exertion, anxiety or nervousness; fever; pulmonary, pleuritic and cardiac conditions causing hypoxia; cerebral disturbance; metabolic acidosis; and hysterical overbreathing (*hyperventilation*). The latter may cause alkalosis and attacks of tetany.

Obstruction in different parts of the respiratory tract may give rise to recognizable varieties of noisy breathing (see Chapter 7). Obstruction in the nasal passages may cause sniffling or bubbling sounds. Paralysis of the soft palate causes an inspiratory snoring noise. Obstruction in the region of the larynx causes inspiratory stridor, as in the whoop of whooping cough. Obstruction in the trachea may produce growling or rattling noises when the lumen is obstructed by mucus. Obstruction in the bronchi may give rise to audible snoring or wheezing noises.

Obstruction of airways in the larynx or larger bronchi characteristically gives rise to inspiratory noises, while obstructions in the small bronchi and bronchioles produces expiratory wheezing. The latter is heard in bronchitis and asthma (*obstructive airways disease*). Alternating periods of cessation of respiration with hyperventilation (*Cheyne–Stokes respiration*) occur in left heart failure and in various cerebral disturbances.

The pattern of breathing may be characteristic of diseases quite distinct from those of the respiratory system. Examples of this are the stertorous breathing after a seizure or severe stroke, the hissing expiration of uraemia, and the 'air hunger' of diabetic ketoacidotic coma, which affects both inspiration and expiration.

ODOURS

The odours of alcohol and of certain drugs, e.g. paraldehyde, are easily recognizable on the breath. That of alcohol does not necessarily mean the patient's condition is due to alcoholic intoxication. The odour of diabetic ketosis has been described as 'sweet and sickly'; that of uraemia as 'ammoniacal or fishy'; and that of hepatic failure as 'mousy', but too much reliance on such delicate distinctions is unwise. *Halitosis* (bad breath) is common in patients whose dental hygiene has been poor, and is associated especially with chronic gingivitis (periodontal or gum disease).

Routine examination

The following is a schema for routine examination (Box 1.7) which should be carried out on patients in hospital. Such a routine may have to be modified according to the needs of the patient, e.g. minimum necessary examination in an acutely ill patient; complete examination of the nervous system in a patient with neurological symptoms (see Chapter 12); or according to the circumstances, e.g. in the doctor's rooms or in the patient's home.

The object of a routine examination is to check the different bodily systems to exclude abnormality. In considering symptoms related to the patient's presenting complaint a more focused and detailed examination is necessary.

BOX 1.7 Schema for routine examination.

- General appearance
- Hair
- Eyes
- Face
- Mouth and pharynx
- Neck
- Upper limbs
- Thorax
  —anteriorly and laterally
  —posteriorly
- Abdomen
- Lower limbs
- Examination of excreta

During the taking of the history and the formal examination the following should be observed.

General
- General appearance (does the patient look healthy, unwell or ill, well cared for or neglected?)
- Intelligence and educational level
- Mental state
- Expression and emotional state
- Build and posture
- Nutrition, obesity, oedema
- Skin colour, cyanosis, anaemia, jaundice, pigmentation
- Skin eruptions, petechiae, spider naevi, vitiligo
- Body hair
- Deformities, swellings
- Temperature, pulse, respiration rate
- Features of endocrine disease, e.g hyperlipidaemia, acromegaly, Cushing's syndrome.

Hair
- Texture and grooming.

Eyes
- Simple tests of visual acuity: compare one eye against the other
- Exophthalmos or enophthalmos
- Ptosis
- Oedema of the lids
- Conjunctivae: anaemia, jaundice or inflammation
- Pupils: size, equality, regularity, reaction to light, accommodation
- Eye movement: nystagmus, strabismus
- Ophthalmoscopic examination of the fundi and ocular chambers.

Face
- Facies
- Jaw movements
- Facial symmetry or asymmetry
- Rash
- Features of endocrine disease or hyperlipidaemia.

Mouth and pharynx (A torch and tongue depressor should be used)
- Breath odours
- Lips: colour and eruptions
- Tongue: protrusion and appearance
- Teeth and gums (if patient has dentures, notice whether they fit and ask whether they are worn for meals or only for cosmetic reasons)
- Buccal mucous membrane: colour and pigmentation
- Pharynx:
  —Movement of soft palate
  —State of tonsils.

Neck
- Movement, pain and range
- Veins
- Lymphatic glands
- Thyroid
- Carotid pulses and bruits.

Upper limbs
- General examination of arms and hands
- Fingernails: clubbing or koilonychia
- Pulse: rate, rhythm, volume and character
- State of arterial wall of radials and brachials
- Axillae: lymph glands
- Blood pressure
- Muscles: muscle wasting, fasciculation
- Tests for power, tone, reflexes and co-ordination
- Cutaneous sensation: check all modalities to exclude root or nerve lesions
- Joints: movement, pain and swelling.

Thorax
Anteriorly and laterally
- Type of chest, asymmetry if any
- Breasts and nipples
- Respiration: rate, depth and character
- Pulsation
- Dilated vessels
- Position of trachea by palpation
- Look for and palpate apex beat
- Palpate over precordium for thrills
- Palpate respiratory movements
- Estimate tactile vocal fremitus
- Percuss the lungs
- Auscultate the heart sounds
- Auscultate the breath sounds
- Estimate vocal resonance, cervical and axillary glands.

Posteriorly (patient sitting)
- Inspect and palpate respiratory movement
- Estimate tactile vocal fremitus
- Percuss the lung resonance

- Auscultate the breath sounds
- Estimate vocal resonance
- Note movements and deformities of the spine
- Palpate from behind: cervical glands, thyroid
- Look for sacral oedema.

Abdomen

- Inspection: size, distension, symmetry
- Abdominal wall: movement, scars, dilated vessels
- Visible peristalsis or pulsation
- Pubic hair
- Hernial orifices
- Palpation: tenderness, rigidity, hyperaesthesia, splashing, masses, liver, gallbladder, spleen, kidneys, bladder
- Percussion: masses, liver, spleen, bladder
- Auscultation: bowel sounds, murmurs
- Impulse on coughing at hernial orifices
- Inguinal glands
- Genitalia: penis, scrotum, spermatic cord; female genitalia, examine if relevant
- Abdominal reflexes
- Rectal examination when indicated
- Gynaecological examination when indicated.

Lower limbs

- General examination of legs and feet
- Stance, balance and gait
- Oedema
- Varicose veins
- Muscles: muscle wasting, fasciculation
- Tests for power, tone, reflexes (including plantar response) and co-ordination
- Joints: movement, pain and swelling
- Peripheral pulses
- Temperature of feet

Examination of excreta

- Urine, sputum, stools, vomit: examination by naked eye, and measure or estimate amount
- Test urine for specific gravity, sugar, protein and blood.

Writing out the history and examination

The history and examination can be recorded in several different ways. The aim is to write a complete yet concise record of a patient's illness. For easy reference this is best done in note form, with important facts marked with an asterisk or underlined.

It is helpful to record routine details of the patient's marital status, children, age, occupation, financial and racial status, and the family history and past medical history first. The patient's presenting complaint and the history of the presenting illness then fall naturally into context with this background information. This approach is particularly pertinent when taking and recording a history of symptoms likely to be psychogenic, or related to potentially serious or difficult problems, e.g. the consequences of head injury or of cancer and its treatment. Try not to be constantly engaged in writing notes while the patient is talking about their problems but, rather, maintain contact with the patient during this time.

The initial statement concerning the physical findings should describe the patient briefly, without any hint of judgemental comment, in order to try to picture the patient. For example, 'well nourished, muscular man', or 'emaciated frightened', or 'jaundiced, breathless co-operative woman', or 'confused, agitated and restlessly wandering patient'. Significant general features should also be noted at this point, especially the general state of health and nutrition, the presence or absence of anaemia or jaundice, or of lymphadenopathy, and features of systemic illness such as abnormalities in the skin, e.g. nailbed infarcts, ecchymoses, vitiligo, etc.

The physical examination, whatever the order in which it is carried out, should be written out under systems. A short statement of the findings under each system should be included. The absence of signs, as well as of symptoms, can be as important as their presence. Simple line drawings can often convey more information than much writing. The minimum statement about a patient's cardiovascular system, for example, might read as in Table 1.4.

Pulse 76 regular, peripheral pulses normal
Neck veins not distended. No peripheral oedema
BP 130/80
Apex beat not displaced
Heart sounds I and II heard in all areas
No murmurs, lungs clear

Table 1.4   Example of CVS statement.

The case notes should conclude with a list of tentative diagnoses and a list of investigations planned and arranged. The plan of management should be outlined, and those features to be used as an index of progress should be indicated.

The *progress notes* should discuss the diagnosis, the patient's symptoms and signs, the results of investigations and any changes in management. Progress notes should clearly state the results of investigations, the development of the plan of management, the treatment plan and the clinical progress. The nature of information given to the patient and to the patient's family and friends must be documented, and special instructions or plans noted. If any discussion has occurred with the patient, or family, concerning resuscitation or decisions related to this, should it prove necessary, this should be carefully and frankly noted (see section on ethical issues, Chapter 21).

The distinction between the patient's problem and the diagnosis, discussed earlier in this chapter, is sometimes stressed by the adoption of a format of case-recording in which the patient's problems are enumerated in each follow-up note, with attention to treatment and management of each problem individually. Although somewhat inclined to repetition, this problem-oriented method of medical record-keeping serves to remind the clinician to attend to all of a patient's problems individually. Certainly, it is relevant to distinguish the patient's subjective problems from the diagnosis at the outset, since the former must be relieved, if at all possible, even if the diagnosis is such that cure is not feasible.

Presenting a case

The value of a student's or doctor's notes on a patient is greatly enhanced if they can be communicated in concise form to other students or doctors. Students should therefore practise making a short summary of their findings, emphasizing both important positive findings and relevant negative ones. This summary should begin with the name, age, sex and occupation of the patient, and end with a brief statement of the problem.

In addition, the student should practise oral presentation of cases at every opportunity. This is an essential skill in explaining clinical problems to other physicians and surgeons; the ultimate test is the ability to communicate a difficult problem to a senior colleague on the telephone. A logical approach to the relevant aspects of the case, with only brief attention to negative data, is essential. The history and findings on examination should be communicated in temporal, coherent order, making an interesting and easily grasped story. If you have the opportunity use an overhead projector, or a blackboard to present visually the most important points in the history, examination and investiga-

tion. In presenting a case, always speak as though to a single other person, rather than to a group. Try to communicate.

Interpretation of clinical data

The object of history-taking, physical examination and ancillary investigations is the making of a diagnosis and the planning of management. In the past this was often taken to mean the detection of a disease process, e.g. 'This patient has Hodgkin's disease'. If no disease process was detected the complaints were described as 'functional'. This was illogical since all disease involves some disorder of function. Nonetheless, many consultations are concerned with bodily disorders that are the expression of mental distress, rather than of serious physical illness. The detection and alleviation of these problems is as important as the diagnosis of an organic disease process. Furthermore, the patient's own concept of their disease, and their reaction to it has to be assessed alongside the doctor's diagnosis. Ultimately, it is the patient's symptoms that must be relieved.

One should begin the process of making a diagnosis by asking oneself broad questions such as: 'What is this person's problem?' and: 'Is there a disability?' If it is decided that there is a disability, one should ask:

• How far can this person's disability be explained by their environment, i.e. in geographical, socioeconomic and cultural terms?
• How far can this person's disability be explained by their own attitude and mental make-up, i.e. in psychological terms?
• How far can this person's disability be explained by a disease process or processes, i.e. in pathological terms?

Although it is axiomatic that one should try to account for all of a patient's symptoms by one disease process, a surprising number of patients in fact have more than one, e.g. coronary artery disease and hiatus hernia, both of which may produce central chest pain; and still more have a disease process which either does not explain the symptoms at all or does not explain all the symptoms, e.g. weakness and tiredness in a patient with mild angina pectoris or mild anaemia. Moreover, an apparently simple event may have a complex medical background. For instance, an old lady gets out of bed, trips and breaks her wrist. It is possible that she was hurrying to the lavatory as she had cystitis, she tripped because her vision was impaired by cataract, and that the wrist fracture occurred because her bones were weakened by osteoporosis.

In making a diagnosis one should try to account for a person's total disability and should not be dismayed if this involves more than one item. Thus the diagnosis in an old lady with multiple symptoms might well be:

- Loneliness
- Depression
- Mild degenerative osteoarthritis

or in a young man with dyspepsia:

- Impending marriage
- Anxiety state
- Duodenal ulcer.

A diagnosis of this kind, which lists the patient's problems and is not confined to labelling organic disease, gives a true picture of the state of affairs. The patient's complaint forms but one part of the patient. Always view the patient as a whole. Will the patient be restored to full mental and physical health when this symptom has resolved?

Diagnosis

The diagnostic process is a complex mental task in which the clinical data are weighed in the clinician's mind against the doctor's previous experience, and his or her formally acquired knowledge of the medical literature. There is no substitute for knowledge, but knowledge can only be used appropriately when its significance is understood in relation to everyday clinical experience. An experienced clinician will arrive at a diagnosis on the basis of apparently minimal clues, because it is clear to that clinician that certain aspects of the patient's history, or physical signs, have especial significance. The way in which a patient describes upper abdominal pain may be more important than the precise characteristics of the pain in suggesting a diagnosis of cardiac or oesophageal pain. On the other hand, the experienced doctor will recognize that it is possible to be misled by over-reliance on clinical intuitions, and investigation should be used as a check on diagnostic

accuracy, as well as in quantifying an abnormality for planning management. The role of modern, computerized imaging cannot be overestimated in this regard.

All clinicians are constantly updating their own database, i.e. their memory of patients and their clinical features, in relation to the acquisition of factual knowledge derived from textbooks and medical journals. There is always something new to be learned in medicine, even for the most experienced doctor. Computer-based diagnostic systems and reference databases are evolving tools in this process of informing clinicians, but they are not substitutes for learning, for wisdom and, above all, for clinical skills and easy patient relationships.

Assessment of functional impairment after injury or illness

In disease of any bodily system it is useful to be able to assess the residual problem faced by the patient. In many different diseases, therefore, rating scales have been designed in order to try to provide some relatively objective measurement. These are weighted in relation to the most important residual problems found in the disorder under assessment. For example, rheumatoid arthritis rating scales are particularly weighted toward stiffness, limitation of mobility of joints, ability to carry out tasks of daily living such as dressing, toileting and feeding and joint pain; in cardiopulmonary disease the rating scales are concerned with breathlessness, exercise tolerance, sputum production and chest pain; and in multiple sclerosis most of the scales in common use rely heavily on impairment of self-caring, incontinence, visual impairment and a quantified clinical examination of the nervous system.

Clearly, these rating scales are not comparable one with another and, since they are ordinal in character, it is difficult to make statistical comparisons between two different assessments made on the same patient at two different times, although this is often done in assessing a patient's response to a treatment. Most of these rating scales were devised with specific research aims in mind, rather than for everyday clinical use, although several are now used routinely in the clinic. Despite these theoretical difficulties in handling rating scales, such scales have proven very useful in clinical practice, since they provide a relatively standardized assessment of a patient's clinical state at any given time.

In considering data from rating assessments it is well to remember that they often include assessments of *clinical impairments*, *disabilities* and *handicaps*, without separating these different concepts, which may overlap or even duplicate each other (Box 1.8).

BOX 1.8 Impairment, disability and handicap: definitions.

- An *impairment* is the absence or abnormality of a basic biological function, for example hand movement, or vision.
- A *disability* is a lack of a normal functional ability, whether physical or psychological, and represents a lack of normal interaction between the patient and their environment. Disability is easier to assess than impairment.
- A *handicap* is the disadvantage resulting from a disability. It thus often consists of dependency on others, or on some piece of equipment, and can be modified or even overcome by suitable manipulation of the environment. Measurement of handicap may not always be relevant, since it can be modified by social changes.

Functional rating scales are becoming more and more important in clinical practice, since they form one method of assessing the value of medical or other interventions in disease states.

CHAPTER 2

The psychiatric assessment

Introduction

The prevalence of psychiatric disorder in the community is of such magnitude that every doctor must be able to carry out a psychiatric assessment. The range of presenting problems is wide, and many patients with emotional disturbance may present, not with overt psychiatric symptoms, but with 'more respectable' physical symptoms. In some patients physical and psychiatric illness may coexist or there may be a direct causal relationship between the two, as in the depressed patient who takes a drug overdose, or the elderly man with a postoperative confusional state. On the other hand, physical and psychiatric illnesses may be unrelated, as in the chronic schizophrenic who develops a neoplastic lesion. In addition, every patient's reaction to illness will be influenced by their emotional state and this will itself affect the course of the illness.

As in physical illness, the approach to diagnosis and treatment of a psychiatric disorder depends on an adequate formulation of the problem. This necessitates following the basic steps of history-taking, examining the patient and, when necessary, arranging appropriate investigations. In psychiatry exact measurements are often not readily available. Emphasis is therefore placed on the history and examination, and further investigations consist mainly of clarification of this information by interview and observation, and from other sources of information. In addition, specific psychological investigations, including measures of the cognitive state and, less frequently, of personality and mood are also used. Laboratory tests and X-rays are used in some cases.

The psychiatric history

Interview technique

As in every medical interview, it is important to put the patient at ease and to establish a relationship in a warm and emphatic way, using words that the patient can understand. On the interview technique will depend not only the accuracy of the information gathered, and therefore the adequacy of the formulation, but also the patient's compliance in any treatment suggested. In no branch of medicine are interviewing skills so important as in psychiatry. The doctor's ability to communicate is doubly important as psychiatric patients, by the very nature of their disturbances, may be particularly difficult to interview. Even for the most well-adjusted person the interview itself may involve being asked searching and potentially embarrassing questions. Awareness of these difficulties is helpful to the interviewer.

BOX 2.1 The psychiatric history.

- Reason for referral
- Presenting complaints
- History of present illness
- Family history
- Personal history
  —Childhood
  —Schooling
  —Occupation
  —Psychosexual and marital experiences
  —Forensic
  —Past medical history
  —Past psychiatric history
  —Drug and alcohol abuse
  —Pre-morbid personality
  —Social circumstances

History-taking scheme

The psychiatric history should be carried out systematically under several headings (Box 2.1). Taking a psychiatric history often requires more than one interview, the number depending on many factors, including the amount of information to be gathered and the rapport established between the patient and doctor. Obviously the above scheme must be adapted to meet the needs of the patient, and different aspects may receive different degrees of emphasis in different patients.

History of present illness

The patient must be given the opportunity to tell the doctor what is worrying him or her. Getting patients to talk about themselves requires the doctor to be patient, relaxed, sympathetic and, above all, to be a good listener. The patient must feel that the doctor has respect for their problem. It is often useful to write down the patient's complaints verbatim since they may constitute a summary of the disorder.

Initially the patient should do most of the talking. The doctor can clarify the problem later if necessary by asking leading questions. For each symptom the following points should be elicited (Box 2.2).

BOX 2.2 The history of illness.

- The complaint itself
- Date and time of onset
- Aggravating and relieving factors
- Consistency of the symptom complex
- Severity
- Definitions
- Site and radiation of physical symptoms
- Associated symptoms
- Any previous history of related problems

The date and circumstances of onset of the symptoms. This should include any precipitating factors or recent stresses. Since the illness may have been present for some time before the onset of the presenting symptoms it may only be by asking the patient when they were last well that the true date of onset of the illness can be decided.

Relieving and aggravating factors.

Consistency. Any variation from day to day or during the day should be determined. This includes searching for any periodicity such as diurnal mood variation; patients with a depressive illness often feel worse in the morning.

Severity. This is often best assessed by asking the patient how the symptom interferes with normal life.

Definition. It is important to clarify what the patient means by symptoms. Confusion may mean one thing to the layman and another to the doctor. Abnormal beliefs or experiences may not be clearly described but the doctor must be absolutely sure about them if the correct diagnosis is to be reached.

Site and radiation. This is mostly relevant when the patient complains of physical symptoms but may be important when the patient is hearing voices; hearing them outside or inside the head may have a different significance.

Associated symptoms. It is important to ask in detail about any other symptoms associated with the major presenting complaint and, at this time, it is relevant to ask about sleep, appetite and weight.

Sleep disturbance may be related to physical problems, such as pain or breathlessness, or to psychological problems. Examples of the latter include insomnia occurring in the presence of anxiety or drug withdrawal; early morning waking and nightmares with depression; excessive sleep with drugs or organic illness; reversed sleep pattern, i.e. increasing during the day and decreased at night, in acute confusional states; and disturbed sleep with affective or organic illness. Sleep disturbance of recent onset is usually highly significant whereas chronic sleep impairment, although distressing to the patient, is usually of less importance in diagnosis.

Appetite is decreased in anorexia nervosa but may be increased in anxious patients who eat for comfort. In depression, appetite may decrease or increase. It is an alteration of pattern that is important. Associated with loss of appetite there may be a *loss of weight* as in depression, anorexia nervosa or self-neglect, and when appetite is increased there may be *weight gain*, which also occurs during treatment with some psychotropic drugs.

Previous history. It is important to find out about any history of similar symptoms, type of treatment and the patient's response to it.

Family history. Similar symptoms in family members and their response to treatment should be asked about.

Family history

The patient's family background is important in many psychiatric disorders. For example, in schizo-

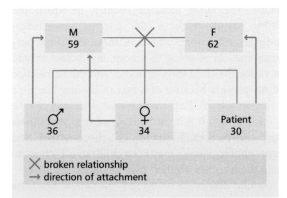

X broken relationship
→ direction of attachment

Fig. 2.1 Diagram of personal relationships. The patient is aged 30 years. The older two siblings, aged 34 and 36 years were closer to their mother, and the patient was close to her father. The parents were separated.

phrenia and the affective psychoses genetic factors may be relevant. Environmental factors are often complex. The loss of a mother in early life predisposes to depression in later life; failure of bonding may lead to difficulties with relationships in adult life and overprotective parents may produce anxious children. This aspect of the history must be covered in some detail, including information mainly about parents and siblings and also, when relevant, about members of the non-nuclear family.

For each parent, if alive, one should ask about age and physical and psychiatric health, both present and previous. If dead, then the age of the parent at the time of death, the cause of death and the patient's age and reaction to the bereavement need to be ascertained, as well as the parents' health while they were alive. The parents' occupations and personalities, and their relationship with each other and with the patient, including any separations in childhood from the patient are all relevant. Children whose parents have had a bad marriage are themselves vulnerable to the development of psychosexual and marital difficulties. For each sibling similar details should be obtained, including information about their marital status. By this stage, some idea of the family atmosphere, interfamily relationships and the position of the patient within the family will have been gained, though it may be necessary to ask directly to obtain this information. It is useful to draw a family tree to facilitate the assimilation and display of the information gathered. This can vary from a simple diagram of the family members with their ages to the use of symbols to denote the emotional relationships between the various family members (Fig. 2.1). As long as the symbols are used

consistently and a reference key is provided it does not matter what symbols are used. For example, in the family shown in Fig. 2.1, the parents were divorced and the elder two siblings were closer to their mother, and the youngest to his father, as indicated by arrows. In some cases it may be relevant to ask about other members of the family, e.g. in instances in which the patient is brought up by, or is particularly close to, a grandparent, or in which a grandparent or parental sibling lives or has lived in the nuclear family home. Finally, the family psychiatric and medical history should be discussed both in the nuclear and in the wider family. This enquiry should include psychiatric disturbance, alcoholism, suicide and epilepsy. An unexplained death in the family may hint at suicide. If any member of the family has had psychiatric treatment, the date and place of this treatment should be ascertained.

Personal history

The question to be answered is: Why have *these* symptoms occurred in *this* patient at *this* time?

This requires familiarity with the patient's earlier circumstances; for example, a severely anxious child with a fear of going to school and inability to separate from his or her parents may well develop symptoms of anxiety (such as agoraphobia) in later life, whereas a person with a long history of difficulty in coping with authority may present later with antisocial behaviour. A systematic scheme of enquiry such as that detailed below helps to ensure that important areas are not omitted, though the weight placed on different aspects of the personal history may differ from patient to patient. A visual display of the information by means of a life chart (Fig. 2.2) may help to clarify the relationship between different areas of the patient's life and illuminate the cause of the current symptoms.

CHILDHOOD

This is the logical place to start the personal history. Begin with questions about the patient's birth. Was it planned, what was the length of gestation? Find out about the mother's health during pregnancy and the nature of the delivery. Note the infantile and childhood milestones, and inquire about neonatal or feeding difficulties; most people are only aware of these if their parents have told them of any difficulties in these areas.

In later childhood, neurotic traits may become

apparent such as particular fears, physical symptoms at times of stress, or periods of unhappiness. These and additional traits such as bed-wetting, temper tantrums, and periods of physical or emotional disorder must be considered in the light of relationships with peers, the atmosphere at home, separations from and relationships with family members, and any bereavement or other major life event. Child abuse, physical, sexual and/or psychological should be asked about tactfully and sympathetically when appropriate, either when asking about childhood, family history or psychosexual history.

ADOLESCENCE

Assessment of adolescence includes questions that usually arise when dealing with the psychosexual history. Relevant areas of enquiry are peer and family relationships, episodes of disturbance, whether anti-social or emotional, and difficulties in growing up. Adolescence is interrelated with *schooling* and *occupation*.

SCHOOLING

It is usual to ask about dates of starting, leaving and changing schools, academic achievement, relationships with peers and teachers, any difficulties in learning or behaviour and periods of non-atten-

dance. The latter includes *truancy*, in which the child, usually without the parents' knowledge, indulges, often with others, in more enjoyable pastimes instead of going to school, and *school refusal*, in which the child stays at home with the knowledge of his parents because of a fear of leaving home or going to school. Enforced *absence* is usually due to illness, although it must be remembered that illness may also be a manifestation of school refusal, and agoraphobic parents may keep children off school to help them cope with their own anxieties.

Similar details are required if the patient has gone on to higher education.

OCCUPATION

A comprehensive work history entails asking about every job the patient has had since leaving school. Enquiry should concentrate on duration of job, level of achievement and promotion, attendance and ability, enjoyment or difficulties, relationship with peers and superiors, reasons for leaving and the duration of any period of unemployment.

If the person has had numerous jobs this may become a repetitive and tedious process. In these cases a shortened approach can be used by asking about the number of jobs, the length of time unem-

Date	Age	Social history	Family history	Psychosexual history	Medical history	Psychiatric history
1952	0					
1957	5					
1962	10	School	Parents' divorce		Pain in chest	Difficulties at school
1967	15					
1972	20	Secretary		Marries (leaves home)	Pain in back	Relieved by Diazepam
1977	25			First child born		Puerperal depression
1982	30	Part-time work		Second child born	Pain in back	Sleep and appetite impaired, lethargy
1992	40			Marital stress	Headache	Sleep disturbance, anxiety, feelings of inability to cope

Fig. 2.2 Life chart of a 40-year-old married mother of two from a broken home referred to the Orthopaedic Department with backache, for which no cause could be found. Associated symptoms included sleep disturbance, poor appetite and lethargy. Given this patient's background, in particular the divorce of her parents, one would not be surprised if she were vulnerable in psychosexual areas, and this is shown clearly in the chart to be the case by the development of emotional disturbance at the time of her marriage and the birth of her first child. One would therefore anticipate that the birth of her second child would also be a traumatic time for her. The presentation with physical symptoms—pain in the back—as a manifestation of psychiatric disorder is consistent both with her symptomatology after her parents' divorce, and at the time of her marriage, and the presence of the associated symptoms of sleep and appetite disturbance and lethargy, all common manifestations of emotional upset. The life chart clearly displays these links.

ployed in total and in the last five years, the longest job, the highest level of achievement, any difficulties at work including being dismissed from a job, general relationship with colleagues and employers, and the general work record, while asking in more detail about the present job.

Where relevant, military service can be dealt with in much the same way as any other occupation.

PSYCHOSEXUAL HISTORY

This is usually the most difficult area to assess, relying as it does on asking highly personal questions which may be as embarrassing for the doctor as the patient. It is important not to allow this potential difficulty to harm the doctor–patient relationship. However, failure to ask these questions may result in the omission of a vital piece of information with serious effects on the overall assessment. Although in some cases it may be necessary to leave some of the questions to later interviews, sensitive and skilful interviewing usually enables adequate exploration of this area in the first interview. Shaping the enquiry so as to lead from easy to difficult questions, for example by taking a menstrual history before the sexual one, and asking questions in such a way as to make the patient feel their sexual behaviour is normal, for example: 'How old were you when you first started to masturbate?' rather than: 'Have you ever masturbated?' facilitates the acquisition of information. It may be tactful with some patients to use less emotionally laden wording, such as 'physical relationship' instead of 'sexual relationship'.

The *sexual history* should encompass the following points: puberty; menstrual history; sex education; masturbation and fantasies; relationships with members of the opposite sex, especially their duration, intensity and sexual contact and enjoyment; engagement; marriage (see below); any homosexual feelings and experiences; and, where appropriate, deviant sexual experiences and fantasies, including sexual abuse in childhood or adolescence.

The *marital history* includes the relationship with the spouse from the time of meeting through the development of their relationship, engagement and marriage. Note the age and occupation of the spouse; the parents' attitude towards him or her; the quality of the marriage, including any areas of disagreement, overt disharmony or periods of separation; their current sexual relationship, both its frequency and enjoyment, and any extramarital affairs. Enquire about pregnancies, terminations and miscarriages, stillbirths and live births with details of the

ages and behaviour of the children and any difficulties with them. If the couple have been together for a long time and there are no children, then it is important to know why. Is it from choice because both husband and wife are career-oriented, or through a dislike of children or fear of pregnancy, suggesting possible psychosexual difficulties? Failure to conceive despite trying may have repercussions on the emotional state of the partners and their relationship. Similarly, if there is only one child to a long-standing marriage or if there are large gaps between the birth of children it is worth asking the patient whether there is any reason for this.

When the patient is not married but is in a stable relationship the same questions should be asked as for the married patient, including future intentions as far as marriage or staying together are concerned. When the patient has been married before, the previous marriage and its ending by death or divorce should also be assessed. Finally, if the patient is neither married nor in a stable relationship it is worth asking about any desires for the future and whether there is a feeling of any difficulties in this area.

FORENSIC HISTORY

This encompasses any and all confrontations with the law and includes juvenile delinquency as well as antisocial behaviour later on in life. Details of offences committed and punishment received should be noted.

PAST MEDICAL HISTORY

It is important to ask in chronological order about any illness or operations in childhood or during adult life; about periods of hospitalization or incapacity and any resulting disability and interference with the patient's life; the reaction of the patient and family to these episodes and any remaining medical problems, including current symptoms and medication. It is, for example, illuminating to find out that the patient who now presents with physical symptoms has had a number of previous episodes of similar symptoms at times of stress and has recovered when the stress was resolved, or that the anxious patient awaiting surgery has always reacted badly in the past to major illnesses or operations. It is useful here to ask about the frequency and nature of contact with the family doctor.

PAST PSYCHIATRIC HISTORY

This includes any episodes of emotional upset, from that thought not severe enough to need medical attention, through the minor neuroses treated by the family doctor, to severe psychiatric disorders needing expert psychiatric treatment, whether as outpatient, day-patient or in-patient on a voluntary or compulsory basis. Ask about circumstances, precipitating factors, place of treatment, duration and response to treatment and any continuing symptoms or medication. It is often worth asking if the patient has ever taken psychotropic medication in the past, whether prescribed by the family doctor or obtained in other ways, not necessarily as any form of drug abuse but, perhaps, from other members of the family. Finally, it is also worth asking about contact with any voluntary organizations, such as the Samaritans, or with social services.

ALCOHOL ABUSE

Alcohol abuse (Box 2.3) may lead to physical, psychiatric and social sequelae and it affects an increasingly large number of people. Yet it is a problem only too frequently neglected in the medical history. All patients should be asked whether they drink and, if so, roughly how much and in what circumstances, remembering that the answers frequently bear little resemblance to actual alcohol consumption.

BOX 2.3 Features that suggest alcohol abuse.

- Excessive weekly intake
- Inability to stop drinking
- Craving for alcohol
- Secret drinking and drinking alone
- Morning drinking
- Drinking to steady nerves, or to steady 'morning shakes'
- Amnesia for events during a drinking binge
- Conviction for drunken driving, or other alcohol-related crime
- Violent behaviour
- Marital problems
- Alcohol-related physical illness

Where there is any suspicion of alcohol-related problems a thorough and systematic drinking history must be obtained. One way of doing this is to construct a daily account of the patient's drinking habits including how they feel when they wake up in the morning, how much sleep they have had, whether they remember what happened the night before, and if they have withdrawal symptoms on getting up in the morning, such as shaking, nausea, retching, anxiety or craving for alcohol. Detailed questions about the content, time, place, type and circumstances of first and all subsequent drinks and whether the patient drinks alone or in company are often reveal-

ing. When dealing with the first drink of the day it is worth asking about the speed at which it is drunk, as people with physical dependence often gulp rather than sip their first drink. Another helpful pointer to the current level of drinking is the amount of money the patient spends on drink, especially when related to their income.

Having dealt with the current drinking habit it is useful to take a more longitudinal perspective on the drinking history, covering such points as any family history of drinking, the age when the patient started drinking and when their alcohol consumption increased, the pattern of drinking, whether daily or in bouts, the type of alcohol consumed, and any precipitating factors, e.g. whether related to stress or mood. Personal difficulties caused by drinking—including its impact on the family; physical or psychiatric illness; loss of work or being drunk at work, or anti-social behaviour—and previous treatment or periods of abstinence or reduction in alcohol intake are important. A history of serious medical or social complications, such as delirium tremens, anti-social behaviour resulting in encounters with the police, or alcohol-related marital problems are especially important.

It is also important, for treatment, to ascertain whether the patient feels he or she is drinking too much and would like to cut down or even stop drinking, and what sort of help might be necessary, or acceptable to achieve this.

DRUG ABUSE

This term implies not only drugs of addiction, whether major, e.g. heroin, or minor, e.g. cannabis, but also prescribed drugs, commonly benzodiazepines, and non-prescribed drugs not normally considered addictive, such as cough linctus or analgesics. An assessment similar to that outlined above for alcohol abuse should be used. Information concerning the route of drug intake and the source of the drugs should be obtained, if possible.

PERSONALITY

Personality disorder is one of the commonest diagnoses used in psychiatry. Personality is defined as the sum of those characteristics that make a person into the individual he or she is (Box 2.4).

Personality may change with illness, for example, disinhibition occurs with frontal lobe brain damage. However, to ascertain in what sort of person this illness has developed, it is necessary to assess pre-morbid personality. This is most reliably assessed from

---

BOX 2.4 Characteristics of personality.

- Behaviour
  —actions and reactions
- Attitude to self
- Relations with others
  —social
  —sexual
- Attitude to authority
- Level of independence
- Mood, e.g. usually happy, cheerful, sad, etc.
- Fantasy life
- Religious beliefs and moral attitudes
- Interests and hobbies

---

an informant familiar with the patient before the onset of the illness. If such an objective opinion is unavailable it is worth asking the patient how others see them, for example: 'Would other people say you were a worrier?' Some features of personality, for example, histrionic behaviour, will be obvious during the interview and others will already have been elicited in the history. Though many of the characteristics which make up the personality overlap (e.g. manipulative behaviour is both a manifestation of behaviour itself and a way of relating to others), they are best dealt with separately.

BEHAVIOUR

The behaviour exhibited by the patient can be considered in terms of actions and reactions.

Actions include level of achievement, histrionic or manipulative behaviour, deliberate self-harm or aggression towards others, disinhibition, obsessional behaviour (e.g. tidiness, being houseproud, perfectionist, conscientious or checking) and alcohol or drug abuse. Many of these will have been covered in the occupational, past psychiatric, forensic, and alcohol or drug abuse history.

Reactions can occur to stressful events, such as illness, bereavement and other losses, or examinations, promotion at work, failure and disappointment, and ability to cope with change (see sections on family, occupational and past medical histories above). Types of reaction include being panicky, unflappable and slow to react, short-tempered and easily angered, or placid. Both actions and reactions can be assessed by considering the following headings.

Attitude to self
- Self-interested or thoughtful about others
- Level of self-esteem and self-criticism
- Self-consciousness and sensitivity
- Acceptance of abilities and achievements

- Self-confidence, whether high or low and constantly needing reassurance.

Relationship to others
Social
- Ease of making and keeping social relationships
- Introverted or extroverted
- Suspiciousness
- Assertiveness
- Warm and affectionate or cold and undemonstrative
- Tolerant or authoritarian and intolerant
- Relationships at work and with the family.

Psychosexual
- Level of psychosexual development, especially the capacity to make sexual relationships
- Direction of sexual attraction
- Areas of difficulty.

Attitudes to authority
- Well-adjusted and accepting
- Anxious and uncertain
- Generally tolerant or intolerant.

Level of independence
- Has the patient left home?
- Still living with parents?
- Accepting of responsibility for their actions
- Capable of making decisions?

Usual mood
- Prone to anxiety and if so, about what, e.g. illness, work or family
- Pessimistic or optimistic
- *Cyclothymic*, i.e. swinging from elation to depression without reaching illness proportions
- Calm or irritable
- Bottles up or shares feelings and emotions
- Easy-going or short-tempered and easily angered.

Religious beliefs and moral attitudes
- Which religion
- Whether practising or not
- Whether tolerant of beliefs and attitudes of others
- Ability to show regret or remorse and limit actions according to conscience.

Interests or hobbies
- What types
- Time spent on them
- Passive spectator or active participant
- Social or solitary pastimes
- Energetic or sedentary.

Fantasy life
- Sexual fantasies
- Non-sexual fantasies
- Dreams
- Nightmares.

SOCIAL CIRCUMSTANCES

Ask the patient about their place and type of abode, satisfaction with the accommodation and with other members of the household, relationships with neighbours, current social contacts, financial problems and, if not already noted, any current or recent stresses including bereavement.

SUMMING UP

At the end of the history it is important to sum up to the patient what you have understood the problem to be. Ask whether you have grasped it in its entirety, left out any important areas or perhaps even totally failed to understand what he or she has been trying to put over. Besides clarifying the history it also shows the patient that you have been listening, and have understood.

The examination

This can be subdivided into physical and psychiatric examination.

Physical examination

Physical examination of patients presenting with symptoms suggestive of psychiatric disorder is often both relevant and necessary. The combination of psychiatric symptoms and physical disease is common. Acutely anxious patients may have signs of thyrotoxicosis. Evidence of liver disease may suggest alcoholism. Needle marks in the arms point to drug abuse; scars of slashed wrists or other signs of self-mutilation may point to psychiatric illness.

Psychiatric or mental state examination

This should be covered systematically (Box 2.5).

BOX 2.5 Examination of the mental state.

- Appearance and behaviour
- Speech
- Mood
- Thought content
- Abnormal beliefs
- Abnormal experiences
- Cognitive state
- Intelligence
- Insight and rapport
- Specific tests of cerebral function
  —questionnaires
  —structured interview schedules

APPEARANCE AND BEHAVIOUR

The patient's appearance and behaviour often reveal the underlying psychiatric disorder. Important points to look for include dress, personal hygiene and general grooming. Note the shabbily dressed elderly man with food stains on his clothes, perhaps indicative of an underlying dementia or schizophrenic illness.

Facial expression is one of the outward signs of the patient's mood. For example, tearfulness or poverty of expression occur in depression, elation in mania, tenseness in anxiety, perplexity or blunting in schizophrenia. The *affect* may be inappropriate, such as the schizophrenic patient who laughs when relating upsetting material; it must be remembered, none the less, that anxious people may also laugh in similar circumstances. The emotional expression may be abnormally labile as in mania or organic brain disease.

The way the patient sits gives important hints to an underlying pathology; is he or she relaxed and obviously at ease, or sitting tensely and fidgeting? The agitated depressive or the excited manic or schizophrenic may be so agitated that he gets up from the seat and paces up and down the room. The demented or confused patient may leave the chair because they do not understand what is going on, or because they feel threatened in the presence of delusions of persecution. The catatonic patient may appear to sit in a peculiar position, whereas the patient with retarded depression may show no movement during the interview and the anxious, overcontrolled patient may hold their body rigidly. The patient may appear to drift off to sleep repeatedly, suggesting either a confusional state with fluctuating levels of consciousness or over-sedation.

The way the patient walks on the way to and from the interview room may show signs of ataxia due to organic brain disease, drug effect or excess alcohol consumption. In the latter the breath will smell of alcohol. There may be signs of hysterical ataxia, which may improve with suggestion or exhortation, or ataxia due to malingering, in which the limp varies from moment to moment and is most marked when the patient knows they are being watched.

There may be other abnormal movements, such as dystonia caused by major tranquillizers, choreiform movements in Huntington's chorea, or tic-like mannerisms, odd postures or other bizarre disorders of movement seen in patients with catatonia due to schizophrenia or organic brain disease. These include perseveration of posture so that the patient's limbs can be moved into an abnormal position which is maintained despite being freely allowed to revert to the previous posture. When this movement is met by a waxy resistance it is termed *waxy flexibility*. The patient may keep on starting and stopping certain purposeful actions, for example when shaking hands with the interviewer, or show *negativism*, in which he or she opposes the examiner's intention. In *echopraxia* the interviewer's actions are copied; these abnormal postures and movements often occur in organic brain disease as well as in non-organic catatonia. There may be signs of slowing or retardation of movement, even, at times, to the extent of stupor which, in the case of catatonia, may be interspersed with periods of violent excitement. Stupor is commonly caused by organic disorders but may also be a result of functional psychoses, such as schizophrenia and depression. Further, stupor may be hysterical in nature, or due to a very high level of anxiety following extreme stress; or it may be simulated by malingerers.

The patient's behaviour during the interview may be disinhibited, as in the manic patient who strips or the patient with organic brain disease who starts to urinate or masturbate during the interview. The patient may be manipulative or seductive and may threaten violence if their wishes are not met. There may be verbal aggression or physical violence, the latter against either the interviewer or objects in the room. On the other hand, the patient may appear to be unduly submissive or self-critical, or may show little or no eye contact with the interviewer. They may appear to be suspicious of questions due to an underlying personality disorder or paranoid illness. The patient may also seem to be paying little attention to the interviewer or to be listening to someone else when there is no one else in the room; this suggests that he or she is experiencing *auditory hallucinations*, i.e. hearing voices. The patient may even be talking to or arguing with these voices. Undue terror without any obvious cause or attempts to touch or shoo away non-existing objects suggests that the patient is experiencing *visual hallucinations*.

It must, however, always be remembered that bizarre behaviour or inability to relate to the interviewer may be signs of subnormal intelligence. Finally, obsessional patients may bring with them lists of their symptoms to present to the interviewer.

SPEECH

It is important to assess the form of speech as well as its content. Does the patient speak at all or is he or she mute and, if so, is this deliberate, organic, hyster-ical or part of a depressive or catatonic stupor? In the mute patient it is important to assess all aspects of speech production including the ability to produce sounds and communicate non-verbally. If the patient does speak, is this spontaneous or only in answer to questions, without monosyllabic or fuller and more elaborate replies? Is speech unduly slow as in depressive illness or so quick and continuous that it is impossible to interrupt, as in hypomania and mania? Are there long pauses before the patient replies or are there arrests of speech in mid-sentence, e.g. in schizophrenia?

Are the words normal or are there neologisms as in some types of schizophrenia or organic brain disease? Is there evidence of *dysphasia* (see page 282) or *dysarthria* (page 281)? Where the words are normal, are the phrases and sentences normal and do they fit together, or does the patient seem to jump from topic to topic; if the latter occurs, is it possible to understand the link between topics, as in flight of ideas in mania, or is there no recognizable link as in *formal thought disorder* in schizophrenia? Is the link, if present, not one of content but of form as in rhyming or punning, usually features of mania? Is there evidence of *echolalia*, in which the patient repeats what the interviewer says, or *perseveration*, when the patient continues with the same theme even if this is no longer appropriate? As an example of the latter, a 60-year-old man, replying to the question 'How old are you?' answers '60, 61, 62, 63, 64, 65, 66' and so on; when asked the subsequent question 'What year were you born?' he answers '1960' and to the next question 'What year is it?' now also answers '1960' (perseveration of a theme of 60). Both echolalia and perseveration are found in organic brain disease and in some types of schizophrenia.

When the speech is abnormal, samples of it should be written down verbatim, or recorded on tape, as this is the only reliable way of recording the abnormality for future assessment. Two doctors may differ in what they call formal thought disorder and therefore writing in the case notes: 'There was evidence of formal thought disorder' is not very helpful. A recorded sample of the patient's speech used gives much less room for disagreement.

MOOD

Mood has both a *subjective* component, which is reflected in the way the patient describes their emotional state, and an *objective* component, i.e. what the interviewer sees, for example, tears.

The subjective and objective components of mood are usually but not always congruent. An example of incongruence is the smiling face of some severely depressed patients. Subjective mood is assessed by asking the patient how he feels in himself, what his mood is, or what his spirits are like. If necessary, leading questions such as 'Are you anxious or depressed?' may be used. Abnormal mood includes most commonly depression and anxiety but also elation, irritability, anger and perplexity. When the mood is abnormal it should be evaluated in detail in the same way as any other presenting symptom.

Depression

This may be mild and influenced by daily activities, or severe. The clinical features are characteristic (Box 2.6). In severe depression symptoms may be worse in the morning, and associated with early morning waking, appetite and weight disturbance, lethargy, loss of concentration, and loss of interest and enjoyment in life. There may also be ideas of worthlessness, self-deprecation, poverty, guilt, persecution, bodily ill-health, nihilism and other morbid ideas. These may sometimes be delusional in intensity (see section on abnormal experiences, page 39). The patient may be agitated or retarded, sometimes even to the point of stupor, and they may be mute or, in lesser cases, show retardation of speech.

> **BOX 2.6 Features of depression.**
>
> - Loss of interest/enjoyment in life
> - Lethargy
> - Poor concentration
> - Early morning waking
> - Appetite and weight disturbance
> - Ideas of worthlessness, guilt, persecution, nihilism
> - Self-deprecation
> - Retardation, leading to depressive stupor
> - Retardation of speech, or muteness
> - Paradoxical agitation and delusional state

The depressed patient may see no future, feel despairing and hopeless, and have thoughts of suicide. Suicidal ideation must always be sought for in depressed patients. Not only is it incorrect that discussing suicide with patients encourages them to commit suicide, but failure to discuss it may lead to tragedies that could have been prevented (Box 2.7). It can be asked for directly or led up to by a series of questions such as: 'How do you see the future?' 'Have you felt it would be nice to escape or be able to

> **BOX 2.7 Features suggesting a risk of suicidal behaviour.**
>
> - Previous self-harm, especially poison, stabbing, hanging or jumping from heights or under vehicles.
> - Continuing suicidal thoughts
> - Current depressive or schizophrenic psychosis
> - Male sex, aged >40 years
> - Social isolation, especially in adolescence or the recently bereaved or divorced
> - Chronic painful illness
> - Alcoholism and drug abuse
> - Family history of suicide

sleep and not wake up?' 'Do you feel at times that you would rather be dead or that you are such a burden to others that they would be better off if you were dead?' 'Have you had thoughts of suicide, however fleeting?' 'Have you made any plans?' Where it is felt that the patient is suicidal but denies it, it is worth asking the question: 'What stops you killing yourself' or: 'What do you have to live for?' Some patients admit to having suicidal thoughts but deny that they would do anything because of the impact it would have on the family or because it is against their religion or they do not have the courage. Suicide, however, is not a respecter of family feelings, religious beliefs or personal bravery. Homicidal thoughts may also be present, as in some mothers with puerperal depressive illnesses who kill their children because they are convinced they have passed on some terrible illness and death is better for them than a life of suffering.

Anxiety

Patients with anxiety states may present with *somatic* symptoms related mainly to autonomic nervous system arousal or hyperventilation (Box 2.8), or to

> **BOX 2.8 Somatic symptoms of anxiety.**
>
> - Headaches and other muscular aches and pains
> - Palpitations
> - Tremor
> - Breathlessness
> - Chest pain
> - Urinary frequency
> - Faintness and lightheadedness
> - Fatigue
> - Pins and needles
> - Diarrhoea
> - Dry mouth
> - Abdominal discomfort
> - Flushes
> - Sweating

psychic symptoms (Box 2.9), or both. The anxiety may be free-floating or situation-dependent as in phobic disorders (e.g. agoraphobia), social phobias and other specific phobias.

The patient may complain of panic attacks with sudden surges of anxiety, with physical symptoms and the desire to run away, sometimes coupled with an inability to move.

Elation

Elated patients usually describe themselves as being on top of the world, feeling happier than they have ever done before. This is a feature of hypomania and mania when it is associated with overactivity, pressure of speech with flight of ideas, sleep impairment, irritability and grandiose ideas. Manic patients may also have moments of tearfulness or the mental state may show signs of both depression and elation, as in mixed affective states.

Other abnormal states

Irritability may occur in many psychiatric disorders, especially anxiety states and hypomania, and in situational and relationship disturbances, such as marital problems. It may also be part of the usual mood in some personalities, such as the intolerant person who does not suffer fools gladly. *Anger* may be related to a specific person or situation or may be part of an underlying psychiatric disturbance, in particular when ideas of persecution are present. Perplexity is usually found in schizophrenic patients who are suspicious that something is going on but cannot quite put their finger on what it is.

THOUGHT CONTENT

The patient should be asked what their main worries are and whether they are preoccupied by any thoughts, e.g. morbid thoughts or *obsessional ruminations*. The latter are thoughts that the patient recognizes as his or her own, realizes are silly and tries to resist, but is unable to do so. They occur in obsessive compulsive neuroses and may be associated with *obsessional rituals*—acts which the patient feels compelled to carry out, even though they recognize them as being absurd. In obsessional rituals the patient realizes that the compulsion comes from within, unlike delusions of influence (see page 40) in which the impulse is felt to come from outside forces. An example of obsessional rumination is the man who knows that his spouse is not unfaithful but has doubts about her which continuously run through his mind and which he is unable to suppress. Common obsessional rituals include hand-washing; the patient may wash his or her hands 40 or 50 times a day with disinfectant and strong detergents until they are raw. Obsessional checking is another common manifestation; for example, the woman who switches off her bedroom lights before leaving the house, gets to the bottom of the stairs and has to go back up again to check the lights are off, goes back down to the front door, has to go back again to check that the lights are off, gets to the bottom of the path and has to return, goes a few steps down the road and has to return and so on. In neither case is the patient able to stop these obsessional rituals without being consumed by extreme anxiety.

ABNORMAL BELIEFS

These vary from *delusions* (Box 2.10), in which the patient has false and unshakeable beliefs which are out of keeping with the social milieu from which he or she comes, to *overvalued ideas*, in which the patient has false beliefs which, although of major concern to him or her, are not completely unshakeable. These abnormal beliefs include misinterpretations, in which the patient concocts false explanations for various normal events which may or may not be delusional in extent. Abnormal ideas should be written down verbatim and asked about in detail.

Though abnormal beliefs usually denote the presence of a psychiatric illness, they may also occur in certain situations in normal people, as in the case of *ideas of reference*, in which the person feels that what others are saying refers to him or her or that they are laughing behind his or her back. This is commonly seen in sensitive people, especially in anxiety-provoking situations, such as parties where most of the other guests are strangers.

Delusions may be primary, like sudden bolts from heaven, or secondary. In the latter their existence is understandable in terms of the rest of the patient's psychopathology, as in affective psychoses. Primary delusions may be *delusional ideas*—fully formed delusions that suddenly enter into the patient's mind, as in the person who for no reason suddenly believes that their food is being poisoned. This is often preceded by a *delusional mood*, in which the patient feels that there is something going on and that things are not quite right, but is unable to elaborate this feeling. In *delusional perceptions* the object is perceived normally but is interpreted in a delusional way, e.g. the man who sees an ashtray on the table, recognizes it as an ashtray but believes that it has been put there to show people that he is a spy. This is not understandable in terms of the rest of the patient's psychopathology. If it were understandable, it would be a *delusional misinterpretation*, which is a secondary delusion. Primary delusions should be diagnosed with extreme caution as, by the time the patient has presented, it may be very difficult to differentiate primary from secondary.

Delusions of persecution
Also called *paranoid delusions*, these are probably the most common delusions and may occur alone or with other abnormal mental signs. They occur in organic psychoses, such as confusional states, dementia, and alcohol- and drug-induced psychoses, and associated with various organic illnesses such as some endocrine disorders and systemic lupus erythematosus. They also occur in functional psychoses such as paranoid schizophrenia, paraphrenia of the elderly, depressive illness and mania; in stress-induced, psychogenic psychoses or hysterical pseudopsychoses; and in some people with paranoid personality developments.

Delusions of grandeur
These delusions occur in the now uncommon syphilitic general paralysis of the insane and in mania and schizophrenia. Patients believe they are on a 'special mission' or are Napoleon or Christ.

Delusions of poverty and other depressive delusions
Depressed patients may insist that they are destitute and have no clothes. Other common depressive delusions include *self-deprecation, worthlessness* and *guilt*, 'I have done something terrible and should be in prison and not in hospital.' Delusions of ill-health, often even potentially fatal, may occur and persist despite every assurance of the patient's physical health. These delusions occur in depression, schizophrenia and abnormal personality development. Some people develop isolated abnormal ideas about their own appearance which may sometimes be delusional in intensity, e.g. their nose is too long or their hair is falling out. These patients often have sensitive personalities, some of them may be depressed and some may become schizophrenic with time.

Nihilistic delusions
These occur mainly in severe depressive illnesses but can also occur in schizophrenia and organic brain disease. The patient with nihilistic delusions says that they are dead or that part of their body is dead. This may lead to self-harm. A rare delusion is of *infestation*, when the patient believes that their house is infested by insects. Delusions of infestation occur in depression, in schizophrenia, or in organic illness.

Delusions of love
Erotomania is another name for this symptom, in which the patient is convinced that someone is in love with him or her, despite the other person having shown no signs of this. They may act upon this misguided belief and pester the individual so that a legal injunction may be necessary to restrain them. These delusions may occur in schizophrenia and occasionally in abnormal personality development.

Delusions of infidelity
With these the patient is morbidly jealous of their spouse, and is convinced that they are having an extramarital affair. He or she may go to extreme lengths to confirm these abnormal beliefs, often pressing the spouse to admit their errant ways. These arguments may lead to violence that can end in murder. These delusions occur in people with suspicious personalities, especially when associated with alcohol abuse, and in schizophrenia and affective psychoses.

Delusions of influence (passivity or alienation phenomenon)
This is one of Schneider's first-rank symptoms, those symptoms which in the absence of organic brain

disease are highly suggestive of schizophrenia (see Box 2.11).

Delusions of influence occur when the patient says that their mind or body is being controlled by outside forces such as laser beams transmitted by a neighbour. When the mind rather than the body is affected, the patient may complain that thoughts are being forced either into or out of their head. Another form of thought alienation is *thought broadcast*, in which the patient's thought leaves their head, travels through the air and enters into other people's heads so that when the patient thinks something, everyone else thinks the same. Alienation may also affect perception, as in patients who experience somatic hallucinations which they say are being caused by other people or by external forces. These are known as '*made*' experiences (see section on tactile hallucinations, page 42).

ABNORMAL EXPERIENCES

These may be divided into *abnormal perceptions* and *abnormal experiences* of the self or the environment.

Abnormal perceptions

These vary in type and may occur with any of the sensory modalities of hearing, vision, smell, taste and touch (Box 2.12). Objects may be distorted while remaining recognizable or they may be a new perception, as in illusions or hallucinations. Distortions in *intensity*, either increased or decreased, may be due to

functional or organic disorders; in *quality*, e.g. colour, are often due to toxic substances; or in *form*, e.g. micropsia (when the object appears smaller or further away) or macropsia, may be due to organic lesions of the visual pathway (see Chapter 10).

Illusions occur when the object is real but perception is disturbed. They are usually related, in the psychiatric sense, to disorders of the perceptual environment of the object, thereby leading to decrease in visual clarity coupled with a state of high emotion in the perceiver. A common example is the experience of walking through a lonely alley on a dark night and perceiving a tree in the distance to be the figure of a man. Vision is impaired by the poor illumination and the lonely alley induces a feeling of fear, thus leading to the illusion. Illusions are common in psychiatric illness, particularly acute confusional states. They most often affect the visual and, to a lesser extent, the auditory modalities. An example of the latter is the woman with puerperal depressive illness who hears the nurses talking outside her room without hearing clearly what they are saying but thinks they are talking about her, saying how ill she is.

Hallucinations occur in the absence of an appropriate object yet the patient still insists that he or she has perceived something. The commonest hallucinations are auditory and visual but, as in any abnormal perception, they can occur in all sensory modalities. They may be due to organic disease of the nervous system or to extreme environmental disturbances as in sensory deprivation. In certain instances they may be non-pathological phenomena, as in *hypnagogic* and *hypnopompic* hallucinations experienced by a person going to sleep or waking up. Hypnagogic hallucinations also occur in narcolepsy.

In psychiatric illness, hallucinations occur in organic and functional psychoses, e.g. in schizophrenia and affective illnesses, severely raised levels of anxiety due to hyperventilation, grief reactions, and hysterical illnesses. They are occasionally displayed by malingerers. They may occur wherever the patient is or may only be present in certain places. Thus the paranoid patient who hears the neighbours' voices plotting against him or her at home does not hear them while in hospital, yet they return when the patient is at home again.

Hallucinations may occur in any of the perceptional modalities.

Auditory hallucinations. The patient may complain of hearing noises, music, distant mumbling which he cannot identify, words, phrases or more elaborate speech. If the patient hears voices rather than sounds they may sometimes be able to recognize them as belonging to someone they know. The voices may be talking to the patient, or talking about him or her (see below). They may be persecutory, neutral or pleasing. The patient may talk back to the voices, or may appear to be listening to them intently. In some cases the voices direct the patient to certain actions which they may feel duty-bound to follow.

Second-person voices with distressing content— 'You stink, you're horrible, go kill yourself'—are found in severe depressive illnesses. Third-person voices, which discuss or argue about the patient or comment on what he or she is doing, are suggestive of schizophrenia in the absence of organic brain disease (see Table 2.1), as is hearing one's own thoughts spoken out loud (*echo de pensées*). In grief reactions, the bereaved person may hear the footsteps or other stigmata of the dead person.

Visual hallucinations. Visual hallucinations may vary in complexity from simple flashes of light to sophisticated 'visions' of peoples or animals. They occur more commonly in organic psychoses, especially acute confusional states, than in functional psychoses, whereas the opposite is true with auditory hallucinations. They may be frightening, as in the case of hallucinations of spiders, insects and rats which occur in delirium tremens, or pleasing as with Lilliputian hallucinations, in which the patient sees tiny people. They may coexist with auditory hallucinations as in temporal lobe epilepsy.

Olfactory hallucinations. These may occur in temporal lobe epilepsy, when an unpleasant smell may be the initial symptom of the attack; in schizophrenia, as in the patient who said that people were making cars emit noxious smells at him; and in depressive illnesses, in which the patient insists that they emit a foul odour which they can smell.

Hallucinations of taste. These are rare in psychiatric practice but characteristically occur in temporal lobe epilepsy.

Tactile and somatic hallucinations. In cocaine psychosis patients may complain that insects are crawling over them (*formication*). Other patients insist that they are experiencing odd sensations in various parts of their body which are produced by other people, as in the man who complained that his

neighbour's laser gun was producing a cold feeling which travelled up his legs. This is another first-rank symptom of schizophrenia in the absence of organic brain disease (Box 2.11). These hallucinations may have a sexual content, as in the patient who insisted that someone was having intercourse with her and she could feel it happening all the time.

Other hallucinations and illusions. Some people complain that, when alone, they feel the presence of someone else beside them. This may occur in grief reactions; as illusions when the patient is frightened; as a manifestation of hysteria; in organic brain disease and schizophrenia. Finally, vestibular hallucinations may occur, usually in acute organic brain disease, such as the patient with delirium tremens who has the sensation of flying through the air.

Abnormal experiences of self and environment

Déjà vu. This may occur in normal people but it is usually associated with temporal lobe epilepsy, and is characterized by the patient feeling that they have been in their current situation before.

Capgras' syndrome. In this syndrome, which occurs most commonly in schizophrenia but may also occur in dementia, the patient asserts that people are not who they claim to be, but are their double.

Depersonalization. This symptom is often a manifestation of heightened anxiety levels. The patient does not feel his or her normal self and may describe this unpleasant experience as if floating above their own body looking down on it. The patient may also complain that they have lost the capacity to feel at an emotional level. This may be one of the most marked symptoms in depressed patients.

Derealization. This often accompanies depersonalization. The patient says that their surroundings feel unreal or grey or colourless.

COGNITIVE STATE

In elderly people or where organic brain disease is suspected, e.g. acute confusional states, this assessment is extremely important. Semiquantitative tests of cognitive function based on the general approach described here are often used, e.g. the Mental Status Questionnaire (MSQ) (Table 2.1) and the Mini-mental State Examination (Table 2.2).

Level of consciousness

An assessment of the level of alertness of the patient or, if unconscious, of the level of unconsciousness may be made. Some patients appear to have fluctuating levels of consciousness; the mental state may then fluctuate between lucidity and gross abnormality. This is a manifestation of an acute confusional state. For a full account of the examination of the unconscious patient see Chapter 13.

Orientation

The patient's orientation in time, place and person should be formally assessed by direct questioning and the patient's answers written down verbatim. Disorientation is an important sign of organic brain disease, whether chronic or acute, but may also occur in chronic, disinterested, institutionalized schizophrenics and in hysterical dissociative states.

Time. Ask about the day, date, month, year and time of day. If the patient does not know the month, ask about the season. All patients should know the year and either the month or season and the approximate time of day, e.g. morning, afternoon, evening or night. Long stays in hospital, where one day is much like the next, however, are not conducive to an awareness of which particular day it is or the exact date of the month.

Place. The patient should know where they are, e.g. home or hospital, and approximately where it is situated, e.g. what town or part of the town. Depending on how long they have been in the place where interviewed, whether at home or in a hospital ward, they should know the way to such places as the bathroom or toilet. Some patients with acute confusional states may say they are in hospital but that the hospital is part of their own home.

Person. If disorientation is suspected the patient should be asked their name and address.

Attention and concentration

The patient's behaviour during the interview will have shown whether they are easily distracted or have been paying attention to and concentrating on the questions you have asked. This can be tested more formally by asking the patient to subtract serial sevens from 100 or, as this may be difficult even for normal people, serial threes from 20. Tasks such as recounting the months of the year and days of the week backwards or repeating a sequence of dig-

its (digit span) forwards are also useful. Repetition of digits backwards (e.g. doctor says 165 to which the patient should reply 561) is dependent not only on attention and concentration but also on the ability to register the numbers 165 and remember them long enough to reverse them and is thus a test of immediate memory. Normal people should be able to manage seven digits forward and five backwards; telephone numbers in most large cities consist of seven digits. Another useful test is to ask the patient to spell 'WORLD' backwards; the impaired patient often transposes the central letters of the word.

Memory

In chronic organic brain disease, memory for recent events is diminished, whereas early in the illness the patient often remains able to remember events which have happened in the past and is thus able to give a coherent account of the family and early personal history. Some patients with memory impairment, as in *Korsakoff's psychosis*, which is usually due to vitamin B deficiency following poor nutrition or associated with heavy drinking, may attempt to cover their disability by *confabulating*. An example is the alcoholic with Korsakoff's psychosis seen after a 6-week stay in hospital, who when asked how long he had been an in-patient stated that he had come in that day and been at work the day before, which he then described in great detail down to what he had for his dessert in the staff canteen. Confabulation is not invention, but consists of the inappropriate recall of recent or distant past experiences.

In the case of head injuries or in epileptic attacks, an attempt should be made to assess the presence of *retrograde* and *anterograde amnesia*, if any, in some detail. Memory impairment may be simulated for gain by some manipulative patients, some of whom may give approximate answers. For example, if the date is Monday 15 November 1993 they may say it is Tuesday 14 October 1983 and then correct themselves to Sunday 16 December 1995. *Hysterical amnesia* may occur in dissociative states in which there is a sudden total loss of memory. In contrast, in *organic amnesia* long-term memory and personal identity are usually spared until the later stages of the disorder. This is so even in dementing illnesses. Patients who are disinterested or depressed may appear to have memory impairment and in the latter case, called *depressive pseudodementia*, the aetiology may only become apparent when the depression lifts and the memory improves.

Past memory will already have been assessed while asking about the family and personal history, but recent memory will need more specific testing. A useful approach is to ask the patient about recent television programmes, such as the events in a popular soap opera, or the fortunes of a favourite football team. Other recent events will include details about the hospital itself, and how the patient got there. Current affairs should also be asked about, such as the names of top politicians and details of any recent happenings of major importance. A less direct question is to ask the patient what has been going on in the world or in this country recently.

A more systematic approach to memory testing is to ask the patient to repeat a name and address immediately and again after about 5 minutes, or to give them a sentence—for example, 'The one thing a nation needs in order to be rich and great is a large, secure supply of wood'—and see how many repetitions are necessary for accurate reproduction. Where relevant, visual as well as auditory memory should be tested. This can be done by giving the patient a picture depicting a series of objects and a few minutes later asking them to recall as many of the objects as they can.

The patient's answers to all specific questions about memory should be recorded verbatim.

INTELLIGENCE

An idea of the patient's level of intelligence is one of the most important pieces of information to be obtained from the interview. Not only will this help to determine suitable treatment (e.g. for psychotherapy the patient must be articulate and intelligent) but it will also affect the interpretation of the mental state examination itself. In the subnormal patient bizarre behaviour and abnormal ideas occurring as part of a *normal* fantasy life may be mistaken for psychiatric illness, when it represents only an attention-seeking device. An approximate assessment of intelligence can be obtained from the educational and occupational history and from an assessment of general knowledge. Alternatively this can be tested more formally (see below). It is useful to enquire whether the patient can read and write, although this may correlate more with education than intelligence, and to see whether the patient is able to solve simple mathematical problems, especially where these are related to daily activities, e.g. shopping.

INSIGHT

It is important to make an assessment of the patient's insight into his or her problems and this may be considered at a number of different levels. First, there is the patient who has no insight at all and does not accept that he or she is ill. Such lack of insight is one of the hallmarks of a psychotic illness where the patient is out of touch with reality. Secondly, the patient may accept that he or she is ill but perceives the illness on physical rather than a psychiatric basis, as occurs with hysterical disorders and some anxiety states. Often a full explanation as to the causes of the symptoms will lead to insight, though this is not always the case. Such patients may deny there are any problems in any areas of their life despite there being obvious spheres of difficulty. Thirdly, there is the patient who accepts the need of psychiatric help but is unable fully to unravel the complexities of their problems.

RAPPORT

The rapport established in the interview between the doctor and patient depends not only on the interview technique but also on the personality and mental attitude of the two participants. The doctor must not force his or her own personality and attitudes on to the patient. The way the patient relates to the doctor (see section on behaviour, page 36) offers an insight to the patient's internal psychological state, enabling the doctor to make an evaluation of such points as dependence, relationships to others, especially those in authority, including parent figures, mood and paranoid ideation. With the patient suffering from a psychotic illness the doctor may feel that meaningful contact has never really been achieved. With the neurotic patient or in the absence of personality problems the doctor–patient relationship forms an important element in psychotherapy. The patient may *displace* on to the doctor feelings for other important people in their life. For example, anger more appropriately directed towards a spouse or parent may instead manifest itself in the interview setting, with the doctor the recipient of this displaced emotion. Finally, the patient may *project* their feelings on to the doctor. An angry patient may not overtly show this anger but may leave the doctor feeling angry; similarly depression and elation may be transmitted to the doctor in the interview. Thus noting how the doctor feels during the interview may give valuable added information for the assessment of the patient's mental state.

FURTHER TESTS OF CEREBRAL FUNCTION

In patients in whom organic brain disease is suspected, a more detailed assessment of cerebral function should be carried out. In addition to the above, this includes an assessment of speech, both verbal and written; spatial, visual, motor and numerical abilities; awareness of body image; and presence of released primitive reflexes. These comprise part of the neurological examination (see Chapter 12).

Further investigations

In psychiatry this consists of information gathering, clarification and continuing assessment of the mental state, laboratory investigations, psychological testing, social enquiry and occupational therapy assessment.

Information gathering

Many patients will need more than one interview to take a full psychiatric history. Other sources of information are needed to clarify and validate parts of the history. Spouse, family, friends and people at work or school may be able to help, but before they are contacted this should be discussed with the patient and verbal or, in some cases, written consent obtained. In addition to separate interviews with the patient, spouse and family, it is often necessary to bring them together in order to carry out diagnostic and therapeutic marital and family interviews. These interviews often provide information unavailable from either party on their own as well as affording an opportunity to see how the couple or family relate to each other. In addition, when feeding back your conclusions, it allows you to give all concerned parties the same information at the same time, thus avoiding potentially divisive miscommunication. If the other informant cannot be interviewed in person it may still be possible to do so by telephone or by letter.

It is obviously important to obtain detailed medical records from the family doctor and from any hospital concerned; the grounds for previous diagnoses can be scrutinized and the response to past treatment assessed. Conditions in the patient's home may be assessed by a social worker, who may be able to see relatives who refuse to see a doctor. The patient's problems can be further assessed by suggesting that a diary of the symptoms, daily activities and emotional state would be helpful. This often indicates links which may illuminate the aetiology of the current disorder. When one is dealing with a specific behavioural disorder, e.g. nervous diarrhoea, overeating or aggressive behaviour, more systematic behavioural analysis may be necessary.

Mental state evaluation

The evaluation of the mental state is a continuous process and should be assessed at each interview. If the patient is admitted to hospital their behaviour on the ward should be observed and documented. This includes an account of the way they relate to other patients, to staff and visitors, and whether there are any signs of sleep or appetite disturbance or other abnormal behaviour.

Questionnaires and structured interview schedules may aid quantitative assessment of the mental state and may be useful in evaluating progress.

One commonly used test is the *Mental Status Questionnaire* (MSQ) (Table 2.1). This consists of ten simple questions that relate to alertness, orientation for time and space, and recent and long-term memory. Normal subjects achieve 9 or 10 correct answers; scores less than 8 imply some degree of mental confusion. Patients with severe confusion score less than 3. The *Mini-mental State Examination* (Table 2.2) differs from the MSQ in that it is more detailed and scores are, to some extent, dependent on educational level. The test has subcategories related to orientation, registration, attention, recall and language. The maximum score is 30, and scores

---

1 What is the name of this place (where are we now)?
2 What is the address of this place?
3 What is the date?
4 What month is it?
5 What year is it?
6 How old are you?
7 When is your birthday?
8 What year were you born?
9 Who is the Prime Minister?
10 Who was the previous Prime Minister?

Each question is scored 0 for incorrect, and 1 for a correct response. Normal subjects score 9 or 10; scores less than 8 imply a degree of mental confusion.

Table 2.1 Mental Status Questionnaire (MSQ).

Orientation—1 point for each correct answer	
What is the:	
time	
date	
day	
month	
year	5 points
What is the name of this:	
ward	
hospital	
district	
town	
country	5 points
Registration	
Name three objects	
Score 1, 2, 3 points according to how	
many are repeated	
Re-submit list until patient word perfect	
in order to use this for a later test of	
recall	
Score only first attempt	3 points
Attention and calculation	
Have the patient subtract 7 from 100 and	
then from the result a total of five times.	
Score 1 point for each correct subtraction	5 points
Recall	
Ask for three objects used in the	
registration test, one point being	
awarded for each correct answer	3 points
Language	
1 point each for two objects correctly	
named (pencil and watch)	2 points
1 point for correct repetition of 'No ifs,	
ands and buts'	1 point
3 points if three-stage commands	
correctly obeyed 'Take this piece of paper	
in your right hand, fold it in half, and	
place it on the floor'	3 points
1 point for correct response to a written	
command such as 'close your eyes'	1 point
Have the patient write a sentence. Award	
1 point if the sentence is meaningful, has	
a verb and a subject	1 point
Test the patient's ability to copy a	
complex diagram of two intersected	
pentagons	1 point
Total score 30	

Table 2.2   Mini-mental State Examination.

lower than 21 are associated with cognitive impairment. Neither the MSQ nor the Mini-mental State Examination are capable of differentiating multifocal from diffuse organic brain disease, but both provide useful baseline assessment of a patient's cognitive performance capacity.

The *face/hand test* is also useful in differentiating organic brain disorders from functional brain disease, e.g. psychoses. The patient sits with their eyes closed and their hands on their knees. The examiner strokes the patient's cheek and, at the same time, one hand. Alternate combinations of face and hand may be touched in random sequence and, each time, the patient is asked to report the contacts. Incorrect answers are associated with organic brain disease.

Neuropsychological testing

Psychological tests can be used to assess the patient's cognitive state, behaviour, personality and thinking process. Tests can be given to assess the level of intelligence, either briefly with the Mill Hill test and the Raven's Progressive Matrices test or in more detail with the WAIS (Wechsler Adult Intelligence Scale). In behavioural disorders it is useful to carry out a thorough behavioural analysis; this must be designed to be relevant to the individual problem. These investigations require specialized skills and are best carried out by the clinical psychologist.

CHAPTER 3

The skin, nails and hair

Introduction

The skin is a large organ of the human body. Forming a major interface between man and his environment, it covers an area of approximately $2\,m^2$ and weighs about $4\,kg$. The structure of human skin is complex (Figs 3.1 and 3.2), consisting of a number of layers and tissue components with many important functions (Box 3.1). Reactions may occur in any of the components of human skin and their clinical manifestations reflect, among other factors, the level in the skin in which they occur.

Dermatology is a visual clinical specialty. The accurate diagnosis of most skin lesions requires an adequate history, careful examination of the patient and, occasionally, laboratory investigation.

BOX 3.1 Functions of the human skin.

- Protection: physical, chemical, infection
- Physiological: homeostasis of electrolytes, water and protein
- Thermoregulation
- Sensation: specialized nerve endings
- Lubrication and waterproofing: sebum
- Immunological: Langerhans cells, lymphocytes, macrophages
- Vitamin D synthesis
- Body odour: apocrine glands
- Psychosocial: cosmetic

History

The history should include detailed questions concerning the present skin condition including the site of onset, mode of spread and duration. The clinician needs to know about any personal history or family history of skin disease, including atopy. Any history of past general medical conditions should be noted, and a careful drug history obtained, including any use of 'over-the-counter' preparations. A social and occupational history should be recorded and, in some circumstances, it is important to obtain details of recent travel, and the sexual history.

Examination

The *whole skin* including hair, nails and assessable mucosae should be fully exposed, preferably in natural light. Sometimes a magnifying lens is useful.

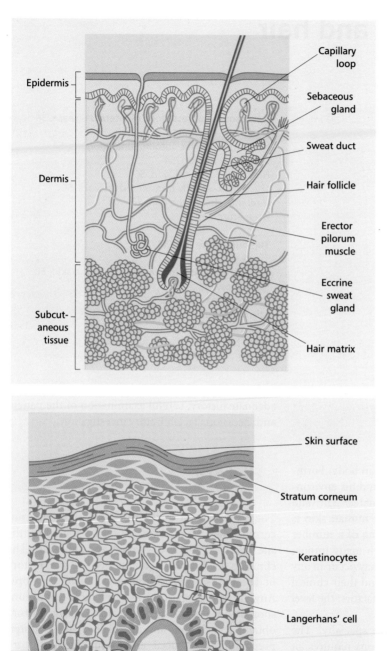

Fig. 3.1 The anatomy of the full thickness of the skin in section.

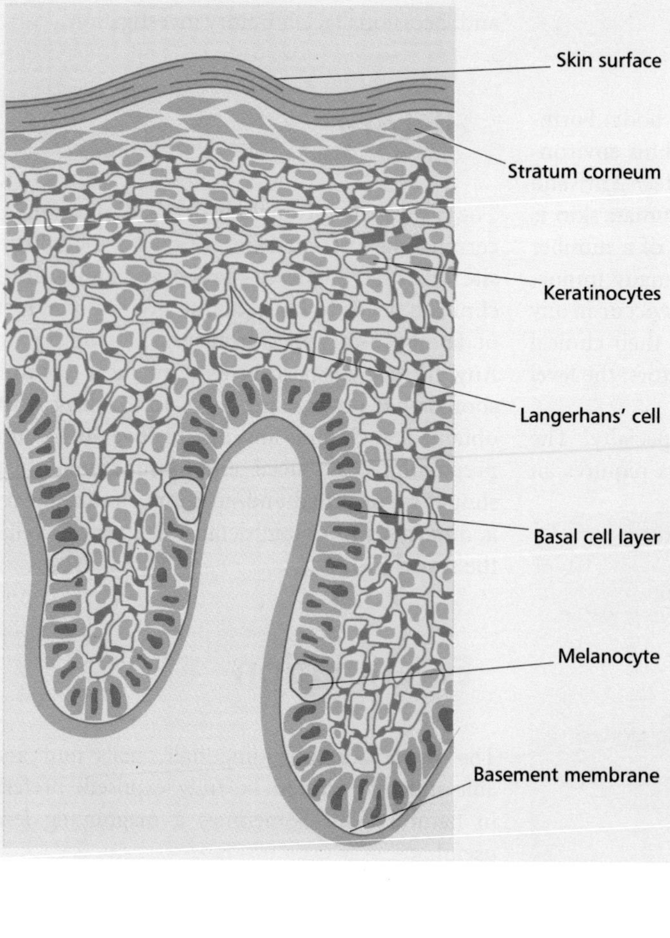

Epidermis

Capillary loop

Sebaceous gland

Sweat duct

Dermis

Hair follicle

Erector pilorum muscle

Eccrine sweat gland

Subcutaneous tissue

Hair matrix

Fig. 3.2 The anatomy of the epidermis.

Skin surface

Stratum corneum

Keratinocytes

Langerhans' cell

Basal cell layer

Melanocyte

Basement membrane

Colour and pigmentation

Before inspecting any rash or lesion notice the colour of the skin. The normal skin colour varies, depending on lifestyle and light exposure as well as constitutional and ethnic factors.

Pallor has many causes, and can be either *temporary*, due to shock, haemorrhage and intense emotion; or *persistent*, due to anaemia or peripheral vasoconstriction, as is seen in patients with severe atopy—an inherited susceptibility to develop asthma, eczema and hay fever. Although pallor is usual in anaemia, it is important to remember that not all pale persons are anaemic and that conjunctival mucosal colour is a better indication of anaemia than skin colour. A pale skin resulting from diminished pigment is also characteristic of *hypopituitarism* and *hypogonadism*. Normal skin contains varying amounts of brown melanin pigment. Brown pigmentation owing to the presence of haemosiderin is always pathological. A congenital generalized absence of pigment in the skin is known as *albinism*; if it is localized it is known as *piebaldism*. Patches of white and darkly pigmented skin are seen in *vitiligo* (Fig. 3.3). In this disorder there is a complete absence of melanocytes. Several autoimmune endocrine disorders are associated with vitiligo.

Abnormal redness is seen after overheating, extreme exertion, sunburn and in febrile, exanthematous and inflammatory skin disease. *Flushing* is a striking redness, usually of the face and neck, which may be transient or persistent. Local redness may be due to *telangiectasia*, especially on the face. *Cyanosis* is a blue or purple-blue tint due to the presence of excessive reduced haemoglobin, either locally, as in impaired peripheral circulation, or generally, when oxygenation of the blood is defective. The tint of *methaemoglobinaemia* is more leaden than ordinary cyanosis; it is caused by drugs, such as dapsone, and certain poisons.

Jaundice varies from the subicteric, lemon-yellow tints seen in *pernicious anaemia* and *acholuric jaundice*, to various shades of yellow, orange or dark olive-green in *obstructive jaundice*. Jaundice, which stains the conjunctivae, must be distinguished from the orange-yellow of *carotenaemia*, which does not. Slight degrees of jaundice cannot be seen in artificial light.

Increased pigmentation may be racial, due to sunburn or connected with various diseases. In *Addison's disease* there is a brown or dark-brown pigmentation, affecting exposed parts and parts not normally pigmented, such as the axillae and the palmar creases; the lips and mouth may exhibit dark bluish-black areas. Note, however, that mucosal pigmentation is a normal finding in a substantial proportion of negroid people.

More or less *generalized pigmentation* may also be seen in the following:

- *haemochromatosis*, in which the skin has a peculiar greyish-bronze colour with a metallic sheen, due to excessive melanin and iron pigment;
- *chronic arsenic poisoning*, in which the skin is finely dappled and affects covered more than exposed parts;
- *argyria*, in which the deposition of silver in the skin produces a diffuse slatey-grey hue; and
- occasionally, the *cachexia* of advanced malignant disease.

In pregnancy there may be pigmentation of the nipples and areolae, of the linea alba and sometimes, a mask-like pigmentation of the face (*chloasma*). Chloasma may also be induced by oral contraceptives containing oestrogen. A similar condition, *melasma*, may be seen in Asian and African males.

Localized pigmentation may be seen in pellagra and in scars of various kinds, particularly those due to X-irradiation therapy. Venous hypertension in the legs is often associated with chronic purpura, leading to haemosiderin pigmentation. The mixture of punctate and fresh purpura and haemosiderin may produce a golden hue on the lower calves and shins. Pigmentation may also occur with chronic infestation by body lice. *Erythema ab igne*, a reticular pattern of pigmentation of the legs of women who habitually sit too near a fire, used to be

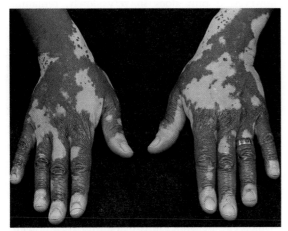

Fig. 3.3 Vitiligo: a disorder of cutaneous pigmentation that is often autoimmune in origin and associated with other autoimmune disorders.

common. When seen on the belly or back it indicates prolonged use of a hot water bottle to relieve pain, e.g. from malignant disease. *Livedo reticularis*, a web-like pattern of reddish-blue discoloration, mostly involving the legs, occurs in autoimmune vasculitis, especially in systemic lupus erythematosus and Sneddon's syndrome, when it is associated with cerebral stroke. The lesions of lichen planus are slightly raised, flat-topped, and have a violaceous hue (Fig. 3.4).

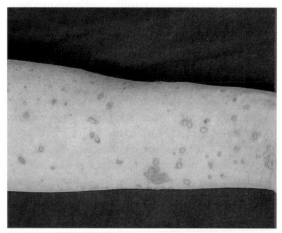

Fig. 3.4   Flat-topped papules of lichen planus.

Skin lesions and eruptions

Skin eruptions and lesions should be examined with special reference to their morphology, distribution and arrangement. The terminology of skin lesions is summarized in Boxes 3.2 and 3.3. Colour, size, consistency, configuration, margination and surface characteristics should be noted.

MORPHOLOGY OF SKIN LESIONS

Inspection and palpation

Assessment of morphology requires visual and tactile examination. Do not be afraid to feel the lesions. You will rarely be exposed to any danger in doing so, with the exception of herpes simplex, herpes zoster, syphilis and human immunodeficiency virus (HIV) disease. If infections such as these are suspected it is wise to wear disposable plastic gloves when examining open or bleeding cutaneous lesions. Begin palpation of the skin. Pass the hand gently over it, pinching it up between the forefinger and thumb, and note the following points:

- Is it smooth or rough, thin or thick?
- Is it dry or moist?

BOX 3.2 Primary skin lesions: a glossary of dermatological terms.

Macule	Non-palpable area of altered colour
Papule	Palpable elevated small area of skin (< 0.5 cm)
Plaque	Palpable flat-topped, discoid lesion (> 2 cm)
Nodule	Solid, palpable lesion within the skin (> 0.5 cm)
Papilloma	Pedunculated lesion projecting from the skin
Vesicle	Small fluid-filled blister (< 0.5 cm)
Bulla	Large fluid-filled blister (> 0.5 cm)
Pustule	Blister containing pus
Weal	Elevated lesion often white with red margin due to dermal oedema
Telangiectasia	Dilatation of superficial blood vessel
Petechiae	Pinhead-sized macules of blood
Purpura	Larger petechiae, which do not blanch on pressure
Ecchymosis	Large extravasation of blood in skin (bruise)
Haematoma	Swelling due to gross bleeding
Poikiloderma	Atrophy, reticulate hyperpigmentation and telangiectasia
Erythema	Redness of the skin
Burrow	Linear or curved elevations of the superficial skin due to infestation of female scabies mite
Comedo	Dark horny keratin and sebaceous plugs within pilo-sebaceous openings

- Is there any visible sweating, either general or local?

The elasticity of the skin should be investigated. If a fold of healthy skin is pinched up, it immediately flattens itself out again when released. Sometimes, however, it only does so very slowly, remaining creased for a considerable time. This is found frequently in healthy old people but may be an important sign of dehydration, e.g. in prolonged vomiting and diarrhoea, or in the subacute presentation of diabetes mellitus.

Subcutaneous oedema

When oedema (see Chapter 1) is present, firm pressure on the skin with a finger produces a shallow pit that persists for some time. In some cases no pitting is produced, especially when the oedema is of very long standing. The best place to look for slight degrees of oedema in cardiac disease is behind the malleoli at the ankles in patients who are ambulant, and over the sacrum in those who are confined to bed. The pressure of the finger should be maintained

BOX 3.3 Secondary skin lesions which evolve from primary lesions.

Scale	Loose excess normal and abnormal horny layer
Crust	Dried exudate
Excoriation	A scratch
Lichenification	Thickening of the epidermis with exaggerated skin margin
Fissure	Slit in the skin
Erosion	Partial loss of epidermis which heals without scarring
Ulcer	At least the full thickness of the epidermis is lost. Healing occurs with scarring
Sinus	A cavity or channel that allows the escape of fluid or pus
Scar	Healing by replacement of fibrous tissue
Keloid scar	Excessive scar formation
Atrophy	Thinning of the skin due to shrinkage of epidermis, dermis or subcutaneous fat
Stria	Atrophic pink or white linear lesion due to changes in connective tissue

for 20–30 seconds, or small degrees of oedema will be overlooked. Pitting is minimal or absent in oedema due to lymphatic obstruction, where the skin is usually thickened and tough.

Subcutaneous emphysema
Air trapped under the skin gives rise to a characteristic crackling sensation on palpation. It starts in, and is usually confined to, the neighbourhood of the air passages. On rare occasions it may result from the clostridial infection of soft tissues after injury or gunshot wounds (*gas gangrene*).

DISTRIBUTION OF SKIN LESIONS
Consider the distribution of an eruption by looking at the whole skin surface.

• Is it *symmetrical* or *asymmetrical*? Symmetry often implies an internal causation whereas asymmetry may imply external factors.

• Is the eruption *centrifugal* or *centripetal*? Certain common diseases such as chickenpox and pityriasis rosea are characteristically centripetal whereas erythema multiforme and erythema nodosum are centrifugal. Smallpox, now eradicated, was also centrifugal. A disease may exhibit a *flexor* or *extensor* bias in its distribution: atopic eczema in childhood is characteristically flexor whereas psoriasis in adults tends to be extensor.

• Are only exposed areas affected, implicating sunlight or some other external causative factor?

• If sunlight is suspected, are areas normally in shadow involved?

• Are the genitalia involved?

• Localized distributions may point immediately to an external contact as cause, for example contact dermatitis from nickel earrings, lipstick dermatitis, etc.

Swelling of the eyelids is an important sign. Without redness and scaling, bilateral periorbital oedema may indicate acute nephritis, nephrosis or trichinosis. If there is irritation, contact dermatitis is the probable diagnosis. Dermatomyositis often produces swelling and heliotrope erythema of the eyelids, without scaling of the skin. In Hansen's disease (leprosy) the skin lesions may be depigmented or reddened, with a slightly raised edge; they are also anaesthetic to pin-prick testing (Fig. 3.5) and mainly located in skin that is normally cooler than body temperature.

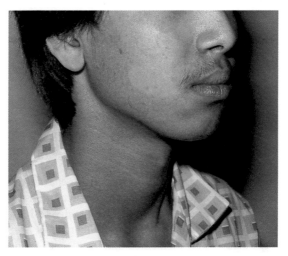

Fig. 3.5 Hansen's disease. There is a depigmented area of anaesthetic and slightly pink skin on the exposed cheek. In this lepromatous lesion acid-fast bacilli were found in scrapings.

CONFIGURATION OF SKIN LESIONS
Once the morphology of individual lesions and their distribution has been established, it is useful to describe their configuration on the skin (see Box 3.4).

The hair

Hair colour and texture are racial characteristics that are genetically determined. The yellow-brown mongol race has black straight hair, the negroids black, curly hair and the white caucasians fair, brown, red

BOX 3.4 Configuration of individual lesions.

Nummular/discoid	Round or coin-like
Annular	Ring-like
Circinate	Circular
Arcuate	Curved
Gyrate/serpiginous	Wave-like
Linear	In a line
Grouped	Clustered
Reticulate	Net-like

or black hair. Secondary sexual hair begins to appear at puberty and has characteristic male and female patterns. Common baldness in men is genetically determined but requires adequate levels of circulating androgens for its expression. It occurs in women only in old age.

Growth

Unlike other epithelial mitotic activity which is continuous throughout life, the growth of hair is cyclic (Fig. 3.6), the hair follicle going through alternating phases of growth (*anagen*) and rest (*telogen*). Anagen in the scalp lasts 3–5 years; telogen is much shorter at about 3 months. *Catogen* is the conversion stage from active to resting and usually lasts a few days. The length of the anagen phase determines the length to which hair in different body areas can grow. On the scalp there are about 100 000 hairs. As many as 100 hairs may be shed from the normal scalp every day as a normal consequence of growth cycling. These proportions can be estimated by looking at plucked hairs (trichogram); the 'root' of a telogen hair is non-pigmented and visible as a white, club-like swelling. Normally 85% of scalp hairs are in anagen and 15% in telogen.

Alopecia

Hair loss (alopecia) has many causes. It is convenient to subdivide alopecia into localized and diffuse types. In addition, the clinician should determine whether the alopecia results in scarring and, therefore, permanent hair loss (Box 3.5).

BOX 3.5 Causes of alopecia.

Non-scarring	*Scarring*
Alopecia areata	Burns, radiodermatitis
Trichotillomania	Aplasia cutis
Traction alopecia	Lupoid erythema
Scalp ringworm (human)	Necrobiosis
	Sarcoidosis
	Pseudopelade
	Kerion

Any inflammatory or destructive disease of the scalp skin may destroy hair follicles in its wake. Thus, burns, heavy X-ray irradiation or herpes zoster infection in the first division of the trigeminal nerve may cause a scarring alopecia. Alopecia in the presence of normal scalp skin may be patchy and localized as in traction alopecia in nervous children, ringworm infections (tinea capitis) or autoimmune alopecia areata. Secondary syphilis is a rare cause of a patchy 'moth-eaten' alopecia.

Scalp hair loss at the temples and crown, with growth of male-type body hair is characteristic of women with virilizing disorders. Metabolic causes of diffuse hair loss in women include hypothyroidism and severe iron-deficiency anaemia. Antimitotic drugs may affect the growing hair follicles, producing a diffuse loss of anagen hairs, which are pigmented throughout their length. Dramatic

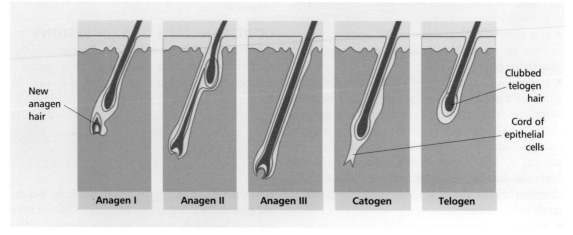

New anagen hair

Clubbed telogen hair

Cord of epithelial cells

Anagen I   Anagen II   Anagen III   Catogen   Telogen

Fig. 3.6 Hair follicle growth stages.

metabolic upsets, such as childbirth, starvation and severe toxic illnesses may precipitate follicles into the resting phase, producing an effluvium of telogen hairs 3 months later when anagen begins again. This is called *telogen alopecia*. The root of a telogen hair is non-pigmented and has a white club-like shape.

The nails

The nails should be examined carefully. The structure of the nail and nail bed is shown in Figs 3.7 and 3.8. The nail consists of a strong, relatively inflexible, keratinous nail plate over the dorsal surface or the end of each digit protecting the finger tip.

Nail matrix abnormalities

Thimble pitting of the nails is characteristic of psoriasis, but eczema and alopecia areata may also produce pitting. A severe illness may temporarily arrest nail growth; when growth starts again transverse ridges develop. These are called *Beau's lines* and can be used to date the time of onset of an illness.

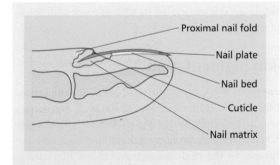

Fig. 3.7   Structure of the nail (lateral view).

Inflammation of the cuticle or nail fold (*chronic paronychia*) may produce similar changes. The changes described above arise from disturbance of the nail matrix.

Nail and nailbed abnormalities

Disturbance of the nail bed may produce thick nails (*pachyonychia*) or separation of the nail from the bed (*onycholysis*). This may occur in psoriasis, but may be idiopathic. Tetracyclines may induce separation when the fingers are exposed to strong sunlight

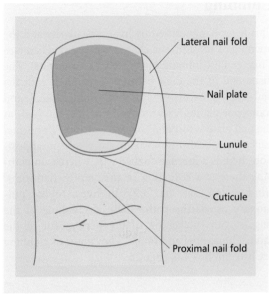

Fig. 3.8   Structure of the nail (dorsal view).

(*photo-onycholysis*). The nail may be destroyed in severe lichen planus or epidermolysis bullosa (a genetic abnormality in which the skin blisters in response to minor trauma). Nails are missing in the inherited nail-patella syndrome. *Splinter haemorrhages* under the nails may result from trauma, psoriasis, rheumatoid arthritis or other 'collagen vascular' diseases, bacterial endocarditis and trichinosis.

The nail in systemic disease

In iron-deficiency states, the fingernails and toenails become soft, thin, brittle and spoon-shaped. They lose their normal transverse convex curvature, becoming flattened or concave (*koilonychia*). The 'half and half' nail, with a white proximal and red or brown distal half, is seen in some patients with chronic renal failure. *Whitening* of the nail plates may be related to hypoalbuminaemia, as in cirrhosis of the liver. Some drugs, notably antimalarials, antibiotics and phenothiozines may discolour the nail. *Nail fold telangiectasia* or erythema is a useful physical sign in dermatomyositis, systemic sclerosis and systemic lupus erythematosus. In dermatomyositis the cuticle becomes ragged. In systemic sclerosis loss of finger pulps may lead to curvature of the nail plates. An impaired peripheral circulation, as in Raynaud's phenomenon can lead to thinning and longitudinal ridging of the nail plate, sometimes with partial onycholysis.

Clubbing

This is probably caused by hypervascularity and the opening of anastomotic channels in the nail bed (see Chapter 1). Clubbing may rarely be congenital. The distal end of the digit becomes expanded, with the nail curved excessively in both longitudinal and transverse planes. Viewed from the side, the angle at the nail plate is lost and may exceed 180°. In normal nails, when both thumb nails are placed in apposition there is a lozenge-shaped gap, whereas in clubbing there is a reduction in this gap (Schamroths' window test, see Fig. 3.9). In hypertrophic pulmonary osteoarthropathy there is clubbing of the fingers with thickening of the periosteum of the radius, ulna, tibia and fibula. The causes of clubbing are listed in Box 1.6, page 20.

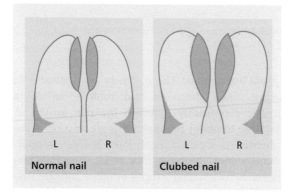

Fig. 3.9   Schamroths' window test.

Cutaneous manifestations of internal disease

Genodermatoses (lesions of inherited origin)

White macules shaped like small ash leaves which are present at birth may be the first sign of *tuberous sclerosis*. Sometimes they are difficult to see by natural light but show up under the Wood's light (ultraviolet light). They should be looked for in infants with seizures. Pigmentation of the lips is a feature of *Peutz–Jeghers syndrome*, genetically determined, in which multiple polyps of the stomach or colon appear which may later undergo malignant transformation. *Café au lait* type macules are often the first sign of neurofibromatosis: (NF1); they may be mul-

tiple. Another valuable sign of von Reckinghausen's disease is bilateral freckling of the axillary skin. The characteristic soft neurofibromata may be solitary or few, or hundreds may be scattered over the body. *Icthyosis* (scaly fish skin) is usually present from childhood and is genetic, but if ichthyosis is acquired in adult life, a search should be made for malignancy or other underlying disease.

Non-organ-specific autoimmune disorders

Several of the so-called collagen vascular diseases may have characteristic eruptions. *Systemic lupus erythematosus*, seen in females between puberty and the menopause, may show a symmetrical 'butterfly' erythema of the nose and cheeks. In *polyarteritis nodosa*, reticular livedo of the limbs, with purpura, vasculitic papules and ulceration occur. In *scleroderma* (systemic sclerosis), acrosclerosis of the fingertips with scarring, ulceration and calcinosis follows a Raynaud's phenomenon of increasing severity. *Dermatomyositis* often presents with a heliotrope discoloration and oedema of the eyelids, and with fixed erythema over the dorsa of the knuckles and fingers and over the bony points of the shoulders, elbows and legs. There is usually weakness of the proximal limb muscles. Dermatomyositis in the middle-aged is associated in 10% of cases with internal malignancy.

Skin pigmentation

Acanthosis nigricans is a brownish velvety thickening of the axillae, groins and sides of the neck. Sometimes there is thickening of the palms and soles, and warty excrescences may develop on the skin, eyelids and oral mucosa. In the middle-aged, acanthosis nigricans is strongly associated with internal malignancy but benign minor forms are seen in obese young women, especially Arabs, and in children with endocrinopathies characterized by insulin resistance. Patchy *depigmented macules* which are hypoanaesthetic and associated with enlargement of the peripheral nerves are features of certain types of leprosy.

Generalized, severe persistent *pruritus* in the absence of obvious skin disease may be due to systemic disease (Box 3.6). However, in old people with dry skin it is common and of no systemic significance. Diabetes mellitus has a number of skin manifestations: of these pruritus vulvae, pruritus ani, balanoposthitis and angular stomatitis are due to

(a)

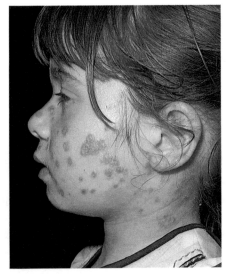

(b)

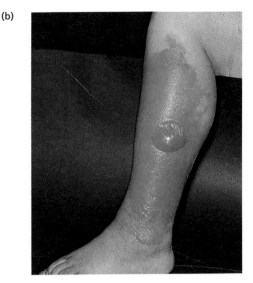

Fig. 3.10   (a) Impetigo. (b) Erysipelas.

Candida overgrowth. Boils, follicular pustules or ecthyma are staphylococcal. Impetigo and erysipelas, a streptococcal infection, are uncommon (Fig. 3.10). *Eruptive xanthomata* are a rare feature of uncontrolled diabetes mellitus. *Necrobiosis lipoidica diabeticorum* produces reddish-brown plaques, usually on the shins, with central atrophy of the skin. It has to be distinguished from peri-tibial myxoedema (which is hypertrophic, not atrophic), the dermatoliposclerosis of chronic venous disease in the legs and the epidermal hypertrophy of chronic lymphatic obstruction.

Neuropathic ('perforating') ulcers are found on pressure points of the heel, ball of foot, or toes and are characteristically painless. *Arteriopathic ulceration* resulting from large vessel disease is seen on the foot, and due to small vessel disease on the calves. *Spider naevi* consist of a central arteriole feeding a cluster of surrounding vessels. Many young people have up to seven on the face, shoulders or arms. In older age-groups pregnancy, the administration of

oestrogens (as in oral contraceptives) and liver disease may cause multiple lesions. Pregnancy and liver disease may also produce erythema of the thenar and hypothenar eminences ('liver palms'). *Leuconychia* is also seen in liver disease.

Erythema nodosum is a condition in which tender, painful, red nodules appear, typically on the shins. They fade slowly over several weeks, leaving bruising, but never ulcerate. Sarcoidosis and drug sensitivity are the commonest causes but other systemic disorders should be considered (Box 3.7).

BOX 3.7 Causes of erythema nodosum.

- Sarcoidosis
- Sulphonamides
- Streptococcal infection
- Tuberculosis
- Inflammatory bowel disease
- Behçet's disease
- Other infections, e.g. leprosy, systemic mycoses, toxoplasmosis, lymphogranuloma venereum

---

BOX 3.6 Causes of pruritus in systemic disease.

- Iron deficiency anaemia
- Diabetes mellitus
- Thyrotoxicosis or hypothyroidism
- Renal failure
- Hepatic failure
- Obstructive jaundice
- Lymphoma and other malignancies
- Drugs: cocaine, morphine, etc.
- Parasites, e.g. onchocerciasis, etc.
- Psychogenic

Xanthomata are yellow or orange papules or nodules in the skin due to dermal aggregations of lipid-loaded cells. Different patterns of hyperlipoproteinaemia may induce varying patterns of xanthomatosis. Thus, the type IIa (hypercholesterolaemia) pattern typically causes tuberose xanthomata on the extensor aspects of the knees and elbows and on the buttocks, sometimes associated with tendon xanthomata. Widespread eruptive xanthomata are more characteristic of hypertriglyceridaemia. White deposits of lipid (*arcus senilis*) in the cornea may have a similar explanation but may be a normal feature in those over 60 years. Flat lipid deposits around the eyes (*xanthelasma*) may be due to hyperlipidaemia but are also seen in the middle-aged and elderly without any general metabolic upset.

Carotenaemia produces an orange-yellow colour of the skin, especially of the palms and soles. It occurs in those who eat great quantities of carrots and other vegetables, in hypothyroidism, in diabetic patients, and also in those taking β-carotene for the treatment of porphyria.

Haemorrhage in the skin

Aggregations of extravasated red blood cells in the skin cause *purpura* (see Fig. 3.11). Purpura may be punctate, from capillary haemorrhage, or may form larger macules according to the extent of haemorrhage and the size of vessels involved. The Hess test for capillary fragility involves deliberately inducing punctate purpura on the forearm by inflating a cuff above the elbow at 100 mmHg for 3 minutes (see Chapter 18). Sensitivity to drugs may cause widespread 'capillaritis'.

The term *ecchymosis* implies a bruise, usually with cutaneous and subcutaneous haemorrhage causing a palpable lump. A frank fluctuant collection of blood is a *haematoma*.

Unlike erythema and telangiectasia, purpura cannot be blanched by pressure. It must not be confused

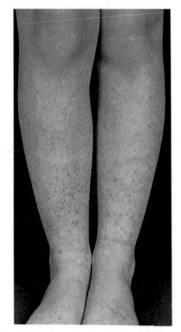

Fig. 3.11 Purpura in Henoch–Schönlein disease.

with senile haemangioma (cherry angioma or Campbell de Morgan spot), which is common in later life on the trunk and has no pathological significance. Haemorrhage into the thick epidermis of the palm or sole due to trauma (e.g. 'jogger's heel') may induce brown or almost black macules which take weeks to disappear, inviting confusion with melanoma.

The skin in sexually transmitted diseases

The skin is involved in various sexually transmitted diseases. The *primary chancre* of syphilis may occur on the genitalia of either sex, at or near the anus, on the lip or, rarely, elsewhere. The rash of secondary syphilis is brownish-red, maculopapular and typically involves the palms and soles. It does not itch. Other manifestations of the *secondary stage* are condylomata lata around the anogenital area, snail-track ulceration and 'mucous patches' in the mouth. There may be low-grade fever, lymphadenopathy and splenomegaly.

Septicaemia is a rare complication of gonorrhoea, which particularly occurs in pregnant women, presenting with pustular skin lesions. Recurrent type II herpes simplex is common on the penis; it occurs less often on the buttocks where relapses may be heralded by a radiating neuralgia. Genital viral warts are common in both sexes. They are particularly important in females because there is evidence that certain viral subtypes are responsible for chronic cervical dysplasia with malignant potential.

AIDS and other HIV-related syndromes have many cutaneous manifestations including disseminated Kaposi's sarcoma (see Fig. 17.5), candidiasis molluscum contagiosum, seborrhoeic dermatitis, folliculitis and oral hairy leucoplakia (Fig. 3.12).

Viral infection of the skin

Several of the commonest viral infections and illnesses of childhood are characterized by fever and a distinctive rash (*exanthem*), including measles, varicella and rubella. In *measles*, upper respiratory symptoms are quickly followed by a characteristic maculopapular erythematous rash. In *rubella* (German measles), the rash is more transient, micropapular and associated with occipital lymphadenopathy and only slight malaise. The exanthem of *varicella* (chickenpox) is papulovesicular and centripetal, and there may be lesions in the

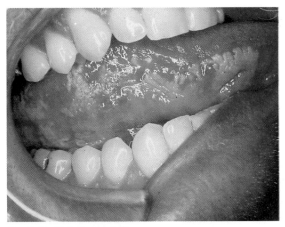

Fig. 3.12   Hairy leucoplakia.

mouth. In *herpes zoster* (Fig. 3.13) and *herpes simplex* infections there is a non-follicular papulovesicular rash in which the vesicles are planted in an inflamed base. The rash is painful. In herpes zoster the rash follows a segmental distribution, in the skin of a dermatome. The vesicular lesion becomes encrusted (Fig. 3.14) and, later, secondary infection may occur.

Other less common viral infections associated with a rash include *erythema infectiosum*, due to a parvovirus, in which the exanthem on the face gives a 'slapped-cheek' appearance, and *roseola infantum*, a disease of toddlers, which mimics rubella.

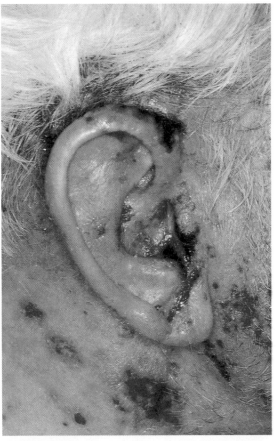

Fig. 3.14   Herpes zoster vesicles on the ear lobe involving the C2 dermatome.

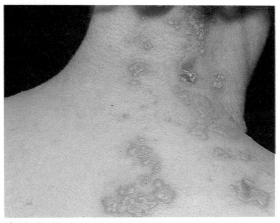

Fig. 3.13   Herpes zoster.

Drug eruptions

In the last 30 years, eruptions caused by drugs have become common. Most, but not all, such rashes are due to allergic hypersensitivity.

Drug rashes can mimic almost every pattern of skin disease. Thus urticaria may be caused by penicillin; a measles-like (morbilliform) rash may be induced by ampicillin, especially when given in infectious mononucleosis; eczema-like rashes are seen with methyldopa and phenylbutazone therapy: whereas gold and chloroquine rashes mimic lichen planus. Generalized exfoliative dermatitis may be induced by sulphonylureas, indomethacin and allopurinol.

Drugs which may sensitize the skin to sunlight (*phototoxic reaction*) include tetracyclines, sulphonamides and nalidixic acid. Acne-like rashes may follow high-dose prednisolone therapy, and are common with phenytoin therapy. Certain cytotoxic drugs and sodium valoproate cause hair loss. Both erythema nodosum and erythema multiforme may be induced by sulphonamides, including co-trimoxazole. Laboratory tests are of almost no value in the diagnosis of drug eruptions. Careful history-taking and knowledge of the common patterns of drug reactions usually allow accurate diagnosis.

Tumours in the skin

Exposure to the sun may result, after many years, in the development of skin tumours, e.g. squamous or basal cell carcinoma, or melanoma. These tumours are especially common in fair-skinned people. *Basal cell carcinoma* arises especially on the face, near the nose, or on the forehead (Fig. 3.15). The lesion may be ulcerated with a firm, rounded edge, or papular. *Melanomas* occur especially on skin that has been burned by the sun, e.g. torso, ears, forearms. They may be pigmented or unpigmented, and may develop rapidly in a mole that has been present for many years. *Seborrhoeic keratosis* is a raised pigmented lesion found in the elderly (Fig. 3.16).

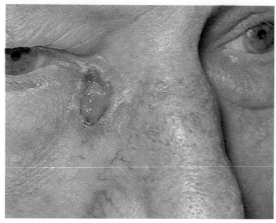

Fig. 3.15 Basal cell carcinoma.

Special techniques in examination of the skin

The skin is uniquely available to the examining physician. There are a number of diagnostic procedures.

Skin biopsy

Under ideal circumstances the skin biopsy provides a wealth of information. The site, timing and technique of the biopsy can be absolutely critical. Inter-

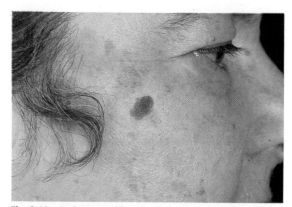

Fig. 3.16 A pigmented basal cell papilloma (seborrhoeic keratosis) on the face. This is a benign lesion.

pretation, particularly of inflammatory dermatosis, is best carried out by a dermatopathologist.

Tzanck preparation

This technique is useful for rapid diagnosis of vesicular infections or blistering eruptions such as pemphigus. The intact blister is opened and the base gently scraped. The material obtained is smeared onto the microscope slide, allowed to air-dry and then stained. Viral lesions will show typical multinucleated giant cells and pemphigus will show acantholytic cells.

Microscopical examination

Microscopical examination is useful in the diagnosis of scabies, pediculosis and fungal infection (tinea and candidiasis).

SCABIES

Scabies is caused by the mite *Acarus (Sarcoptes) scabei*. The female *Acarus* is larger than the male and burrows in the epidermis, depositing eggs. These burrows should be looked for between the fingers, on the hands or wrists and sides of the feet. They can be recognized with the naked eye as short dark lines terminating in a shining spot of skin. The eggs lie in the dark line, the *Acarus* in the shining spot. It may be picked out by means of a flat surgical needle and placed on a slide under the microscope for more detailed examination.

PEDICULOSIS

Three forms of pediculosis or louse infestation occur: *Pediculus capitis* on the head, *Pediculus corporis* on the trunk and *Pediculus pubis* on the pubic and axillary hairs. The eggs or nits of *P. pubis* and *P. capitis* adhere to the hairs. From their position on the hairs one can judge roughly the duration of the condition, for they are fixed at first near the root of the hair, and are carried up as the hair grows, so the higher the nits are, the longer the pediculi have been present. *P. corporis* should be looked for in the seams of the clothes, especially where the clothes come into contact with the skin, e.g. over the shoulders. The bites of the parasite produce haemorrhagic spots, each with a dark centre and a paler areola. Marks of scratching should be looked for on parts accessible to the patient's nails. *P. pubis* is venereally acquired and causes intense pubic itching. The nits are laid on the pubic hair and the lice themselves are easily visible.

P. corporis is seen only in the grossly deprived, in vagrants, in those living rough, and in conditions of war and social upheaval. In contrast, *P. capitis* is common in schoolchildren, however clean they and their families may be, and is endemic in many schools.

FUNGUS INFECTIONS
Fungus may grow in the skin, nails or hair and can cause disease (ringworm or tinea).

Skin
The skin between the toes, the soles of the feet and the groins are the commonest sites of fungal infection. The lesions may be scaly or vesicular, tending to spread in a ring form with central healing (Fig. 3.17); macerated, dead-white offensive-smelling epithelium is found in the intertriginous areas such as the toe clefts.

Nails
Discoloration, deformity, hypertrophy and abnormal brittleness may result from fungus infection.

Hair
Ringworm of the scalp is most common in children. It presents as round or oval areas of baldness covered with short, broken-off, lustreless hair stumps. These hair stumps may fluoresce bright green under Wood's ultraviolet light. Some fungi do not produce fluorescence with Wood's light, however, and these can be detected only by microscopy and culture (Fig. 3.18).

Microscopical examination for fungus infection
Scales from the active edge of a lesion are scraped off

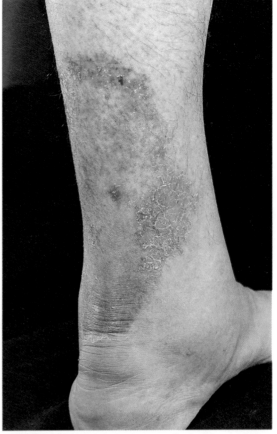

Fig. 3.17   Tinea rubrum (ringworm infection).

lightly with a scalpel, or the roofs of vesicles are snipped off with scissors. The material is placed in a drop of 10–20% aqueous potassium hydroxide solution on a microscope slide, covered with a coverslip and left for 30 minutes to clear. It is then examined under the light microscope with the 8-mm or 4-mm objective using low illumination. The mycelia are

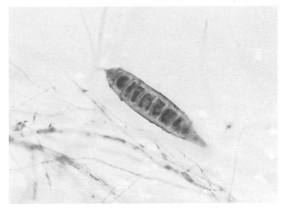

Fig. 3.18   Lactophenol blue preparation showing macronidia of *Microsporum* spp. isolated from skin scrapings from a patient with ringworm.

recognized as branching, refractile threads which boldly transgress the outlines of the squamous cells. Nails are examined in much the same way but it is necessary to break up the snippings and shavings into small fragments. These are either heated in potassium hydroxide or are left to clear in it overnight before being examined.

A scalp lesion is cleaned with 70% alcohol or with 1% cetrimide: infected stumps and scales are removed by scraping with a scalpel. The hairs are cleaned in potassium hydroxide in the same way as skin scales. Examination under the microscope reveals spores on the outside of the hair roots, and mycelia inside the hair substance. The species of fungus responsible may be established by culture on Sabouraud's glucose–agar (see Chapter 20).

Wood's light

Wood's light lamp emits long-wave ultraviolet light at a peak of 360 nm. Wood's light examination is performed in a darkened room and is useful in identifying fluorescence of fungi and corynebacterial infection (erythrasma), elevated porphyrins in urine or localization of pigmentary abnormalities.

Patch testing

This is an important and valuable tool for diagnosis of suspected allergic dermatitis due to contact (contact dermatitis).

The formulation of the allergens is critical and various standard contact allergen batteries have been developed in different countries and clinics to include the commonest culprits. Patch testing is simple but results are not always easy to interpret. Allergens are placed in shallow aluminium wells of 1 cm^2 and applied in strips to the patient's back for 48 hours for initial reading and a second reading at 96 hours. This ensures that any delayed type hypersensitivity e.g. Coombe's Type IV reaction to an allergen can be identified.

CHAPTER 4

The endocrine system and metabolic disorders

Introduction

The endocrine system comprises the classical endocrine organs:
- Pituitary
- Thyroid
- Parathyroid
- Adrenal
- Pancreatic islet cells
- Gonads.

Metabolic disorders are conditions which can be attributed to:
- Biochemical abnormality
- Enzyme defect
- Abnormal receptor mechanism.

Examples of metabolic disorders include the various forms of hyperlipidaemia, abnormalities of carbohydrate metabolism and several disorders of bone integrity.

It is useful to consider disorders of the endocrine system and metabolic disorders together because the mechanisms involved in endocrine and metabolic homeostasis are closely allied in terms of functional integration. The mode of presentation of these disorders does not fit neatly into a system-based model. The symptoms are rarely specific to a particular system and, frequently, a constellation of otherwise non-specific symptoms suggests the diagnosis.

The history

For diagnostic purposes the history consists of:
- Presenting symptoms
- History of the development of the illness
- Family history.

Presenting symptoms

There are a number of symptom complexes that particularly suggest an endocrine or metabolic cause. These are described below.

THIRST AND POLYURIA

Excessive thirst (*polydipsia*) and increased urine output (*polyuria*) are the most important presenting symptoms of diabetes mellitus. They are sometimes referred to as primary diabetic symptoms and they occur when the renal tubular glucose concentration is increased to the point that it exceeds the maximal tubular capacity for glucose reabsorption, causing an osmotic diuresis. Therefore, people with an increased renal threshold for glucose may be asymptomatic despite hyperglycaemia. Polydipsia and polyuria may also be due to failure of renal concentrating capacity due to deficiency of antidiuretic hormone (*neurogenic diabetes insipidus*) or a failure of antidiuretic hormone action (*nephrogenic diabetes insipidus*). The latter may be inherited or may occur

61

secondary to impairment of antidiuretic hormone action by hypercalcaemia or hypokalaemia. Sometimes, apparent polydipsia and polyuria may be due to increased fluid intake, which at its most extreme may be vastly excessive (*psychogenic polydipsia*). The distinction between psychogenic polydipsia and diabetes insipidus is important. Generally, nocturnal polyuria is not a feature of psychogenic polydipsia but this is not an absolute distinction, and further investigation of urine concentrating capacity is usually required.

WEIGHT LOSS

Loss of weight is a feature of decreased food intake or increased metabolic rate. Sometimes both factors may operate to reduce body weight, as in the *cachexia* of malignant disease. Thyroid overactivity (*hyperthyroidism*) is nearly always associated with a combination of weight loss and increased appetite although, occasionally, the latter may be stimulated more than the former so that a paradoxical increase in weight occurs. Weight loss is rarely the sole presenting symptom of hyperthyroidism and other clinical features predominate, particularly in younger patients (Box 4.1). Vitiligo may be an associated feature in autoimmune thyroiditis with hyperthyroidism. In the elderly, however, hyperthyroidism may be indolent and may simulate malignant disease with a gradual weight loss. Cardiac arrhythmias are a frequent feature in the elderly. The weight loss of thyrotoxicosis must be distinguished from that due to *anorexia nervosa*. The latter is characterized by a long history of low body weight in the absence of other features of ill-health. The disorder particularly occurs in young girls. Any form of weight loss may be associated with amenorrhoea.

BOX 4.1 Clinical features of hyperthyroidism.

- Weight loss
- Atrial fibrillation
- Tachycardia, heart failure
- Eye signs
  —Lid lag
  —Lid retraction
  —Exophthalmos
- Sweating
- Thyroid gland enlargement and bruit
- Fine distal tremor
- Thinning of hair
- Proximal weakness; cannot rise from squat
- Chorea

Other endocrine conditions in which weight loss is a major feature are listed in Box 4.2. The rapid weight loss which occurs at the onset of insulin-dependent diabetes is the single most important clinical feature in distinguishing it from the non-insulin-dependent form of the disease (type 2 diabetes mellitus).

BOX 4.2 Endocrine and metabolic diseases in which weight loss is a clinical feature.

- Hyperthyroidism
- Type 1, insulin-dependent diabetes mellitus
- Hypopituitarism
- Adrenocortical failure (Addison's disease)
- Anorexia nervosa

WEIGHT GAIN OR REDISTRIBUTION

Increase in body weight (Box 4.3) is a predictable result of a reduction in metabolic rate. Weight gain is therefore a common feature of *primary hypothyroidism*. However, obesity is rarely a consequence of specific endocrine dysfunction. In the majority of patients 'simple obesity' is due to a long-standing imbalance between energy intake and expenditure; the problem frequently presents in childhood and is present in more than one family member. Glucocorticoid hormone excess (*Cushing's syndrome*) results in an increase in body fat predominantly involving abdominal, omental and interscapular fat (truncal obesity) with paradoxical thinning of the limbs due to muscle atrophy.

BOX 4.3 Conditions in which increased body weight is a feature.

- Simple obesity: energy intake/expenditure imbalance
- Primary hypothyroidism
- Cushing's syndrome
- Hypothalamic lesions

MUSCLE WEAKNESS

Symptomatic muscular weakness in the absence of neurological disease is a feature of several metabolic disorders, including thyrotoxicosis, Cushing's syndrome and vitamin D deficiency. In all these conditions the *metabolic myopathy* (Box 4.4) causes symmetrical proximal weakness, mainly involving the shoulder and hip girdle musculature. There is often associated muscle wasting. The major symptom is difficulty in climbing stairs, boarding a bus or rising from a sitting position. Virtually all patients with hyperthyroidism have proximal weakness. This may be subclinical, but can usually be demonstrated by asking the patient to rise from the squatting position. The proximal myopathy of *vitamin D deficiency* is often painful, in contrast to the other causes. The differential diagnosis of painful proximal muscular weakness includes polymyositis and polymyalgia rheumatica, as well as spinal root or plexus disease.

BOX 4.4 Conditions in which metabolic myopathy is a feature.

Painless
- Hyperthyroidism
- Cushing's syndrome
- Acromegaly
- Iatrogenic steroid myopathy

Painful
- Vitamin D deficiency
- Osteomalacia
- Hypothyroidism

COLD INTOLERANCE

An abnormal sensation of cold which is out of proportion to that experienced by other individuals may indicate underlying *hypothyroidism* (Boxes 4.5 and 4.6). This symptom differs from the localized vasomotor symptoms in the hands found in Raynaud's phenomenon and is rather non-specific, especially in the elderly patient.

BOX 4.5 Conditions in which temperature intolerance is a feature.

- Intolerance to cold
  —hypothyroidism
- Intolerance to heat
  —hyperthyroidism

BOX 4.6 Clinical features of hypothyroidism

- Weight gain
- Sallow complexion and fine skin
- Thinning of scalp and lateral eyebrow hair
- Cold intolerance
- Deepened, gruff voice
- Slow physical and mental activity
- Unsteadiness and slightly slurred speech
- Tingling in toes and fingers
- Aching muscles with cramp
- Mild proximal weakness
- Slow pulse and shortness of breath
- Angina pectoris

HEAT INTOLERANCE

The increased metabolic rate of thyrotoxicosis may be associated with heat intolerance in which, at its most extreme, the patient finds comfortable an ambient temperature which others find unpleasantly cold. This is an important symptom, highly specific for thyroid overactivity which, in part, may explain some of the seasonal variation in presentation of the condition.

INCREASED SWEATING

Some individuals experience excessive sweating (*hyperhidrosis*) as a constitutional abnormality, characterized by onset in childhood or adolescence and, sometimes, by a family history. A more recent increase in sweat secretion, on the other hand, may be an early indication of thyroid overactivity. Paroxysmal sweating is a common feature of anxiety. Increased catecholamine secretion from a phaeochromocytoma of the adrenal medulla is a rare cause of hyperhidrosis. Intermittent sweating after meals (gustatory hyperhidrosis) may occur in patients with autonomic dysfunction. Growth hormone excess (acromegaly) also increases sweating, perhaps because of hypertrophy of sweat glands, and this feature can be used to assess activity of the disease in the clinic. Increased sweating should be distinguished from flushing which occurs physiologically at the time of the natural menopause. Flushing may be a presenting feature of serotonin-secreting carcinoid tumours of the gut.

TREMOR

A fine rapid resting tremor is one of the cardinal clinical features of thyrotoxicosis. This must be distinguished from the coarser and more irregular tremor of anxiety which is usually associated with a cool peripheral skin temperature, in contrast to the warm skin of the thyrotoxic patient. Tremor due to neurological disease is of greater amplitude, slower rate, and may be present at rest, as in Parkinson's disease, or on movement, as in cerebellar intention tremor. It therefore rarely simulates thyrotoxic tremor.

PALPITATIONS

A sensation of increased heart rate or force of contraction may be a feature of thyrotoxicosis, but is more likely to be due to anxiety. Awareness of the heart beat while lying down is normal. Other causes of rapid heart rate include paroxysmal tachyarrhythmias. The sensation of intermittent forceful cardiac contraction, sometimes described by the patient as a missed beat, is often due to the compensatory pause following an ectopic beat, and is usually a normal phenomenon.

POSTURAL UNSTEADINESS

Dizziness, or a sensation of faintness on standing, should prompt measurement of lying and standing blood pressure. Postural hypotension, a fall of diastolic blood pressure on standing, occurs with reduced blood volume. In the absence of obvious bleeding or gastrointestinal fluid loss one should consider adrenal insufficiency as the cause. Postural hypotension is frequently due to autonomic neuropathy, especially in long-standing diabetes mellitus. It is also a common complication of any hypertensive drug therapy for essential hypotension. The drug history is particularly important in the elderly patient with dizziness.

VISUAL DISTURBANCE

Several endocrine conditions may cause visual symptoms. Decreased visual acuity may occur from space-occupying lesions compressing the optic nerve. For example, severe dysthyroid eye disease and orbital or retro-orbital tumours may present in this way. *Bitemporal hemianopia* (bilateral loss of part or all of the temporal fields of vision), often asymmetrical or incongruous, is a major feature of suprasellar extension of pituitary adenomas compressing the optic chiasm, but may occur in other tumours in this location. Double vision (*diplopia*) on lateral or upward gaze, often results from medial or lateral rectus muscle tethering in dysthyroid eye disease (see Figure 10.2). Apparent magnification of vision (*macropsia*) can occur in hypoglycaemia.

FASTING SYMPTOMS

Tachycardia, sweating and tremor, occurring intermittently, especially when fasting, are suggestive of hypoglycaemia. These symptoms resemble those associated with the increased sympathetic drive found in states of fear or with excess secretion of noradrenaline, as in phaeochromocytoma. In severe persistent hypoglycaemia these symptoms may progress to decreased consciousness. This is a serious emergency implying neuroglycopenia sufficient to impair brain function. Spontaneous or fasting hypoglycaemia can be due to:

- autonomous insulin production due to an insulinoma;
- glucocorticoid deficiency, with or without thyroxine and growth hormone deficiency, e.g. primary adrenal failure or hypopituitarism;
- inappropriate insulin, or excessive sulphonylurea drug administration in a diabetic patient; or
- rarer causes of hypoglycaemia, e.g. hepatic failure

and rapidly growing malignant lesions, especially retroperitoneal sarcomas.

CRAMPS AND 'PINS AND NEEDLES'

Intermittent cramp and 'pins and needles' (*paraesthesiae*), especially if bilateral, can be due to a decreased circulating ionized calcium level. This may occur in hypoparathyroidism or be associated with a fall in the ionized component of serum calcium, due to an increased extracellular pH (*alkalosis*). The latter may occur with any alkalosis, but is particularly well-recognized in hyperventilatory states (respiratory alkalosis) and hypokalaemia (metabolic alkalosis). Refractory cramping symptoms after correction of hypocalcaemia can be due to an associated hypomagnesaemia. However, the differential diagnosis of paraesthesiae in the hands includes median nerve compression at the wrist (carpal tunnel syndrome), a syndrome that is usually accompanied by typical sensory and motor disturbance suggestive of a lesion in the median nerve (see Chapter 12).

NAUSEA

This is a rare symptom of endocrine disease. It is an important presenting feature of adrenal insufficiency in which typically it is maximal in the morning and may be associated with vomiting. Similar symptoms may occur with severe hypercalcaemia and may be the sole manifestation of this condition. These two conditions should be considered early in the differential diagnosis of a patient presenting with upper gastrointestinal symptoms in the absence of demonstrable structural disease. Occasionally, thyrotoxicosis may present with nausea and vomiting, although looseness of stools is the more common gastrointestinal manifestation of this condition.

DYSPHAGIA

Difficulty in swallowing is an unusual manifestation of endocrine disease but may be the presenting feature of multinodular thyroid enlargement with retrosternal extension. Smaller goitres only rarely result in dysphagia. Severe hyperthyroidism with generalized weakness may be associated with a reversible myopathy of the pharyngeal musculature and consequent dysphagia.

NECK PAIN AND SWELLING

Superficial discomfort in the neck may lead to the incidental finding of thyroid enlargement. However, it should be borne in mind that modest degrees of thyroid enlargement are very common, whereas pain arising from the thyroid is comparatively unusual. The most common cause of local discomfort and tenderness in the neck is inflammatory lymphadenopathy. Severe tenderness of the thyroid itself, especially when accompanied by fever and signs of thyrotoxicosis suggests a diagnosis of viral subacute thyroiditis (de Quervain's thyroiditis). Occasionally autoimmune thyroiditis may give rise to pain and tenderness, which mimics a viral thyroiditis but is less severe. A sudden onset of localized pain and swelling in the thyroid is indicative of bleeding into a pre-existing thyroid nodule and is a recognized complication of multinodular goitre. The symptoms are self-limiting. Painless enlargement of the thyroid gland (*goitre*) presents either because of pressure effects, resulting in dysphagia progressing to tracheal compression and stridor, or cosmetic disturbance. The underlying cause of thyroid enlargement is often difficult to establish. The family history and subsequent investigation may point to autoimmune thyroiditis or dyshormonogenesis. A history of rapid enlargement of the gland, especially in an elderly patient, suggests an anaplastic thyroid carcinoma. Coexisting severe diarrhoea points towards a diagnosis of medullary carcinoma of the thyroid. In the differential diagnosis goitrogenic drugs, for example lithium, should be considered, as should residence in iodine-deficient areas. Previous exposure to neck irradiation, or to radioactive iodine, in childhood, may also be important.

IMPOTENCE

Decreased erectile potency may be a consequence of primary abnormalities, such as:

- decreased blood supply to the penis, e.g. atherosclerosis;
- neural dysfunction, e.g. autonomic neuropathy complicating diabetes;
- testosterone deficiency, e.g. hypopituitarism and primary testicular failure;
- drug therapy, e.g. certain anti-hypertensives;
- psychological factors; or
- a combination of several causes.

It is often difficult to distinguish with certainty between impotence due to organic and psychological factors, although total erectile failure and the absence of nocturnal and morning erections suggest a physical cause. Impotence in a diabetic patient should not be assumed to be inevitably due to autonomic neuropathy and other causes should be considered. A reduction in testicular size points towards an endocrine aetiology but is not invariably found in hypopituitarism. Most importantly, it should be recognized that male impotence is often complicated by a psychological disturbance, which may serve to exacerbate the problem.

GYNAECOMASTIA

Mild breast enlargement in the male may occur as a temporary phenomenon in puberty and may persist for several years. Gynaecomastia in the adult male may result from:

- excess oestrogen stimulation;
- reduction in circulating androgen;
- antagonism of androgen action; or
- androgen insensitivity (Box 4.7).

Clinical assessment of the patient with gynaecomastia should therefore include enquiry concerning any change in libido and examination of thyroid status, the genitalia, the muscles and for stigmata of chronic liver disease (Box 4.7).

BOX 4.7 Causes of gynaecomastia.

Increased oestrogen/testosterone ratio
- Chronic liver disease
- Thyrotoxicosis
- Phenytoin therapy

Androgen receptor antagonists
- Spironolactone; digoxin

Inherited androgen receptor defects
- Testicular feminization syndrome
- Primary and secondary hypogonadism
- Tumour production of human chorionic gonadotrophin (HCG)
- Oestrogen production of Leydig cell tumour of testis
- X-linked spinal muscular atrophy (Kennedy syndrome); Klinefelter phenotype

---

AMENORRHOEA

Perhaps the most common cause of failure of onset of menses (*primary amenorrhoea*) is physiological delay of puberty, a diagnosis which can only be made with certainty in retrospect. Important pathological causes include:

- hypothalamic–pituitary dysfunction, for example due to tumours;
- ovarian failure, for example, due to failure of normal ovarian development or to cytotoxic chemotherapy;
- thyroid dysfunction; and
- defects in lower genital tract development.

Important diagnostic pointers in the history include symptoms suggestive of thyroid disease, or any visible disability which might indicate compression of the optic chiasm due to a hypothalamic or pituitary tumour. *Secondary amenorrhoea* has similar causes. In addition, marked weight loss may lead to amenorrhoea, as in anorexia nervosa or inflammatory bowel disease. Amenorrhoea, or infrequent scanty periods, may occur in women subject to excessively rigorous physical training programmes.

GALACTORRHOEA

Occasionally physiological lactation may persist after breast-feeding following childbirth has ceased. Inappropriate lactation is usually bilateral. There are a number of causes, such as:
- prolactin-secreting tumours of the pituitary gland;
- idiopathic galactorrhoea, in which there is an apparent increased sensitivity to normal levels of serum prolactin;
- hyperprolactinaemia due to hypothyroidism;
- hyperprolactinaemia due to dopamine antagonist drugs; and
- hyperprolactinaemia due to lactotroph-disinhibiting lesions of the hypothalamic–pituitary region.

Inappropriate secretion of breast milk should therefore always prompt enquiry for symptoms referable to the thyroid and pituitary glands, and a thorough drug history should be taken.

EXCESS HAIR GROWTH

An increase in growth of facial and body hair in adult females is a relatively common symptom which may be due to increased circulating androgens. However, it is most commonly a normal, racially determined characteristic. Pathological causes of hirsutism include:
- polycystic ovary syndrome;
- late presentation of congenital adrenal hyperplasia;
- androgen-secreting ovarian or adrenal tumours.

The history is vital in the clinical assessment. If symptoms commenced shortly after the age of the menarche, then a tumour source of androgen is unlikely. A regular menstrual cycle is good evidence against severe androgen excess, suggesting that hirsutism is constitutional and not pathological. Increased libido on the other hand, suggests an increased androgen secretion, which may be either ovarian or neoplastic in origin.

BOWEL DISTURBANCE

Constipation and abdominal distension may be features of hypothyroidism or pan-hypopituitarism. Diarrhoea may occur as part of autonom-

ic neuropathy involving the gut in diabetes mellitus. Peptic ulceration may occur in the Zollinger–Ellison syndrome, in which gastrin-secreting tumours of the gut result in increased gastric acid secretion.

SKIN CHANGES

A striking pallor occurs in primary testicular failure and in pan-hypopituitarism. Excessive pigmentation occurs in Cushing's syndrome, with increased sebum production causing greasy skin and acne on the face and shoulders. In carcinoid tumours of the gut or lung increased 5-hydroxyindol acetic acid secretion results in a violaceous cyanosis-like skin discoloration. A variegate, patchy rash is a feature of porphyria, an inherited abnormality of haem metabolism. In hypoadrenalism there is pallor with pigmentation of the conjunctival membrane beneath the lids, and of the inside of the mouth, and axillae. In hypothyroidism the skin appears pale, sallow, or even slightly yellow, and the scalp and lateral eyebrow hair are thinned. In hyperthyroidism the skin is dry and hot, but often not flushed. In hypocalcaemia the nails are friable. In uraemia the skin is pale, or yellow and slightly pigmented, and in terminal uraemia a 'uraemic frost' may appear on the skin.

Vitiligo, a patchy depigmentation of the skin, is common in many autoimmune disorders particularly autoimmune hyperthyroidism, a vitamin B_{12} deficiency.

Family history

The family background of endocrine or metabolic disease may be particularly useful in the evaluation of several of the more common disorders. It is also particularly important in the assessment of less common, inherited disorders of metabolism.

DIABETES MELLITUS

In comparison with insulin-dependent diabetes, non-insulin-dependent diabetes has a strong hereditary component. Therefore a family history may be useful in the initial assessment of patients with diabetes, and also of patients with premature vascular disease in whom there may be an abnormality of glucose tolerance.

THYROID DISEASE

Autoimmune hypothyroidism and hyperthyroidism frequently show familial aggregation. Dyshormonogenetic goitre is also often inherited.

RENAL CALCULI

Primary hyperparathyroidism, an important cause of renal stones, may be familial, occurring either as an isolated disorder or as a part of the syndrome of multiple endocrine neoplasia (type 1).

ATHEROMA

Large-vessel atheromatosis, particularly affecting the coronary circulation, may manifest a strong familial component. This is of considerable importance in the context of hereditary disorders of lipoprotein metabolism, especially familial hypercholesterolaemia (type A).

The examination

General assessment

This should begin with observation of the general appearance. Start by assessing the state of nutrition and with measurement of weight and height. The body mass index (BMI) is calculated from the formula:

$$\text{BMI} = \frac{\text{Weight (kg)}}{\text{Height (m)}^2}.$$

The normal range for the BMI in men is 20–25 and in women is 18–24. The BMI is useful in the assessment of obesity and malnutrition (see page 79).

The distribution of fat should be noted. Concentration of fat in the intra-abdominal and interscapular regions with relative sparing of the limbs (truncal obesity) is characteristic of Cushing's syndrome and is accompanied by a typical moonfaced plethoric appearance (Fig. 4.1) due to a combination of increased subcutaneous fat and thinning of the skin.

Patients with growth hormone hypersecretion, resulting from somatotroph pituitary adenomas, also demonstrate a classical facial appearance with increased fullness and coarsening of soft tissues, including the lips and tongue, which may be accompanied by overgrowth of the zygoma, orbital ridges and mandible (prognathism) in patients with longstanding disease (Fig. 4.2). Acromegaly in young people causes continuation of growth beyond the normal time of cessation of growth at about age 16–18 years, and consequent increase in height. Increased adiposity in a child who is growing poorly suggests the possibility of growth hormone deficiency or hypothyroidism.

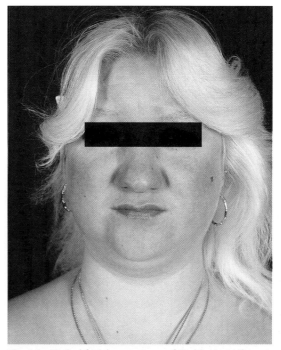

Fig. 4.1 Typical facial appearance of Cushing's syndrome. Note the increased fat deposition and plethoric appearance with thinning of the skin.

The skeletal proportions should be noted; a long-limbed appearance may indicate delayed epiphysial fusion due to hypogonadism (*eunuchoidism*) or the connective tissue abnormality, Marfan's syndrome. A eunuchoid body habitus is confirmed by demonstrating that the leg length (top of symphysis pubis to ground) exceeds the sitting height or that the span exceeds the total height. Shortening of the limbs occurs with a variety of skeletal dysplasias.

The cytogenetic disorder Turner's syndrome (karyotype 45X0), which is characterized by gonadal dysgenesis and the variable presence of other visceral abnormalities, has a typical phenotypic appearance including short stature, failure of secondary sexual development, decreased or absent secondary sexual hair, an increase in the normal angulation between the humerus and the lower arm, a low posterior hair line and an exaggerated fold of skin between the neck and shoulder. It is most important that accurate wall-mounted stadiometers be used in the assessment of normal growth and its possible disorders.

The hands should be carefully examined for evidence of finger-clubbing which, among other things, may be a rare manifestation of thyrotoxic Graves' disease (*thyroid acropachy*). Palmar erythema may also be found in thyrotoxicosis of any cause as well as

(a)

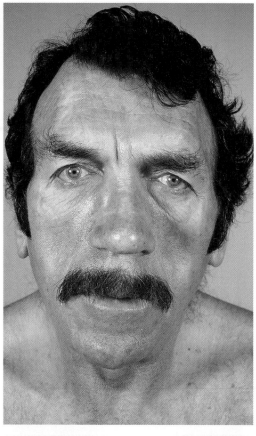

thyroidism; Fig. 4.3). Palmar contractures are a relatively common incidental finding and a recognized feature of chronic liver disease but also may occur in patients with long-standing diabetes mellitus. The latter is frequently associated with subtle phalangeal flexural contractions (*cheiroarthropathy*).

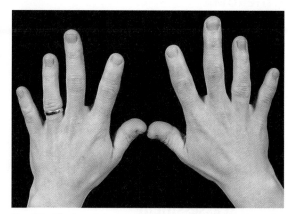

Fig. 4.3 The hands in pseudohypoparathyroidism. Note the characteristic shortening of the 4th and 5th metacarpals.

Subcutaneous deposits of triglyceride-rich lipoproteins in the palmar skin creases (*palmar xanthomata*) are pathognomonic of increased intermediate density lipoprotein (WHO type III hyperlipidaemia).

The skin

A careful external examination may yield specific diagnostic information in addition to that evident on the initial general examination. Pigmentation, especially buccal, circumoral or palmar may indicate the increased secretion of adrenocorticotrophic hormone which occurs with adrenal failure (*Addison's*

(b)

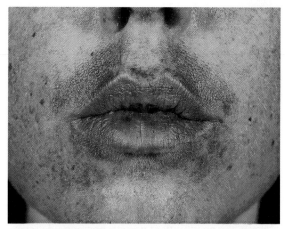

Fig. 4.4 Circumoral pigmentation in a patient with hypersecretion of adrenocorticotropic hormone (ACTH).

Fig. 4.2 The facial (a) and hand (b) appearance of acromegaly. There is overgrowth of the facial skeleton, coarsening of features and an increase in soft tissues most obvious in the hands.

in patients with chronic liver disease or rheumatoid arthritis.

A unique selective shortening of the fourth and fifth metacarpals may be found as the major somatic manifestation of a group of recessively inherited disorders of parathormone action (*pseudohypopara-*

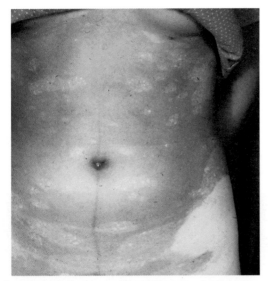

Fig. 4.5 Extensive areas of depigmentation (vitiligo) in a patient with organ-specific autoimmune disease.

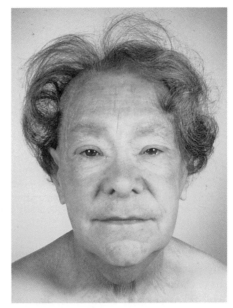

Fig. 4.7 The facial appearance of hypothyroidism. The patient demonstrates periorbital puffiness and coarsening of scalp hair. Courtesy of Dr P.G. Kopelman.

disease; Fig. 4.4); patches of depigmentation, or vitiligo (Fig. 4.5), may also be found in Addison's disease or other organ-specific autoimmune disorders. Violaceous striae, arising as a result of stretching of thin skin with exposure of the dermal capillary circulation, suggest the possibility of glucocorticoid excess (Fig. 4.6) and abnormal dryness of the skin and the coarseness of the hair are found in hypothyroidism (Fig. 4.7). Localized thickening of the dermis due to mucopolysaccharide and inflammatory cell deposition, particularly on the anterior aspects of the legs, when it is known as pretibial myxoedema, is one of the classical but relatively rare extrathyroidal manifestations of Graves' disease. An ulcerating skin lesion also demonstrating a predilection for the anterior tibial region is necrobiosis lipoidica diabeticorum (Fig. 4.8); this lesion is associated with marked skin atrophy and is specific to diabetes mellitus.

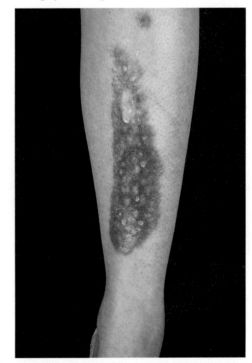

Fig. 4.8 Necrobiosis lipoidica diabeticorum. The ulceration occurs typically in atrophic skin on the anterior tibial region.

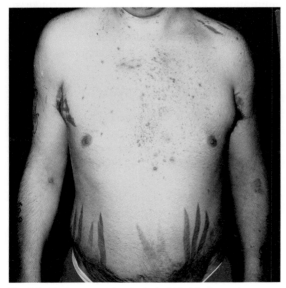

Fig. 4.6 Violaceous striae typical of Cushing's syndrome.

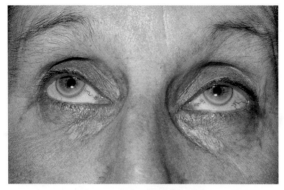

Fig. 4.9 Subcutaneous cholesterol deposition on the medial aspect of the eyelids (xanthelasma). Courtesy of Dr G.A. Hitman.

The examination of the skin may also demonstrate the presence of xanthelasmata, subcutaneous deposits of cholesterol just medial to the eyelids (Fig. 4.9) which are suggestive but not diagnostic of hypercholesterolaemia. The latter may also be manifest by the presence of xanthomata on the achilles or patellar tendons.

In the female, dermatological examination should also include attention to any abnormality of hair distribution, either excess hair growth in an androgen-dependent distribution (*hirsutism*) or hair loss in a male pattern, both of which may indicate increased circulating androgen and should prompt examination for evidence of virilization (see below).

The thyroid

The neck should be examined for evidence of thyroid enlargement. Significant thyroid enlargement is usually evident on inspection. Remember that the thyroid gland always moves on swallowing. The normal thyroid may be palpable in thin patients and it should be remembered that the right lobe is slightly larger than the left; therefore diffuse thyroid enlargement, as in Graves' disease, is often apparently asymmetrical. A prominent fat pad between skin creases in the neck may easily be mistaken for thyroid enlargement.

Palpation of the thyroid gland is best carried out from behind the patient with the fingers encircling the neck; the landmarks for palpation are the laryngeal cartilage, just below which is the cricoid cartilage and the isthmus of the thyroid. The following points should be addressed.

• Is the gland diffuse and smooth as in thyroid stimulating hormone (TSH)-mediated or autoimmune thyroid enlargement? If so is it soft as in dyshormonogenesis or the diffuse goitre of puberty, or is it firm or even hard as in autoimmune thyroiditis? A bruit heard over the thyroid indicates increased blood supply and is frequently found in untreated Graves' disease; this should not be confused with a transmitted bruit from the carotid.

• Are two or more areas of nodularity palpable, suggesting a multinodular goitre (Fig. 4.10) and if so does it extend downward behind the sternum (*retrosternal goitre*)? Is the patient clinically thyrotoxic, indicating autonomous thyroxine production within one or more nodules?

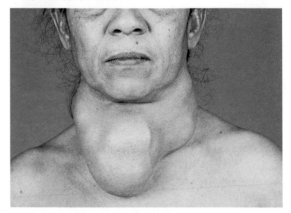

Fig. 4.10 A large multinodular goitre. Note the asymmetrical growth of the nodules.

• Is the palpable abnormality a single focal nodule suggesting a simple cyst, adenoma or carcinoma. Is there any lymphadenopathy which might be associated with the latter?

• Is the goitre firm and asymmetrical?

• Are there features of local pressure effects or local infiltration, e.g. a hoarse voice from recurrent laryngeal nerve involvement?

• Is there weight loss and debility? These features suggest lymphoma or anaplastic carcinoma.

The cardiovascular system

Particular attention should be paid to any postural drop in blood pressure. This may indicate a depleted extracellular fluid volume, for example in patients with adrenal insufficiency, or autonomic dysfunction, the commonest cause of which is diabetes mellitus. Additional indicators of the latter include failure of reflex bradycardia during the Valsalva manoeuvre and loss of beat-to-beat variation in cardiac cycle length determined by ECG. A hyperdynamic circulation, sinus tachycardia or atrial fibrillation may be found in thyrotoxicosis; this may progress to cardiac decompensation and cardiac failure.

The breasts and genitalia

The breasts should be examined for mass lesions and, if suggested by the history, for galactorrhoea. In the male any tendency to gynaecomastia should be noted (Fig. 4.11). This may range from minor degrees of subareolar glandular enlargement to substantial breast prominence; breast enlargement associated with generalized adiposity should not be confused with true gynaecomastia.

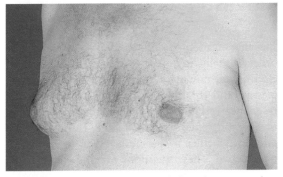

Fig. 4.11 Gynaecomastia. There is slight enlargement of both breasts in this man.

Genital examination in the male should document testicular volume. This is particularly important in the assessment of pubertal development for which volume should be measured by comparison with calibrated ovoids (Prader orchidometer). Prepubertal testicular volume is less than 4 ml whereas increased volume implies pubertal gonadotrophin stimulation. Testicular atrophy in the adult male indicates hypogonadism, due either to primary testicular failure, hypothalamic–pituitary dysfunction or chronic liver disease. Tumours of Leydig cells are usually palpable and should be sought in any patient with gynaecomastia.

Examination of the external genitalia in the female is important when androgen hypersecretion is suspected. Enlargement of the clitoris is a feature of excess androgen secretion.

Ambiguity of the external genitalia is indicative of fetal androgen excess in the karyotypic female and testosterone or dihydrotestosterone deficiency or resistance in the male; these conditions are rare and require specialized investigation.

The eyes

The hypercalcaemic patient should be carefully examined for corneal calcification, evident as a narrow band on the medial or lateral border of the

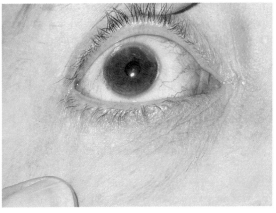

Fig. 4.12 Corneal calcification (band keratopathy) in a patient with long-standing hyperparathyroidism.

cornea (Fig. 4.12); this usually indicates long-standing hypercalcaemia and a diagnosis of primary hyperparathyroidism.

In patients with thyroid disease the presence of exophthalmos (*proptosis*) should be noted. This may be unilateral or bilateral and may be associated with apparent ophthalmoplegia due to tethering of the extraocular muscles, particularly the medial and inferior rectus muscles, such that diplopia occurs on upward or lateral gaze (*dysthyroid eye disease*; Fig. 4.13). These ocular signs are especially important in the diagnosis of autoimmune thyroid disease (*Graves' disease*). It must be remembered that

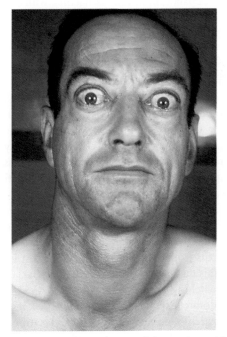

Fig. 4.13 Lid retraction and proptosis in a patient with thyrotoxic Graves' disease.

unilateral proptosis may also occur with an orbital tumour. Lid retraction, evident as a wide-eyed staring expression, and lid lag, in which depression of the upper lid lags behind the eye in a downward gaze, are due to increased activity of the sympathetic innervation of levator palpebri superioris and are not specific to Graves' disease. Any degree of corneal exposure due to failure of complete lid apposition should be documented.

Visual acuity should be measured both with and without a pinhole to correct for any refractive error. Reduced acuity may be a feature of optic nerve compression in severe dysthyroid eye disease or of asymmetrical pressure on the optic chiasm due to hypothalamic–pituitary space-occupying lesions. In the latter, assessment of the visual fields may reveal a bitemporal hemianopia; this is frequently incomplete and incongruous reflecting the asymmetrical growth of the tumour. Examination of the optic discs with the ophthalmoscope may show pallor indicating neural atrophy resulting from long-standing pressure on the optic nerve.

In the diabetic patient retinoscopy may show characteristic microvascular changes of two main types:
• small haemorrhages and exudates, either scattered (background retinopathy) or surrounding the macula (maculopathy), all associated with reduction in pinhole-corrected visual acuity; and
• areas of pallor, indicating ischaemia, with or without the formation of fronds of new vessels (proliferative retinopathy).

The nervous system

Examination of the nervous system reveals a rapid fine tremor in thyrotoxicosis. Proximal weakness with or without wasting of the shoulder and hip girdle musculature (*proximal myopathy*) is a typical feature of thyrotoxicosis, glucocorticoid excess and vitamin D deficiency. Osteomalacic myopathy is often associated with myalgia.

Hypocalcaemia is associated with increased neural excitability which may be demonstrated by gentle percussion over the proximal part of the facial nerve (as it exits from the parotid gland). The test is positive if this manoeuvre evokes involuntary facial muscular twitching (*Chvostek's sign*).

Tendon reflexes will be abnormally brisk in thyrotoxic patients and may show a slow relaxation phase in hypothyroidism. Both hypothyroidism and acromegaly may give rise to nerve entrapment syndromes particularly of the median nerve at the wrist (*carpal tunnel syndrome*).

Long-standing diabetes mellitus is frequently complicated by peripheral neuropathy with sensory loss in a stocking distribution, exaggeration of the foot arch and increased plantar prominence of the metatarsal heads due to muscle imbalance. This complication may culminate in plantar trophic ulceration.

Investigation

The investigation of endocrine and metabolic disorders usually involves: (a) the measurement of electrolytes, minerals, metabolites or hormones in plasma; and (b) isotopic, radiological or magnetic resonance imaging of specific endocrine glands. In investigating endocrine disease one is usually interested in whether a specific gland is overactive or underactive. These questions may be answered by basal hormone measurements, serum-free thyroxine and thyroid-stimulating hormone in thyrotoxicosis and hypothyroidism, but in many instances the lack of a clear distinction between basal hyposecretion, normal secretion and hypersecretion necessitates the use of stimulation tests and suppression tests.

Endocrine stimulation tests

These are designed to demonstrate how much hormone a gland can secrete in response to a near maximal stimulus. Examples include:
• *insulin tolerance testing* in which carefully controlled insulin-induced hypoglycaemia stimulates

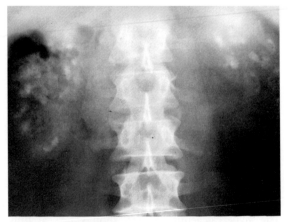

Fig. 4.14 Widespread renal calcification typical of nephrocalcinosis in a patient with long-standing hyperparathyroidism.

Fig. 4.15 Computerized tomography of the pituitary (axial view and sagittal reconstruction) demonstrating a large pituitary adenoma with marked suprasellar and sphenoidal sinus extension.

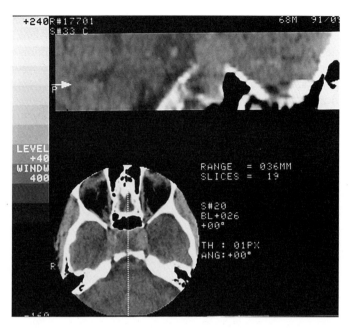

hypothalamic–pituitary secretion measured by serum growth hormone, cortisol and prolactin;

• *tetracosactrin testing* in which an injection of a synthetic adrenocorticotropic hormone (ACTH) analogue is used to assess adrenocortical reserve; and

• *oral glucose tolerance test* which is an indirect test of insulin secretion and action is determined by the rise and subsequent fall in the plasma glucose level following an oral glucose load.

Endocrine suppression tests

These test whether a physiological feedback mechanism is intact or if secretion of the hormone in ques-

tion has become at least partly autonomous. For example, the suppression of plasma cortisol by the synthetic glucocorticoid dexamethasone is incomplete in Cushing's syndrome and suppression of serum growth hormone by an oral glucose load fails to occur in acromegaly.

Endocrine imaging

Plain X-ray imaging is of limited value in the investigation of endocrine disorders. However, lateral

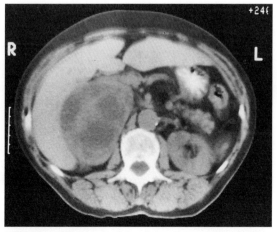

Fig. 4.16 Axial CT scan of the abdomen in a patient with a right adrenal medullary phaeochromocytoma. Note the extensive tumour mass with areas of hypodensity indicating episodes of partial tumour infarction.

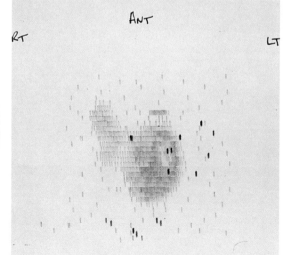

Fig. 4.17 Technetium-labelled isotope scan of the thyroid in a patient with a focal thyroid nodule. Note the focal area of uptake corresponding to the palpable lesion with surrounding inactivity indicating autonomous function within the nodule.

and anteroposterior views of the pituitary fossa can be useful in demonstrating abnormal calcification in the fossa or gross expansion of the fossa due to large intrasellar or suprasellar tumours. Plain abdominal radiology may show renal calcification (*nephrocalcinosis*; Fig. 4.14) in patients with long-standing hypercalcaemia or renal tubular acidosis.

CT imaging is useful in assessing the pituitary (Fig. 4.15), adrenal glands (Fig. 4.16) and thorax. However, MR imaging of the pituitary offers definite advantages over CT in terms of improved precision in detecting small intrasellar tumours and better definition of the lateral border of the pituitary and the cavernous sinus.

Isotopic imaging is particularly useful for demonstrating autonomous function within endocrine tumours. This technique is applicable to the thyroid gland (radio-labelled pertechnetate; Fig. 4.17), the adrenal cortex (radio-labelled selenocholesterol) and the adrenal medulla (radio-labelled meta-iodobenzylguanidine).

CHAPTER 5

The gastrointestinal tract and abdomen

Introduction

The human gastrointestinal tract is a complex system of serially connected organs approximately 8 m in length extending from the mouth to the anus which, together with its connected secretory glands, controls the passage, processing, absorption and elimination of ingested material. Symptoms of gut disorders are often vague, and signs of abnormality few unless the disease is advanced. Careful analysis of the clues provided both from the gut itself and from the effect of gut disease on the body as a whole are required if diagnosis is to be achieved.

Symptoms of gastrointestinal disease

In normal health there is awareness of the functional state of the gut, and this can be related to body needs. For example, thirst and hunger are common symptoms and the latter may be associated with epigastric discomfort or pain. The state of hydration can be subjectively assessed by awareness of the sensation of dryness of the mouth. Swallowing is normally perceived, and there is temperature sensation in the upper and mid-oesophagus, as well as in the mouth. The normal gastric motility can, to some extent, be perceived, and it is common for people to experience vigorous peristaltic contractions in the gut. The movement of gas and fluid in the gut, called borborygmi, can also be perceived. The experience of a sensation of fullness in the colon and rectum prior to defaecation, or during constipation and the call to stool are, similarly, aspects of the normal sensation of gut activity.

During illness, or sometimes following the ingestion of spicy foods, epigastric discomfort, or fullness, and intestinal hurry, may occur. These symptoms also reflect normal activity in the gut.

The common symptoms of gastrointestinal disease are listed in Box 5.1.

> **BOX 5.1 Common symptoms of gastrointestinal disease.**
>
> - Dysphagia
> - Heartburn
> - Indigestion
> - Flatulence
> - Hiccups
> - Vomiting
> - Constipation
> - Diarrhoea
> - Abnormal stools
> - Abdominal pain
> - Abdominal distension
> - Weight loss
> - Bleeding
> - Haematemesis
> - Rectal bleeding
> - Melaena

Symptoms of oesophageal disease

Disease of the oesophagus can cause the following symptoms.

Dysphagia, the sensation of something sticking in the throat or chest during swallowing, may be due to oesophageal stricture from benign or malignant causes. Dysphagia is a potentially serious symptom that should always be investigated.

Heartburn is due to acid reflux from the stomach into the lower part of the oesophagus. It causes pain in the epigastrium, chest and neck and may be difficult to distinguish from angina pectoris. It occurs particularly at night when the patient lies flat in bed, or after bending or stooping when abdominal pressure is increased. Alcohol often induces heartburn.

Painful swallowing, without difficulty in swallowing, is usually due to local infection. It is common in patients with AIDS in whom candida or herpes simplex often occur in the oesophagus.

Symptoms of stomach disease

In disease of the stomach the following symptoms may occur.

Dyspepsia, or indigestion, includes heartburn, pain, distension, nausea or 'an acid feeling' occurring after eating or drinking. The patients may also use this term to describe an inability to digest food. The symptom is subjective, frequent, and usually benign in origin, although sometimes associated with peptic ulceration.

Flatulence describes excessive wind. It is associated with belching, abdominal distension and the passage of flatus per rectum. It is only infrequently associated with organic disease of the gastrointestinal tract, but usually represents a functional disturbance in which excessive air is swallowed. Certain foods produce relatively large amounts of gas, for example legumes, resulting in increased flatulence.

Hiccups are due to repeated sudden diaphragmatic contraction, often triggered by upper gastrointestinal irritation, but occasionally due to brainstem disease.

Vomiting is a neurogenic response triggered by chemoreceptors in the brainstem or reflexly through irritation of the stomach. Vomiting consists of a phase of nausea, followed by hypersalivation, pallor, sweating and hyperventilation. Retching, an involuntary effort to vomit, then occurs followed by expulsion of gastric contents through the mouth and sometimes through the nose. Most nausea and vomiting of gastrointestinal origin is associated with local pain in the abdomen. Painless vomiting should suggest neurological disease.

Other symptoms

Other symptoms associated with gastrointestinal problems include the following.

Constipation is a subjective complaint. Patients feel constipated when they sense that they have not adequately emptied their bowel by defaecation. The term is sometimes used to describe the passage of hard stools, irrespective of stool frequency. The passage of formed stool less frequently than twice a week is usually taken to indicate an abnormality of bowel frequency in clinical practice.

Diarrhoea is common as a result of dietary indiscretion or from viral or bacterial infection. Diarrhoea may consist of watery stools of large volume, bloody diarrhoea, or frequent loose motions.

Chronic diarrhoea should raise the possibility of malabsorption with steatorrhoea. *Steatorrhoea* is the passage of pale, bulky stools containing excessive fats that commonly float in water and are difficult to flush away.

Abdominal pain may occur in the upper abdomen, in the hypochondrium, in the lower abdomen, or in the rectum. The important features of abdominal pain are its site, intensity, character of duration and frequency, together with aggravating and relieving factors and associated features (see page 104).

Abdominal distension has many causes. It may relate to flatulence, or more commonly to functional bowel disease in which the viscera are enlarged because their contractivity is diminished from disease of the bowel musculature, or its innervation. Distension is also a feature of steatorrhoea and malabsorption. It may result from ascites, or from enlargement of the viscera, for example in liver disease.

Weight loss is a feature of malabsorption, but may also result from loss of appetite (*anorexia*) or from starvation. It is a common feature of systemic diseases such as cancer, but is a late feature of cancer usually implying metastases.

Haematemesis results from bleeding in the upper gastrointestinal tract, causing the vomiting of blood or blood products.

Rectal bleeding results from bleeding in the rectum or anal canal, most commonly from piles but sometimes from anal or rectal carcinoma.

Melaena, the passage of dark, partially digested blood, implies bleeding from a site more proximal than the gastrointestinal tract, usually in the upper colon or small intestine.

Jaundice (see below) implies disease of the liver or the biliary tract. It may also occur from excessive haemolysis. It causes yellowness of the skin and conjunctiva, and may be associated with other cutaneous and systemic features of liver disease, often with dark urine (see Chapters 1, 6 and below).

General signs

Certain systemic features of gastrointestinal disease may be evident on general examination (see Chapter 1). Particular note must be taken of the hands for clubbing, a clue to malabsorption or chronic liver impairment, and for palmar erythema and leuconychia which indicate liver disease. Other general signs which point to a diagnosis of liver disease include jaundice, spider naevi, gynaecomastia, loss of secondary sexual hair, testicular atrophy and parotid swelling. Pruritis and scratch marks should suggest chronic cholestasis. A facial appearance resembling Cushing's syndrome may also be found with chronic alcohol abuse.

Inflammatory bowel disease occasionally presents with extra-intestinal manifestations, e.g. arthritis, especially in the large joints, uveitis and skin rashes, including erythema nodosum and pyoderma gangrenosum. The nutritional state of the patient must be carefully assessed, since if food intake is normal the nutritional state is an index of the functional integrity of the gastrointestinal tract.

Assessment of the nutritional state

Assessment of the nutritional state of a patient is an important part of the clinical examination. While gross malnutrition is usually easy to recognize, lesser degrees of body tissue depletion may be difficult to detect, particularly if oedema is also present, as in hypoalbuminaemia associated with severe protein loss, severe malabsorption, or kwashiorkor. Malnutrition may be due to starvation, to maldigestion of food or to malabsorption of the products of the process of digestion.

There are several ways to assess the nutritional state. The most important are the clinical history, including dietary history, and the physical examination, including anthropometric measurements. Other more subtle indices of malnutrition include muscle function tests and evaluation of creatinine excretion and serum levels of albumin. Anaemia, hypoalbuminaemia, ferritin and iron-binding capacity and the prothrombin time are also useful indices of malnutrition.

History

If starvation is excluded, patients likely to be at risk of malnutrition are those with reduced intake due to poor appetite or inability to eat. Malnutrition may also develop in patients with gastrointestinal failure and when metabolic needs exceed energy intake, as in hyperthyroidism.

Depressed appetite may accompany any severe illness, particularly malignancy and chronic renal or cardiac failure, in which nausea is often an accompanying problem. Other common causes include mental depression, viral illness, such as flu, which often causes transient loss of appetite, and chronic drug or alcohol abuse. Drug addicts may spend all their available income on drugs and neglect food. Alcoholics obtain calories from their drink but often develop protein and vitamin malnutrition syndromes. Malnutrition due to inability to eat (*dysphagia*) may occur in patients with neurological disturbances such as strokes, and in patients with oropharyngeal or oesophageal disease. A history of diarrhoea or steatorrhoea with progressive weight loss despite a good appetite should lead to consideration of alimentary disorders such as coeliac disease, bacterial overgrowth syndromes, or inflammatory bowel disease.

Increased metabolic needs arise in severely ill patients, particularly those with fever, burns or cancers, or following major trauma, including surgery. Hyperthyroidism must also be remembered as a cause of weight loss despite good appetite.

Dietary history

A simple evaluation of diet is valuable in the assessment of any patient and is mandatory in all patients who appear malnourished. General questions about frequency of meals, types of food eaten, and methods of food preparation give a clue to dietary habits but are occasionally misleading if patients are elderly or impoverished. Recent changes in appetite or dietary patterns should be noted.

It is important to enquire whether the patient avoids certain foodstuffs for any reason. Do they follow, for instance, a strict diet, or have they been advised to avoid any foods in order to relieve gastrointestinal symptoms? Patients with gluten sensitivity, for example, will have been advised to avoid wheat products, while patients with intestinal lactase deficiency will avoid milk. A strict vegetarian or vegan diet may lead to vitamin B_{12} deficiency. Excessive dietary fibre intake leads to flatulence, bulky stools, increased bowel frequency and uncomfortable bowel distension. Low dietary fibre intake may be associated with constipation or difficult defaecation. In anorexia–bulimia, a disorder usually affecting young women, there are cyclic changes in appetite, food intake and dietary fads develop in association with a pathological aversion to body habitus and self.

Physical examination

In the general assessment of nutritional status careful attention must be given to the presence and distribution of body fat, the muscle bulk and the presence of oedema. Loss of muscle mass is common in *malnutrition*. Wasting of the temporalis muscles produces the characteristic gaunt appearance of the starved. Additional clues to poor nutrition are a dry, cracked skin, loss of scalp and body hair, and poor wound healing. In malnutrition the limb muscles are thin, the distal reflexes may be difficult to elicit, and the subcutaneous fat is atrophic. In *obesity* there is an increase in the proportion of fat in the body, largely in the subcutaneous compartment. In *protein–calorie malnutrition* there is a deficiency of protein with relatively good carbohydrate intake; the blood albumin level is reduced, and there may be oedema so that the body weight may be an unreliable indicator of malnutrition.

The nutritional state can be assessed semiquantitatively by measuring skinfold thickness with skin calipers, as an estimate of fat stores. A more accurate estimate of nutritional status is obtained by comparing weight with height: the Quetelet (body mass) index.

SKINFOLD THICKNESS

The skinfold thickness can be measured at standard sites, such as the biceps, triceps, infrascapular and supra-iliac regions, using a Harpenden calliper or similar device. The calliper is designed so that the jaws of the device remain parallel and constant pressure is exerted between them at different skinfold thicknesses. The triceps skinfold, midway between acromion and olecranon is the most commonly used site. The skinfold thickness is measured in the vertical plane with the arm hanging relaxed by the side of the body. Normal values are shown in Table 5.1.

Skinfold measurements vary between the same observer by 0.3–0.6 standard deviations. If the arm circumference is measured at the same site, and it is

	Standard	80%	60%
Adult males	12.5	10.0	7.5
Adult females	16.5	13.0	10.0
Nutritional state	Normal nutrition	Moderate depletion	Severe depletion

Table 5.1 Skinfold thickness: Normal triceps skinfold thickness measured by Schofield's callipers (mm). The 80% and 60% ranges are associated with nutritional depletion.

assumed that the arm and muscle circumference are circular and circumferential respectively, a cross-sectional area for muscle and fat can be derived.

QUETELET (BODY MASS) INDEX

The relationship between body weight and height provides a simple estimate, in adult subjects, as to whether weight is appropriate for height. The normal range of the index, calculated by the following formula, is 10–25:

$$\text{Quetelet body mass index} = \frac{\text{weight (kg)}}{\text{height (m)}^2}.$$

The Quetelet index correlates well with three other, more technical methods of measuring body fat: total body water, body densitometry and whole body potassium measurements.

Nutritional intervention will be needed in practice if the Quetelet index is less than 18 or if weight loss

---

BOX 5.2 Health penalties of disturbed nutrition.

Malnutrition
- Reduced ability to perform physical and mental work
- Reduced exercise tolerance
- Impaired respiratory function
- Impaired immunity
- Poor wound and fracture healing
- Increased surgical risk
- Amenorrhoea
- Osteoporosis
- Specific deficiency syndromes

Obesity
- Increased mortality indices
- Reduced quality of life
- Reduced physical fitness and mobility
- Hypertension and ischaemic heart disease
- Diabetes mellitus
- Osteoarthritis
- Hiatus hernia
- Gall stones
- Increased operative risk
- Increased risk of cancer, e.g. cancer of breast

---

during an illness is greater than 10%. Patients with a Quetelet index greater than 30 are so obese that weight loss is advisable. In malnourished children retardation of growth in height tends to lag behind that of weight and 'catch-up' growth occurs when

malnutrition is corrected. The relation between weight and height in children should always, therefore, be compared with age, using the centile charts of normal ranges (Chapter 15). In *marasmus* there is severe growth retardation and wasting with a normal serum albumin, no oedema and a relatively alert child. In *kwashiorkor* growth retardation is not so severe, skin and hair changes are present, the albumin is low, there is oedema, and the child is miserable.

There are health penalties for malnutrition and for obesity (Box 5.2).

Composition of the body

The body can be considered to be composed of stores of different nutrients, which can be utilized during fasting or starvation, and increased during times of plenty (Table 5.2).

	kg	kcal/g	kcal stored
Water	42	0	0
Fat	10	9	90 000
Protein	10	4	40 000
Glycogen:			
muscle	0.15	4	600
liver	0.075	4	300
Circulating glucose, fatty acids,			
triglycerides, etc			113

Table 5.2 Body composition in health (calculated for a 70-kg man)

The composition of the body has been studied directly in cadavers. It can also be assessed in life, using methods that are restricted to clinical research rather than clinical practice. The lean body mass (LBM) can be calculated from measurement of the total body water (TBW), determined by a labelled water dilution method, according to the formula:

$$\text{Lean body mass} = \frac{\text{Total body water (litres)}}{0.73}.$$

Lean body mass can also be calculated by body densitometry and by gamma neutron activation analysis of total body nitrogen, calcium and other elements.

The body's composition changes with increasing age as shown in (Table 5.3).

| | Newborn | 10 years | | Adult | |
		M	F	M	F
Weight (kg)	3.4	31	31	72	58
LBM (kg)	2.9 (85%)	27 (87%)	26 (81%)	61 (85%)	42 (72%)
Fat (kg)	0.5 (15%)	4 (13%)	6 (19%)	11 (15%)	16 (28%)

Table 5.3 Body composition at different ages.

The mouth and throat

The examination of the mouth and throat is conducted with the patient sitting up either in bed, with the head resting comfortably back on pillows, or in a chair. A bright torch, a tongue depressor (spatula) and a pair of latex gloves are essential. The lips, teeth, gums, tongue, palate, fauces and oropharynx are then visualized systematically, and finally palpation of the sides of the tongue, floor of mouth and tonsillar regions is carried out.

Inspection

THE LIPS

Look closely at the philtrum (the shallow depression running from nose to upper lip) for the tell-tale scar of a repaired cleft lip. When present, particularly if associated with 'nasal speech', inspect the palate carefully for signs of a cleft. Next, look at the corners of the mouth for cracks or fissures (*angular stomatitis*). The cracks are reddish-brown, moist, superficial, linear ulcers radiating from the angles of the mouth. In children their origin is infective (*perleche*); they are common in the elderly when ill-fitting or deficient dentures result in overclosure of the mouth. Cheilosis is also seen in severe iron-deficiency anaemia; it also occurs in vitamin B_2 (riboflavin) deficiency.

Observe any desquamation or inflammation of the lips (*cheilitis*). This is common and self-limiting in cold weather. Grouped vesicles on the lips on a red base with crusted lesions are seen in herpes simplex labialis commonly associated with coryza. This infection is usually of short duration and the lack of induration and ulceration serves to distinguish it from other more serious conditions. Recurrent actinic cheilitis with small blisters and exfoliation, however, is a premalignant condition found in people constantly exposed to the sun and wind, such as farmers and fishermen.

Look for any ulcer on the lips. *Carcinoma* (epithelioma) usually occurs on the lower lip away from the midline; the ulcer is indolent, flat and shallow, although in time the edge may become heaped up and induration may be felt. Epithelioma must be differentiated from keratoacanthoma, pyogenic granuloma and the chancre of primary syphilis. A *keratoacanthoma* (molluscum sebaceum) is a lesion due to overgrowth of the stratum granulosum of the skin. It usually presents as a firm, rounded nodule sometimes with ulceration; it is more common on the upper lip and heals spontaneously without treatment. *Pyogenic granuloma* is a soft red raspberry-like nodule on the upper lip which often follows minor trauma. The upper lip is the commonest site of an extragenital chancre, which appears as a small, round lesion that is firm and indurated. A 'snail-track ulcer' in secondary syphilis has a serpiginous outline and greyish-white non-purulent exudate. In both epithelioma and chancre enlarged, painless cervical nodes are commonly felt. *Rhagades*, white scars at the angles of the mouth that extend into the mouth, due to cheilosis associated with congenital syphilis, are now only of historical interest. A crack in the middle of the lower lip in cold weather is a common, painful problem, but is of no sinister significance.

Very occasionally multiple small brown or black spots are seen on the skin around the mouth (*circumoral pigmentation*) which may also extend on to the lips and buccal mucosa. This pigmentation constitutes one of the triad of cardinal features of the Peutz–Jeghers syndrome and signifies underlying small bowel polyposis, a condition inherited as a Mendelian dominant. On the buccal mucosa the pigmentation may look very like that seen in Addison's disease. Look carefully at the lips and tongue for telangiectasia (page 17). Their presence may signal the existence of others elsewhere in the intestine, which occasionally bleed.

Now gently grasp the lower lip with the index finger and thumb of both hands and evert it fully, to display the mucous surface of the lip. Two lesions are commonly seen in this site: aphthous ulcers and retention cysts. *Aphthous ulcers* are small, superficial, painful ulcers with a white or yellow base and a narrow halo of hyperaemia (Fig. 5.1). Such ulcers are

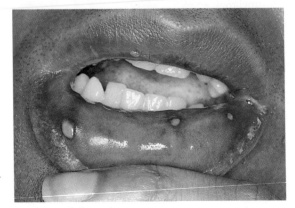

Fig. 5.1 Aphthous ulcers.

also seen on the tongue, buccal mucosa and palate. *Retention cysts* of the mucous glands of the lips and buccal mucosa appear as round, translucent swellings, elevated from the surface with a characteristic white or bluish appearance. They are also found on the mucous surface of the lower lip.

THE TEETH

Ask the patient to grimace so as to show the teeth. If the patient wears dentures, ask him or her to remove them and open the mouth widely. Using a tongue depressor to retract first the lips and then the cheeks, note the number of teeth present and look for decay (*caries*). The tooth most commonly missing is an impacted unerupted third mandibular molar (wisdom tooth). Inspect both the buccal and lingual aspects of the teeth. It is said that lack of teeth may cause indigestion but many edentulous people suffer no indigestion whether they wear dentures or not. Look for any changes in the following.

Colour

Tartar deposition occurs mainly on the lingual aspect of the lower incisor and canine teeth and consists of precipitated calcium salts of saliva which is stained brown in smokers. The chewing of betel nuts may also discolour the plaque of teeth a reddish-brown. Children up to the age of 8 treated with tetracycline (and children of expectant mothers so treated after the 14th week of pregnancy) are at risk of acquiring permanent staining of both the deciduous and permanent teeth. This takes the form of disfiguring horizontal bands, which may be yellow or grey and must not be mistaken for bands of hyperplasia on the enamel due to exanthematous fevers or any serious illness occurring during the development of the crowns. In endemic fluorosis, chalk-white patches appear on the teeth or the teeth present a dull, unglazed appearance, sometimes with pitting and brown staining (*Maldon teeth*).

Shape

Ill-formed hypoplastic teeth have a broad, concave biting edge, whilst some notching of the incisors is seen in those who persistently bite cotton or hold hairclips between their teeth. This must not be mistaken for *Hutchinson's teeth*—a manifestation of congenital syphilis, but a very rare finding nowadays. In this condition the two central upper permanent incisors are rounded in section and notched at their biting edge. They may also be broader near the gum than at the crown, so as to be peg-shaped. The first

permanent molars may be dome-shaped. The two central upper incisors are sometimes lost in leprosy. Patients who habitually induce vomiting, e.g. in anorexia nervosa, may show evidence of gastric acid-induced erosion of the inner surface of the incisors.

Ridging

Transverse ridging is sometimes seen in the permanent teeth of those who had vitamin C and D deficiency in infancy.

Enlargement of the lower jaw in acromegaly leads to alteration of the bite, so that the lower teeth may close outside the upper ones.

THE GUMS

Examine the gums at the same time as the teeth. Pink, healthy gums adhere closely to the necks of the teeth and have a sharp border. With increasing age *gingival recession* occurs, so making the teeth appear longer and exposing the cementum below the enamel. This makes it easier for infection to gain a hold.

In *chronic marginal gingivitis*, the gums are retracted, frequently bleed easily and lose their characteristic stippling. Sometimes pus can be squeezed from them (*pyorrhoea alveolaris*).

Acute herpetic gingivostomatitis due to the simplex virus occurs most commonly in infants and children. Many small vesicles appear on the gums, cheeks, palate, tongue and lips. The vesicles rupture to produce shallow ulcers with a yellowish floor and bright red margins. *Vincent's gingivostomatitis*, an infection due to fusiform spirochaetes, characteristically destroys the interdental papillae. A thick, felted, greenish-grey slough is formed and halitosis is present. In patients exposed to lead compounds, a *stippled blue line* can often be observed running along the edge of the gum, especially opposite those teeth showing gingivitis. Similar lines may be produced by bismuth or mercury but these are uncommon signs. The gums in scurvy are swollen, irregular in outline, red, spongy and bleed easily. Hypertrophy of the gums may occur in pregnancy and in patients treated for long periods with phenytoin. Haemorrhages may be observed in the buccal mucous membrane in thrombocytopenic purpura and acute leukaemia.

Pus can form in a carious tooth to form an alveolar or dental abscess with throbbing pain, exacerbated by tapping the affected tooth. Localized swelling of the gum and swelling of the face (if pus has escaped through the lateral alveolar margin) are signs associated with this condition. Ill-fitting dentures can produce a granuloma or an ulcer on the gum at the point of pressure where the denture does not fit properly. Such a lesion has to be differentiated from a carcinomatous ulcer arising in the gum; the latter presents the same macroscopic features as malignant ulcers elsewhere in the mouth.

Epulis is a general term used to describe any swelling arising in the gum of the maxilla or mandible.

THE TONGUE

Ask the patient to protrude the tongue. Inability to do so fully (*ankyloglossia*) is seen, very rarely, in infants due to tongue-tie (a congenitally short frenulum linguae) or in advanced malignancy of the tongue involving the floor of the mouth. When carcinoma involves the side of the tongue (the commonest site) and the floor of the mouth, slight deviation towards the affected side may occur. Slight deviation is not uncommon and may be due to asymmetry of the jaws. In hemiplegia, deviation towards the paralysed side may be found. In lesions of the hypoglossal nerve or its nucleus there may be fasciculation of the affected side; later this side may be wasted and deeply grooved (*lingual hemiatrophy*). The tongue is large in acromegaly, cretinism, myxoedema, lymphangioma and amyloidosis.

Tremor of the tongue may be due to nervousness, thyrotoxicosis, delirium tremens or parkinsonism.

Next examine the dorsum of the tongue.

Colour

Is the tongue pale, red or discoloured? Pallor is seen in severe anaemia. Discoloration is most often due to the ingestion of coloured foods, e.g. red wine or coloured sweets.

Moistness

The state of the tongue gives some indication of the state of hydration of the body, provided the patient is not a mouth breather. A dry, brown tongue may be found in the later stages of any severe illness, but is found particularly in advanced uraemia and acute intestinal obstruction.

Fur

Furring of the tongue is of little value as an indication of disease. It is often found in heavy smokers. A brown fur, the 'black hairy tongue', is due to a fungus infection and is of no special significance, though frequently a source of great alarm to its possessor. The tongue of scarlet fever at first shows bright red papillae standing out of a thick white fur.

Later the white coat disappears leaving enlarged papillae on a bright red surface—the 'strawberry tongue'. Hairy leucoplakia is a common feature in patients with HIV infection. In chronic superficial glossitis, areas of *leucoplakia* (whitish opaque areas of thickened epithelium) are separated by intervening smooth and scarred areas; there are no normal papillae to be seen and the fissures run mainly in a longitudinal direction.

The papillae

Generalized atrophy of the papillae produces a smooth or bald tongue which is characteristic of vitamin B_{12} deficiency but may also sometimes be found in iron-deficiency anaemia, coeliac disease and other gastrointestinal disorders and deficiency states, especially pellagra. In severe cases smoothness may be associated with wrinkling of the mucous membrane, which has then to be distinguished from fissuring of the tongue seen in chronic superficial glossitis due to syphilis, and congenital fissuring of the tongue or 'scrotal tongue', which is common and of no pathological significance. In *congenital fissuring* the papillae are normal but the surface is interrupted by numerous irregular but more or less symmetrical folds which tend to run mainly horizontally. In *median rhomboid glossitis* a lozenge-shaped area of loss of papillae and fissuring is seen in the midline anterior to the foramen caecum. It feels nodular and may be mistaken for a carcinoma. It must also be distinguished from a lingual thyroid but this is situated posterior to the foramen caecum. *Geographical tongue* is another harmless anomaly characterized by localized irregular red areas of desquamated epithelium and filiform papillae surrounded by a whitish-yellow border; the papillae change in distribution and give the appearance of a map. The 'false geographical tongue' with a similar appearance occurs chiefly in children with fever.

The sides and undersurface

Ask the patient to open the mouth wide and protrude the tongue fully to one side. Then retract the cheek with a spatula. This displays the side and lateral undersurface well. Some patients find this impossible to do, so wrap a gauze swab around the tip of the tongue and with index finger and thumb gently pull the tongue out and to one side. Benign ulcers in this site are common and may be inflammatory or traumatic in origin, very often due to ill-fitting dentures or broken carious teeth; such ulcers tend to be painful, superficial and lack induration. However, in an elderly patient any ulcer at this site must be regarded as malignant until proved otherwise by biopsy; it is the most frequent site of carcinoma in the mouth and presents as a hard, indurated ulcer with everted raised edges.

Now ask the patient to retract the tongue fully and slightly elevate the tip with the mouth wide open. This displays the undersurface of the anterior tongue and floor of the mouth. Note the frenulum linguae and the orifice of the submandibular duct opening on either side of the base of the frenulum. The ampulla of each duct lies just proximal to the orifice and is a common site for calculi formed in the submandibular salivary gland to lodge. The calculus is seen as a white or yellow bleb distending an oedematous hyperaemic ampulla.

A small ulcer on the frenulum is sometimes seen in persistent coughing and particularly in whooping cough. Sublingual varicosities are common in the elderly. Two types of cyst may be found in the floor of the mouth:
- *ranula*, which forms a bluish-white translucent swelling of variable size and is due to blockage of the duct of a mucous gland; and
- *sublingual dermoid cyst*, a round opaque swelling lying beneath the mucosa either above or below the mylohyoid, which is due to sequestration of epidermal tissue beneath the skin along the embryological lines of fusion of the mouth.

THE BUCCAL MUCOSA
Inspect the buccal mucosa. Retract the cheek with a spatula. Note the opening of the parotid duct, which is seen as a tiny swelling opposite the upper second molar tooth. In the catarrhal stage of measles, before the appearance of the rash, small bluish-white spots, surrounded by a red areola, may be seen opposite the molar teeth. These are known as *Koplik's spots*. In the same position irregular areas of dots of slate-grey or blue pigmentation are seen in Addison's disease.

Aphthous ulcers, mucus retention cysts and *papillomata* present the same appearance on the buccal mucosa as elsewhere in the mouth. Mouth ulcerations (see Box 5.3)—either aphthous or larger, more chronic lesions—are well-recognized manifestations of inflammatory bowel disease, particularly Crohn's disease. Mouth ulcers in association with genital ulcers indicate Behçet's syndrome. White opalescent patches (rather like white paint) of *leucoplakia* may also be seen on the inner aspect of the cheek; these should be differentiated from lichen planus, an oral manifestation of a skin disease, but in this case look

elsewhere, especially on the arms and legs, for similar lesions. *Thrush* (monilial stomatitis), a fungal infection due to *Candida albicans*, presents as a different sort of white patch. It is seen as small white points raised somewhat above the surrounding surface, which is usually redder than normal. As the infection gains hold so the lesions coalesce and may form extensive sheets throughout the mouth. Patches of thrush are apt to be mistaken for small milk curds, but curds can be easily detached, while thrush patches can be removed only with difficulty and then tend to leave behind a raw surface. Thrush is common in debilitated children, beneath unclean dentures and in patients on cytotoxic or immunosuppressive drugs. It is also seen frequently on surgical wards, especially in ill patients with sepsis in the postoperative period and those treated with broad-spectrum antibiotics, which destroy the normal bacterial flora of the mouth and thus allow the fungi to flourish. Oropharyngeal candidiasis is also a feature of cellular immunodeficiency states including AIDS.

BOX 5.3 Causes of mouth ulcers.
- Inflammatory bowel disease
- Behçet's disease
- Leucoplakia
- Lichen planus
- Thrush (candidiasis)
- Idiopathic aphthous ulcers
- Koplik's spots (measles)
- Malignant erosion

THE PALATE, FAUCES, TONSILS AND PHARYNX
Ask the patient to put the head right back and keep the mouth wide open. Inspect the hard and soft palates and note the position of the uvula. Get the patient to say 'ah', which raises the soft palate and increases visibility of the fauces, tonsils and oropharynx. (For abnormalities of movement of the soft palate during phonation see page 222.)

If a good view of these structures has not been obtained, introduce a spatula to depress the base of the tongue and, if necessary, another spatula to retract the anterior pillar of the fauces to view the tonsils properly.

Again look for any ulcers, erythema or vesicles. *Vesicles* confined to one side of the hard palate which progress to painful oval ulcers are characteristic of herpes zoster of the maxillary division of the trigeminal nerve (fifth cranial); this disorder usually occurs in older patients and is accompanied by a characteristic skin rash in the corresponding dermatome on the face. Herpes zoster infection of the glossopharyngeal nerve (ninth cranial) produces similar lesions in the pharynx.

Malignant ulcers do occur on the hard palate but much less frequently than elsewhere in the mouth, and present the same appearances. Ectopic salivary gland tissue may be present in the mouth; the hard palate is the commonest site. Tumours of this tissue present as a smooth, hard swelling projecting from the surface of the hard palate, sometimes with central ulceration.

If a hole is seen in the hard palate it is usually due to one of the following:
● imperfect closure or breakdown after repair of a cleft palate;
● radionecrosis of bone following radiotherapy for treatment of local carcinoma; or
● tertiary syphilis with formation of a gumma.

Petechiae on the palate are common in glandular fever but they are also features of any form of thrombocytopenia, rubella and streptococcal tonsillitis. Oral lesions may be the presenting feature of *glandular fever*: enlarged tonsils are covered with a white exudate which tends to become confluent; there is oedema of the fauces and soft palate; and erythema of the oropharynx. This contrasts with the yellow punctate follicular exudate seen in *streptococcal tonsillitis*. Whenever a membranous exudate is seen, *diphtheria* should spring to mind and, as in all cases of mouth infection, a swab should be taken for bacteriological examination. The membrane in diphtheria varies in colour from white to green and often starts on the tonsil before spreading to the fauces and pharynx.

Finally, look at the pharynx. The presence on its surface of a number of small round or oval swellings, somewhat like sago grains, is so common as to be almost normal in appearance. In pharyngitis these are much increased.

Notice any vesicles or ulcers. In *chickenpox* (herpes varicella) oral lesions may be apparent before the characteristic rash appears. There is erythema of the pharyngeal and buccal mucosae, followed by vesicles which progress to oval or round ulcers with a white slough. In *herpangina* (Coxsackie virus infection) which is also common in the young, similar lesions may be seen in the oropharynx, soft palate and uvula.

In the *common cold* (coryza), mucopus may be noticed on the posterior wall of the pharynx running down from the nasopharynx. Less common nowadays are a peritonsillar abscess (*quinsy*) and retropharyngeal abscess. The latter forms a smooth, tense, tender swelling which bulges forwards from the posterior wall of the oropharynx.

THE BREATH

Carious teeth, infection or ulceration of the gum, stomatitis, and retention and decomposition of secretion in the follicles of enlarged tonsils are the commonest sources of offensive breath. Characteristic odours may be recognized:
● in ketosis, the breath smells of acetone;
● in uraemia, there is a fishy or ammoniacal odour;
● in hepatic failure, the odour is described as 'mousy';
● in suppurative conditions of the lung the breath may have a putrid smell;
● in bronchiectasis the odour has been compared to that of apple blossom with a hint of stale faeces.
● Paraldehyde and alcohol also impart their characteristic smells to the breath.

Palpation

Palpation forms an important, frequently neglected part of the examination of the mouth, particularly in patients who complain of oral symptoms or in whom unexplained cervical lymphadenopathy is found. Although not a routine part of physical examination, palpation in the mouth is imperative in anyone with a solitary or suspected ulcer in the oral cavity and bimanual palpation provides further information about such things as swellings in the floor of the mouth or cheek.

Impress on the patient that you will be as gentle as possible. Put on a disposable glove or finger cot, and ask the patient to remove any dentures and to open the mouth widely. With the tongue elevated and to one side, place the index finger of the right hand beneath the tongue on one side of the frenulum and run the finger back along the floor of the mouth. Even a small calculus can easily be felt in any part of the submandibular duct. Then come forwards, running the finger along the lingual side of the tongue to the midline and return on the buccal side of the gum towards the lower molar teeth. Now run the finger up the mucosa covering the ascending ramus of the mandible, and examine both palatal and buccal aspects of the gum of the upper jaw.

If an ulcer is present, try and decide whether any induration is present or not. To perform bimanual examination, with the index finger already inside the mouth, place the fingertips of the left hand flat beneath the mandible, or over the cheek, outside the mouth, and exert gentle pressure between your right index finger and the fingers of the left hand.

Now palpate the tongue and feel the dorsum and the lateral and undersurfaces with the index finger; it sometimes helps for the patient to protrude the tongue to one or other side to do this and, if necessary, the tongue can be held in a gauze swab between finger and thumb of the other hand.

Palpation of the posterior third of the tongue, fauces and tonsils is the least pleasant part for the patient as it usually causes gagging, and it is thus left until last. As before, the index finger is used and run over these structures as rapidly as possible. Feel for irregularity, ulceration and particularly induration, in order to detect a small or hidden carcinoma. Any abnormality felt in these sites in a patient with symptoms demands illuminated head lamp and laryngeal examination (Chapter 9).

The abdomen (see Figs 5.2 and 5.3)

It is helpful when recording in notes or communicating information to colleagues to think of the abdomen as divided into regions (Fig. 5.4). The two *lateral vertical* planes pass from the femoral artery below to cross the costal margin close to the tip of the ninth costal cartilage. The two *horizontal* planes, the subcostal and interiliac, pass across the abdomen to connect the lowest points on the costal margin, and the tubercles of the iliac crests respectively.

Remember that the area of each region will depend on the width of the subcostal angle and the proximity of costal margin to iliac crest, in addition to other features of bodily habitus which naturally vary greatly from one patient to the next.

Inspection

The patient should be lying supine with arms loosely by the patient's sides, on a firm couch or mattress, the head and neck supported by enough pillows, normally one or two, sufficient for comfort (Fig. 5.5). A sagging mattress makes examination, particularly palpation, difficult. Make sure there is a good light, that the room is warm and that your hands are warm. A shivering patient cannot relax and vital signs, especially on palpation, may be missed.

Stand on the patient's right side and expose the abdomen by turning down all the bedclothes except the upper sheet. The clothing should then be drawn up to just above the xiphisternum and the sheet folded down across the upper thighs to expose the groins and genitalia. This point is important; many are the patients who present with intestinal

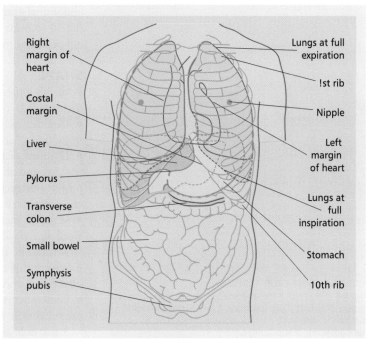

Right margin of heart

Costal margin

Liver

Pylorus

Transverse colon

Small bowel

Symphysis pubis

Lungs at full expiration

!st rib

Nipple

Left margin of heart

Lungs at full inspiration

Stomach

10th rib

Fig. 5.2 Anterior view of external relations of the abdominal and thoracic organs.

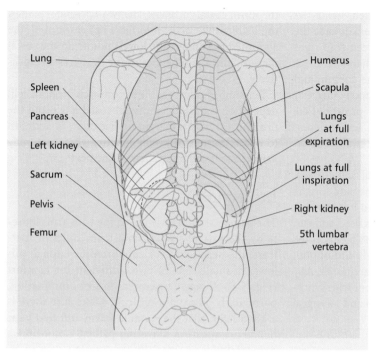

Fig. 5.3 Posterior view of the external relations of the abdominal and thoracic organs. The liver is not shown.

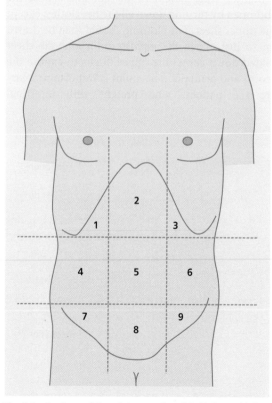

Fig. 5.4 Regions of the abdomen. 1 and 3: Right and left hypochondrium; 2: epigastrium; 4 and 6: right and left lumbar; 5: umbilical; 7 and 9: right and left iliac; 8: hypogastrium or suprapubic.

obstruction due to a strangulated femoral or inguinal hernia where the diagnosis has been missed initially due to lack of proper exposure of the groins in an effort to save embarrassment. However, once full inspection has taken place the sheet may be pulled up to the level of the symphysis pubis to allay anxiety.

Inspection is an important and neglected part of abdominal examination. It is well worthwhile spending 30 seconds observing the abdomen from different positions to note the following features.

SHAPE

Is the abdomen of normal contour and fullness, or distended? Is it scaphoid (sunken)?

● *Generalized fullness* or *distension* may be due to fat, fluid, flatus, faeces or fetus.

● *Localized distension* may be symmetrical and centred around the umbilicus, as in the case of small bowel obstruction, or asymmetrical as in gross enlargement of the spleen, liver or ovary.

● Make a mental note of the site of any such swelling or distension; think of the anatomical structures in that region and note if there is any movement of the swelling, either with or independent of respiration.

● Remember that chronic urinary retention may cause palpable enlargement in the lower abdomen.

A *scaphoid* abdomen is seen in advanced stages of

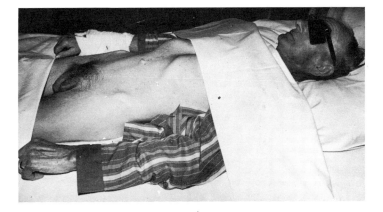

Fig. 5.5 Position of the patient and exposure for abdominal examination. Note that the genitalia must be exposed.

starvation and malignant disease, particularly carcinoma of the oesophagus and stomach.

THE UMBILICUS

Normally the umbilicus is slightly retracted and inverted. As it is at the centre of the abdomen, one's eyes inevitably come to rest on it at the same time as noting the general shape of the abdomen. If it is everted then an umbilical hernia may be present and this can be confirmed by feeling an expansile impulse on palpation of the swelling when the patient coughs. The hernial sac contains omentum, bowel or fluid. A frequent finding in the umbilicus of elderly obese women is a concentration of inspissated desquamated epithelium and other debris (*omphalolith*).

MOVEMENTS OF THE ABDOMINAL WALL

Normally there is a gentle rise in the abdominal wall during inspiration and a fall during expiration; the movement should be free and equal on both sides. In *generalized peritonitis* this movement is absent or markedly diminished, which helps to limit further spread of infection within the peritoneal cavity and the pain of peritoneal irritation (the 'still, silent abdomen'). To aid the recognition of intra-abdominal movements shine a light across the patient's abdomen. Even small movements of the intestine may then be detected by alterations in the pattern of shadows cast over the abdomen.

Visible pulsation of the abdominal aorta may be noticed in the epigastrium and is a frequent finding in nervous, thin patients. It must be distinguished from an aneurysm of the abdominal aorta, where pulsation is more obvious and a widened aorta is felt on palpation.

Visible peristalsis of the stomach or small intestine may be observed in three situations:

● *Obstruction at the pylorus.* Visible peristalsis may occur where there is obstruction at the pylorus produced either by fibrosis following chronic duodenal ulceration or, less commonly, by carcinoma of the stomach in the pyloric antrum. Peristalsis will be seen as a slow wave either passing across the upper abdomen from left to right hypochondria or, if gross gastric dilatation is present, passing down to the suprapubic region and ascending to terminate in the right epigastrium. In pyloric obstruction, a diffuse swelling may be seen in the left upper abdomen but, where obstruction is long-standing with severe gastric distension, this swelling may occupy the left mid and lower quadrants. Such a stomach may contain up to 2 litres of fluid and, on shaking the abdomen, a splashing noise is usually heard ('*succussion splash*'). This splash is frequently heard in healthy patients for up to 3 hours after a meal, so enquire when the patient last ate or drank.

In congenital pyloric stenosis of infancy not only may visible peristalsis be apparent but the grossly hypertrophied circular muscle of the antrum and pylorus may be felt as a 'tumour' to the right of the midline in the epigastrium. Both these signs may be elicited more easily after the infant has been given a feed.

● *Obstruction in the distal small bowel.* Peristalsis may be seen where there is intestinal obstruction in the distal small bowel or coexisting large and small bowel hold-up produced by distal colonic obstruction, with an incompetent ileocaecal valve allowing reflux of gas and liquid faeces into the ileum. Not only is the abdomen distended and tympanitic (hyperresonant) but the distended coils of small bowel may be visible in a thin patient and tend to stand out in the centre of the abdomen in a 'ladder pattern'.

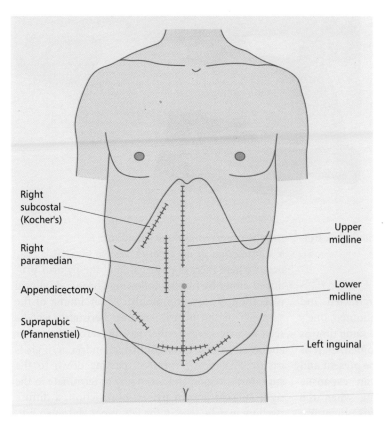

Right
subcostal
(Kocher's)

Right
paramedian

Appendicectomy

Suprapubic
(Pfannenstiel)

Upper
midline

Lower
midline

Left inguinal

Fig. 5.6 Some commonly used abdominal incisions. The midline and oblique incisions avoid damage to the innervation of the abdominal musculature and the later development of incisional hernia.

• *As a normal finding* in very thin, elderly patients with lax abdominal muscles or large, wide-necked incisional herniae seen through an abdominal scar.

SKIN AND SURFACE OF THE ABDOMEN

In marked abdominal distension the skin is smooth and shiny. *Striae atrophica* or *gravidarum* are white or pink wrinkled linear marks on the abdominal skin. They are produced by gross stretching of the skin with rupture of the elastic fibres and indicate a recent change in size of the abdomen, such as is found in pregnancy, ascites, wasting diseases and severe dieting. Wide purple striae are characteristic of Cushing's syndrome and excessive steroid treatment.

Note any *scars* present, their site, whether they are old (white) or recent (red or pink), linear or stretched (and therefore likely to be weak and contain an incisional hernia). Common examples are given in Fig. 5.6.

Look for *prominent superficial veins*, which may be apparent in three situations (Fig. 5.7): thin veins over the costal margin; occlusion of the inferior vena cava; and venous anastomoses in portal hypertension. However, small, thin veins over the subcostal margins are common and usually of no significance. *Inferior vena caval obstruction* not only causes oede-

ma of the limbs, buttocks and groins, but in time distended veins on the abdominal wall and chest wall appear (Fig. 5.7(b)). These represent dilated anastomotic channels between the superficial epigastric and circumflex iliac veins below, and the lateral thoracic veins above, conveying the diverted blood from long saphenous vein to axillary vein; the direction of flow is therefore upwards. If the veins are prominent enough, try to detect the direction in which the blood is flowing (Fig. 5.8). Distended veins around the umbilicus (caput medusae) are uncommon but, if present, signify *portal hypertension* (Fig. 5.7(c)), other signs of which include splenomegaly and ascites. Distended veins represent the opening up of anastomoses between portal and systemic veins and are seen in other sites, such as oesophageal varices and piles.

Pigmentation of the abdominal wall may be seen in the midline below the umbilicus, where it forms the linea nigra and is a sign of pregnancy. Erythema ab igne is a brown mottled pigmentation produced by constant application of heat, usually a hot water bottle or heat pad, on the skin of the abdominal wall. It is a sign that the patient is experiencing severe pain.

Finally, inspect both groins, and the penis and

(a)

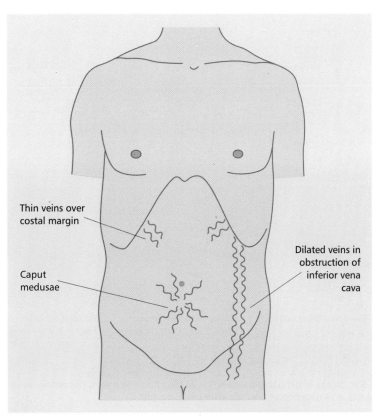

Fig. 5.7 (a) Veins of the abdominal wall. The veins shown represent venous drainage channels that dilate when there is obstruction in the inferior vena cava (b) or in the liver (c).

Thin veins over costal margin

Caput medusae

Dilated veins in obstruction of inferior vena cava

(b)

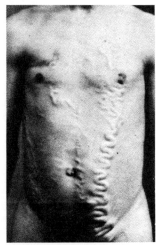

(c)

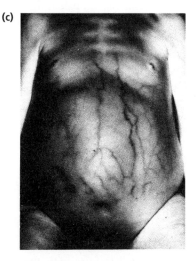

scrotum of a male, for any swelling and to ensure that both testes are in their normal position. Then bring the sheet up just to cover the symphysis pubis.

Palpation

Palpation forms the most important part of the abdominal examination. Tell the patient to relax as best they can and to breathe quietly, and assure them that you will be as gentle as possible. Enquire about the site of any pain and come to this region last. These points, together with unhurried palpation with a warm hand, will give the patient confidence and allow the maximum amount of information to be obtained. It is helpful to have a logical sequence to follow and, if this is done as a matter of routine, then no important point will be omitted. The scheme below is suggested.

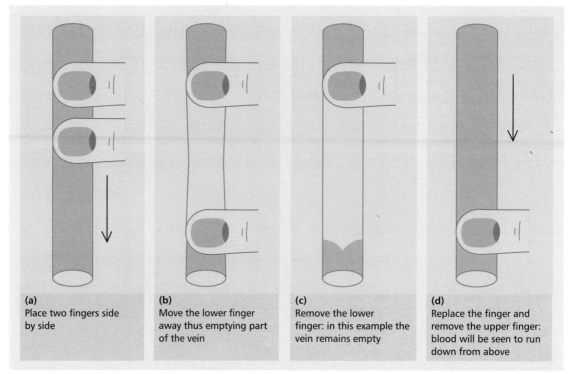

(a)
Place two fingers side by side

(b)
Move the lower finger away thus emptying part of the vein

(c)
Remove the lower finger: in this example the vein remains empty

(d)
Replace the finger and remove the upper finger: blood will be seen to run down from above

Fig. 5.8 A way of detecting the direction of blood flow in a vein. The venous valve prevents retrograde reflux (c) and the vein fills in its direction of flow (d), after emptying (a, b).

• Start in the left iliac region, palpating lightly, and work anticlockwise to end in the suprapubic region; repeat this using deeper palpation and with both hands if necessary;
• next feel for the left kidney;
• feel for the spleen;
• feel for the right kidney;
• feel for the liver;
• feel for the urinary bladder;
• feel for the aorta and para-aortic glands, and common femoral vessels;
• if a swelling is palpable, spend time eliciting its features;
• palpate both groins; and
• examine the external genitalia.

Start by placing the right hand flat on the abdomen in the left iliac fossa with the wrist and forearm in the same horizontal plane where possible, even if this means bending down or kneeling by the patient's side (Fig. 5.9).

The art is to 'mould' the relaxed right hand to the abdominal wall, not to hold it rigid. The best movement is gentle but with firm pressure with the fingers held almost straight with slight flexion at the metacarpophalangeal joints.

Always avoid sudden poking with the fingertips

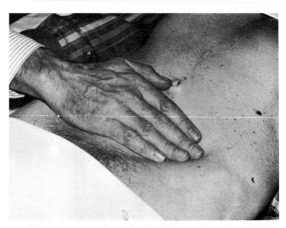

Fig. 5.9 Correct method of palpation. The hand is held flat and relaxed and 'moulded' to the abdominal wall.

(Fig. 5.10). Try and visualize the normal anatomical structures beneath the examining hand, and gently palpate each quadrant of the abdomen, noting any area of tenderness or localized rigidity. If necessary, repeat the palpation more slowly and deeply; in an obese or very muscular patient, putting the left hand on top of the right will allow you to exert increased pressure (Fig. 5.11).

A small proportion of patients find it impossible to relax their abdominal muscles when being

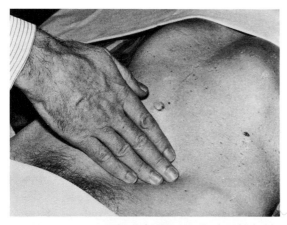

Fig. 5.10 Incorrect method of palpation. The hand is held rigid and mostly not in contact with abdominal wall.

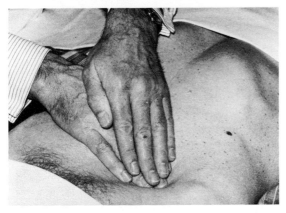

Fig. 5.11 Method of deep palpation in an obese, muscular or poorly relaxed patient.

examined. In such cases it may help to ask them to breathe deeply, to bend their knees up or to distract their attention in other ways. No matter how experienced the examiner, little will be gained from palpation of a poorly relaxed abdomen.

LEFT KIDNEY

The right hand is placed anteriorly in the left lumbar region whilst the left hand is placed posteriorly in the left loin (Fig. 5.12).

Ask the patient to take a deep breath in, press the left hand forwards, and the right hand backwards, upwards and inwards. The left kidney is not usually palpable unless either low in position or enlarged. Its lower pole, when palpable, is felt as a rounded firm swelling between both right and left hands (i.e. bimanually palpable) and it can be pushed from one hand to the other.

SPLEEN

Like the left kidney, the spleen is not normally palp-

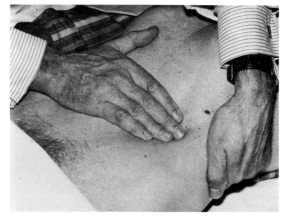

Fig. 5.12 Palpation of the left kidney.

able. It has to be enlarged to two or three times its usual size before it becomes palpable, and then is felt beneath the left subcostal margin. Enlargement takes place in a superior and posterior direction before it becomes palpable subcostally. Once the spleen has appeared in this situation, the direction of further enlargement is downwards and towards the right iliac fossa (Fig. 5.13). Place the flat of the left hand over the lowermost rib cage posterolaterally, and the right hand beneath the costal margin well out to the left. Ask the patient to breathe in deeply, press in deeply with the fingers of the right hand beneath the costal margin, at the same time exerting considerable pressure medially and downwards with the left hand (Fig. 5.14). Repeat this manoeuvre with the right hand being moved more medially beneath the costal margin on each occasion (Fig. 5.15). If enlargement

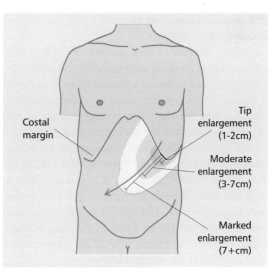

Costal margin

Tip enlargement (1-2cm)

Moderate enlargement (3-7cm)

Marked enlargement (7+cm)

Fig. 5.13 The direction of enlargement of the spleen. The spleen has a characteristic notched shape and the organ moves downwards during full inspiration.

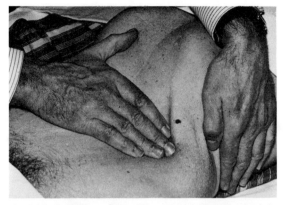

Fig. 5.14 Palpation of the spleen. Start well out to the left.

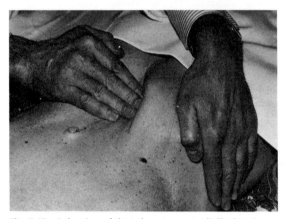

Fig. 5.15 Palpation of the spleen more medially than in Fig. 5.14.

of the spleen is suspected from the history and it is still not palpable, turn the patient half on to the right side, ask them to relax back on to your left hand, which is now supporting the lower ribs, and repeat the examination as above.

In minor degrees of enlargement, the spleen will be felt as a firm swelling with smooth, rounded borders. Where considerable splenomegaly is present, its typical characteristics include a firm swelling appearing beneath the left subcostal margin in the left upper quadrant of the abdomen, which is dull to percussion, moves downwards on inspiration, is not bimanually palpable, whose upper border cannot be felt (i.e. one cannot 'get above it'), and in which a notch can often, though not invariably, be felt in the lower medial border. The last three features distinguish the enlarged spleen from an enlarged kidney; in addition there is usually a band of colonic resonance anterior to an enlarged kidney.

RIGHT KIDNEY

Feel for the right kidney in much the same way as for

the left. Place the right hand horizontally in the right lumbar region anteriorly with the left hand placed posteriorly in the right loin. Push forwards with the left hand, ask the patient to take a deep breath in and press the right hand inwards and upwards (Fig. 5.16).

The lower pole of the right kidney, unlike the left, is commonly palpable in thin patients and is felt as a smooth, rounded swelling which descends on inspiration and is bimanually palpable.

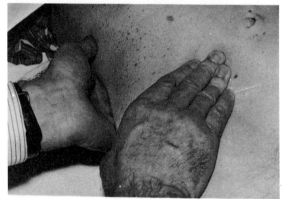

Fig. 5.16 Palpation of the right kidney.

LIVER

Sit on the couch beside the patient. Place both hands side-by-side flat on the abdomen in the right subcostal region lateral to the rectus with the fingers pointing towards the ribs. If resistance is encountered move the hands further down until this resistance disappears. Ask the patient to breathe in deeply and, at the height of inspiration, press the fingers firmly inwards and upwards (Fig. 5.17).

If the liver is palpable it will be felt as a sharp, regular border which rides beneath the fingers. Repeat

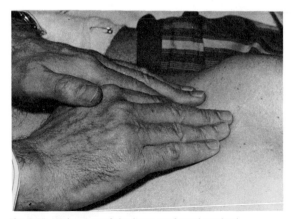

Fig. 5.17 Palpation of the liver: preferred method.

this manoeuvre working from lateral to medial regions to trace the liver edge as it passes upwards to cross from right hypochondrium to epigastrium. Another commonly employed though less accurate method of feeling for an enlarged liver is to place the right hand below and parallel to the right subcostal margin. The liver edge will then be felt against the radial border of the index finger (Fig. 5.18). The liver is often palpable in normal patients without being enlarged. If a liver edge is indefinitely felt, try to percuss in the right hypochondrium, keeping your hand still as the patient breathes deeply. Movement of the lower border together with dullness with respiration is further supporting evidence of hepatic enlargement. Hepatomegaly is described as being so many centimetres palpable below the right costal margin.

Try and make out the character of its surface, i.e. whether it is soft, smooth and tender as in heart failure, very firm and regular as in obstructive jaundice and cirrhosis, or hard, irregular, painless and sometimes nodular as in advanced secondary carcinoma. In tricuspid regurgitation the liver may be felt to pulsate. Occasionally a congenital variant of the right lobe projects down lateral to the gallbladder as a tongue-shaped process, called Riedel's lobe. Though rare, it is important to be aware of this because it may be mistaken either for the gallbladder itself or the right kidney.

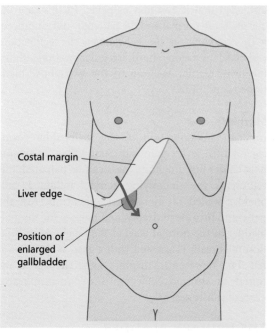

Fig. 5.19   Palpation of an enlarged gallbladder, showing how it merges with the inferior border of the liver so that only the fundus of the gallbladder and part of its body can be palpated.

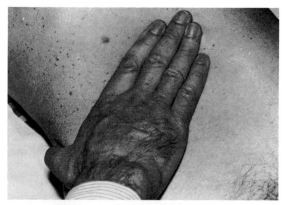

Fig. 5.18   Palpation of the liver: alternative method.

GALLBLADDER

The gallbladder is palpated in the same way as the liver. The normal gallbladder cannot be felt. When it is distended, however, it forms an important sign and may be palpated as a firm, smooth, rough or globular swelling with distinct borders, just lateral to the edge of the rectus abdominis near the tip of the ninth costal cartilage. It moves with respiration. Its

upper border merges with the lower border of the right lobe of the liver, or disappears beneath the costal margin and therefore can never be felt (Fig. 5.19). When the liver is enlarged or the gallbladder grossly distended, the latter may be felt not in the hypochondrium, but in the right lumbar or even as low down as the right iliac region.

The ease of definition of the rounded borders of the gallbladder, its comparative mobility on respiration, the fact that it is not normally bimanually palpable and that it seems to lie just beneath the abdominal wall helps to identify such a swelling as gallbladder rather than a palpable right kidney. This distribution may prove difficult, however, especially when the gallbladder lies in the mid or lower parts of the abdomen.

The gallbladder can usually be palpated in the following clinical situations. In *all* these situations the swelling is painless.

● In *carcinoma of the head of the pancreas* and other causes of malignant obstruction of the common bile duct, the ducts become dilated, as does the gallbladder. The patient is also deeply jaundiced.

● In *mucocele of the gallbladder*, a gallstone becomes impacted in the neck of a collapsed, empty, uninfected gallbladder and mucus continues to be secreted into its lumen. Finally, the uninfected wall is so

distended that it becomes palpable. In this case the bile ducts are normal and the patient is not jaundiced.
• In *carcinoma of the gallbladder*, the gallbladder will be felt as a stony, hard, irregular swelling, unlike the firm, regular swelling of the two above-mentioned conditions.

Murphy's sign

In acute inflammation of the gallbladder (*acute cholecystitis*) severe pain is present. Often an exquisitely tender but indefinite mass can be palpated; this represents the underlying acutely inflamed gallbladder walled off by greater omentum. Ask the patient to breathe in deeply, and palpate for the gallbladder in the normal way; at the height of inspiration the breath is arrested with a gasp as the mass is felt. This represents Murphy's sign. The sign is *not* found in chronic cholecystitis or uncomplicated cases of gallstones.

THE URINARY BLADDER

Normally the urinary bladder is not palpable. When it is full and the patient cannot empty it (retention of urine), a smooth firm regular oval-shaped swelling will be palpated in the suprapubic region and its dome (upper border) may reach as far as the umbilicus. The lateral and upper borders can be readily made out, but it is not possible to feel its lower border, i.e. the swelling is 'arising out of the pelvis'. The fact that this swelling is symmetrically placed in the suprapubic region beneath the umbilicus, that it is dull to percussion, and that pressure on it gives the patient a desire to micturate, together with the signs above, confirm such a swelling as the bladder (Fig. 5.20).

In women, however, the palpable bladder has to be differentiated from a gravid uterus (firmer, mobile side to side and vaginal signs different), a fibroid uterus (may be bosselated, firmer and vaginal signs different) and an ovarian cyst (usually eccentrically placed to left or right side).

THE AORTA AND COMMON FEMORAL VESSELS

In most adults the aorta is not readily felt but with practice it can usually be detected by deep palpation a little above and to the left of the umbilicus. In thin patients, particularly women with a marked lumbar lordosis, the aorta is more easily palpable. Palpation of the aorta is one of the few occasions when the fingertips are used as a means of palpation. Press the extended fingers of both hands, held side by side, deeply into the abdominal wall in the position shown in Fig. 5.21; make out the left wall of the aorta and note its pulsation. Remove both hands and repeat the manoeuvre a few centimetres to the right. In this way the pulsation and width of the aorta can

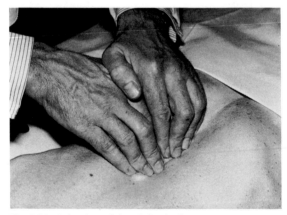

Fig. 5.21 Palpation of the abdominal aorta.

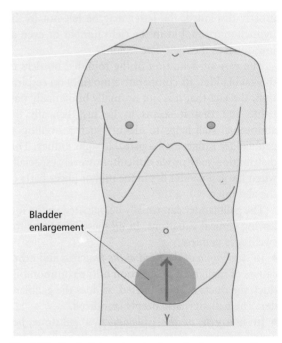

Fig. 5.20 Physical signs in retention of urine; a smooth, firm and regular swelling arising out of the pelvis which one cannot 'get below' and which is dull to percussion.

be estimated. It is difficult to detect small aortic aneurysms; where a large one is present, its width may be assessed by placing a finger on either side of it and its expansile character noted by the fact that when pulsation occurs, the width between each finger increases (Fig. 5.22).

The common femoral vessels are found just below the inguinal ligament at the midpoint between the

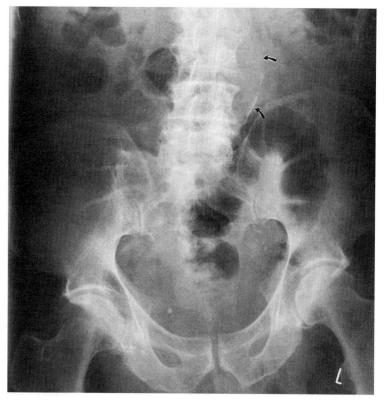

anterior superior iliac spine and symphysis pubis. Place the pulps of the right index, middle and ring fingers over this site in the right groin and palpate the wall of the vessel. Note the strength and character of its pulsation and then compare it with the opposite femoral pulse (Fig. 5.23).

Lymph nodes lying along the aorta (para-aortic nodes) are palpable only when considerably enlarged. They are felt as rounded, firm, often confluent, fixed masses in the umbilical region and epigastrium along the left border of the aorta.

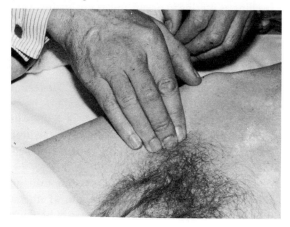

Fig. 5.23 Palpation of the right femoral artery.

CAUSES OF CONFUSION ON PALPATION

In many patients, especially those with a thin or lax abdominal wall, faeces in the colon may simulate an abdominal mass. The pelvic colon is frequently palpable, particularly when loaded with hard faeces. It is felt as a firm, tubular structure some 12 cm in length, situated low down in the left iliac fossa, parallel to the inguinal ligament. The caecum is often palpable in the right iliac fossa as a soft, rounded swelling with indistinct borders. The transverse colon is sometimes palpable in the epigastrium. It feels somewhat like the pelvic colon but rather larger and softer, with distinct upper and lower borders and a convex anterior surface.

In the epigastrium, the muscular bellies of rectus abdominis lying between its tendinous intersections can mimic an underlying mass and give rise to confusion. This can usually be resolved by asking the patient to tense the abdominal wall, when the 'mass' may be felt to contract.

WHAT TO DO WHEN AN ABDOMINAL MASS IS PALPABLE

When a swelling in the abdomen is palpable make sure first that it is not a *normal* structure, as described above. Next consider whether it could be due to enlargement of the liver, spleen, right or left kidney, gallbladder, urinary bladder, aorta or para-aortic nodes.

Now palpate the swelling again. The aim of examination is to decide the organ of origin and the pathological nature of the mass. In doing this it is helpful to bear in the mind the following points.

Site

First make sure that the swelling does indeed lie in the abdominal cavity and not in the anterior abdominal wall. Ask the patient to lift their head and shoulders off the pillow and press firmly against their forehead. Now feel the swelling again. If it disappears or becomes much less obvious, then it lies within the peritoneal cavity, whereas if it remains the same size it must be within the layers of the abdominal wall.

Note the region occupied by the swelling. Think of the organs that normally lie in or near this region and consider whether the swelling could arise from one of these organs. For instance, a swelling in the right upper quadrant most probably arises from the liver, right kidney, hepatic flexure of colon or gallbladder.

Now, if the swelling is in the upper abdomen, try and determine if it is possible to 'get above it', that is, to feel the upper border of the swelling as it disappears above the costal margin, and similarly, if it is in the lower abdomen, whether one can 'get below it'. If one cannot 'get above' an upper abdominal swelling, a hepatic, splenic, renal or gastric origin should be suspected. If one cannot 'get below' a lower abdominal mass the swelling probably arises in the bladder, uterus, ovary or occasionally upper rectum.

Size and shape

As a general rule, gross enlargement of the liver, spleen, uterus, bladder or ovary presents no undue difficulty in diagnosis. On the other hand swellings arising from the stomach, small or large bowel, retroperitoneal structures such as the pancreas, or the peritoneum (see section on mobility, below), may be difficult to diagnose. The larger a swelling arising from one of these structures, the more it tends to distort the outline of the organ of origin. For example, the characteristic outline of the kidney is retained early on, but when there is a large renal mass this outline is lost and recognition becomes difficult.

Surface, edge and consistency

The pathological nature of a mass is suggested by a number of features. A swelling that is hard, irregular in outline and nodular is likely to be a *neoplasm*, whilst a regular, round, smooth, tense swelling is likely to be *cystic*, but remember degeneration and softening with cyst formation occurs not infrequently in malignant tumours. A solid, ill-defined and tender mass suggests an inflammatory lesion as in Crohn's disease of the ileocaecal region.

Mobility and attachments

Considerable information can be gained from eliciting the mobility or fixity of an abdominal mass. Swellings arising in the liver, spleen, kidneys, gallbladder and distal stomach all show downward movement during inspiration, due to contraction of the diaphragm. One cannot, however, move such structures with the examining hand. In contrast, swellings originating in structures that have a mesenteric or other broad base of attachment are not influenced by respiratory movements but *can* be made to move freely by palpation, e.g. tumours of the small bowel and transverse colon, cysts in the mesentery, and large secondary deposits in the greater omentum.

When, on the other hand, the swelling is completely fixed it usually signifies one of three things:
- a mass of retroperitoneal origin, e.g. pancreas;
- part of an advanced tumour with extensive spread to the anterior or posterior abdominal walls or abdominal organs; or
- a swelling resulting from severe chronic inflammation involving other organs, e.g. diverticulitis of the sigmoid colon or a colovesical attachment or fistula.

In the lower abdomen, the side-to-side mobility of a fibroid or pregnant uterus rapidly establishes such a swelling as uterine in origin and as not arising from bladder or ovary.

IS IT BIMANUALLY PALPABLE OR PULSATILE?

Bimanually palpable swellings in the lumbar region are usually renal in origin. Just occasionally, however, a posteriorly situated gallbladder or a mass in the posteroinferior part of the right lobe of the liver may give the impression of being bimanually palpable.

Finally, try to decide whether a swelling exhibits *pulsation*. It is often difficult to be certain whether a swelling in the upper abdomen that is pulsatile is merely transmitting pulsation from the underlying aorta or whether it is truly expansile in nature. The best way to determine this is to place two fingers on the swelling and observe what happens to them in systole. If the fingers remain parallel, then the pulsation is transmitted. If, however, the fingers tend to separate, then true expansile pulsation is present and the swelling is arterial, and may be an aneurysm (see page 94).

Percussion

Details of how to percuss correctly are given on page 147. In the abdomen only light percussion is necessary—a resonant (tympanitic) note is heard throughout except over the liver, where the note is dull. Percussion is particularly useful for confirming the presence of an enlarged liver or spleen suspected on palpation. The absence of dullness over the suspected mass makes the diagnosis of hepatomegaly or splenomegaly unlikely.

DEFINING THE BOUNDARIES OF ABDOMINAL ORGANS AND MASSES

Liver
The upper and lower borders of the right lobe of the liver can be mapped out accurately by percussion. Start anteriorly, at the fourth intercostal space, where the note will be resonant over the lungs, and work vertically downwards. In the normal liver the upper border is found at about the fifth intercostal space, where the note will become dull; this dullness extends down to the lower border at or just below the right subcostal margin. The normal dullness over the upper part of the liver is reduced in severe emphysema, in the presence of a large right pneumothorax and when there is gas or air in the peritoneal cavity. The latter, occurring in a patient with severe abdominal pain, indicates perforation of a viscus (unless the patient has recently undergone laparotomy). This sign, however, is not one that should be relied on as there has to be a large volume of air or gas present to reduce the normal liver dullness, and this is not usually the case.

Percussion just below the right costal margin is useful in hepatomegaly. Ask the patient to breathe deeply while you percuss lightly, keeping the finger parallel to the rib margin. As the liver descends during inspiration a change in percussion note from resonance to dullness signals the edge of the liver. The upper margin of the liver can also be assessed, so giving a direct measure of hepatic size, normally 12–15 cm in height, i.e. extending to the fifth rib, or just below the right nipple in men.

Spleen
Percussion over an enlarged spleen provides rapid confirmation of the findings detected on palpation (page 91 and Fig. 5.14). Dullness extends from the left lower ribs into the left hypochondrium and left lumbar region. The lower border of an enlarged spleen is readily mapped out; splenic dullness gives way to the resonance of surrounding bowel.

Bladder
The findings in a patient with retention of urine are usually unmistakable on palpation (page 94 and Fig. 5.20). The dullness on percussion provides reassurance that the swelling is cystic or solid and not gaseous; its superior and lateral borders can be readily defined from adjacent bowel, which is resonant.

Other masses
The boundaries of any localized swelling in the abdominal cavity, or in the walls of the abdomen, can sometimes be defined more accurately by percussion than palpation. The dullness of a solid or cystic mass contrasts with the tympanitic note of surrounding loops of bowel.

DETECTION OF ASCITES AND ITS DIFFERENTIATION FROM OVARIAN CYST AND INTESTINAL OBSTRUCTION
Three common causes of diffuse enlargement of the abdomen are:
- the presence of free fluid in the peritoneum (*ascites*);
- a massive ovarian cyst; and
- obstruction of the large bowel, distal small bowel, or both.

Percussion rapidly distinguishes between these three, as can be seen in Fig. 5.24. Other helpful symptoms or signs which are usually present are as follows.
Gross ascites
- Dull in flanks
- Umbilicus transverse and/or hernia present
- Shifting dullness positive
- Fluid thrill positive.
Large ovarian cyst
- Resonant in flank.
- Umbilicus vertical and drawn up
- Large swelling felt arising out of pelvis which one cannot 'get below'.

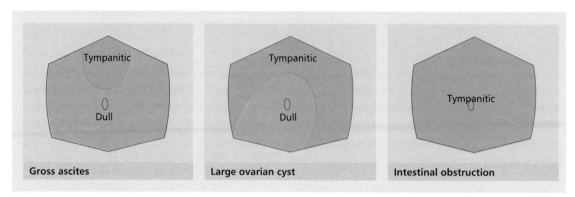

Fig. 5.24 Diffuse enlargement of the abdomen.

Intestinal obstruction
- Resonant throughout
- Colicky pain
- Vomiting
- Constipation
- Increased and/or 'noisy' bowel sounds.

It is unwise and difficult to diagnose *ascites* unless there is sufficient free fluid present to give generalized enlargement of the abdomen. Two signs—shifting dullness and a fluid thrill—which present either singly or together, make the diagnosis of ascites certain. Useful as these two signs are, they can be elicited in only about half the cases of ascites. Absence of shifting dullness or of fluid thrill or both does *not* exclude a diagnosis of ascites.

To demonstrate *shifting dullness*, lie the patient supine and percuss laterally from the midline, keeping your fingers in the longitudinal axis, until dullness is detected; in normal individuals dullness is detected only over the lateral abdominal musculature. Then, keeping your hand on the abdomen, ask the patient to roll away from you, on to the left side. Percuss again in this new position; if the previously dull note has now become resonant then ascitic fluid is probably present. To confirm its presence, repeat the manoeuvre on the left side of the abdomen.

To elicit a *fluid thrill* the patient is again laid on their back. Place one hand flat over the lumbar region of one side, get an assistant to put the side of their hand firmly in the midline of the abdomen, and then flick or tap the opposite lumbar region (Fig. 5.25). A fluid thrill or wave is felt as a definite and unmistakable impulse by the detecting hand held flat in the lumbar region. The purpose of the assistant's hand is to dampen any impulse that may be transmitted through the fat of the abdominal wall. As a rule a fluid thrill is felt only when there is a large amount of ascites present which is under tension.

Auscultation

Auscultation is a useful way of listening for bowel sounds and deciding whether they are normal, increased or absent, and of detecting bruits in the aorta and main abdominal vessels.

The stethoscope should be placed on one site on the abdominal wall (just to the right of the umbilicus is best) and kept there until sounds are heard. It

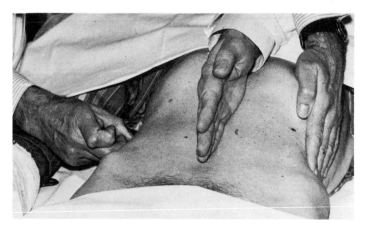

Fig. 5.25 Eliciting a fluid thrill.

should not be moved from site to site. Normal bowel sounds are heard as intermittent low- or medium-pitched gurgles interspersed with an occasional high-pitched noise or tinkle.

In *simple acute mechanical obstruction of the small bowel* the bowel sounds are excessive and exaggerated. Frequent loud low-pitched gurgles (*borborygmi*) are heard, often rising to a crescendo of high-pitched tinkles and occurring in a rhythmic pattern with peristaltic activity. The presence of such sounds occurring at the same time as the patient experiences bouts of colicky abdominal pain is pathognomonic of small bowel obstruction. In between the bouts of peristaltic activity and colicky pain, the bowel is quiet and no sounds are heard on auscultation.

In an obstructed loop of bowel, when strangulation and, later, gangrene supervene, however, peristalsis ceases, and the bowel sounds rapidly become less frequent and stop altogether. In *generalized peritonitis* bowel activity rapidly disappears and a state of *paralytic ileus* ensues, with gradually increasing abdominal distension. The abdomen is 'silent' but one must listen for several minutes before being certain that such a state exists. Frequently towards the end of this period a short run of faint, very high-pitched tinkling sounds is heard. This represents fluid spilling over from one distended gas- and fluid-filled loop to another and is characteristic of ileus.

A *succussion splash* may be elicited by palpation (page 87) and also on auscultation. It may be heard in pyloric stenosis, advanced intestinal obstruction with grossly distended loops of bowel and in paralytic ileus. Lie the patient supine and, using the palm of the right hand, place the stethoscope over the epigastrium. Then roll the patient from side to side to agitate any fluid and gas in the stomach. A splashing sound, like the noise made by a hot water bottle partially filled with water and air, will be heard if the stomach is distended with fluid.

Vascular bruits may also be heard in the abdomen. Place the stethoscope lightly on the abdominal wall over the aorta, above and to the left of the umbilicus, and listen for a bruit. Do likewise over each iliac artery in the corresponding iliac fossa, and over the common femoral arteries in each groin. If a bruit is heard it is a significant finding which indicates turbulent flow in the underlying vessel, either due to stenosis or to aneurysm. Very occasionally bruits may be heard in the epigastrium when there is stenosis of the coeliac axis or superior mesenteric artery,

or on either side of the midline in the mid-abdomen in patients with hypertension due to stenosis of the renal artery (see Chapter 8). A bruit may also be heard over a hepatoma because of increased blood flow within the tumour.

The groins

Once the groins have been inspected, ask the patient to turn their head to one side and cough. Look at both inguinal canals for any expansile impulse. If none is apparent, place the left hand in the left groin so that the fingers lie over and in line with the inguinal canal; place the right hand similarly in the right groin (Fig. 5.26). Now ask the patient to give a loud cough and feel for any expansile impulse with each hand. When a patient coughs, the muscles of the abdominal wall contract violently and this imparts a definite, though not expansile, impulse to the palpating hands which is a source of confusion to the inexperienced. Trying to differentiate this normal contraction from a small, fully reducible inguinal hernia is difficult, and the matter can usually be resolved only when the patient is standing up.

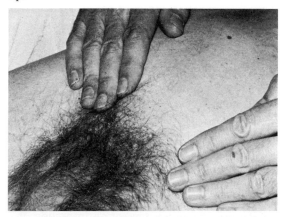

Fig. 5.26 Palpating the groins to detect an expansile impulse on coughing.

The femoral vessels have already been felt (page 94 and Fig. 5.23) and auscultated (page 188). Now palpate along the femoral artery for enlarged inguinal nodes, feeling with the fingers of the right hand, and carry this palpation medially beneath the inguinal ligament towards the perineum. Then repeat this on the left side. If the patient complains of a lump in the groin they should be examined lying down *and standing up*.

The male genitalia

The examination of the genitalia is important in men presenting with abnormalities in the groin, and in many acute or subacute abdominal syndromes. Thus disease of the genitalia may lead to abdominal symptoms, such as pain or swelling.

Disposable gloves should be worn if there is any suspicion of venereal infection. A detailed description is given in Chapter 17.

What to do if a patient complains of a lump in the groin

A lump in the groin or scrotum is a common clinical problem in all age-groups. Most lumps in the groin are due either to herniae or enlarged inguinal nodes; inguinal herniae are considerably more common than femoral with an incidence ratio of 4:1. In the scrotum, hydrocele of the tunica vaginalis or a cyst of the epididymis are common causes of painless swelling; acute epididymo-orchitis is the most frequent cause of a painful swelling.

Examination of the groins and scrotum is part of a general examination and must not be conducted in isolation. Generalized diseases such as lymphoma may present as a lump in the groin. Usually the diagnosis of a lump in the groin or scrotum can be made simply and accurately. Remember that the patient should be examined not only lying down, but also standing up.

Ask the patient to stand in front of you, get him to point to the side and site of the swelling and note whether it extends into the scrotum. Get him to turn his head to one side and give a loud cough; look for an expansile impulse and try to decide whether it is above or below the crease of the inguinal ligament. If an expansile impulse is present on inspection, it is likely to be a hernia, so move to whichever side of the patient the lump in the groin is on. Stand beside and slightly behind the patient. If the right groin is being examined place the left hand over the right buttock to support the patient, the fingers of the right hand being placed obliquely over the inguinal canal. Now ask the patient to cough again. If an expansile impulse is felt then the lump must be a hernia.

Next decide whether the hernia is *inguinal* or *femoral.* The best way to do this is to determine the

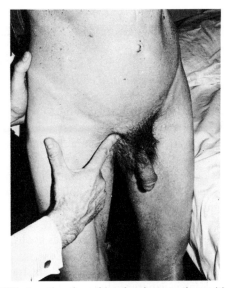

Fig. 5.27 Locating the pubic tubercle. Note the position of the examiner, at the side of the patient, with one hand supporting the buttock.

relationship of the sac to the pubic tubercle. To locate this structure push gently upwards from beneath the neck of the scrotum with the index finger (Fig. 5.27) but do not invaginate the neck of the scrotum as this is painful. The tubercle will be felt as a small bony prominence 2 cm from the midline on the pubic crest. In thin patients the tubercle is easily felt but this is not so in the obese. If difficulty is found, follow up the tendon of adductor longus, which arises just below the tubercle.

If the hernial sac passes *medial to and above* the index finger placed on the pubic tubercle, then the hernia must be inguinal in site; if it is *lateral to and below*, then the hernia must be femoral in site.

If it has been decided that the hernia is inguinal then one needs to know these further points:

What are the contents of the sac? Bowel tends to gurgle, is soft and compressible, while *omentum* feels firmer and is of a doughy consistency.

Is the hernia fully reducible or not? It is best to lay the patient down to decide this. Ask the patient whether the hernia is reducible and if so get him to reduce it himself to confirm this. It is more painful if the examiner reduces it.

Is the hernia direct or indirect? Again, it is best to lay the patient down to decide this. Inspection of the direction of the impulse is often diagnostic, especially in thin patients. A direct hernia tends to

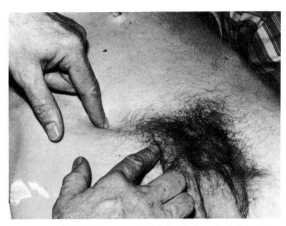

Fig. 5.28 Left hand: palpation of the pubic tubercle; index finger occluding the deep inguinal ring. Right hand: index finger on the pubic tubercle.

bulge straight out through the posterior wall of the inguinal canal, whilst in an indirect hernia the impulse can often be seen to travel obliquely down the inguinal canal. Another helpful point is to place one finger just above the mid-inguinal point over the deep inguinal ring (Fig. 5.28). If a hernia is fully controlled by this finger then it must be an indirect inguinal hernia.

Apart from a femoral hernia, the differential diagnosis of an inguinal hernia includes a large hydrocele of the tunica vaginalis, a large cyst of the epididymis (one should be able to 'get above' and feel the upper border of both of these in the scrotum), an undescended or ectopic testis (there will be an empty scrotum on the affected side), a lipoma of the cord, and a hydrocele of the cord.

In considering the *differential diagnosis of a femoral hernia*, one must think not only of an inguinal hernia but of a lipoma in the femoral triangle, an aneurysm of the femoral artery (expansile pulsation will be present), a saphen-ovarix (the swelling disappears on lying down, has a bluish tinge to it, there are often varicose veins present and there may be a venous hum), a psoas abscess (the mass is fluctuant, and may be compressible beneath the inguinal ligament to appear above it in the iliac fossa), and an enlarged inguinal lymph node. Whenever the latter is found, the feet, legs, thighs, scrotum, perineum, and the pudendal and perianal areas must be carefully scrutinized for a source of infection or primary tumour.

The examination is completed by following the same scheme in the opposite groin.

What to do when the patient complains of a swelling in the scrotum

It is easier and better to examine the patient first lying down and afterwards standing up. *Inspection, palpation* and *transillumination* are the three keys to rapid, accurate diagnosis. After inspection of the scrotum and groins, try and answer the following questions.

Can I 'get above' the swelling? Palpate the neck of the scrotum between fingers and thumb. If fingers and thumb cannot be approximated so that only the spermatic cord is palpable, then the swelling in question is not confined to the scrotum but is descending from the groin and is therefore an inguinoscrotal hernia, i.e. one cannot 'get above' it. (Very rarely an infantile hydrocele occurs which leads to the same signs though the testis is impalpable.) If fingers and thumb can be approximated so that one can 'get above' the swelling, that swelling can only be arising from the cord, the epididymis or the testis.

Is the swelling cystic or solid? Is the testis palpable separately from the swelling? Palpate the swelling in the same way as the testis and scrotal contents (page 402), which will give a good indication whether the swelling is cystic or solid.

What does it look like when transilluminated? Tense the scrotal skin gently over the swelling and place a bright torch *behind* the swelling. If it transmits light then it must be a cystic swelling and is either a *cyst of the epididymis* (a spermatocele) or a *hydrocele of the tunica vaginalis*. The former lies above and a little behind the testis and the testis is palpable separately from the swelling. In the latter the testis is not palpable separately from the swelling, i.e. it is enclosed within the tunica vaginalis and therefore surrounded by fluid.

If the cyst is not translucent then its consistency is solid. Palpate the epididymis and testis again. Enlargement of the epididymis is found in inflammation (*epididymitis*): if it is tender it is acute; if it is painless it is chronic (and usually tuberculous). Enlargement of the testis is found in *orchitis* (usually acute), when it is therefore tender or, rarely, as a result of *malignancy*.

Is it visible only when the patient is standing? A swelling that is not apparent lying down but appears on standing and which feels soft and rather like palpating a bag of worms is a *varicocele*, i.e. varicosity of the veins of the pampiniform and/or cremasteric plexi.

The female genitalia

These are described in Chapter 14. As in men, examination of the genitalia may be an important part of the examination of the gastrointestinal system in acute abdominal disorders.

The anus and rectum

Few other regions of the body reveal such a wealth of physical signs and diagnoses on inspection and digital examination as the perianal area, anus, anal canal and rectum.

The left lateral position is best for routine examination of the rectum (Fig. 5.29). Make sure that the buttocks project over the side of the couch with the knees drawn well up, and that a good light is available. Put a disposable glove on the right hand and stand slightly behind the patient's buttocks, facing the patient's feet. Tell the patient what you are about to do and that you will be as gentle as possible.

Inspection

Separate the buttocks carefully and inspect the perianal area and anus. Note the presence of any abnormality of the perianal skin, e.g. inflammation, which may vary in appearance from mild erythema to a raw, red, moist, weeping dermatitis, or in chronic cases thickened white skin with exaggeration of the

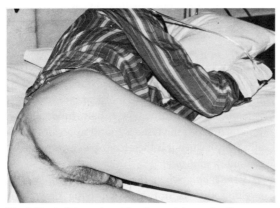

Fig. 5.29   Left lateral position for rectal examination.

anal skin folds. The latter form *anal skin tags*, which may follow not only *severe pruritus* but also occur when prolapsing piles have been present over a period of time. Tags should not be confused with *anal warts* (condylomata acuminata), which are sessile or pedunculated papillomata with a red base and a white surface. Anal warts may be so numerous as to surround the anal verge, and even extend into the anal canal. Note any 'hole' or dimple near the anus with a tell-tale bead of pus or granulation tissue surrounding it, which represents the external opening of a *fistula-in-ano*. It is usually easy to distinguish a fistula-in-ano from a *pilonidal sinus*, where the opening lies in the midline of the natal cleft but well posterior to the anus.

The following acutely painful anorectal conditions can usually be diagnosed readily on inspection. An *anal fissure* usually lies directly posterior in the midline. The outward pathognomonic sign of a chronic fissure is a tag of skin at the base (sentinel pile). The fissure can easily be demonstrated by gently drawing apart the anus to reveal the tear in the lining of the anal canal.

A *perianal haematoma* (thrombosed external pile) occurs as a result of rupture of a vein of the external haemorrhoidal plexus. It is seen as a small (1 cm), tense, bluish swelling on one aspect of the anal margin and is exquisitely tender to the touch. In *prolapsed strangulated piles*, there is gross swelling of the anal and perianal skin, which looks like oedematous lips, with a deep red or purple strangulated pile appearing in between, and sometimes partly concealed by, the oedema of the swollen anus. In a *perianal abscess*, an acutely tender, red fluctuant swelling is visible which deforms the outline of the anus. It is usually easy to distinguish this from an *ischiorectal abscess* where the anal verge is not deformed, the signs of acute inflammation are often lacking and the point of maximum tenderness is located midway between the anus and ischial tuberosity.

Note the presence of any ulceration. Finally, if rectal *prolapse* is suspected, ask the patient to bear down and note whether any pink rectal mucosa or bowel appears through the anus, or whether the perineum itself bulges downwards. Downward bulging of the perineum during straining at bending down, or in response to a sudden cough, indicates weakness of the pelvic floor support musculature, usually due to denervation of these muscles. This sign is often found in women after childbirth, in women with faecal urinary incontinence and in patients with severe chronic constipation.

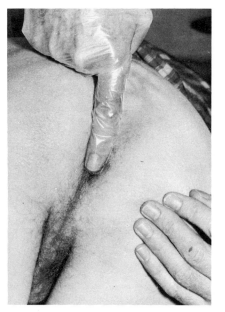

Fig. 5.30 Correct method for insertion of the index finger in rectal examination. The pulp of the finger is placed flat against the anus.

Digital examination (palpation)

Put a generous amount of lubricant on the gloved index finger of the right hand, place the *pulp* of the finger (not the tip) flat on the anus (Figs 5.30 and 5.31) and press firmly and slowly in a slightly backwards direction. After initial resistance the anal

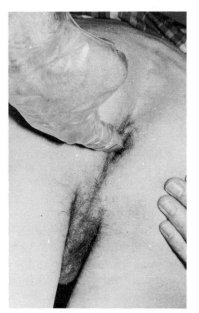

Fig. 5.31 Incorrect method of introduction of finger into the anal canal.

sphincter relaxes and the finger can be passed into the anal canal. If severe pain is elicited attempting this manoeuvre then further examination should be abandoned as it is likely the patient has a fissure and unnecessary pain will be caused.

Rotate the finger through 360 degrees in the canal and feel for any thickening or irregularity of the wall of the canal. Assess the tone of the anal musculature; it should normally grip the finger firmly. If there is any doubt ask the patient to contract the anus on the examining finger or to cough. The latter induces a brisk contraction of the external anal sphincter which in the normal patient will be readily appreciated. In the old and infirm with anal incontinence or prolapse almost no appreciable contraction will be felt. With experience it is usually possible to feel a shallow groove just inside the anal canal which marks the dividing line between the external and internal sphincter. The anorectal ring may be felt as a stout band of muscle surrounding the junction between the anal canal and rectum.

Now pass the finger into the anorectum. The examiner's left hand should be placed on the patient's right hip and later it can be placed in the suprapubic position to exert downward pressure on the sigmoid colon. Try to visualize the anatomy of the rectum, particularly in relation to its anterior wall. The rectal wall should be assessed with sweeping movements of the finger through 360 degrees, 2, 5 and 8 cm inwards or until the finger cannot be pushed any higher into the rectum. Repeat these movements as the finger is being withdrawn. In this way it is possible to detect malignant ulcers, proliferative and stenosing carcinomas, polyps and villous adenomas. The hollow of the sacrum and coccyx can be felt posteriorly. Laterally, on either side, it is usually possible to reach the side walls of the pelvis. In men one should feel anteriorly for the *rectovesical* pouch, *seminal vesicles* and the *prostate*. Normally the rectovesical pouch and seminal vesicles are not palpable. In a patient with a pelvic abscess, however, pus gravitates to this pouch, which is then palpable as a boggy, tender swelling lying above the prostate. If the pouch contains malignant deposits, hard irregular nodules may be felt. In infection of the seminal vesicles, these structures become palpable as firm, almost tubular swellings deviating slightly from the midline just above the level of the prostate.

In men, assessment of the *prostate gland* is important. It forms a rubbery, firm swelling about the size of a large chestnut. Run the finger over each lateral lobe, which should be smooth and regular. Between the two lobes lies the median sulcus, which is palpable as a faint depression running vertically between each lateral lobe. Though it is possible to say on rectal examination that a prostate is enlarged, accurate assessment of its true size is not possible. In carcinoma of the prostate, the gland loses its rubbery consistency and becomes hard, whilst the lateral lobes tend to be irregular and nodular and there is distortion or loss of the median sulcus.

In women, the cervix is felt as a firm, rounded mass projecting back into the anterior wall of the rectum. This is often a disconcerting finding for the inexperienced. The body of a retroverted uterus, fibroid mass, ovarian cyst, malignant nodule or a pelvic abscess may all be palpated in the pouch of Douglas (recto-uterine pouch), which lies above the cervix. This aspect of rectal examination forms an essential part of pelvic assessment in female patients.

On withdrawing the finger after rectal examination look at it for evidence of mucus, pus and blood. If in doubt wipe the finger on a white swab. Finally make sure to wipe the patient clean before telling him or her that the examination is completed.

The acute abdomen

Diagnosis and management of acute abdominal disorders depends on information derived both from the history and from the examination.

History

The patient usually presents with *acute abdominal pain*. In considering this symptom, its site, severity, radiation, character, time and circumstances of onset, and any relieving features are all important.

SITE

Ask the patient to point to the site of maximal pain with one finger. If pain is experienced mostly in the *upper abdomen* think of perforation of a gastric or duodenal ulcer, cholecystitis or pancreatitis. If pain is located in the *mid-abdomen*, disease of the small bowel is likely. Pain in the *right iliac fossa* is commonly due to appendicitis and pain in the *left iliac fossa* to diverticulitis. In women *low abdominal pain* of acute onset is often due to salpingitis, but rupture of an ectopic pregnancy should also be considered; the menstrual history is thus important. The coexistence of *severe back and abdominal pain* indicates a

ruptured abdominal aneurysm or a dissecting aneurysm. When the parietal peritoneum is irritated, pain is felt at the site of the affected organ, but when the visceral peritoneum is predominantly involved pain is often referred in a somatic distribution. For example, in acute appendicitis pain is felt near the umbilicus at first but later, with parietal peritoneal involvement, moves towards the site of the appendix, usually in the right iliac fossa.

SEVERITY

Try to assess the severity of the pain. Ask whether it keeps the patient awake. In women who have had children, compare the severity with labour pains. Sometimes comparison to the pain of a fractured bone is useful.

RADIATION

If pain radiates from the right subcostal region to the shoulder or to the interscapular region, inflammation of the gallbladder (cholecystitis) is a likely diagnosis. If pain begins in the loin but then is felt in the lumbar region a renal stone or renal infection should be considered. Pain beginning in the loin and radiating to the groin is likely to be due to a ureteric calculus and umbilical pain radiating to the right iliac fossa is usually due to appendicitis. Central upper abdominal pain, later radiating through to the back, is common in pancreatitis.

CHARACTER AND CONSTANCY

Constant severe pain felt over many hours is likely to be due to infection. For example, diverticulitis or pyelonephritis can present in this manner. *Colicky pain*, on the other hand, i.e. pain lasting a few seconds or minutes and then passing off, leaving the patient free of pain for a further few minutes, is pathognomonic of small bowel obstruction. If such pain is suddenly relieved after a period of several hours of severe pain, perforation of a viscus should be considered. Large bowel obstruction produces a more constant pain than small bowel obstruction, but colic is usually prominent.

MODE OF ONSET

In obstruction from mechanical disorders such as that due to biliary or ureteric stone, or obstruction of the bowel from adhesions or volvulus, the onset of colicky pain is usually sudden. It is often related to activity or movement in the previous few hours. In infective and inflammatory disorders the pain usually has a slower onset, sometimes over several days, and there is no relation to activity. Recent ingestion of a rich, heavy meal often precedes pancreatitis. Alcohol excess or the ingestion of aspirin or steroid therapy are often observed as precipitating features in patients presenting with perforated peptic ulcer or with haematemesis.

RELIEVING FEATURES

Abdominal pain relieved by rest suggests an infective or inflammatory disorder. If the patient cannot keep still and rolls around in agony then ureteric or biliary colic are likely diagnoses.

VOMITING

A history of vomiting is not in itself very helpful because vomiting occurs as a response to pain of any type. However, effortless projectile vomiting often denotes pyloric stenosis or high small bowel obstruction. In peritonitis the vomitus is usually small in amount but vomiting is persistent. There may be a faeculent smell to the vomitus when there is low small bowel obstruction. Persistent vomiting with associated diarrhoea strongly suggests gastroenteritis (see section on examination of vomit, page 106).

MICTURITION

Increased frequency of micturition occurs both in urinary tract infections and in other pelvic inflammatory disorders as well as in patients with renal infections or ureteric stones. In the latter, haematuria commonly occurs.

APPETITE AND WEIGHT

In patients with a chronic underlying disorder, such as abdominal cancer, there may be a history of anorexia and weight loss, although weight loss also occurs in a variety of other disorders. Sudden loss of appetite clearly indicates a disorder of sudden onset.

OTHER FEATURES

It is important to note whether there have been previous episodes of abdominal pain and whether or not they have been severe. A tendency to improvement or worsening of the patient's symptoms after the onset is also important in deciding on management. The patient may have noticed swellings at the site of a hernial orifice, indicating the likelihood of an obstructed hernia, or there may be a history of blunt or penetrating abdominal trauma. Sometimes the patient may be aware of increasing abdominal distension, a phenomenon indicating intestinal obstruction or paralytic ileus probably associated with an inflammatory or infective underlying bowel disorder. Food poisoning may be suggested by a history of ingestion of unusual foods such as shellfish or a meal in unfamiliar surroundings. The menstrual history should never be forgotten, particularly in relation to the possibility of an ectopic pregnancy. Enquiry should always be made as to a purulent vaginal discharge, indicating salpingitis, or of discharge of mucus, pus or blood from the rectum, suggesting ulcerative colitis.

Examination

A detailed explanation of the findings in the very large number of causes of an acute abdomen is out of place in this book. The student should consult an appropriate textbook of surgery. What is intended here is an explanation of the terms used and of the findings on palpation in acute inflammatory conditions of the peritoneum. The physical signs found on inspection and on auscultation (page 98) have already been discussed.

GUARDING

Guarding is an involuntary reflex contraction of the muscles of the abdominal wall overlying an inflamed viscus and peritoneum, producing localized rigidity. It indicates localized peritonitis. What is felt on examination is spasm of the muscle, which prevents palpation of the underlying viscus. Guarding is seen classically in uncomplicated acute appendicitis. It is very important to distinguish this sign from voluntary contraction of muscle.

RIGIDITY

Generalized or 'board-like' rigidity is an indication of diffuse peritonitis. It can be looked upon as an extension of guarding, with involuntary reflex rigidity of the muscles of the anterior abdominal wall. It is quite unmistakable on palpation, as the whole abdominal wall feels hard and 'board-like', precluding palpation of any underlying viscus. The least downward pressure with a palpating hand in a patient with generalized rigidity produces severe pain. It may be differentiated from voluntary spasm by getting the patient to breathe: in voluntary spasm the abdominal wall will be felt to relax during expiration.

REBOUND TENDERNESS

Rebound tenderness is elicited by palpating slowly and deeply over a viscus and then suddenly releasing the palpating hand. If rebound tenderness is positive, then the patient experiences pain. This sign is explained by the fact that gradual stretching of the abdominal wall by deep palpation followed by sudden release of this pressure stimulates the parietal peritoneum which, if inflamed, produces pain. Rebound tenderness is not always a reliable sign and should be interpreted with caution, particularly in those patients with a low pain threshold.

RADIOLOGY

A plain X-ray of the abdomen is an important immediate investigation in the diagnosis of the acute abdomen, especially in suspected perforation or obstruction (Fig. 5.32).

Examination of vomit

The character of the vomit varies with the nature of the food ingested and the absence or presence of bile, blood or intestinal obstruction. In pyloric stenosis the vomit is apt to be copious and sour-smelling, to contain recognizable food eaten many hours before and to exhibit froth on the surface after standing.

The presence of much mucus gives vomit a viscid consistency. The appearance of the vomit in haematemesis varies in relation to the site and severity of the bleeding (see page 10). If bleeding is copious the vomit may present the appearance of pure blood, or it may be dark red and contain clots. Such bleeding may come from a gastric ulcer or from the oesophageal varices of portal hypertension. More commonly the blood is altered to a blackish or dark brown colour by being in contact with gastric juice. The dark brown colour is due to the conversion of haemoglobin into haematin. The altered blood gives to the vomit an appearance often compared to that of 'coffee grounds'. The taking of preparations of iron or red wine may produce a similar appearance in the vomit. Vomit which contains dark green bile may resemble vomit which contains blood; however, on diluting with water the green colour of the bile becomes more apparent while blood remains dark. Remember that blood in vomit may have come from the nose or lungs and been swallowed; bright red blood that is 'vomited' nearly always originates from the naso- or oropharynx and not from the stomach. Faeculent vomit, characteristic of advanced intestinal obstruction, is brown in colour, rather like vom-

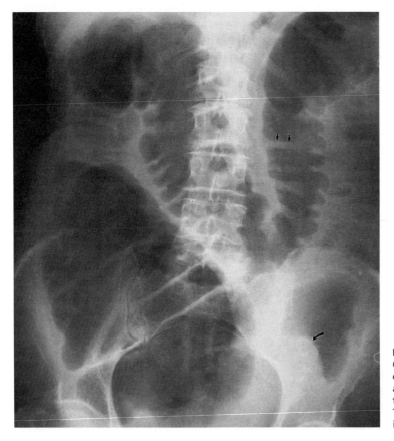

Fig. 5.32 Plain X-ray of the abdomen. Obstruction of the large bowel due to carcinoma of the sigmoid colon (curved arrow). The two small arrows indicate the transverse haustrae of the colon. The colon is dilated with gas, indicating obstruction.

ited tea. Its main hallmark, however, is its typically faecal odour. Vomit containing formed faeces is rare but indicates a communication between the stomach and transverse colon, i.e. gastrocolic fistula.

Examination of faeces

Examination of the faeces is an investigation of great importance all too easily omitted. No patient with bowel disturbance has been properly examined until the stools have been inspected. The white surface of a bedpan makes an ideal background for the detection of blood, pus and mucus.

Naked eye inspection

THE AMOUNT
Note whether the stools are copious or scanty, and whether they are hard, formed, semi-formed, or liquid.

COLOUR
Black stools may be produced by blood or the ingestion of iron or bismuth. In haemorrhage occurring high up in the intestine the altered blood makes the stools dark, tarry-looking and very offensive, and all chemical tests for blood are strongly positive. *Pallor* of the stools may be due to lack of entrance of bile into the intestine, as in obstructive jaundice; to dilution and rapid passage of the stool through the intestine as in diarrhoea; or to an abnormally high fat content as in malabsorption.

ODOUR
The stools in jaundice are often very offensive. Cholera stools, on the other hand, contain very little organic matter, and are almost free from odour. The stools of acute bacillary dysentery are almost odourless, while those of amoebic dysentery have a characteristic odour, something like that of semen. Melaena stools have a characteristic smell.

ABNORMAL STOOLS
Watery stools are found in all cases of profuse diarrhoea and after the administration of purgatives. In cholera the stools—known as *rice-water* stools—are colourless, almost devoid of odour, alkaline in reaction and contain a number of small flocculi consisting of shreds of epithelium and particles of mucus. Purulent or pus-containing stools are found in severe dysentery or ulcerative colitis, or in cases where an abscess has found its way into the intestines. Slimy stools are due to the presence of an excess of mucus, and point to a disorder of the large bowel. The mucus may envelop the faecal masses or may be intimately mixed with them.

Bloody stools vary in appearance according to the site of the haemorrhage. If the bleeding takes place high up, the stools look like tar. In an intussusception they may look like redcurrant jelly. If the haemorrhage is from the large intestine, the blood is less intimately mixed with faecal matter, and may even be of a bright colour. In haemorrhage from the rectum or anus it may merely streak the faecal masses. A massive duodenal bleed, however, may be red in colour when gastrointestinal transit time is brief.

The stools of bacillary dysentery consist at first of faecal material mixed with blood and pus, later of blood and pus without faecal material. Those of amoebic dysentery characteristically consist of fluid faecal material, mucus and small amounts of blood. The stools of steatorrhoea are very large, pale and putty-like or porridge-like and sometimes frothy. They are apt to stick to the sides of the lavatory pan and are difficult to flush away. If formed, they usually float.

Chemical examination

HEMA-CHEK SLIDE TEST FOR OCCULT HAEMORRHAGE
This test paper contains orthotolidine and strontium peroxide. A blue colour is produced when the test paper and developer are in contact with faeces containing blood.

A thin smear of faeces is made on the paper test 'slide' provided. The flap is closed and the paper 'slide' turned over. The flap is opened at the back and one or two drops of Hema-Chek developer are placed on the test area. A blue colour develops within 30 seconds if blood is present.

This test can be used on patients on a normal diet, but it may not detect small amounts of gastrointestinal bleeding.

This test is of value in indicating the presence of gastrointestinal bleeding, but may be negative in the presence of lesions which bleed intermittently or slightly, particularly those situated in the upper gastrointestinal tract. Spectroscopic methods and isotopic methods using radioactive chromium-labelled red cells that can localize the source of bleeding in the gut are also available.

TESTS FOR FAECAL FAT

Fat is present in food as neutral fat or triglyceride. It is split to greater or lesser degrees by lipases, mainly of the pancreas, into glycerol and fatty acids. Some of the fatty acids, if unabsorbed, combine with bases to form soaps. Fat may, therefore, be found in the faeces as neutral fat, fatty acids and soaps.

The estimation of the proportion of split and unsplit fats present has been found unreliable as a method of distinguishing pancreatic from non-pancreatic steatorrhoea because of the effects of bacterial activity on neutral fats.

For the estimation of the fat in the stools, the patient may be placed on a diet containing 50 g of fat per day. The fat present in the stools collected over at least 3 days is then estimated and should not exceed 6 g/day (11–18 mmol/day). It has been found that equally reliable results are obtained if the patient eats a normal diet, provided a 3–5 day collection is made. The radioactive-labelled triolein (^{14}C) ingestion/absorption test enables accurate assessment of fat transport across the gut mucosa without quantitative faecal fat measurement.

Aspiration of peritoneal fluid

Aspiration of peritoneal fluid (*paracentesis abdominis*) is undertaken for diagnostic and therapeutic purposes. It is essential first to make sure that the bladder is empty; if there is any doubt a catheter should be passed before paracentesis is attempted.

The patient should be lying flat or propped up at a slight angle. An abdominal binder or many-tailed bandage should be placed in position around the patient's back before paracentesis is begun. The aspiration is usually performed in the right iliac fossa, a little outside the midpoint of a line drawn from the umbilicus to the anterior superior iliac spine.

With suitable sterile precautions, the skin at the point chosen should be infiltrated with local anaesthetic and the anaesthetic then injected down to the parietal peritoneum. If the puncture is made simply for diagnostic purposes, a 10-ml syringe and a suitable needle can be used. If it is intended to drain the peritoneum, a trocar and flanged cannula (which can be fixed to the skin with adhesive tape) should be employed. A tiny incision should be made in the anaesthetized area of the skin and then the trocar and cannula inserted. Resistance is felt as the trocar perforates the parietal peritoneum. The trocar is then withdrawn from the cannula and the fluid drained into a bottle via a tube connecting the cannula to the bottle. The binder is then secured over the abdomen, which helps to promote drainage. The rate of flow, which should not be too fast, can be controlled by means of a clip on the tubing. When aspiration is complete, the cannula should be withdrawn. The puncture wound is sealed with a plastic dressing and a dry dressing applied. Therapeutic drainage should, however, be avoided if possible as diuretics are preferable.

The fluid withdrawn is sent for bacteriological and cytological examination (Fig. 5.33) and chemical analysis. Transudates, such as occur in heart failure, cirrhosis and the nephrotic syndrome, normally have a specific gravity less than 1.018 and a protein content under 25 g/litre; i.e. less than two-thirds the concentration of albumin in the plasma. Exudates occurring in tuberculous peritonitis or in the presence of secondary deposits usually have a specific gravity above 1.018 and more than 1.0 g/litre of protein. The distinction, however, is somewhat unreliable. Tubercle bacilli and an exudate of lymphocytes are characteristic features of the peritoneal fluid in tuberculous peritonitis. Blood-stained fluid strongly suggests metastases. Malignant cells may also be demonstrated in the latter condition, and in malignant ascites the fluid recurs rapidly after paracentesis. In ascites due to cirrhosis the finding of 500 or more neutrophils per mm^3 fluid and an unexpectedly high protein content suggests the onset of a secondary bacterial peritonitis.

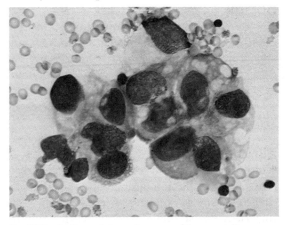

Fig. 5.33 Ascites cytology. A group of tumour cells showing random orientation and large abnormal nucleoli indicating malignancy. Ascitic fluid from patient with ovarian carcinoma. May–Grünwald–Giemsa stain. × 160.

Special techniques in the examination of the GI tract

There are a number of common and important methods of examining the oesophagus, stomach and duodenum, the small and large intestine, the liver, gallbladder and pancreas.

Examination of the oesophagus, stomach and duodenum

In the last 10–15 years the development of the fibre-optic endoscope with video imaging has revolution-ized the inspection of the upper gastrointestinal tract (Fig. 5.34). With this instrument it is possible to inspect directly as far as the duodenal loop using only light sedation and local pharyngeal anaesthesia. Because of the ability to photograph and biopsy any suspicious lesions, this technique is the investigation of choice for demonstrating structural abnormalities in the upper gut.

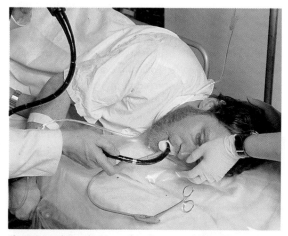

Fig. 5.34 The technique of endoscopy of the upper gastrointestinal tract. The endoscope tube is swallowed, with its attached illumination and photographic accessories. Light sedation is used by some gastroenterologists, but this is often unnecessary.

Suspected cases of oesophagitis, peptic stricture or ulcer (Fig. 5.35), neoplasia and oesophageal varices are readily confirmed by endoscopy, while therapeutic endoscopy is supplanting surgery in many cases of bleeding oesophageal varices and oesophageal stricture. In inoperable cancer of the oesophagus, palliative prostheses can be inserted endoscopically.

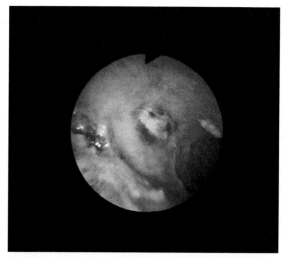

Fig. 5.35   An acute gastric erosion seen by endoscopy.

Endoscopy, using lasers for photocoagulation, is also developing a role in the management of gastrointestinal bleeding and obstructing tumours.

Oesophageal function studies

The oesophageal phase of swallowing can be assessed by barium swallow. Slowing or arrest of transit of the food bolus in the oesophagus can be demonstrated during fluoroscopy (page 111). In special clinical applications manometric studies of swallowing are used to localize functional abnor-malities in the co-ordination of oesophageal peri-stalsis, e.g. achalasia and oesophageal spasm. In patients with epigastric discomfort or fullness (*heartburn*), related to eating or to lying supine, reflux of acid from the stomach into the lower oesophagus should be suspected. This is common in people with hiatus hernia, or other causes of incompetence of the lower oesophageal sphincter. Acid reflux can be detected by monitoring the pH in the lower oesophagus during a 24-hour period. A sudden fall of pH in this region will be accompa-nied by typical heartburn pain. The pH measuring probe, attached to an oesophageal line, is placed in the lower oesophagus, 5 cm above the oesopha-gogastric junction, for 24 hours and the pH recorded continuously. The patient indicates when pain is experienced by pressing an electronic marker on the monitor tape recorder. This investi-gation has found a major clinical application in the differential diagnosis of acid reflux pain from car-diac pain.

Gastric secretory studies and serum gastrin levels

Measurement of acid secretion by the stomach was formerly much used for the assessment of patients with peptic ulcer disease, and for the diagnosis of hyperacidity caused by the rare gastrin-secreting tumours (Zollinger–Ellison syndrome). However, measurement of acid secretion is not useful in the assessment of patients with peptic ulceration as, in most patients with duodenal ulceration, acid secretion is within the normal range and in many patients with Zollinger–Ellison syndrome acid secretion capacity overlaps with that of patients with idiopathic peptic ulcer disease.

In normal subjects the *basal acid output* is no more than a few millilitres per hour, containing up to 10 mmol/litre of hydrogen ion. The *maximal acid output*, measured during 1 hour after the administration of pentagastrin (6.0 µg/kg body weight), a synthetic analogue of the naturally occurring human hormone, gastrin, may reach 27 mmol/litre/h in males, and 25 mmol/litre/h in females. Patients with gastric ulcer or carcinoma have low maximal acid output.

In most patients with Zollinger–Ellison syndrome the ratio of basal to maximum acid secretion is increased to more than 0.6. In these patients the level of gastrin in the serum is increased above 100 ng/litre, and this is currently the best available screening test for this disorder. Serum gastrin levels are also increased in renal failure, pernicious anaemia, after vagotomy and during cimetidine therapy.

Tests for *Helicobacter pylori*

In recent years the role of infection by *Helicobacter pylori* in the pathogenesis of gastric and duodenal ulceration has become increasingly well-documented, although the association of this infection with peptic ulceration is not fully understood. *H. pylori* is a small, 3×0.5 µm Gram-negative spiral bacillus that appears wavy under the microscope. The organism is found in the antrum in about 60% of patients with gastritis or gastric ulceration, and in almost all patients with duodenal ulceration. *H. pylori* can be detected by microscopy or culture of gastric mucosal biopsies obtained during endoscopic examination of the stomach and duodenum, but the most convenient test depends on the ability of the organism to break down urea to ammonia.

H. pylori is rich in urease. In a simple clinical test the gastric biopsy is placed in contact with a pellet or solution containing urea and a coloured pH indicator. The colour of the substrate changes when the pH is greater than 6, indicating the conversion of urea to ammonia by urease in *H. pylori*. A variant of this method utilizes ^{14}C- or ^{13}C-labelled urea, given to the patient by mouth. The patient's breath is monitored for radiolabelled carbon dioxide, indicating breakdown of the ingested urea by urease containing organisms in the upper gastrointestinal tract. Serological and saliva-based tests for *H. pylori* are also becoming available.

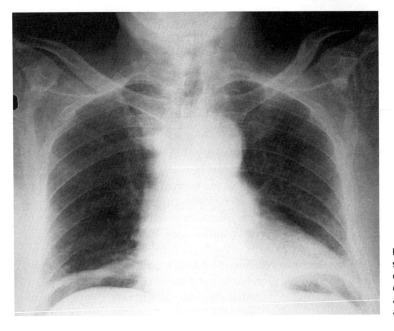

Fig. 5.36   Plain X-ray of the chest showing gas under the right and left diaphragms after perforation of the duodenal ulcer. The patient was admitted in shock with abdominal pain and rigidity.

Gadiology of the upper gastrointestinal tract

PLAIN RADIOGRAPHS

Plain radiographs of the chest and abdomen with the patient supine and in the erect position are of great value in cases of suspected peritonitis due to perforation of a gastric or duodenal ulcer, when gas may be seen under the diaphragm, usually on the right side (Fig. 5.36).

BARIUM SWALLOW

The direct observation of the passage of a radio-opaque barium solution through the pharynx and oesophagus into the stomach remains an important investigation of dysphagia. In addition to structural abnormalities such as neoplasia or stricture, disorders of motor function can be detected which might otherwise escape diagnosis. Lack of progress of barium through the lower oesophageal sphincter on swallowing in a patient with dysphagia indicates the presence of *achalasia*, a disorder of neuromuscular co-ordination of the oesophageal body and failure of the lower sphincter to relax. The oesophagus may be grossly dilated and unable to contract.

The barium-filled crater of a chronic gastric ulcer may be seen in the stomach as a projection from the wall (profile view) or as a rounded deposit (*en face* view) with, in either case, mucosal folds radiating towards the crater. A duodenal ulcer is usually seen *en face* with a stellate appearance of the mucosal folds. Often no definite crater is seen, but the cap is deformed as a result of scarring, characteristically producing a trefoil deformity, sometimes with pseudo-diverticula. In pyloric stenosis there is an increased amount of resting juice present and a grossly enlarged stomach which empties extremely slowly. Polypoid gastric carcinomas cause filling defects in the barium-filled stomach. Malignant ulcers may be difficult to differentiate from simple ulcers, and the radiologist therefore pays particular attention to the mucosal folds and mobility of the wall in the region of the ulcer. Infiltrating tumours produce a rigid conical shape to the stomach with absence of peristalsis and no ulceration. Carcinomas involving the cardia and pylorus cause obstruction and, if small, may be difficult to differentiate from simple lesions.

Small intestine

BARIUM FOLLOW-THROUGH X-RAYS

The small intestine may be studied by taking films of the abdomen at intervals after a barium meal. Abnormalities in the transit time to the colon and in small bowel pattern, e.g. dilatation, narrowing, increase in transverse barring or flocculation, may be demonstrated in malabsorption. Areas of narrowing with proximal dilatation, fistulae and mucosal abnormalities may be produced by Crohn's disease. Small bowel diverticula or neoplasms may also be demonstrated.

SMALL BOWEL ENEMA

This is an alternative to the barium meal and follow-through examination and involves intubating the duodenum and passing small quantities of a non-flocculating barium suspension down the tube. This method is particularly valuable for detecting isolated focal lesions.

RADIOISOTOPE STUDIES

In inflammatory bowel disease the location of the disease, and a measure of its activity, can be obtained by radioisotope studies using indium-labelled white blood cells.

SMALL INTESTINAL ENDOSCOPY AND BIOPSY

Samples of small intestinal mucosa are valuable for histological diagnosis of suspected sprue syndromes. Direct biopsy of the lower duodenum at endoscopy is usually sufficient for diagnosis of coeliac disease but jejunal tissue can also be obtained. Biopsies can also be obtained by endoscopic laparoscopy. After the biopsy has been taken the specimen should be examined immediately by the pathologist under a low-power microscope to assess the general appearance of the intestinal villi.

The small intestinal biopsy is of particular importance in diagnosis of the malabsorption syndrome, where a flat mucosa is seen in place of the usual multiple villi. Serum antibodies to gliadin, reticulin and endomysial antigen are also useful in establishing a diagnosis of coeliac disease.

Colon, rectum and anus

PROCTOSCOPY

The anal canal and lower rectum can be readily visualized with a rigid proctoscope. Place the patient in the position described for rectal examination and gently pass the lubricated instrument to its full depth. Remove the obturator and inspect the mucosa as the instrument is slowly withdrawn. Piles are seen as reddish/blue swellings which bulge into the lumen of the instrument. The internal opening of an anal fistula, an anal or low rectal polyp and a chronic anal fissure are other abnormalities that may be seen.

SIGMOIDOSCOPY

It is often necessary to examine the rectum and colon more fully than is possible by proctoscopy and, in such cases, the sigmoidoscope is employed. Sigmoidoscopy requires skill and experience. In accomplished hands the instrument can be passed for 30 cm. The procedure causes little discomfort and anaesthesia is unnecessary.

Proctitis, polyps and carcinomas may be seen and biopsies taken. Sigmoidoscopy is particularly useful in the differential diagnosis of diarrhoea of colonic origin.

In suspected amoebic dysentery, the mucous membrane should be inspected and portions of mucus and scrapings from the ulcer may be removed and examined microscopically for amoebic cysts.

Urine tests for purgative abuse are useful in the investigation of persistent unexplained diarrhoea. Urine 5HIAA (5-hydroxyindole acetic acid) excretion is increased in carcinoid tumours: diarrhoea is a feature of this syndrome.

BARIUM ENEMA

A plain X-ray of the abdomen should always be taken in patients with suspected perforation or obstruction before considering a contrast study (Fig. 5.32). Barium suspension is introduced via a tube into the rectum as an enema and manipulated around the rest of the colon to fill it. Screening is performed by a radiologist and films taken. The barium is then evacuated and further films taken. By this means, obstruction to the colon, tumours, diverticular disease, fistulae and other abnormalities can be recognized.

Following evacuation, air is introduced into the colon. This facilitates visualization of the mucosa and is especially valuable for detecting small lesions

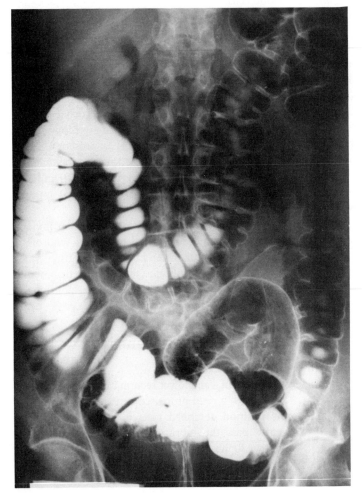

Fig. 5.37 Barium enema with air contrast. The right colon is outlined by barium sulphate, and the rectum, left colon and part of the transverse colon are outlined by air with a thin mucosal layer of barium sulphate. Note the normal haustral pattern in the colon and the smooth appearance of the rectum. The anal canal can also be seen.

Fig. 5.38 Barium enema with air contrast. In this patient with ulcerative colitis, the normal mucosal pattern, and the haustra themselves, have been obliterated. The patient is lying on his right side so that there are clear fluid levels in the barium sulphate suspension in the bowel.

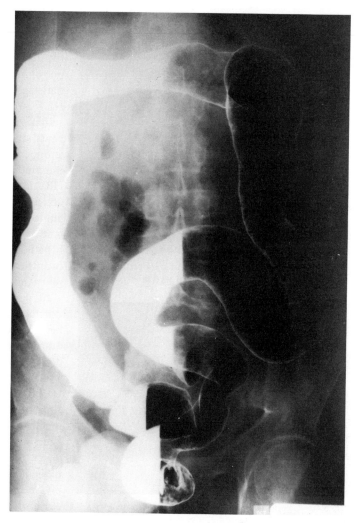

such as polyps and early tumours (Figs 5.37 and 5.38).

FIBRE-OPTIC EXAMINATION OF THE COLON

As in the upper gut the use of flexible fibre-optic instruments has revolutionized the investigation of the colon. Both sigmoidoscopes and colonoscopes are available. The former instrument may be employed in an out-patient setting after a simple enema preparation; the latter requires more extensive colon preparation and sedation but is also an out-patient procedure. These techniques are invaluable for obtaining tissue for diagnosis of inflammatory and neoplastic disease and for removal of neoplastic polyps (Figs 5.39 and 5.40). Dilatation of strictures and laser treatment of obstructing varices can also be managed by endoscopy.

The liver

BIOCHEMICAL TESTS OF LIVER FUNCTION

These are used in the differential diagnosis of jaundice, to detect liver cell damage in other disorders and to monitor the results of surgery of the biliary system and pancreas. These include urinary urobilin, plasma bilirubin, alkaline phosphatase, serum aminotransferases, plasma proteins, and plasma prothrombin. Serum gamma glutamyl transferase levels are especially sensitive of liver dysfunction as, for example, in alcoholism.

Smooth muscle antibodies are present in the blood in chronic hepatitis, and other autoantibody studies are used in the investigation of chronic inflammatory liver disease. Antinuclear and anti-smooth muscle antibodies are found in the blood in primary biliary cirrhosis.

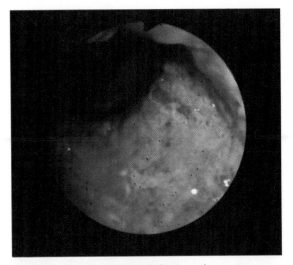

Fig. 5.39 View of colonic epithelium at colonoscopy, revealing the inflammatory changes of ulcerative colitis.

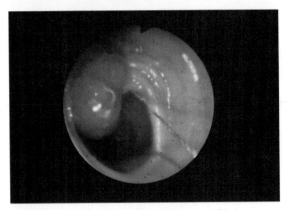

Fig. 5.40 Colonic polyp seen at colonoscopy; this is a premalignant lesion that sometimes has a genetic basis.

Blood copper studies, with measurement of the copper-carrying capacity of serum proteins, are important in the investigation of cirrhosis of unknown cause, in order to exclude Wilson's disease, a disorder of copper transport in the blood in which copper is stored in the liver, leading to cirrhosis. Copper is also stored in the brain in this disorder, causing a progressive encephalopathy with cerebellar ataxia and extrapyramidal features. The blood copper and caeruloplasmin levels are decreased, but urinary copper excretion is increased. Excessive iron storage in the liver can also lead to cirrhosis, and detection of increased ferritin levels (an iron storage protein normally found in the liver) in the blood provide a clue to this diagnosis. Blood transferrin levels are slightly decreased, but blood iron levels are markedly increased, representing free, unbound iron in the circulation.

HEPATITIS

Antibodies to the hepatitis A, B and C viruses can be detected in the blood, and the presence of an effective immune response or of active hepatitis due to one or more of these viruses assessed. During the initial stage of infection with hepatitis B virus (HBV) HBV surface antigen (HBsAg) is present in the serum. After a few weeks or months HBsAg disappears, and levels of anti-HBs and anti-HBcAg (an antibody to a viral core antigen) rise. This is the immune state. In patients who become carriers of HBV infection HBsAg and HBeAg (a viral envelope antigen) persist, with only low levels of antibodies. Some of these patients will develop chronic persistent active HBV hepatitis. Chronic persistence of hepatitis B infection is particularly a problem in countries of the Far East and Asia, and in homosexual men in Western countries.

In patients in whom hepatocellular carcinoma develops as a complication of chronic persistent hepatitis, or in association with hepatic cirrhosis of other causation, alpha fetoprotein becomes detectable in the serum.

ULTRASOUND SCAN

A probe, emitting ultrasonic pulses, is passed across the liver and surrounding areas. Echoes detected from within the patient are received with a transducer, amplified and suitably displayed. This technique is the most commonly used method for noninvasive investigation of the liver. It can detect cirrhosis and small metastases and is of particular value in the diagnosis of fluid-filled lesions such as cysts and abscesses. Fine needles can be inserted into a suspicious lesion under direct ultrasound guidance for cytology and for drainage of fluid-filled lesions.

ISOTOPE SCAN

A radioisotope of technetium or colloidal gold is injected intravenously and taken up by the reticuloendothelial system. A gamma camera is used to show the size and shape of the liver. Abnormal areas take up more or less isotope than normal; examples are primary or secondary hepatic tumours, abscesses and cysts. Technetium-labelled red blood cells can be used to detect the location of sources of bleeding in the gastrointestinal tract.

COMPUTERIZED TOMOGRAPHY (CT) SCANNING

CT can be used to produce cross-sectional images of the liver and other intra-abdominal and retroperitoneal organs. This technique is of great value in the investigation of patients with disease of these organs. MRI is generally not so useful in the study of bowel disorders as CT, since in CT studies the bowel can be outlined with an iodinated ingested radiocontrast agent.

NEEDLE BIOPSY OF LIVER

Percutaneous needle biopsy is the standard technique for obtaining liver tissue for histological examination. Whilst needle biopsy can be conducted under mild sedation and local anaesthesia, it should be carried out only in hospital under supervision and blood should be available for transfusion, if necessary. Generally the method is safe and reliable but there is a tiny but definite mortality from the procedure due to leakage of bile and/or blood into the peritoneal cavity from the puncture site. This risk can be reduced by inserting a 'thrombin plug' at the puncture site in the liver capsule. The procedure should therefore always be regarded as a potentially dangerous investigation and should be performed only by those well-trained in the technique. Contra-indications include patients with a bleeding diathesis, deep obstructive jaundice or ascites.

EXPLORATION OF LIVER FOR LIVER ABSCESS

Liver abscesses due to *Entamoeba histolytica* are nearly always found in the right lobe (Fig. 5.41). When suspected clinically, their presence and position may be demonstrated and localized radiologically or by isotope or ultrasound scanning. Metronidazole (Flagyl) 800 mg three times a day for 10 days is now the first line of treatment and cures the great majority of cases. Where there is a lack of response to treatment after 5 days, exploration by needle aspiration for diagnostic and therapeutic purposes may be performed.

The procedure is conducted under local anaesthesia and strict asepsis. A needle of wide enough bore to admit a thick pus (a lumbar puncture needle is suitable) is selected and a piece of adhesive tape is wound around it 9 cm from its point. The needle is entered either at the site of maximum tenderness or in the right eighth, ninth or tenth intercostal space in the mid-axillary line, and passed medially in a horizontal plane to a maximum depth of 9 cm. By this means the whole of the right lobe of the liver may be explored. When pus is encountered, strong suction has to be employed to remove as much of the pus as possible and this is done with the aid of a two-way syringe. As the pus is removed, it may be replaced by a suitable volume of air (about half the volume of pus removed). The patient is then X-rayed in several positions to determine the exact site and size of the abscess, and to allow the effect of treatment to be followed.

SELECTIVE ANGIOGRAPHY OF COELIAC AXIS AND HEPATIC ARTERY

Angiography is used in the investigation of haematemesis or melaena when an angioma in the bowel is suspected as the cause of bleeding. It is an invasive technique that demands considerable skill on the part of the radiologist. A catheter is passed retrogradely up the aorta from a femoral puncture; its tip is manipulated into the coeliac axis and thus into the hepatic artery. Radiopaque contrast material may then be injected to demonstrate the vasculature.

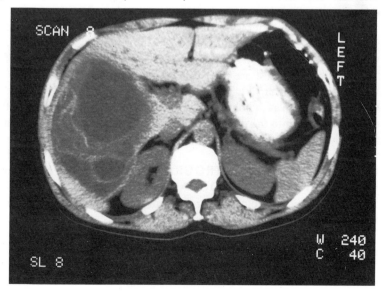

Fig. 5.41 Hydatid cyst of the liver. Several abscesses consisting of low-density lesions can be seen in the right lobe of the liver. The cyst walls are calcified in this unenhanced CT scan.

Gallbladder and bile ducts

The main functions of the gallbladder are to concentrate and store hepatic bile and to empty this bile into the duodenum after appropriate stimuli.

ULTRASOUND

The gallbladder is most easily investigated by ultrasound. It appears as an echo-free structure. If stones are present they are usually easily seen as echo-dense with a characteristic 'acoustic shadow' behind them. Ultrasound detects 90% of gallbladder stones but only about 50% of stones in the bile ducts themselves.

ORAL CHOLECYSTOGRAPHY

This procedure depends on the excretion of iodine-containing compounds that have been absorbed from the gut after oral ingestion, by the liver. They are concentrated in the gallbladder, making it opaque. Apart from a non-functioning gallbladder, stones, abnormalities of the wall of the gallbladder, anatomical variations and failure to contract in response to a fatty meal may be demonstrated. Cholecystography is particularly useful in detecting dilatation of the bile duct.

INTRAVENOUS CHOLANGIOGRAPHY

Intravenous cholangiography can be used to demonstrate the bile ducts. The technique depends on the fact that an intravenously administered iodine-containing compound is excreted by the liver in the bile in such a concentration that it is radiopaque and therefore does not depend on the concentrating power of the gallbladder, as in cholecystography. As with cholecystography it cannot be performed in the jaundiced patient. It is particularly used postoperatively, after biliary tract surgery.

Of particular interest are the width of the common bile duct (usually less than 10 mm), the presence of stones seen as radiolucent filling defects, and the entry of dye into the duodenum. A dilated duct nearly always signifies an abnormality.

ERCP (ENDOSCOPIC RETROGRADE CHOLANGIOPANCREATOGRAPHY)

As in the stomach and colon, the structure of the biliary tract is best investigated by endoscopic methods.

Using a special side-viewing duodenoscope, the duodenal papilla is identified and a cannula passed through it into the common bile duct. Radiopaque contrast fluid is then injected down the cannula and the whole of the biliary system is visualized. The technique is particularly useful in the rapid diagnosis and localization of the different causes of jaundice due to obstruction of the main bile ducts, and in demonstrating the bile ducts where intravenous cholangiography has failed.

PERCUTANEOUS TRANSHEPATIC CHOLANGIOGRAPHY

Percutaneous transhepatic cholangiography is a very useful investigation in patients with jaundice due to obstruction of the main bile ducts. The site of the obstruction due to tumours of the head of the pancreas, or iatrogenic and malignant bile duct strictures, can be accurately localized and differentiated. The information gained prior to laparotomy is of great value to the surgeon. This technique is only used if ERCP fails.

The pancreas

ULTRASOUND AND CT SCANS

These are both useful methods in the diagnosis of pancreatic disease. Each method can differentiate solid from cystic lesions greater than 2.5 cm in size and the success rate in diagnosis is around 70%. Ultrasound is particularly useful in the diagnosis of true and pseudopancreatic cysts and is an essential tool for percutaneous needle biopsy. A plain X-ray is a simple and reliable method for detecting calcification in the pancreas in chronic pancreatitis.

ERCP

The ERCP procedure can display the entire pancreatic duct system. It is therefore valuable not only in the diagnosis of chronic pancreatitis but also in defining those cases which could benefit from surgery.

In patients with cholangiocarcinoma needle biopsy can be performed at ERCP, and brush cytology of the biliary system may also provide histological proof of the diagnosis. A smear of fluid can be stained and examined under the microscope by the pathologist.

Pancreatic function tests are now rarely used in diagnosis, although measurement of the blood amylase level is still valuable in the diagnosis of acute pancreatitis.

CHAPTER 6

The kidneys and the urinary system

Symptoms of renal disease

Renal disease is often revealed by the incidental finding of hypertension proteinuria or raised blood urea or creatinine concentrations. In some cases the underlying disease has been truly asymptomatic; in others the significance of apparently trivial symptoms has been ignored.

The symptom which most often brings a patient to a doctor is *pain*. Pain due to acute bladder or urethral inflammation is called *dysuria*; this is a burning or tingling sensation felt at the urethral meatus or in the suprapubic area during or after micturition. Dysuria with frequent and urgent micturition constitutes the syndrome of cystitis; in severe cases there may be blood in the urine (*haematuria*). Cystitis is extremely common in young women, in whom it is usually related to sexual activity, and in such patients investigation for a serious underlying cause is rarely required. In older women and in men an underlying condition, especially urinary obstruction, must be excluded. In men, perineal or rectal pain suggests infection of the prostate gland (*prostatitis*). Cystitis should be suspected in young children who cry on micturition. Infection of the urine in children may be associated with deformity of the urinary tract and

this requires further investigation. Although symptoms of cystitis in women are often due to bacterial infection, this can be proved in only about half the cases.

Pain due to disease of the kidney is usually felt in the flank, hypochondrium or iliac fossa. Acute obstruction of a kidney causes severe, often colicky pain radiating to the groin and, in the male, to the testicle; chronic obstruction causes less severe discomfort, often none. The pain of acute pyelonephritis and of renal or perirenal abscess is also severe, but constant, and is associated with pyrexial symptoms. If perirenal pus has tracked upwards under the diaphragm the patient may complain of pain in the chest or shoulder; if it has tracked retroperitoneally over the psoas muscle they may be unable to extend the hip and may have to hold it in flexion (Fig. 6.1). Kidneys which are enlarged (e.g. polycystic kidneys) or grossly scarred may cause a dull, nagging flank pain. Acute glomerulonephritis is typically painless. It must be emphasized that severe and progressive damage to the kidneys often occurs without there being any discomfort or other symptoms.

Red urine is usually due to *haematuria* rather than haemoglobinuria. Haematuria may originate in any part of the urinary tract. It is unwise to attribute it to a urinary infection, except in sexually active young women with severe cystitis. Other causes are listed in Box 6.1. It is particularly important not to forget the possibility of an underlying carcinoma and it is often necessary to inspect the bladder with a cystoscope to ensure that a carcinoma is not missed. Occasionally, an attack of renal colic with haematuria culminates in the passage of a stone or of crumbly material—'gravel'. This should be saved for chemical analysis; microscopy may show whether renal papillary tissue is present.

Microscopy of a centrifuged specimen of urine is an essential investigation in patients with haematuria. The presence of haematuria is due to renal disease, probably nephritis, and further investigation of the outflow tract and bladder by endoscopy is unnecessary.

Frequency of micturition often goes unnoticed during the day, because daytime voiding is determined as much by habit and social factors as by necessity. To be called regularly from sleep in order to mic-

> **BOX 6.1   Causes of haematuria.**
>
> - Severe cystitis
> - Glomerulonephritis
> - Carcinoma of kidney
> - Renal tuberculosis
> - Necrosis of renal papilla
> - Benign prostatic enlargement
> - Haemangioma of renal outflow tracts
> - Urethritis

turate is much more easily recognized as abnormal, and this may be due to loss of renal concentrating capacity, urinary infection, bladder obstruction or neurological disease affecting the bladder. Nocturnal micturition (*nocturia*) is frequently the first symptom of chronic renal disease. If a patient complains of frequency try to discover whether large or small quantities of urine are being passed, because there

(a)

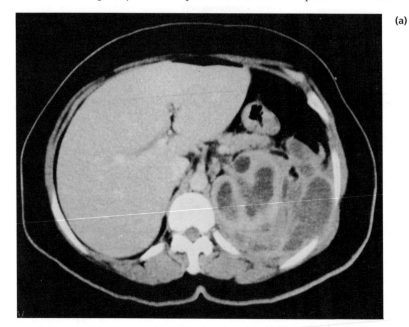

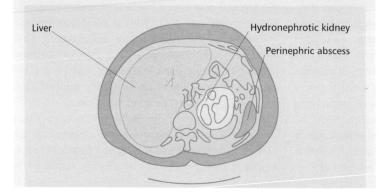

Liver

Hydronephrotic kidney

Perinephric abscess

Fig. 6.1 Computerized tomographic scan of the abdomen. This shows the abdomen, in transverse section, of a patient who had a ureteric calculus obstructing her left kidney and causing hydronephrosis (a), pyelonephritis and perirenal abscess (b). The abscess tracked round the spleen and down into the psoas and iliacus muscles. She had severe constant pain in the left iliac fossa and groin and had to walk in a bent position because rotation of the psoas and iliacus muscles caused flexion of the left hip.

are several important causes of the production of too much urine (*polyuria*; page 124).

In acute glomerulonephritis the volume of urine produced may be very small (*oliguria*), and haematuria often occurs. Unless fluid intake is restricted the patient will develop evidence of salt and water accumulation, such as breathlessness, swelling of face and ankles and hypertension. Acute glomerulonephritis rarely causes complete cessation of urine production (*anuria*); if this occurs, obstruction of both kidneys, or of a solitary functioning kidney, or obstruction at the bladder outlet must be suspected.

The nephrotic syndrome consists of heavy proteinuria, lowering of the plasma concentration of albumin, and oedema. The oedema is due to transfer of fluid from vascular to extravascular compartments, and to a retention of fluid which is not usu-ally so dramatic as to be noticed by the patient, but which is obvious as an imbalance between measured fluid intake and urine output, or from serial weighing of the patient. Remember that day-to-day variations in body weight are due to changes in fluid balance, and not to changes in nutritional status. Heavy proteinuria may cause noticeable frothing of the urine on micturition, and this may antedate other manifestations of the syndrome by several months.

Just as frequency and dysuria are the most common urinary symptoms in young women, so disturbed micturition due to enlargement of the prostate is the most common urinary abnormality in men past middle age. Characteristically, the stream of urine produced on voiding is poor and the patient complains of difficulty in initiating micturition (*hesitancy*) and in stopping it (*terminal dribbling*).

(b)

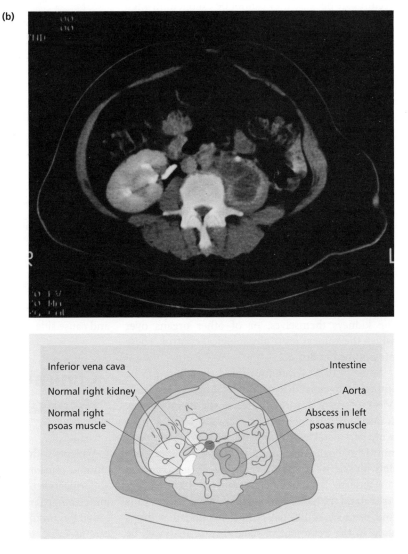

Inferior vena cava

Normal right kidney

Normal right psoas muscle

Intestine

Aorta

Abscess in left psoas muscle

Recurrent haematuria may occur and *acute retention* of urine (an agonizing condition) may supervene. Occasionally a patient presents with uraemia and no antecedent symptoms. All these features may be caused by benign enlargement of the prostate, or by carcinoma of this gland. A benign cause must never be accepted until carcinoma of the bladder or kidney have been excluded.

Urethral discharge is only recognized by men and requires further investigation (see Chapter 17). It is often unaccompanied by pain, but there may be dysuria and frequency.

Uraemia

The term 'uraemia' refers to the numerous symptoms and signs which develop in patients with severe renal failure. Some of these are due to poisons which accumulate because they cannot be excreted through the glomeruli, some to the excessive loss of substances which are normally retained by tubular reabsorption, and others to the breakdown of physiological control which the kidney normally exerts over distant organs.

Certain symptoms cannot be attributed to specific physiological abnormalities. These include tiredness, lack of concentration, irritability, depression and inability to cope mentally and physically with normal daily routines. Nausea, vomiting, diarrhoea and pruritus suggest the condition is advanced, and confusion, fits and stupor are preterminal events. Such symptoms are often what is meant when a patient is said to be 'uraemic' and tend to be markedly improved by any treatment which lowers the blood urea concentration, such as reduction in the dietary protein intake, or artificial kidney treatment.

A number of other symptoms cannot be attributed to more specific disturbances in the function of the kidneys themselves, or of other organs over which the kidneys exert physiological control. These are outlined in Box 6.2

Some of these symptoms of kidney failure can be improved by renal dialysis; others progress despite it. Most of them improve after a successful kidney transplant. Anaemia can be managed by treatment with parenteral erythropoietin, and synthetic vitamin D analogues are useful in managing bone pain and muscle weakness by restoring normal calcium metabolism. It should be remembered that whatever has caused the kidneys to fail may affect other organs and produce additional symptoms; and that drugs used in the treatment of renal disease may well be

BOX 6.2 Possible effects of kidney failure on other systems.

Disturbances of water and electrolyte balance
- Breathlessness due to salt and water overload
- Deep sighing breathing (*Kussmal respiration*) due to acidosis
- Weakness and postural fainting due to hypotension caused by salt and water depletion
- Lethargy and weakness from hypokalaemia.

Disturbances of the erythropoietic system
- Lethargy and breathlessness associated with anaemia due to impaired production of erythropoietin by the kidneys. In advanced cases there is defective coagulation and patients may complain of excessive bruising
- Haemorrhage from the gastrointestinal tract or lungs may occur.

Disturbances of the cardiovascular system
- Cardiac failure or angina associated with fluid overload, hypertension, anaemia, and impaired ventricular function (*uraemic cardiomyopathy*)
- Precordial chest pain due to pericarditis
- Cardiac arrhythmias associated with hyperkalaemia.

Disturbances of the respiratory system
- Breathlessness and haemoptysis from fluid overload or so-called 'uraemic lung'
- Chest pain due to pleurisy.

Disturbances of the musculoskeletal system
- Muscular weakness and bone pain due to impairment of vitamin D activation and to excessive parathyroid gland activity. Rarely, acute pain due to gout may develop, especially in the feet.

Disturbances of the nervous system
- Hypertensive stroke and encephalopathy
- Clouding of consciousness, fits and coma in advanced renal failure
- Impaired sensation or paraesthesiae in the feet, due to peripheral neuropathy in long-standing uraemia.

Disturbances of the eyes
- Pain from conjunctivitis caused by local deposits of calcium
- Visual blurring from hypertensive retinal damage or retinal vascular thrombosis.

poorly excreted and are thereby liable to accumulate and cause side-effects.

Clinical signs in renal disease

In patients with renal disease, especially when there is chronic renal failure, there are often many clinical abnormalities. The examination should proceed by inspection, palpation, percussion and auscultation, followed by consideration of possible eye and ear complications, urine testing, and other special investigations.

Inspection

The skin of a person with chronic uraemia tends to be dry and flaky, and has a pallid, dirty brown appearance. There may be bruises or purpura and scratch marks may be seen, indicating pruritus. If the patient is salt- and water-depleted the skin may be lax, collapsing slowly after it has been pinched between finger and thumb. This sign is difficult to elicit in older persons whose skin may be lax. Rarely, subcutaneous lumps caused by deposits of calcium in patients with overactive parathyroid glands may be found and these may ulcerate. 'Uraemic frost' looks like dandruff on the forehead and is due to

(a)

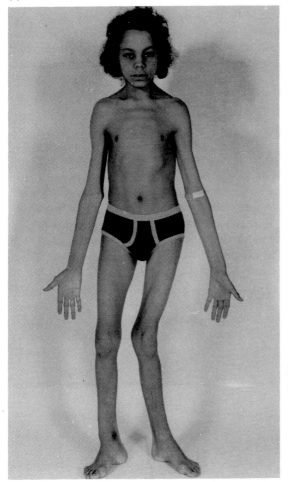

urea crystallizing out from the sweat; it is found in terminal uraemia. In patients undergoing artificial kidney treatment the scars of vascular access surgery may be seen on forearms or ankles, and the veins on the dorsum of the hands and forearms may be dilated as a result of arteriovenous anastomosis constructed in the forearm for vascular access as part of renal dialysis therapy. Pitting oedema of the ankles and sacrum, oedema of the genitals and facial puffiness may denote the presence of nephrotic syndrome.

The *nails* are sometimes opaque and white (*leuconychia*) in nephrotic syndrome or in chronic renal failure. Transverse ridges (Beau's lines) may draw attention to past episodes of severe illness or malnutrition. Splinter haemorrhages in the nailbeds suggest that vasculitis or endocarditis is responsible for acute renal failure. In severe chronic renal failure the mucosae are pale due to anaemia. Throat infection, white deposits in the mouth and ulcers on the lips should be looked for in severely ill patients or those receiving treatment with steroids or cytotoxic drugs; these are due to bacterial, fungal and viral infections respectively. Warts and skin cancers on light-exposed skin are common in immunosuppressed patients with renal transplants.

Growth is impaired and puberty delayed in children with chronic renal failure; renal rickets may cause valgus or varus deformity of the knees ('knock knees' or 'bow legs') and ankles (Fig. 6.2(a) and (b)),

(b)

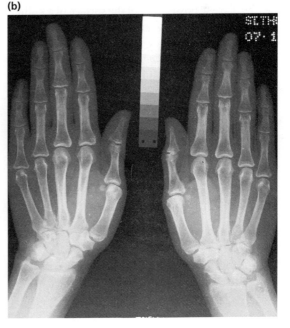

Fig. 6.2 (a) Knock knees and varus deformity of the ankles due to renal osteodystrophy. (b) X-ray of the hands of a patient with chronic renal failure and secondary hyperparathyroidism showing renal osteodystrophy. There is a loss of density of the tips of the digits (acro-osteolysis) with loss of density on either side of the interphalangeal joints and subperiosteal bone resorption. The latter is best seen in the middle phalynx of the index and middle fingers.

swelling of the costochondral junctions ('rickety rosary') and proximal muscle weakness so that the patient cannot stand up from a squatting position without levering up with the arms. Resorption of bone in the terminal phalanges, due to long-standing secondary overactivity of the parathyroid glands, may shorten the fingers (Fig. 6.3), and softening of the vertebrae with consequent curvature of the spine and loss of height, may cause a round-shouldered appearance (*kyphosis*).

The uraemic flap is a coarse, dipping movement of the outstretched fingers, exaggerated by dorsiflexion of the wrists, which is indistinguishable from the *metabolic flap* (asterixis) of hepatic or respiratory failure; it is a preterminal event and denotes an urgent need for artificial kidney treatment. It may be accompanied by sporadic twitching of the limbs, and muscle cramps. Some uraemic and dialysis patients have an uncontrollable desire to move their legs continually ('restless legs').

Palpation

Normal kidneys, especially the right one, which is lower than the left, are sometimes palpable in a thin person with a relaxed abdomen. Otherwise a palpable kidney is likely to be abnormal due to hydronephrosis (unilateral or bilateral), multiple cysts (usually bilateral), tumour (usually unilateral) or infiltration; if one kidney has been removed the other may hypertrophy enough to be palpable. The characteristics of a palpable kidney are described on page 89. Coarse bosselation of the surface of a kidney suggests the presence of multiple large cysts (polycystic kidneys).

The characteristics of a bladder distended because of delayed micturition, obstruction or neuropathy

are described on page 94. In women, fat people and in those who have difficulty in relaxing their abdominal muscles, it is often difficult to detect a large bladder by palpation; dullness on percussion of the suprapubic area is often a more reliable clinical sign.

Tenderness of the kidney or bladder is often due to infection or obstruction or, in the case of the kidney, to infarction, haemorrhage into cysts, or acute rejection of a renal transplant. It should be remembered that a transplanted kidney lies in the iliac fossa, where it can be felt as a firm swelling underneath the skin and anterior abdominal musculature.

Diffuse soft subcutaneous swelling, which indents or pits on finger pressure, is the hallmark of oedema due to overload of salt and water, heart failure or the nephrotic syndrome. In the latter it is more likely to extend to thigh or back, because the patient can more easily lie flat without getting breathless. Patients with vasculitis may present with renal abnormalities and a purpuric rash which can be felt as well as seen because of the perivascular inflammation (Fig. 6.4).

Percussion

Apart from diagnosing pulmonary complications such as pneumonia, the main value of percussion in patients with renal disease is in detecting ascites and pleural effusions in the nephrotic syndrome. Shifting dullness and fluid thrill in the abdomen can be demonstrated in patients undergoing peritoneal dialysis.

Auscultation

Auscultation is helpful in the diagnosis of uraemic pericarditis and pleurisy, characterized respectively

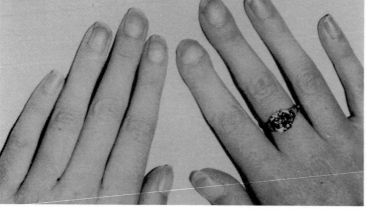

Fig. 6.3 Shortening of the distal phalanges in a patient with severe osteodystrophy.

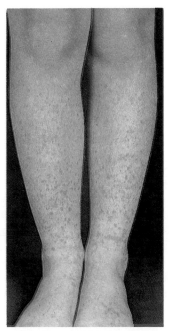

Fig. 6.4 Purpura in Henoch–Schönlein disease.

by pericardial and pleural friction rubs (pages 186 and 151). These may be found in patients undergoing dialysis, and sometimes in conditions, such as systemic lupus erythematosus and vasculitis which involve the kidney, heart or lungs as part of a multisystem inflammatory disorder. Hypertension may occasionally be produced by reduction in blood flow to a kidney caused by stenosis of a renal artery. Attention is drawn to this possibility by a *bruit* heard in the flank posteriorly, or more often, over the renal artery anteriorly when the stethoscope diaphragm is pressed firmly into the relaxed hypochondrium. Even if no bruit can be heard in the flank, an ileo-femoral bruit implies the presence of atherosclerosis and increases the probability of renal artery stenosis.

The eyes

Yellowish deposits of calcium in the sclerae due to parathyroid overactivity may be symptomless, but can cause conjunctivitis. Thin curved white lines just inside the corneoscleral junction are evidence of limbic calcification, caused by hyperparathyroidism (see Fig. 10.14). They must be distinguished from arcus senilis, a broader band at the edge of the cornea, merging with the sclera and most marked superiorly and inferiorly. *Retinal changes* are often seen in patients with renal disease, largely because of its

association with hypertension, diabetes and vascular disorders. Hypertensive and diabetic retinopathy (Figs 10.11 and 10.12) are described on page 235. Thrombosis of retinal artery or vein (Figs 10.13 and 10.15) occurs occasionally in patients with very high or rapidly changing blood pressure. Haemorrhages and exudates may also be seen in vasulitic conditions such as systemic lupus erythematosus and polyarteritis nodosa.

The ears

Alport's syndrome is an hereditary disease causing proteinuria, haematuria, renal failure, ocular abnormalities, and sensorineural deafness which particularly affects the hearing of high-frequency sounds. Deafness may also be associated with other forms of hereditary renal disease.

Urine testing

The urine should be tested in any general medical examination and not just in patients with known renal disease. Testing the urine often leads to the discovery of unsuspected illness, such as diabetes mellitus or renal failure, and jaundice or hypertension. Many tests are better performed on fresh urine by doctor or nurse than on stale urine by the laboratory.

Urine passed into a clean, dry vessel is suitable for chemical tests, which should be done within the hour unless the urine is refrigerated, in which case it should be returned to room temperature before testing. Antiseptics or detergents may cause false results. Special methods of collection, designed to reduce contamination from urethra and vestibule, are desirable for microscopic examination and essential for bacteriological examination.

The urine should be examined physically and chemically. Microscopic and bacteriological examination may be very valuable, but are not done routinely.

Physical examination

Attention should be paid to quantity; colour and transparency; specific gravity; and naked-eye characteristics of the deposit.

QUANTITY

In healthy people the volume of urine passed daily varies from about 700 to 2500 ml. Normally, very much more urine is excreted during the day than during the night, so that sleep is undisturbed by the need to micturate. Urine excretion is increased after food, drink, alcohol, or exposure to cold. Diminished excretion occurs when fluid intake is low and after sweating.

A pathological increase (*polyuria*) occurs in diabetes mellitus and diabetes insipidus, during the elimination of oedema fluid and sometimes in renal failure. Nocturnal polyuria (*nocturia*) is often the first clinical indication of chronic renal failure.

Abnormal reduction of urine output may be due to salt and water depletion from such factors as diarrhoea, vomiting, fever and extensive burns; the sudden lowering of blood pressure; severe heart failure; or acute diffuse disease of the kidney tissue such as occurs in acute glomerulonephritis. Complete cessation of urine output (*anuria*) is uncommon and often results from obstruction.

COLOUR AND TRANSPARENCY

Urochrome and uro-erythrin are pigments which give normal urine its characteristic colour. The exact tint varies; urine darkens on standing due to the oxidation of colourless urobilinogen to coloured urobilin.

Small quantities of blood are often undetectable by inspection, but give the urine a smoky appearance; larger quantities make it brownish or red. The presence of large amounts of haemoglobin from lysed red cells, as after mismatched blood transfusion or in blackwater fever, produces a colour varying from dark red (when it may be confused with the similar but more transparent colour resulting from excessive consumption of beetroot) to brownish or even almost black. Porphyrins darken on standing to a dark brown or red colour, and melanins similarly become dark brown or black.

Bile pigments make the urine brown, with a green tint at the surface when viewed in the specimen glass against the light, and cause a yellow froth when the urine is shaken in a test tube.

The urine is abnormally pale when it is very dilute and in renal failure, when the normal colouring is greatly diminished or absent. However, its concentration cannot be estimated reliably from its appearance.

Various drugs discolour the urine. Some examples are tetracyclines (yellow); anthraquinone purgatives such as senna (orange); desferrioxamine (reddish brown); phenindione (pink); nitrofurantoin and nitridazole (brown); rifampicin and phenazopyridine (red); methylene blue, present in some proprietary pills (green); methyldopa and iron sorbitol (grey or black). Metronidazole therapy causes darkening of the urine.

Urine is normally quite transparent when freshly passed, but pus or phosphates may make it cloudy. Phosphates dissolve when the urine is rewarmed to body temperature. Stale, unrefridgerated urine often appears hazy or musky because of the bacterial proliferation which occurs at room temperature.

SPECIFIC GRAVITY

The concentration of urine is most accurately expressed as its *osmolality*, which depends on the number of osmotically active solute particles per unit of solvent; this may be determined by measuring its freezing point.

It is usually sufficient, however, to measure the specific gravity, which depends on the type as well as on the number of solute particles. This is most easily assessed using a commercial reagent strip. Less conveniently and less hygienically it can be measured with a urinometer, in which case it is essential that there is enough urine to allow the urinometer to float freely in the measuring cylinder; if there is insufficient urine, the urine should be diluted with an equal volume of distilled water and the last two figures of the urinometer reading doubled.

The normal specific gravity, which is proportional to the urinary concentration of urea and sodium, varies from 1.002 to 1.025, depending on the state of hydration of the patient and the time of day—usually being greatest on arising in the morning. It may occasionally rise to 1.035 even in health. If the specific gravity of any urine specimen exceeds 1.018 it may be assumed that renal concentrating capacity is normal.

Approximate correlations between specific gravity and osmolality are given in Fig. 6.5. The specific gravity, when measured with a urinometer, rises by 0.004 for every 1 mg/100 ml glucose present in the urine and by 0.003 for every 1 mg/100 ml protein; it is also increased by excretion of radiographic contrast medium. The increases produced by these heavy molecules are more than expected from the changes in osmolality. The discrepancy is not evident if the specific gravity is measured with a commercial reagent strip.

The specific gravity falls to very low levels in patients with compulsive water drinking and in diabetes insipidus; in certain disorders affecting tubular function the kidneys lose their ability to respond to antidiuretic hormone, even though glomerular func-

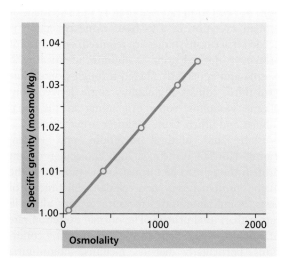

Fig. 6.5 Relationship between specific gravity and osmolality.

tion is preserved (renal diabetes insipidus.

When renal failure develops, the kidneys become less able to concentrate and dilute the urine, until eventually the specific gravity becomes fixed at 1.010, which is the specific gravity of the glomerular filtrate (*isosthenuria*) (Fig. 6.6).

NAKED-EYE CHARACTERISTICS OF THE DEPOSIT

Normal urine is perfectly clear and transparent when voided; but pus, bacteria and precipitated urates and phosphates may make it cloudy. If the opalescence persists after filtration it is due to the presence of bacteria.

Phosphates and urates may precipitate in normal urine. Phosphates produce a white deposit when the urine is alkaline; warming increases their deposition because the urine becomes more alkaline due to the loss of carbon dioxide. Phosphates are not important and dissolve after acidification with acetic acid. Clear urine may become cloudy at room temperature; this is usually due to the precipitation of urates which dissolve on rewarming or adding sodium hydroxide. Although usually of no significance, urate excretion increases when purine breakdown is augmented, as in myeloproliferative disorders and some forms of gout.

Chemical examination

Many of the traditional chemical tests for urinary constituents have been replaced for routine purposes by commercial tablet or reagent 'stick' or 'strip' tests.

In order to avoid false results it is important that the manufacturer's instructions are followed exactly, that the tablets or strips are kept dry and in their closed containers, and that the indicator ends of strips are not handled. The reagent strip should be dipped briefly into the urine and its edge then run against the rim of the urine container to remove excessive moisture. The strip is held horizontally (to prevent the mixing of chemicals from adjacent bands) and the colour changes are compared, at the exact times specified, with the manufacturer's colour charts on the reagent strip container. Most strips test for several constituents of urine, so care must be taken not to confuse the colour bands or to read them at the wrong times. It is difficult to appreciate subtle colour changes in artificial light. (Make sure the strips are fresh and not time-expired).

pH

It is customary to test the pH of the urine with commercial reagent strips, but the result is rarely

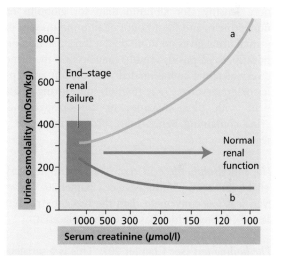

Fig. 6.6 Relationship between renal concentration and diluting capacity, and serum creatinine concentration. The serum creatinine is plotted on a logarithmic scale. This therefore represents linear changes in glomerular filtration rate, such as might occur in progressive renal failure. End stage renal failure is shown on the left of the figure, and normal renal function on the right. Curve a represents maximum concentrating capacity, e.g in water deprivation. The normal kidney can maintain the serum creatinine in the normal range by increasing urine osmolality. In renal failure the urine cannot be concentrated and the serum creatinine rises. Curve b represents the maximum diluting capacity, e.g. after ingestion of large volumes of water. The normal kidney excretes urine of low osmolality. In end-stage renal failure urine osmolality cannot be reduced and the water load is not adequately handled. In end-stage renal function there is isosthenuria, i.e. the urine tends toward an iso-osmolar state (specific gravity 1.010).

important except when a drug has been given with the intention of altering the pH for therapeutic purposes. Normal fresh urine is nearly always slightly acid, except shortly after a meal. Rarely, it is repeatedly neutral or alkaline and, if the patient is not taking alkalis, this may indicate impairment of tubular acidification. This can be confirmed by accurate measurement of the urinary pH after giving ammonium chloride (page 135).

PROTEINS

Before testing for protein, using the salicylsulphonic acid or boiling tests, it is essential that the urine should be absolutely clear; it may be necessary to filter it. This is unnecessary when reagent strips are used.

Tests for protein

Commercial reagent strips. The protein-testing band on commercial reagent strips changes from yellow to various shades of green depending on the concentration of protein in the urine. The test is more sensitive for albumin than for globulin or mucoprotein, and the amount of albumin present in normal urine gives no more than a trace reaction on the strip. False-positive results may occur if the urine is very alkaline, contaminated with certain antiseptics or preservatives (e.g. thymol) and during treatment with phenothiazines or phenazopyridine. Urine containing Bence–Jones protein may give a negative reaction.

The salicylsulphonic acid test. This is simple, very reliable and semiquantitative (see Chapter 20). However, it is less convenient than the reagent strip test described above which has generally replaced it.

The boiling test (see Chapter 20). This is a satisfactory test for protein but is rather messy and unhygienic and less convenient than the other tests.

If proteinuria is detected by salicylsulphonic acid or boiling tests, but not by reagent strip tests, the presence of Bence–Jones protein should be suspected. This should be further investigated by immunoelectrophoretic methods.

Significance of proteinuria

Normally less than 150 mg protein is excreted in the urine over a 24-hour period, and random samples contain less than 20 mg/litre. This is insufficient to cause more than a trace reaction with commercial reagent strips. The tests estimate protein concentra-

tion, not excretion rate. Laboratory measurement of protein excretion in a 24-hour urine collection is needed if accurate studies are required. One-third of protein in normal urine is albumin, identical with plasma and apparently filtered through glomerulus. Two-thirds consist of globulins, some derived from plasma globulins, some originating in the renal tubules and others from the lower urinary tract, e.g. prostatic and urethral secretions and semen; Tamm–Horsfall protein, a high molecular weight protein thought to be formed in the tubules, is the major proteinaceous non-cellular constituent of casts. Some laboratories measure urinary albumin rather than total protein. The normal excretion rate of albumin is less than 20 mg/24 h. In some conditions, particularly diabetes mellitus, albuminuria occurs as an early sign of renal involvement. This microalbuminuria may not be detectable by stick testing at this early stage.

Fever and exercise may transiently increase urinary protein excretion in otherwise healthy people. The term '*orthostatic proteinuria*' denotes the finding of protein in urine collected during the day, but not in the first urine passed after rising in the morning; it is usually of no importance save that it may lead to the mistaken belief that the kidneys are damaged. Persistent proteinuria usually implies renal disease, but gives limited information about its nature and severity. Diseases affecting the lower urinary tract usually cause only slight proteinuria. The absence of proteinuria, of course, does not necessarily imply that the kidneys are normal.

BLOOD AND ITS DERIVATIVES

The term '*haematuria*' indicates that the urine contains intact red cells, '*haemoglobinuria*' that it contains free haemoglobin. Both conditions give positive chemical tests for haemoglobin, but can be differentiated by microscopy of the fresh urine deposit.

Very small numbers of red cells cause no discoloration of the urine. Large numbers give it a peculiar opaque appearance to which the term 'smoky' is applied, and still more produce a brown or red colour, the cells often settling to form a similarly coloured deposit.

Tests for blood

Reagent strips. The reaction is based on the peroxidase-like activity of haemoglobin or myoglobin; a patchy discoloration suggests that the urine contains red blood cells, which may be seen by microscopy of a fresh urine specimen. Stale or infected urine (containing peroxides produced by proliferating bacteria) or the presence of other oxidants (e.g. sodium hypochlorite antiseptic solution) may give a false-positive reaction, and reducing agents, such as ascorbic acid, a false-negative one.

Significance of blood and blood pigments in urine

Menstrual contamination is the most common cause of blood in the urine. Otherwise this is usually due to disease of kidney, ureter, bladder or urethra, although exercise may occasionally cause haematuria in otherwise healthy persons. Non-menstrual haematuria, even in patients treated with anticoagulants, always requires full investigation. Erythrocytes which have passed through the renal tubules tend to be distorted, whereas those coming from the lower urinary tract are undistorted provided the urine is fresh and not unduly concentrated. This can be used to differentiate glomerular from non-glomerular bleeding. The finding of red cell casts is a more easily appreciated, although less sensitive, indication of glomerular bleeding.

Haemoglobinuria may occasionally follow strenuous exertion in normal people. It may also be due to haemolysis within blood vessels (as after mismatched blood transfusion) or in urine (as when blood cells lyse in dilute urine). *Myoglobinuria* is uncommon; it, too, can be produced by hard exercise and by muscle damage, such as found in crush injuries and in certain metabolic myopathies.

Urine which contains blood or haemoglobin must inevitably contain some protein, and it is often difficult to know whether the blood is sufficient to account for all the protein present. If human blood is added to normal urine in an amount sufficient to make it smoky, only a trace of proteinuria is produced. Even when the quantity added is sufficient to render the urine distinctly red, the concentration of protein is only about 0.5 g/litre.

SUGARS

Several reducing sugars may be found in urine. Glucose (*glycosuria*) is much the most important. In normal people glycosuria occurs in amounts too small to be detected by the usual methods. Glycosuria may result from excessive blood glucose levels, as in diabetes mellitus, or from defective tubular reabsorption—'*renal*' *glycosuria*. If a patient with glycosuria also has symptoms of diabetes mellitus this diagnosis may be made with reasonable confidence. In the absence of such symptoms a random estimation of blood glucose concentration may confirm the diagnosis, although a formal glucose tolerance test is sometimes required.

Other reducing sugars which may be found include lactose, fructose, pentose and galactose. *Lactosuria* occurs in late pregnancy and during lactation. *Pentosuria* may be caused by eating large quantities of certain fruits, such as plums, cherries and grapes but, like galactosuria and fructosuria, may be due to a rare inborn error of metabolism. It should be noted that sucrose is not a reducing sugar and artificially loading the urine with this substance does not produce a positive Clinitest reaction.

Reducing substances which are not sugars may occasionally be found in the urine. Thus homogentisic acid (present in alcaptonuria, a rare inborn error of metabolism) and treatment with ascorbic acid, cephalosporins, nalidixic acid, probenecid or aspirin may give a positive result with tests for reducing sugars.

Tests for reducing substances

Reagent strips. These are virtually specific for glucose. Non-glucose reducing sugars give a negative reaction, but false-positive reactions may be given by strong oxidizing agents such as hypochlorite or peroxide-containing antiseptics, bleaches and detergents. The tests are semiquantitative and are highly sensitive unless inhibited by a high concentration of ascorbic acid in the urine.

Clinitest. This is a convenient modification in tablet form of Benedict's test (see Chapter 20). It is not specific for glucose, and is less sensitive for glucose than the reagent strips.

KETONES

Acetoacetic acid and acetone (as well as hydroxybutyric acid, which is not a ketone) may appear in the urine of patients with severe diabetes mellitus, and after starvation or prolonged vomiting and diarrhoea. The ketones may be detected using Rothera's nitroprusside test or more usually, one of its modifications such as Ketostix or Acetest, all of which are very sensitive. Severe ketonuria is implied if the ferric chloride (Gerhardt) test is positive.

Tests for ketones

When testing for ketones the urine must be fresh and unboiled, because acetoacetic acid is easily decomposed by proliferating microorganisms or heat.

Reagent strips. These utilize a modification of Rothera's nitroprusside test and are semiquantitative. A mauve colour denotes the presence of acetoacetic acid. False-positive results may occur if the urine contains bromsulphthalein, phenylketones, phenazopyridine or metabolites of L-dopa. Acetone and hydroxybutyric acid do not react in this test.

Acetest. This is a modification of Rothera's test in tablet form.

BILE PIGMENTS

Bile pigment makes the urine yellow or brownish in colour but this is not specific for bile. A crude test for its presence is to shake the urine in a test tube: a positive result is given by the formation of a stable yellow froth, the stability of which is due to the presence of bile salts, and the colour to bilirubin.

Bilirubin

Bilirubin is the end-product of haem metabolism. It is normally transported in plasma in an unconjugated form which is lipid-soluble, strongly bound to protein and not excreted in the urine. Therefore, the urine of healthy people does not contain bilirubin. During its excretion into the bile, bilirubin is conjugated to a diglucuronide. This is water-soluble, less tightly bound to albumin, and can be excreted in the urine.

The finding of bilirubinuria in a jaundiced patient suggests that the jaundice is due to the accumulation of conjugated bilirubin in the plasma, resulting from hepatocellular damage or hepatic obstruction. Jaundice due solely to unconjugated bilirubin, as in intravascular haemolysis, is not associated with bilirubinuria.

Chlorpromazine·or phenazopyridine in the urine may give a false-positive reaction in both strips and tablet tests, and highly coloured compounds, such as rifampicin and phenazopyridine, may simulate the colour change.

Ictotest. This is based on the coupling of bilirubin with a diazonium salt.

Commercial reagent strips. These are less sensitive than Ictotest.

Urobilinogen and urobilin

Bilirubin secreted by the liver into bile is reduced by intestinal bacteria to urobilinogen, some of which is reabsorbed into the portal circulation to be excreted into bile by the liver again (*enterohepatic circulation*). A small amount reaches the systemic circulation and is excreted into the urine. The colourless urobilinogen oxidizes to pigmented urobilin on standing and, if present in quantity, as in obstructive jaundice, colours the urine orange. Absence of urinary urobilinogen in a patient with obstructive jaundice indicates that the obstruction is so complete that no bile pigment is reaching the intestine. In a patient without jaundice, urobilinogenuria may imply that a normal liver is unable to cope with an unduly large load of urobilinogen as in mild haemolysis or that a damaged liver is unable to excrete the normal amount of urobilinogen coming to it via the enterohepatic circulation as in cirrhosis or early infective hepatitis.

Ehrlich's aldehyde test and reagent strip tests. An excess of urobilinogen in the urine can be detected by Ehrlich's aldehyde test or by the commercial strip test modification of this reaction. The test must be performed on fresh urine because on standing urobilinogen undergoes spontaneous oxidation to urobilin, which does not give the reaction. Porphobilinogen (which is excreted in the urine in certain types of porphyria and condenses to porphyrins on standing, giving stale porphyric urine a port wine colour) also produces a red colour in the test, but the colour is not extracted into the alcohol phase.

In the commercial stick version of Ehrlich's aldehyde test the positive reactions may also be produced by porphobilinogen and para-aminosalicylic acid, and phenazopyridine may give a masking discoloration. Stale urine, in which urobilinogen has already been oxidized to bilirubin, may give a false-negative test.

Microscopical examination

It is customary to examine the deposit from urine which has been centrifuged at 1000–1500 rpm for about 3 minutes. This is useful for qualitative examination, and mid-stream urine (see section on bacteriological examination, page 131) is generally suitable for this purpose. Fragile items, such as casts, may be disrupted by prolonged or rapid centrifugation. Cells and casts also disintegrate rapidly in stale urine, and it is essential to examine a fresh specimen if red, white and epithelial cells are to be distinguished. Unstained cellular elements, especially casts, are not very refractile. They are best seen if the microscope diaphragm is partially closed and the condenser racked down to reduce the cohesion of the illumination.

Quantitive examination of the cellular deposit is best done on uncentrifuged urine in a haemocytometer chamber. Figures 6.7–6.10 illustrate the urinary sediment as seen by phase-contrast microscopy. Readers using ordinary microscopy must not expect to see casts and cells so clearly defined.

ERYTHROCYTES

Haematuria may arise in any part of the urinary tract and may be caused by a medical condition such as glomerulonephritis, a condition requiring surgery, or an acute urinary infection (Box 6.1).

Under the microscope erythrocytes typically appear as roughly circular elements of about 7 μm diameter with clear yellow centres (Fig. 6.7). If the urine is concentrated the erythrocytes become shrunken and crenated, but in dilute urine they enlarge and their biconcave shape changes to a more spherical one. Red cells which have passed through the renal tubules become distorted (*dysmorphic*), and this can be used as a way of distinguishing glomerular bleeding from that arising in the lower urinary tract. Normal urine contains no more than 3 red cells/mm³ of uncentrifuged urine or less than 1 per high power field (hpf) of centrifuged urine. Red cells may be confused with droplets of oil from fingers, or catheter lubricant. However, oil droplets are easily differentiated by their variable size, their higher refractive index and the fact that they are more circular. Yeast cells may mimic erythrocytes, but are more variable in size and budding forms may be seen.

Small numbers of red cells do not discolour the urine, and may not give a positive chemical test for haemoglobin, especially if the urine is fresh.

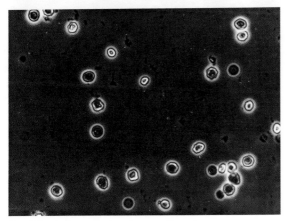

Fig. 6.7 Erythrocytes in urinary sediment.

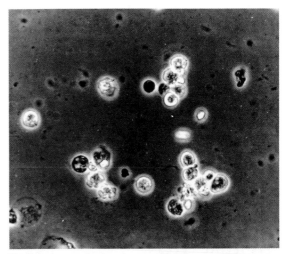

Fig. 6.8 Leucocytes in urinary sediment.

LEUCOCYTES

Leucocytes (Fig. 6.8) are slightly larger than red cells and can usually be recognized by their round shape, lobed nuclei and refractile granular cytoplasm. Their structure is more easily seen if the urine is acidified (which will cause the red cells to disintegrate) but without the use of phase-contrast microscopy or special stains, they cannot be differentiated reliably from renal tubular epithelial cells. When numerous, they tend to form clumps. They degenerate in a matter of hours and must be sought in fresh urine. Urinary leucocyte concentration is closely related to white cell excretion rate. More than 10 leucocyte/mm³ of uncentrifuged mid-stream urine is abnormal in adult women, between 3 and 10 is of doubtful significance; more than 3 leucocytes/mm³ is abnormal in men. The difference between men and women is a result of contamination of the urine by vaginal secretions. Centrifuged urine should not contain more than 5 leucocytes per hpf, although this is a less accurate measure.

An increase in the concentration of leucocytes suggests that the urine is infected, although it may occur without detectable infection, e.g. in patients with renal calculi and, sometimes, in cystitis and urethritis. If pus cells are repeatedly found in apparently sterile urine, tuberculosis of the urinary tract must be considered. The diagnosis of bacterial urinary infection ultimately rests on culture, not microscopy, for infection can be present without any increase in urinary leucocyte concentration. However, sometimes the bacteria can be seen on microscopic examination, even in unstained preparations.

A commercial strip test for leucocytes in urine is

available, based on their content of esterases. It is claimed to correlate well with the presence of 10 or more leucocytes/mm³ urine. Masking discolorations are produced by substances which discolour the urine, notably nitrofurantoin. False-negative reactions are caused by a high specific gravity, high glucose concentration and the presence of tetracycline, certain cephalosporins and oxalic acid.

The presence of a large number of pus cells in the first few millimetres of urine passed by a man, without a corresponding increase in the mid-stream urine, suggests that he has urethritis or (if the specimen has been passed after prostatic massage) chronic prostatitis.

EPITHELIAL CELLS

Renal tubular epithelial cells cannot be differentiated reliably from leucocytes in unstained preparations. A single dose of aspirin may cause large numbers of renal tubular epithelial cells to be shed into the urine.

Transitional epithelial cells from bladder or ureters appear as large oval cells with single nuclei. Polygonal squamous cells, sometimes in sheets, come from urethral or vaginal secretions; if they are present in large numbers the specimen is contaminated and probably unsuitable for culture.

SPERMATOZOA

Spermatozoa are seen at times in urine from males and females and their characteristic appearance is easy to recognize. They have no pathological significance.

PROSTATIC THREADS

Prostatic threads are found when there is chronic inflammation of the prostate, especially after gonorrhoea. They are much larger than casts, being visible to the naked eye as they float in the urine or on its surface.

CASTS

The precipitation of mucoprotein in renal tubules results in the formation of *hyaline casts* (Fig. 6.9). On this basic material erythrocytes (forming red cell casts), leucocytes (forming white cell casts), or tubular epithelial cells (forming epithelial casts or, if they contain lipid droplets, fatty casts) may be deposited. Disintegration of the cellular elements of a cast changes its appearance to that of a granular or waxy cast (Fig. 6.10).

The finding of an occasional hyaline cast is nor-

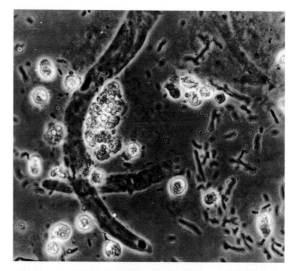

Fig. 6.9 Hyaline casts, leucocytes and bacteria in urinary sediment. Reproduced with permission from *Hand Atlas of the Urinary Sediment* (1971) by E.S. Spencer and I. Petersen, published by Munksgaard, Copenhagen.

mal. Many such casts, or the presence of cellular or granular casts, is evidence that the kidneys are diseased. Red cell casts indicate that the bleeding originates within the kidney from glomerulonephritis. Very broad casts (called 'renal failure casts') are sometimes found and are so shaped because they are formed in tubules which are large and dilated through severe parenchymal disorganization.

Casts are easily missed if the microscopic illumination is too bright and they disintegrate if the urine has been centrifuged too rapidly or for too long. They should be looked for towards the edges of the

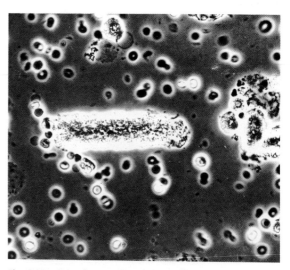

Fig. 6.10 Granular casts in urinary sediment.

coverslip. They are distinguishable from other objects which may be mistaken for them (such as hairs, wool, cotton, masses of urates, prostatic threads and rolled-up epithelial cells) by their shape and characteristic outline. Formed in renal tubules and having taken their shape, casts are always cylindrical. *Hyaline casts* are pale, transparent and homogenous, and can be difficult to distinguish from the background unless phase-contrast microscopy is used; they may be long and narrow with tapering ends and are then sometimes called *cylindroids*. *Cellular casts* are recognized by their constituent cells. *Granular casts* contain fine or coarse granules, consisting of the disintegrated remains of cells.

CRYSTALS

Alkaline urine often contains 'coffin-lid' shaped crystals of ammonium magnesium phosphate (triple phosphate). Conversely, envelope-shaped crystals of calcium oxalate may be found in acid urine, especially after eating asparagus. Uric acid crystals can occur in normal urine, but their presence in large numbers suggests that the patient may have gout; they may crystallize out in various shapes.

Amorphous phosphate or urate debris frequently obscures interesting cellular material; these can be dissolved by acidification or gentle warming respectively. Crystals are usually of no pathological significance, but occasionally are of diagnostic importance, e.g. hexagonal cystine crystals, indicative of cystinuria.

MICROORGANISMS

Bacteria, especially if motile, may be seen during higher power microscopy of fresh unstained, uncentrifuged urine (see Fig. 6.9), but they are more easily seen by Gram-staining the centrifuged deposit. Their finding on microscopy indicates that they are present in very large numbers and, if the specimen is fresh and uncontaminated, strongly suggests that the urine is infected. Urine from women may contain *Trichomonas vaginalis* or yeasts, usually from contamination with vaginal secretion. Occasionally, a true trichomonal or candidal infection occurs in patients with uncontrolled diabetes mellitus. Trichomonads are pear-shaped or round parasites about twice the size of leucocytes and with unipolar flagellae that may be seen with difficulty. Yeasts are slightly smaller than red cells, and may be confused with them, with air bubbles, or with oil droplets.

BILHARZIA

Schistosoma haematobium is best looked for in the last few millimetres of a stream of urine passed in mid-morning. The ova (see Fig. 19.1) measure about 0.12×0.44 mm. A spine projects at one pole. The ova of *S. mansoni* are less often found in the urine and have a lateral spine.

Bacteriological examination

COLLECTION OF SAMPLES

It is only rarely necessary to catheterize a patient in order to obtain urine for culture. A *mid-stream urine* specimen, collected after the vulva or glans penis has been cleaned with tap water, is suitable for most bacteriological purposes. Antiseptic solutions should not be used for cleaning, because they may interfere with the growth of bacteria during culture.

In women the labia are separated by patient or nurse and the vulva is cleaned twice in an antero-posterior direction with swabs soaked in tap water and then with a dry swab. Whilst the labia are still held apart some urine, perhaps 20–50 ml, is passed into a toilet or bowl, but the next portion (mid-stream urine) is collected into a clean, wide-mouthed jar and sent for bacteriological culture. Urine collected in this way is unsuitable for culture if the patient is menstruating heavily, but reasonably satisfactory specimens can be collected after insertion of a vaginal tampon if menstruation is light.

Occasionally, it is important to obtain a specimen free from urethral contaminants. This can be done by *suprapubic aspiration of urine*. The patient is asked not to micturate for several hours so that her bladder is full. After bladder distension has been confirmed by percussion, the suprapubic area is shaved and cleaned with antiseptic. An 'intramuscular' needle is inserted at right angles to the skin surface immediately above the symphysis pubis and urine is aspirated; it may be necessary to use a longer needle if the patient is fat. The technique is safe and, with slight modification, may be used in pregnant women and infants.

The most satisfactory specimen for culture is the first one collected after arising from sleep, for any bacteria in the bladder have been able to multiply undisturbed for several hours. This should be cultured as soon as possible (and certainly within 2 hours of collection) or refrigerated at 4°C immediately, in order to prevent contaminant bacteria multiplying so much that they may be misinterpreted as pathogens. Mid-stream urines, and those obtained by catheterization, should be cultured quantitatively and there are several simple ways of doing this.

SIGNIFICANCE OF BACTERIURIA

In general, the finding of more than 100 000 bacteria/ml (10^8/litre) in a mid-stream urine specimen indicates the presence of urinary infection. Nevertheless, contamination may sometimes produce counts greater than this, and urinary infection may sometimes be present with lower counts. Although urine usually becomes infected with only one species or serotype of bacteria, such a finding does not exclude contamination. However, the detection of more than one kind usually indicates that the urine has been contaminated. In doubtful cases culture of a suprapubic aspirate may be helpful; any growth in such a specimen, other than a few skin contaminants, indicates that there is infection within the urinary tract. In patients with symptomatic infection the urinary leucocyte concentration is usually increased, but this is often not so when the patient has few or no symptoms.

Measurement of renal function

The glomeruli filter off the contents of the plasma except those of high molecular weight or those tightly bound to plasma proteins. The tubules then reabsorb certain solutes, excrete others and reabsorb most of the filtered water. Progressive damage to the kidney by chronic renal disease is associated with destruction of glomeruli. This leads to a reduction in the overall *glomerular filtration rate* which, for practical purposes, can be detected by measuring the blood and creatinine concentrations. At the same time flow of urine through the remaining tubules is increased, which overloads the diluting and concentrating mechanisms. The result is a progressive diminution in the ability of the kidneys to concentrate and dilute urine as renal destruction progresses, until finally the specific gravity becomes fixed at 1.010 (approximately 285 mosmol/kg) which is the specific gravity of the plasma water which has been filtered through the glomeruli (Fig. 6.11).

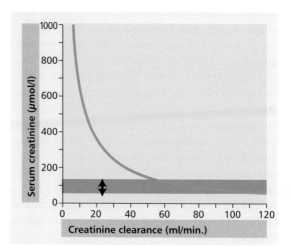

Fig. 6.11 Relationship between creatinine clearance and plasma creatinine concentrations. The normal range of serum creatinine concentration can be maintained only when the renal creatinine clearance is greater than about 60 ml/min. The red area represents the normal range of creatinine concentration.

Concentration of urea and creatinine in the blood

The concentration of urea in the blood depends on a balance between its production from exogenous protein and its excretion by the kidneys. Its level thus varies with protein intake, and may be raised in conditions such as fever and gastrointestinal haemorrhage. In spite of this the plasma urea is widely used as a crude indicator of renal function, and high levels correlate fairly well with the clinical picture of uraemia. The normal range is 2.5–6.6 mmol/litre (15–40 mg/dl).

Creatinine (normally 62–124 µmol/litre or 0.7–1.4 mg/dl) is derived almost entirely from endogenous sources. Its blood concentration correlates with the glomerular filtration rate better than does that of urea because it is less affected by extrarenal factors, such as dietary protein intake.

The relationship between blood urea and creatinine concentrations on the one hand and glomerular filtration rate on the other is hyperbolic, not linear (Figs 6.6 and 6.11). Because of this, glomerular filtration must fall considerably before urea and creatinine concentrations become abnormal. However, in patients with severe renal failure a small change in glomerular filtration rate causes a large rise in urea and creatinine levels. The relationship between glomerular filtration and blood creatinine can be rendered approximately linear by plotting the latter as a reciprocal. This useful mathematical technique enables past and future changes in glomerular filtration rate to be predicted.

Measurement of glomerular filtration rate

The normal glomerular filtration is about 70–170 ml/min, but it depends on sex, weight and surface area. The measured value can be corrected for differences in size by expressing it as the value the patient would have if he or she had a surface area of 1.73 m². This is particularly useful in children. The patient's surface area can be calculated from height and weight, using a nomogram.

Although glomerular filtration rate can be estimated mathematically from plasma creatinine concentration after correction for the patient's gender and weight, it is better to measure it using clearance or radioisotope techniques. *The renal clearance of a substance is the smallest volume of plasma from which the amount of that substance excreted in the urine each minute could have been obtained at the time of the test.* It is calculated from the expression UV/P, where U is the concentration of the substance in the urine (in µmol/litre), V is the volume of urine produced (in ml/min) and P is the plasma concentration of the substance (in µmol/litre). An accurately timed collection of urine must be obtained, traditionally over 24 hours, although an overnight collection is more convenient.

If a substance is excreted by glomerular filtration, and is neither secreted nor reabsorbed by the tubules, its clearance is equal to the glomerular filtration rate. Inulin clearance is considered to be the most accurate measure of glomerular filtration rate but there are practical difficulties in performing the test and other methods are preferred for routine use. The clearance of endogenous creatinine is popular but it overestimates glomerular filtration rate at low filtration rates and in patients with the nephrotic syndrome. Glomerular filtration rate can also be derived from the rate of disappearance of ethylenediaminetetraacetic acid, labelled with radioactive

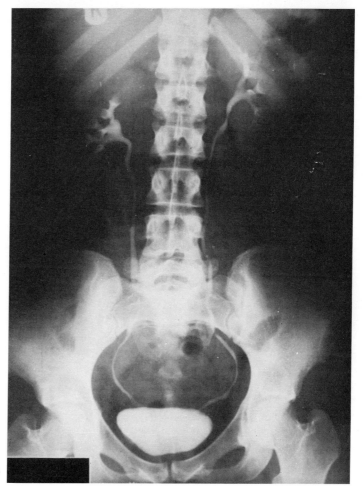

Fig. 6.12 Normal excretion urogram. In this film, taken 15 min after intravenous injection of the iodine-based contrast medium, the calyces of both kidneys, the ureters, and the bladder can be seen.

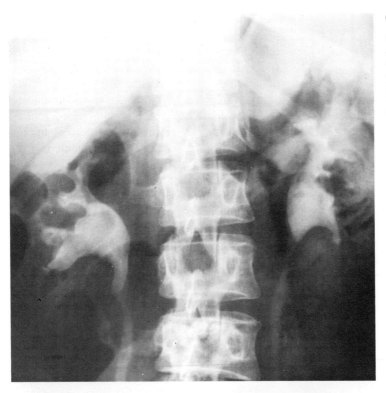

Fig. 6.13   (a) Excretion urogram 5 min after injection of contrast. The ureters are opacified and the calyces also appear to be outlined by contrast (b) Preliminary film, before contrast. injection. The calyces are opacified by large staghorn calculi.

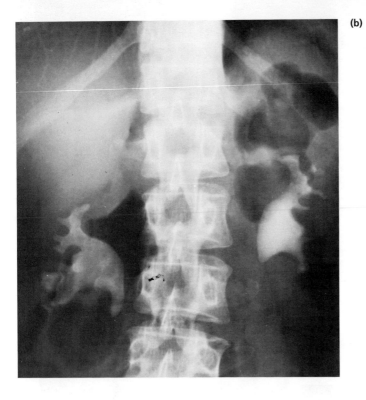

(b)

Fig. 6.14 Excretion urogram. In this film, made 30 min after injection of contrast, the left kidney fails to excrete a detectable concentration of contrast (non-functioning left kidney) and the right kidney shows dilated, hydronephrotic calyces. The right ureter is partially obstructed at the level of the body of the fifth lumbar vertebra. The circular lucency in the bladder is the dilated balloon of a Foley catheter.

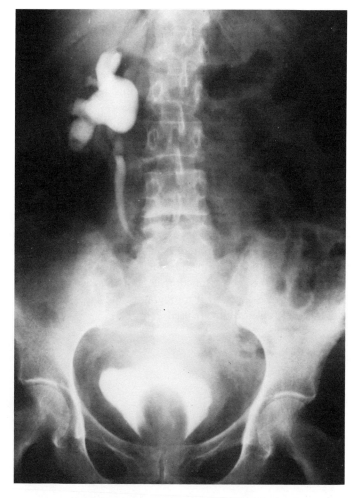

chromium (^{51}Cr–EDTA) or certain other radio-isotopes from the circulation.

Renal concentrating ability

The concentration of the urine, best measured as its *osmolality,* may be as low as 50 mosmol/kg after water loading, or as high as 1400 mosmol/kg after fluid deprivation. If a random specimen of urine has a specific gravity greater than 1.018 (700 mosmol/kg) it can be assumed that concentrating ability is normal. Fluid deprivation for a prolonged period, or injection of vasopressin or an analogue may be used to provide a more accurate test of concentrating ability; urine osmolality of at least 750 mosmol/kg or specific gravity of 1.020 should be attained if concentrating power is normal. In order to produce maximum concentration, fluid depletion for 24–36 hours may be necessary, although the latest specimens are not invariably the most concentrated. Fluid depletion is unpleasant and care must be taken that the patient does not become dehydrated, which may happen easily if the renal concentrating capacity is poor. Fluid deprivation is a slightly more effective stimulus to concentration than vasopressin. The reduction in concentrating and dilating capacity of the kidney as glomerular filtration rate falls is shown in Fig. 6.6.

Renal acidifying ability

If the pH of a random specimen of urine is below 5.5 it can be assumed that renal acidifying ability is normal. In chronic glomerular disease the kidneys usually retain their ability to reduce urine pH below 5.5 until renal failure is advanced. In certain diseases affecting predominantly the renal tubules the urine cannot be adequately acidified, even though the glomerular filtration rate is normal. In order to test for this, ammonium chloride capsules (0.1 g/kg body weight) can be given orally. Normally the urine pH is reduced to less than 5.4. The test should not be done if the patient is already acidotic: in such an event the urine pH should be below 5.4 without further stimulus, and the production of further acidosis may be dangerous. *Renal tubular acidosis* is a cause of renal calculi and nephrocalcinosis, and it is as part of the investigation of these syndromes that this test is most commonly performed.

Radiological and other investigations

EXCRETION UROGRAPHY

This depends on the excretion by the kidney of certain radiopaque organic compounds of iodine, after their intravenous injection (Fig. 6.12, p. 133). It is important in the investigation of renal failure and of suspected structural abnormalities such as calculi or obstruction. When renal function is poor the kidneys are more easily seen if tomographs and large doses of contrast medium are used.

Figure 6.13(a) (p. 134) shows the kidneys, pelvicalyceal systems and upper ureters 5 minutes after injection of contrast medium. Figure 6.13(b) shows how important a pre-injection film is: the pelvicalyceal systems look as if they are filled with contrast medium, but this has not yet been injected! A large calculus (so-called staghorn calculus) has formed a radiopaque cast of the outflow tract of each kidney. Figure 6.14 (p. 135) demonstrates a non-functioning left kidney with hydronephrosis on the right. Further examples of excretion urograms, with clinical correlation are shown in Fig. 6.13.

MICTURATING CYSTOGRAPHY

In this investigation a similar radiopaque medium is instilled into the bladder through a catheter. Cineradiograms are taken of the bladder, its outflow tract and the ureters, as the patient voids the dye. This test is used in the investigation of the bladder outflow tract, especially if vesico-ureteric reflux is suspected.

(a)

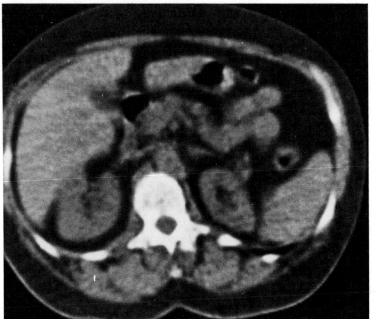

(b)

Fig. 6.15 (a) Computerized tomographic scan with (b) drawing showing normal kidneys.

Liver

Kidney

Hilum

Intestine

Aorta

Spleen

Pelvis of kidney

Kidney

COMPUTERIZED TOMOGRAPHY

The kidneys are easily examined in radiographic 'slices' of the body produced by computerized tomography (CT). This technique is particularly useful for demonstrating collections of fluid (including cysts) and tumours (Figs 6.15 and 6.16). Unlike ultrasound examination, CT scanning is helped rather than hindered by the presence of a lot of fat.

ULTRASOUND EXAMINATION

The kidneys and their gross structure are relatively easily demonstrated, except in obese people, by ultrasound examination, in which echoes reflected from internal structures are used to build up an image. The technique is particularly useful for identifying collections of fluid (including cysts) and diagnosing outflow obstruction. An experienced ultrasonographer can provide much useful information with this technique.

(a)

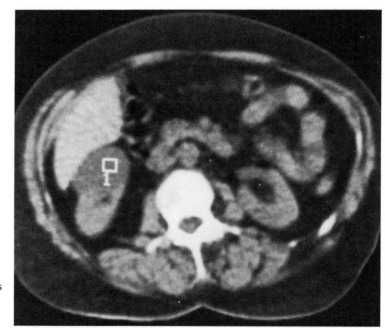

Fig. 6.16 (a) Computerized tomographic scan with (b) drawing showing cyst in right kidney. □ denotes a region of interest (the cyst), in which measurements of tissue density can be made.

(b)

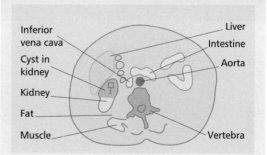

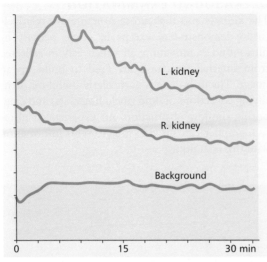

Fig. 6.17 Radioisotope excretion (ordinate) during the 30 min after intravenous injection in a patient with right renal artery stenosis and hypertension. The left kidney achieves more rapid excretion of isotope. The malfunctioning right kidney was the cause of the patient's hypertension.

RADIOISOTOPE INVESTIGATIONS

Radiographic and ultrasound techniques define the structure of organs well, but give comparatively little information about their function. The converse is true of radioisotope investigations. In studies of the urinary tract, radioisotopes (Fig. 6.17) are particularly useful in measuring glomerular filtration rate, indicating the relative contribution of each kidney to overall renal function, diagnosing obstruction, and assessing bladder emptying and the retrograde passage of urine from the bladder towards the kidney (*vesico-ureteric reflux*).

CYSTOSCOPY AND URETHROSCOPY

The interior of the bladder and urethra may be inspected through a cystoscope and urethroscope respectively. The main value of these procedures is in the diagnosis and treatment of tumours of the bladder and in assessing the effects of disease of the prostate.

(a)

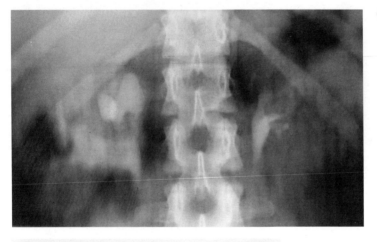

Fig. 6.18 (a) The right kidney is large and the calyces are dilated and clubbed. The left kidney is small. (b) Isotope excretion study showing poor excretion by the left kidney.

(b)

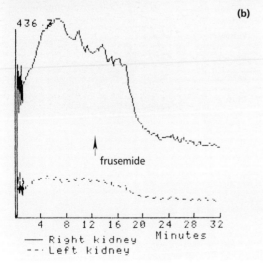

RENAL BIOPSY

By means of a special needle inserted into the back, biopsy specimens of the kidney may be obtained. The technique is of most clinical value in predicting the likely response to steroid therapy of certain patients with the nephrotic syndrome. It may also be valuable in the investigation of acute renal failure and in the diagnosis and assessment of systemic disorders such as amyloidosis and systemic lupus erythematosus and vasculitis. It is essential also in the management of patients after renal transplantation (Box 6.3).

Clinical patterns

In this section two patients are described, together with the results of investigation, in order to illustrate the practical value of the integration of clinical data obtained by examination and by imaging.

Case 1

A 27-year-old woman, found in pregnancy to have a raised blood pressure, with proteinuria, urinary infection and impaired renal function (serum creatinine 144 μmol/litre; creatinine clearance 62 ml/m). After delivery an intravenous urogram (Fig. 6.18a) showed a small left kidney with clubbed calyces and poorly defined outline. The right kidney was large (14 cm long) with clubbed upper pole calyces. The discrepancy in size and function between the two kidneys was confirmed by the [99MTc]DTPA radioisotope scan and the associated time–activity curve (Fig. 6.18b).

(a)

(b)

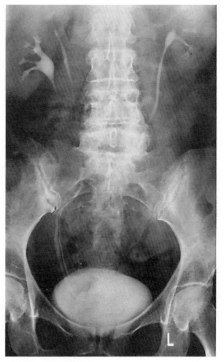

(c)

Fig. 6.19   (a) Intravenous urogram showing a small stone in the right kidney. (b) Injection of radiographic contrast medium. (c) Excretion of medium to reveal a right pelvic–ureteric system.

BOX 6.3 Indications and contraindications to percutaneous needle renal biopsy, and its complications.

Indications
- Nephrotic syndrome
- Renal failure of uncertain cause
- Failure to recover after acute renal failure
- Systemic disease with renal involvement
- To provide diagnosis in unexplained proteinuria or haematuria
- In the management of renal transplantation therapy

Contraindications
- Uncooperative patient
- When there is only one kidney
- When the kidneys are small, in renal failure
- Uncontrolled hypertension
- Bleeding disorder
- Gross obesity

Complications
- Haematuria in 20% (rarely severe)
- Pain in flank or shoulder top
- Perirenal haematuria
- Infection
- Intravenal arteriovenous aneurysm formation

Case 2
A 63-year-old woman who presented with urinary infections, but normal serum urea and creatinine concentrations. An intravenous urogram showed a small stone in the right kidney in the pre-contrast film (Fig. 6.19a), the kidneys being more clearly revealed immediately after injection of radiographic contrast medium (Fig. 6.19b); as this medium is excreted a right duplex pelvic-ureteric system is revealed (Fig. 6.19c).

CHAPTER 7

The respiratory system

Introduction

Lung diseases account for up to a third of deaths in most countries and a major proportion of visits to the doctor and time away from work or school. The symptoms of pulmonary disease may be trivial or extremely distressing; either may indicate serious and life-threatening disease. The functional capacity of the lungs is large compared with everyday needs and therefore diseases may be very advanced before a patient seeks medical advice. The lungs are well-hidden and protected in the thorax, and this can make assessment and diagnosis difficult at times. As with every aspect of diagnosis in medicine the key to success is a clear and carefully recorded history.

Symptoms of respiratory disease

The principal symptoms of lung disease are *cough, sputum production, breathlessness (dyspnoea)* and *chest pain*.

Cough

A cough may be dry or productive of sputum.
● How long has it been present? A cough lasting a few days following a cold has less significance than one lasting several weeks in a middle-aged smoker, which may be the first sign of a malignancy.
● Is the cough worse at any time of day or night? A dry cough at night may be an early symptom of asthma, as may cough which comes in spasms lasting several minutes.
● Is the cough aggravated by anything, such as dust, pollen or cold air? The increased reactivity of the airways seen in asthma, and in some normal people for several weeks after viral respiratory infections may present in this way. Severe coughing, whatever its cause, may be followed by vomiting. In children with whooping cough a spasm of coughing is followed by a characteristic forced inspiration through a narrowed glottis creating a 'whooping' noise which is a form of *stridor* (see below).

Sputum

● Is sputum produced? What does it look like? Children and some adults swallow sputum, but it is always worth asking for a description of its colour and consistency. Yellow or green sputum is usually purulent. Asthmatic people may produce small amounts of very thick or jelly-like sputum, sometimes in the shape of a cast of the airways. Eosinophils may accumulate in the sputum in asthma causing a purulent appearance, even when no infection is present.

Haemoptysis

• Is there any blood in the sputum? The potentially serious significance of blood in the sputum is well-known, and fear often leads patients to not mention it: a specific question is always necessary.
• Is it fresh or altered blood?
• How often has it been seen and for how long? Is the blood seen alone, or is there associated production of purulent sputum?

When severe lung damage in infancy and childhood was common, bronchiectasis was often found in adults. The amount of sputum produced daily often exceeded a cupful. Bronchiectasis is now rare, and chronic bronchitis causes the production of smaller amounts of sputum.

Dyspnoea

Breathlessness is a difficult symptom for many patients to explain and quantify.
• Is the breathlessness only related to exertion? How far can the patient walk at normal pace on the level? This may take some skill to elicit as few people note their symptoms in this form, but a brief discussion about what they can do in their daily lives usually gives a good estimate of their mobility.
• Is the breathlessness intermittent? Exertion may bring on attacks of *asthma*, but asthmatic attacks can also occur at rest, and especially at night, disturbing sleep. Asthmatics can be so resigned to their illness they may not mention this and a specific question is needed. Waking three or more nights per week indicates poorly controlled asthma. In contrast, patients with *emphysema*, and some with chronic bronchitis, will often say that as long as they are sitting or in bed they feel quite normal; it is exercise which troubles them.

Breathlessness that is not related to any organic cause may present as the hyperventilation syndrome. Often this may follow transient problems with breathing, such as mild asthma or a pulmonary embolism, but the cause is obscure in many patients. It can be recognized by the association of other features, such as fatigue, dizziness, anxiety, paraesthesiae of the hand and around the mouth and muscular chest pains, but the precise diagnosis can seldom be made at the first consultation.
• Always ask if the patient hears any noises coming from their chest. Even if a wheeze is not present when you examine the patient, it is useful to know that they have noticed it on occasions. Remember that heart disease causing pulmonary oedema will cause breathlessness which may be worse on lying down (*orthopnoea*).

Pain in the chest

• Chest pain caused by lung disease is usually pleuritic. This means that it is a sharp pain, usually on one side of the chest or the other, and it is made worse by deep breathing or coughing. The pain of pleurisy is often severe, but it may still be very significant diagnostically, even if it is mild. Sometimes pleuritic pain improves when an effusion develops and the lung is no longer rubbing on the pleural surface of the chest wall.
• A constant, and very severe sharp pain may follow rib fracture. This can be caused by an external injury, but sometimes severe coughing leads to fractures of one or more ribs. A spontaneous pneumothorax causes pain on the same side which is not usually pleuritic, but lateral, low down and aching.

Other symptoms and signs

OEDEMA
Swelling of the feet or ankles may develop as a late sign of severe chronic lung disease, because of the development of heart failure. Rarely, it may be the first sign of lung disease, but there is usually a history of breathlessness before oedema develops. Patients will notice difficulty getting their shoes on during the day.

NASOPHARYNX AND LARYNX
Some questions related to the *ear, nose and throat* are often relevant. Recurrent sinusitis and rhinitis may be linked with asthma or, less commonly, with bronchiectasis. A change in the voice may indicate involvement of the left recurrent laryngeal nerve by a carcinoma of the lung. Sometimes patients using inhalers for asthma, and especially inhaled steroids, develop hoarseness or weakness of the voice which improves on changing the treatment. Do not ascribe hoarseness to this cause in older patients, since

carcinoma of the vocal cords can also be present with hoarseness or a change in the quality of the voice. Laryngoscopy is always indicated.

OCCUPATION

Both past and present occupations are important in assessing lung disease. The link with asthma and work is not always clear, although there are many substances encountered in industry which are well-known to cause severe and chronic asthma. A useful question is to ask about symptoms during holidays or longer periods away from work; a weekend is often not long enough for recovery to occur and thus the link with work may be missed.

EXPOSURE TO TOXIC SUBSTANCES AND ALLERGENS

Exposure to asbestos for a few years in youth may lead to mesothelioma or other asbestos-related diseases in later life. Some organic substances can cause an allergic alveolitis; exposure may be at work (*farmer's lung*) or in the home (*bird fancier's lung*). Allergy to pets may be a factor in asthma and rhinitis, but remember that simple avoidance or separation at home may be as effective as complete removal from exposure. In many allergic patients there is a family history of related disorders.

SMOKING

Always record smoking habits. Cigarette smoking is the single most important cause of chronic lung disease and can be relevant to current problems, even if the patient gave up smoking some years earlier. Most emphysema, chronic bronchitis and lung cancer is associated with cigarette smoking.

Physical signs

Physical signs in the chest are usually fairly easy to elicit and often combine to form a clear picture of the abnormalities in the underlying lung. Correlation of this information with the patient's history frequently enables an exact clinical diagnosis to be made. The chest X-ray is a useful extension of the clinical examination, particularly if the latter fails to define the cause of respiratory symptoms. For example, in a middle-aged smoker with a worsening cough and in whom there are no localized physical signs, lung cancer cannot be excluded without the aid of a chest X-ray and perhaps additional investigations.

A number of other non-invasive special investigations such as pulmonary function tests and CT scanning are helpful in reaching a diagnosis in chest disease.

Anatomy

The lungs are well-protected within the thoracic cage; however, the approximate location of the underlying lobes can be deduced from surface markings. This is easier to understand when the appearances on the chest X-ray and the anatomy of the bronchial tree, as seen during bronchoscopy, are also considered.

The *bifurcation of the trachea* corresponds in front with the lower border of the manubrium sterni, that is with the angle of Louis, and behind with the disc between the fourth and fifth thoracic vertebrae. The ribs are best counted downwards from the second costal cartilage. This cartilage articulates with the sternum at the extremity of the angle of Louis, which is a transverse bony ridge at the junction of the body of the sternum and the manubrium sterni and which is easily felt beneath the skin.

A line from the second thoracic spine to the sixth rib in the mammary line corresponds to the upper border of the lower lobe (major interlobar fissure). On the right side a horizontal line from the sternum at the level of the fourth costal cartilage, drawn to meet the line of the major interlobar fissure, marks the boundary between the upper and middle lobes (the minor interlobar fissure). The greater part of each lung, as seen from behind, is composed of the lower lobe; only the apex belongs to the upper lobe. The middle and upper lobes on the right side and the upper lobe on the left occupy most of the area in front. In the axillary regions, parts of all the lobes are accessible. Figures 7.1–7.3 illustrate the bronchial and lobar/segmental anatomy.

The chest X-ray, consisting of posteroanterior and lateral views, enables lesions to be pinpointed fairly accurately in particular lobes, or even segments.

Fibre-optic bronchoscopy enables the anatomy of the bronchial tree to be inspected from inside the chest. This investigation complements clinical and radiographic assessment and enables specific treatment, such as surgery or radiotherapy, to be carried out accurately. A knowledge of the anatomy of the bronchial tree is essential when performing bronchoscopy and interpreting the findings.

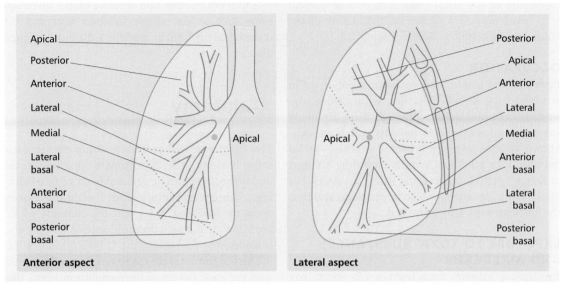

Fig. 7.1   The right lung (anterior and lateral aspects) showing the segmental bronchi. Dashed lines represent interlobar fissures.

General assessment

Even if an examination is specifically directed towards the respiratory system, it is incomplete if there is not also some general examination of the patient. Ideally, the patient should be comfortably resting on a bed, sitting at an angle of 45 degrees and supported by pillows.

The form, physique and general nourishment of the patient should be noted. The patient may be breathless even after the minimal exertion of undressing and this is a valuable observation during the overall assessment. The nature of the *voice* (is it hoarse?) should be noted. The hands should be inspected for *clubbing* (see page 19), *pallor* or *cyanosis*. The lips and tongue should be inspected for central cyanosis (Fig. 7.4). A breathless patient may be using the accessory muscles of respiration (e.g. sternomastoid), which gives an indication of the severity of the breathlessness. Intercostal recession (a drawing-in of the intercostal spaces with inspiration) indicates severe airway obstruction and a very non-compliant lung.

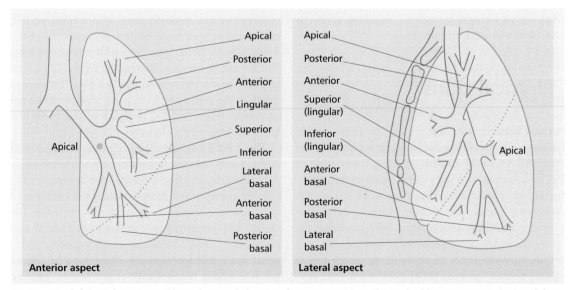

Fig. 7.2   The left lung (anterior and lateral aspects) showing the segmental bronchi. Dashed lines represent the interlobar fissure.

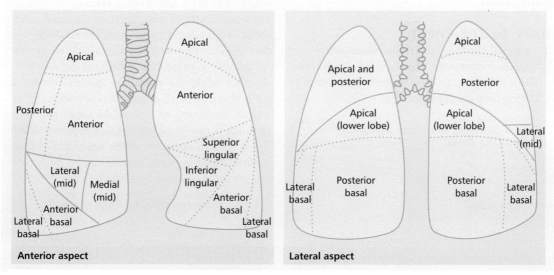

Fig. 7.3 The respiratory segments supplied by the segmental bronchi.

The *venous pulses* in the neck (see Chapter 8) should be inspected. A raised venous pressure is usually indicative of right heart failure but can be due to obstruction of the superior vena cava. In this case the patient often appears plethoric and has a swollen face. If the upper level of the venous pressure can be seen in the neck, venous pulsation is absent. This is usually due to malignancy in the upper mediastinum. If superior vena caval obstruction is present the patient must also be carefully examined for coexistent obstruction of the trachea and major bronchi. If the latter is present there may be an obvious stridor, and peak expiratory flow rate (see below) will be reduced.

The *lymph nodes* in the supraclavicular fossae, cervical regions and axillary regions should be palpated. They are often enlarged secondary to the spread of malignant disease from the chest, and this finding will influence decisions regarding treatment. If malignancy is suspected within the chest, the abdomen must also be examined, paying particular attention to possible enlargement of the liver.

BOX 7.1 Points to note in a general assessment.

- Physique
- Voice
- Breathlessness
- Clubbing
- Cyanosis or pallor
- Intercostal recession
- Use of accessory respiratory muscles
- Venous pulses
- Lymph nodes

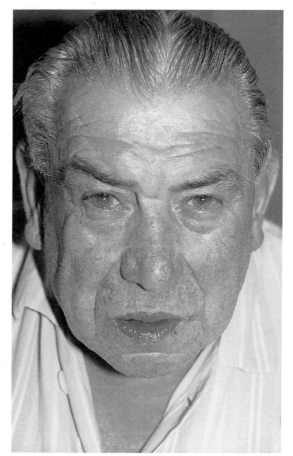

Fig. 7.4 Respiratory failure. The patient is breathless at rest and there is central cyanosis with blueness of the lips and face. The lips are pursed during expiration, a characteristic feature of chronic obstructive airways disease (COAD). This facial appearance is often accompanied by heart failure with peripheral oedema (cor pulmonale).

Inspection

SHAPE OF THE CHEST

The normal chest is bilaterally symmetrical and elliptical in cross-section. The chest may be distorted by disease of the ribs or spinal vertebrae as well as by underlying lung disease (Box 7.2).

> **BOX 7.2 Features to note in assessing the shape of the chest.**
>
> - Kyphosis
> - Scoliosis
> - Flattening
> - Over-inflation

Kyphosis (forward bending) or *scoliosis* (lateral bending) of the vertebral column will lead to asymmetry of the chest and may significantly restrict lung movement. Scoliosis may also lead to displacement of the trachea and apex beat. The spine and rib cage may become particularly immobile in ankylosing spondylitis.

Unilateral apical fibrosis, often secondary to tuberculosis, may produce obvious flattening of the affected side. Severe chronic airflow limitation (Fig. 7.5) often leads to an overinflated and barrel-shaped chest. The ribs are set less obliquely than normal and tend to move upwards because of the pull of the prominent accessory muscles of respiration.

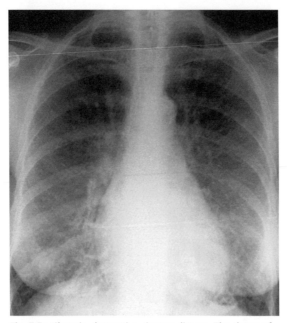

Fig. 7.5 Chronic obstructive airways disease. The shape of the diaphragm is low and flat. The lung fields are hyperinflated, translucent and the mediastinal outline is narrowed. There are areas of emphysema in the right mid and in both lower zones.

MOVEMENTS OF THE CHEST

The normal rate of respiration in a relaxed adult is about 14-16 breaths per minute (Box 7.3). It is seldom possible to count respiration rate accurately if the patient is aware this is being done, but if it is observed while the examiner appears to take the pulse, this usually gives an accurate assessment. It is seldom necessary to count the respiratory rate, although it can be of interest as a repeated nursing observation in some situations. An increased rate of respiration, *tachypnoea*, may be caused by nervousness, exertion, fever or hypoxia.

> **BOX 7.3 Measurements of the chest.**
>
> - Rate of respiration
> - Rhythm of respiration
> - Chest expansion
> - Symmetry

It is often useful to observe respiration during sleep. Some patients may have disorders of breathing during sleep which lead to complete cessation of respiratory effort (*central apnoea*), or continuation of respiratory effort due to obstruction of the upper airways by soft tissues in the region of the pharynx (*obstructive apnoea*), or a combination of the two conditions. In less severe examples there may be reduced ventilation (*hypoventilation*) or partially obstructed ventilation causing snoring. In order to determine the significance of these changes, detailed sleep studies measuring airflow, chest wall movements and blood gases are often necessary.

Cheyne–Stokes breathing is the name given to a disturbance of respiratory rhythm in which there is a gradual deepening and then diminishing respiratory effort and rate, sometimes associated with short periods of complete apnoea. This is often observed in severely ill patients and particularly in severe cardiac failure, narcotic drug poisoning, and neurological disorders (see Chapters 12 and 13).

Measurement of chest expansion is a traditional manoeuvre. It can be easily recorded with a tape measure around the chest at about the level of the nipples. In a fit young man the chest may expand 5–8 cm and in patients with severe emphysema it may expand less than 1 cm. As a measure of lung capacity, it is rather crude and it is better nowadays to perform proper measurements of lung function as well (see page 155).

Asymmetrical expansion of the chest may occur when the underlying lung is abnormal. A pleural effusion, pneumothorax, extensive consolidation or collapse, or fibrosis can all diminish expansion on the affected side. Other physical signs will also be present. A good test of the diaphragm is to ask the patient to sniff vigorously; this requires a sudden diaphragmatic contraction and patients with diaphragmatic weakness even if unilateral, cannot sniff normally (see page 159).

It is important to realize that observing depth and rate of breathing does not always give an accurate clue to the efficiency of breathing. It is quite possible for a patient to be underventilating the alveoli and inadequately oxygenating the blood even though breathing appears to be fast and deep. The ultimate assessment of the efficiency of the lungs depends on blood-gas analysis (see page 155).

Palpation

Before making a systematic examination, it is useful to palpate any part of the chest which presents an obvious *swelling*, or where the patient complains of pain (Box 7.4). Feel gently, as pressure may increase the pain. It is often important, particularly in the case of musculoskeletal pain, to identify a site of tenderness.

BOX 7.4 Points to note on palpation of the chest.

- Swelling
- Pain and tenderness
- Tracheal position
- Cardiac impulse
- Asymmetry
- Tactile vocal fremitus

Pain and tenderness may be due to:
- a recent injury of the chest wall or to inflammatory conditions;
- intercostal muscular pain where, as a rule, localized painful spots can be discovered on pressure;
- a painful costochondral junction;
- secondary malignant deposits in the rib;
- herpes zoster before the appearance of the eruption;
- pleurisy
- cardiac causes, such as myocardial infarction and pericarditis.

The nature of any swelling should be investigated. Fluctuation occurs when an abscess is formed in the chest wall.

The *positions* of the cardiac impulse and trachea should then be determined. Feel for the trachea in the suprasternal notch and decide whether it is central or deviated to one side by its relation to the suprasternal notch and the insertion of the sternomastoids. Avoid heavy-handedness in this situation as it is uncomfortable for the patient if the examiner is rough. A slight deviation of the trachea to the right may be found in healthy people.

Displacement of the cardiac impulse alone may be due to scoliosis (the commoner form, with convexity to the right causing a displacement of the cardiac impulse to the left and vice versa), to funnel depression of the sternum or to enlargement of the left ventricle. In the absence of these conditions a significant displacement of the cardiac impulse or trachea, or of both together, suggests that the position of the mediastinum has been altered by disease of the lungs or pleura. The mediastinum may be 'pushed' away from the affected side by a pleural effusion or pneumothorax. Fibrosis or collapse of the lung will 'pull' the mediastinum towards the affected side; in this condition, only the trachea is displaced.

The possibility of asymmetrical expansion of the chest may be further explored by palpation. If one faces the patient and places the fingertips of both hands on either side of the lower rib cage, so that the tips of the thumbs meet in the midline in front of but not touching the chest, then a deep breath by the patient will increase the distance between the thumbs and indicate the degree of expansion. If one thumb remains closer to the midline, this is confirmation of diminished expansion on that side.

Tactile vocal fremitus is detected by palpation but this is not a commonly used routine examination technique. It is discussed further under auscultation, below.

Percussion

Percussion is a useful technique and can be used to distinguish reliably between the presence of a pneumothorax and a pleural effusion when the physical signs may be otherwise identical (Box 7.5). At first it is worth practising on yourself or on colleagues, as percussion can be rather uncomfortable to the patient if performed repeatedly and inexpertly.

The middle finger (pleximeter finger) of the left hand is placed on the part to be percussed and the back of its middle phalanx is then struck with the tip

BOX 7.5 Points to note on percussion of the chest.

- Resonance
- Dullness
- Pain and tenderness

of the middle finger of the right hand. The movement should be at the wrist rather than the elbow and the percussing finger should be bent so that when the blow is delivered, its terminal phalanx is at right angles to the metacarpal bone and it strikes the pleximeter finger perpendicularly. As soon as the blow has been given, the striking finger must be raised, just as the hammers of a piano fall back from the wires as soon as they have been struck. The blow should be no heavier than is necessary to elicit the resonance of the part being examined and the wrist joint should move loosely. Repeated heavy blows cause discomfort to patients and can even fracture ribs.

The character of the sound produced varies qualitatively and quantitatively. When the air in a cavity of sufficient size and appropriate shape is set into vibration, a resonant noise is produced and there is also a characteristic feeling in the pleximeter finger. The sound and feel of resonance over a healthy lung has to be learnt by practice. In general it is of a low pitch and clear in character.

Some examiners tap with one finger directly on each clavicle before carrying out routine percussion. This will only yield an abnormality if there is gross difference between the two sides and is probably not worth while.

Always systematically compare the percussion note on two equivalent sides of the chest. It is usually sufficient to percuss three or four anterior areas comparing left with right, three or four areas on the back of the chest and two or three in the axillae. The

normal degree of resonance varies from individual to individual, and in different parts of the chest in the same individual, being most resonant below the clavicles and scapulae where the muscles are relatively thin, and least resonant over the scapulae. The lower limits of lung resonance should be determined by percussing from above downwards with the pleximeter finger parallel to the diaphragm. In quiet respiration and on light percussion, the lower border of the right lung lies in the mammary line at the sixth rib, in the mid-axillary line at the eighth rib and in the scapular line at the tenth rib. On heavier percussion some loss of resonance, due to the underlying liver and diaphragm, is found at higher levels and in the mammary line can be detected from the fourth interspace downwards.

On the left side, the lower border overlaps the stomach so there is a transition from lung resonance to tympanitic stomach resonance. Posteriorly, however, the splenic dullness and the dullness of the various solid structures which lie below the lung near the spine are interposed so that the sounds resemble those found on the right. The position of the lower border corresponds fairly closely with that on the right side although it may be slightly lower.

An increase in resonance, or hyperresonance, is difficult to detect. It may be noticeable when the pleural cavity contains air and the lung is collapsed towards the hilum, as in pneumothorax (Fig. 7.6). Sometimes, however, in this situation one is tempted to think that the slightly duller side is the abnormal

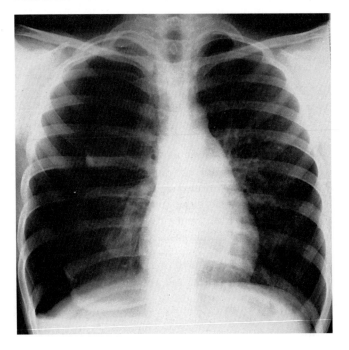

Fig. 7.6 Tension pneumothorax. Large translucent zone in the periphery of the right hemithorax with a collapsed lung lying underneath the heart. The tracheal outline is shifted over to the left. There is a small amount of fluid at the right costophrenic angle, probably owing to a small haemothorax.

side. Further examination and X-ray will reveal the true situation.

Reduction of resonance (dullness to percussion) occurs when the pleura is thickened, when the underlying lung is more solid than usual for any reason, and when the pleural cavity contains fluid. A feeling of resistance to the percussion blow within the finger used for tapping is usually found when there is underlying pleural fluid and this is often called 'stony dullness'. It is easier to detect a unilateral pleural effusion but, of course, effusions may occur bilaterally in many patients (Fig. 7.7).

Percussion is a useful part of chest examination

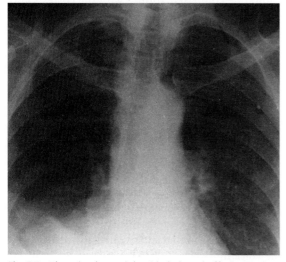

Fig. 7.7 There is a large right-sided pleural effusion and a small left-sided pleural effusion. The appearances were due to secondary effusions from a carcinoma of the breast.

and can usually be done speedily and without any discomfort to the patient. It is of course useful elsewhere, e.g. for percussing the spleen or liver edge, or in demonstrating ascites.

Auscultation

After having listened to the chest, the physician should be able to comment on the *character and intensity of the breath sounds, the presence or absence of any added sounds* and *the character of vocal resonance* (Box 7.6).

The patient should be in the usual position for examining the chest while one listens, usually with a stethoscope diaphragm, to the representative areas anteriorly, posteriorly and in the axillae. It is worth while demonstrating the type of breathing required. This is slightly deeper and faster than normal through the mouth, but if you simply ask the

---

> **BOX 7.6 Points to note on auscultation of the chest.**
>
> - Vesicular breath sounds
> - Bronchial breath sounds
> - Vocal fremitus and resonance
>   —bronchophony
>   —whispering pectoriloquy
>   —aegophony
>   Added sounds
>   —pleural rub
>   —wheezes
>   —crackles

patient to take deep breaths you may find a slow snorting inspiration followed by the breath being held is the result. It is usually better to help the patient to breathe correctly by demonstrating than to keep on saying alternately 'breathe in' and 'breathe out'.

BREATH SOUNDS

Breath sounds have *intensity* and *quality*. The intensity (or loudness) of the breath sounds may be normal, reduced or increased. The quality of the breath sounds is described as either *vesicular* or *bronchial*.

Breath sounds will be of normal intensity when the lung is inflating normally but will be reduced if there is localized airway narrowing, if the lung is extensively damaged by a process such as emphysema, or if there is intervening pleural thickening or pleural fluid. Breath sounds may be of increased intensity in very thin subjects. Bronchial breathing (see below) is often quite loud but it is entirely possible for breath sounds with a bronchial quality to be much quieter than the vesicular sounds heard elsewhere in the chest as, for example, when there is a pleural effusion overlying consolidation. Do not confuse loud breath sounds with bronchial breathing (see below).

Vesicular breath sounds probably originate in the larger airways and, when heard through normal lung, the attenuating and filtering effect of the lung produces rather quiet, low-pitched rustling sounds. There is usually no distinct pause between the end of inspiration and the beginning of expiration. When airway distortion is present, as in asthma, the slowing of expiration prolongs the normal exploratory sound.

Bronchial breath sounds probably originate from the same larger airways but when the lung between these airways and the chest wall is airless as a result of consolidation, collapse or fibrosis, the breath sounds are heard with relatively little loss by filtration and attenuation. The sound resembles that obtained by listening over the trachea, although the noise there is much louder. The quality of the sound is rather harsh and higher frequencies are heard. It becomes inaudible just before the end of inspiration, so that there is a gap before the expiratory sound is heard. The expiratory sound has a more sibilant character than the inspiratory one and lasts for most of the expiratory phase (Fig. 7.8).

The intensity and quality of all breath sounds is so

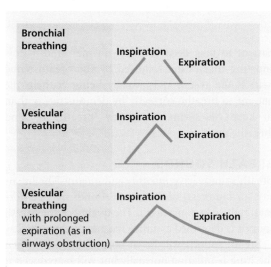

Fig. 7.8 Respiratory sounds. The diagram shows the pattern of inspiration and expiration.

variable from patient to patient and in different situations that it is only by repeated auscultation of the chest of many patients that one becomes familiar with the normal variations and learns to recognize the abnormalities.

VOCAL FREMITUS AND VOCAL RESONANCE

Vibration may be detected by palpation with the palm of the hand placed flat on the chest. The patient is then asked to repeat something like 'ninety-nine' in a clear normal voice. The examining hand perceives distinct vibrations when this is done and this is called *vocal fremitus*. One must determine whether the vibrations in corresponding areas on the two sides of the chest are approximately equal in intensity. Where the heart encroaches on the left lung the fremitus is much diminished. Vocal fremitus is increased when the lung is consolidated or contains a large cavity near the surface, diminished when the corresponding bronchi are obstructed, and totally absent when the lung is separated from the chest wall by pleural effusion or pneumothorax (Figs

7.6 and 7.7). In young persons and women the vocal resonance is different both in character and intensity from that in adult men.

Palpation for vocal fremitus is closely allied to listening to the intensity and character of *vocal resonance*. When the patient repeats 'ninety-nine', the ear perceives not the distinct syllables but a resonant sound, the intensity of which depends on the loudness and depth of the patient's voice and the conductivity of the lungs. The nearer the stethoscope is to a large bronchus, the more intense the sound.

Each point examined on one side of the chest should be compared at once with the corresponding point on the other side. Vocal resonance of normal intensity generally conveys the impression of being produced just at the chest piece of the stethoscope. If it seems to be nearer the ear than this, the resonance is increased. When it appears to be near the earpiece of the stethoscope the increase is marked; this is often described as *bronchophony*.

If the words become clear and seem to be spoken right into the listener's ear, it will generally be found that even whispered words are distinctly heard (*whispering pectoriloquy*). It is useful to ask the patient to whisper something different such as 'one, two, three'. Increased resonance occurs when the lung substance conducts the sound waves set up by the voice more clearly than usual from the bronchi. *Consolidation* is the commonest cause (see Fig. 7.20). Bronchophony and whispering pectoriloquy occur when a moderately large bronchus is surrounded by solid lung reaching to the chest wall, as in lobar pneumonia. Whispering pectoriloquy is also characteristic of a *cavity* of some size communicating with the bronchus, and it may be heard above the level of a pleural effusion. In some cases a certain degree of whispering pectoriloquy is heard in health, in the proximity of the trachea and large bronchi and, particularly, at the right apex.

Vocal resonance is either abolished or much diminished when a layer of fluid separates the lung from the chest wall (except when bronchial breathing is heard; see above) and in pneumothorax. It is also diminished in cases of thickened pleura and of emphysema.

Above the level of a pleural effusion or in some cases over an area of consolidation, the voice may sound nasal or bleating; this is known as *aegophony*.

ADDED SOUNDS

Added sounds are abnormal sounds that arise in the pleura or in the lung. Sounds resembling pleural friction rubs may be produced by movement of the stethoscope on the patient's skin or of the examiner's hands or clothes against the stethoscope. Sounds arising in the patient's muscles may resemble adventitious sounds; in particular the shivering of a cold patient makes any attempt at auscultation useless. The stethoscope rubbing over hairy skin may produce sounds resembling crepitations (fine crackles, see below). Crepitous sounds may occur in the region of a broken rib.

The *pleural rub* is characteristic of pleural inflammation and occurs at a stage when there is usually pain. It has a creaking or rubbing character and in some instances, is palpable. Coarse crepitations may sometimes be confused with a pleural rub, but unlike crepitations the rub does not change in character after coughing and the association with localized pain is usually characteristic.

Other added sounds arise in the lung. They should be referred to as *wheezes* and *crackles.* Older terms such as *rales* to describe coarse crackles, *crepitations* to describe fine crackles, and *rhonchi* to describe wheezes are poorly defined, have led to confusion, and are best avoided.

Wheezes are musical sounds associated with airway narrowing. The loudest most obvious wheeze is the stridor associated with laryngeal spasm or tracheal stenosis. The noise is often inspiratory and expiratory and it is usually fairly obvious that it originates from the upper airways. As one listens to the chest further away from the centre, the sound decreases.

A fixed *monophonic* wheeze can be generated by localized narrowing of a single bronchus, as may occur in the presence of a tumour or foreign body. It may be inspiratory or expiratory or both and may change in intensity with position.

Widespread *polyphonic wheezes* particularly heard in expiration are characteristic of diffuse airflow obstruction, especially in asthma and bronchitis. These wheezes are probably related to dynamic compression of the bronchi, which is accentuated in expiration when airway narrowing is present.

Sometimes, in spite of widespread airflow obstruction, patients do not wheeze. This paradoxical absence of wheezing can lead to misleading assessment of patients with severe asthma whose chest may become quiet when their asthma is at its worst. Presumably, when airway obstruction is severe the very low air flow rates generated do not produce any sounds and there may also be physical obstruction of small airways with viscid mucus.

Crackles are short, explosive sounds often described as bubbling or clicking noises. When the large airways are full of sputum, a coarse rattling sound may be heard even without the stethoscope. Crackles are not, however, usually produced by moistness in the lungs, even though this may seem to be the explanation in pulmonary oedema. It is more likely that they are produced by sudden changes in gas pressure related to the sudden opening of previously closed small airways.

Crackles during expiration at the beginning of inspiration are common in patients with airflow obstruction. The sounds are low-pitched, scanty and loud, and may clear with coughing. They are usually of very little diagnostic significance.

A series of inspiratory crackles at the end of inspiration is typical of pulmonary oedema and fibrosing alveolitis. They may also be heard on re-expansion of a previously deflated lung, as when there has been abdominal distension or with resolving pneumonia. Late inspiratory crackles heard particularly at the bases indicate delayed airway opening, as occurs when the lung is stiff in interstitial pulmonary fibrosis (fibrosing alveolitis) or when the small bronchi are oedematous, as in pulmonary oedema.

Sputum

When sputum is being produced, patients should always be asked to describe its appearance and amount. It is often best to ask the patient roughly how much they would bring up over 24 hours using a familiar measure, such as a tablespoon. Some patients, and particularly children, swallow sputum but usually they can describe whether or not it is yellow or green, or contains blood. Hospital inpatients should have a sputum pot and this must be inspected.

Mucoid sputum is characteristic in patients with chronic bronchitis when there is no active infection. It is clear and sticky and not necessarily produced in a large volume. A particularly tenacious form of mucoid sputum may be produced by asthmatics, and sometimes they cough up casts of the bronchial tree, particularly after an attack. Patients who have bronchopulmonary aspergillosis may bring up black sputum or sputum with black parts in it; this is the fungal element of the *Aspergillus* (Fig. 7.9).

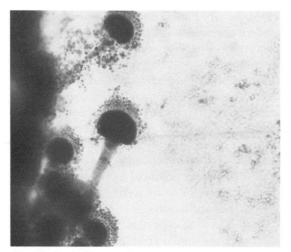

Fig. 7.9 *Aspergillus* spp. from bronchial aspirate, after culture on Saburaud's medium.

Sputum may become *mucopurulent* or *purulent* when infection is present, although occasionally there is a yellow tinge to sputum which has a lot of eosinophils in it in association with asthma (Box 7.7). Generally, however, purulent sputum indicates bacterial infection which may be part of bronchitis, pneumonia (see Fig. 7.20), bronchiectasis or a lung abscess (Fig. 7.10). In these last two conditions the quantities may be large and the sputum is often foul-smelling.

White or pink *frothy sputum* may be brought up by patients in gross pulmonary oedema (Fig. 7.11).

Blood may be coughed up alone or sputum may be more or less blood-stained. It is sometimes difficult for the patient to describe whether or not the blood

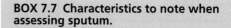

BOX 7.7 Characteristics to note when assessing sputum.

- Mucoid
- Purulent
- Frothy
- Blood-stained
- Rusty

has originated from the chest or whether it comes from the gums or nose, or even from the stomach. The patient should always be asked about associated conditions such as epistaxis, or the subsequent development of melaena, which occurs in the case of upper gastrointestinal bleeding. Usually, however, it is clear that the blood originates from the chest and in most patients this is an indication for further investigation, including chest X-ray and bronchoscopy if necessary. Pulmonary causes of haemoptysis include carcinoma (Figs 7.12 and 7.13(a) and (b)), tuberculosis (Fig. 7.14(a) and (b)), pulmonary embolus (Fig. 7.15) and bronchiectasis, or there may be a cardiac cause such as mitral stenosis.

In certain special circumstances the sputum can have a characteristic appearance. In lobar pneumonia it is classically rusty, small in quantity and very viscid. In the rare instance when a liver abscess ruptures into the lung, there may be bright yellow or green sputum. When an amoebic liver abscess discharges into the lung, the sputum is said to have the appearance of anchovy sauce. When sputum is particularly foul-smelling, the presence of anaerobic organisms must be considered.

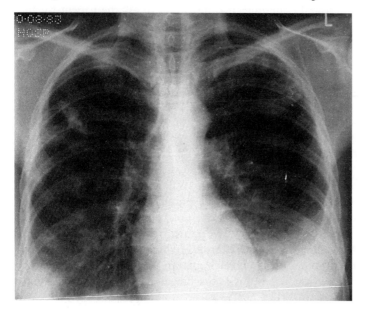

Fig. 7.10 There are multiple cavities in both lung fields with fluid levels throughout the upper mid and lower zones. There are also quite large pleural reactions. The appearances are those of multiple pulmonary pyogenic abscesses with involvement and reactive change of the pleura. The patient also has a confluent area of opacification in the left lower lobe consistent with a pneumonia.

Fig. 7.11 Cardiac failure. The heart is enlarged. There are some Kerley B lines present at both bases with some opacification in the mid zones and bases consistent with some interstitial oedema.

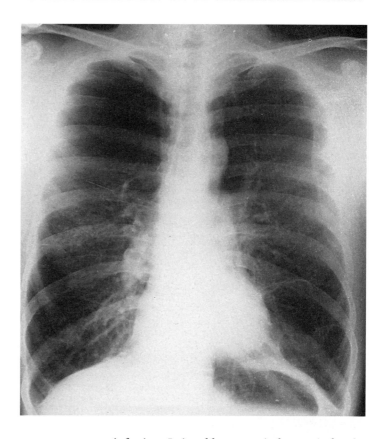

SPUTUM EXAMINATION

Sputum may be examined in the laboratory for the presence of pus cells and organisms and may be cultured in an attempt to identify the causative agent of

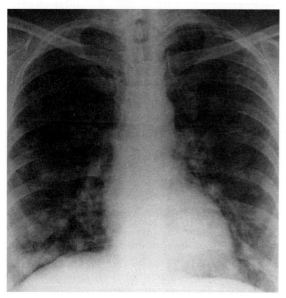

Fig. 7.12 Multiple pulmonary opacities throughout both lung fields. The opacities are variable in size and are well-defined. The appearances are typical for multiple secondaries.

an infection. It is seldom practical to wait for the results of such examinations and most clinical decisions have to be based on the clinical probability of a particular infection being present. A laboratory test may subsequently give useful confirmation or indicate unsuspected infections.

Sputum examination for malignant cells is useful in reaching a diagnosis of carcinoma of the lung. Special staining and subsequent culture for acid-fast bacilli is needed when tuberculosis is suspected.

Sometimes sputum is found to contain fungi, yeasts or the characteristic dumbbell-shaped asbestos bodies.

Lung function tests

The physiological function of the lung can be accurately determined by lung function testing. Many sophisticated tests are possible but even the simplest equipment can produce useful information. It is of particular value to perform lung function tests in order to give an objective assessment of lung performance. To attempt to treat diseases like asthma without performing even the simplest measures of lung function is analogous

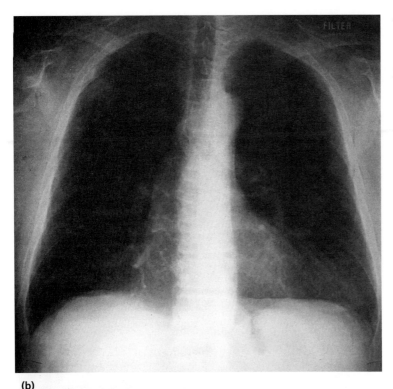

(a)

Fig. 7.13 (a) There is a space-occupying lesion lying in the upper outer aspect of the right upper lobe. The appearances must be presumed to be a primary carcinoma until proven otherwise. The rest of the lung fields appear translucent consistent with some underlying obstructive airways disease. The mediastinal and heart outlines appear normal. (b) CT scan—same patient. This cut through the mediastinum shows some pre-tracheal lymphadenopathy secondary to the space occupying lesion in the right upper lobe which was shown to be an adenocarcinoma of the lung. The example highlights the importance of CT in showing lymphadenopathy that is not detectable on plain X-ray.

(b)

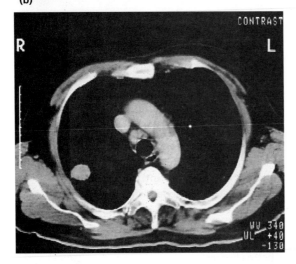

to treating hypertension without measuring blood pressure.

The commonest reason for performing a lung function test is to reach a diagnosis when a patient is complaining of breathlessness. In addition, these tests can be most useful for following the progress of a disease and for testing objectively the effects of treatment. It is of value to measure lung function prior to anaesthesia and surgery, particularly if thoracic surgery leading to lung resection is planned. Sometimes useful medicolegal information can be obtained from lung function tests.

SPIROMETRY

There are many types of spirometer available and all record similar information. Figure 7.16 shows the typical trace obtained by a deep inspiration followed by the fastest possible, and maximal, expiration. Trace (a) shows that the normal forced vital capacity (FVC) is fully exhaled in under 3 s; more than three-quarters is exhaled in the first second. In addition to measuring the vital capacity in litres, the volume expired in the first second, or the first expiratory volume at 1 s (FEV_1) can be measured and the ratio of FEV_1:FVC can be calculated. This is normally greater than 70%.

Trace (b) shows the findings when diffuse airflow obstruction is present. The rate at which the air can be exhaled is diminished throughout expiration. The length of expiration is prolonged and FEV_1 is much reduced. This is an *obstructive* pattern and is seen in asthma, chronic bronchitis and emphysema. In patients with asthma this obstruction may be reversible by treatment with bronchodilators or even corticosteroids.

Trace (c) shows a *restrictive* pattern. This patient has a reduced lung volume, perhaps as a result of pulmonary fibrosis or chest wall deformity, but there is no obstruction to airflow and FEV_1 is normal.

A popular instrument for assessing airflow obstruction is the peak flow meter (Fig. 7.17). There is

(a)

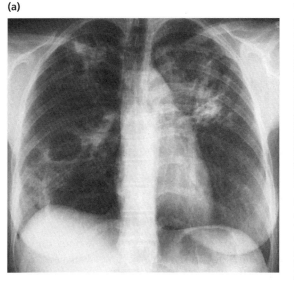

(b)

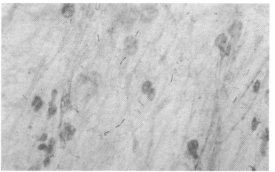

Fig. 7.14 (a) Chest X-ray. There is widespread opacification in both upper lobes with cavitation and further cavitation is seen in the apical segment of the right lower lobe. The appearances are those of a cavitating pneumonia and distribution is typical for tuberculous disease. (b) *Mycobacterium tuberculosis* seen as rods in Ziehl–Neelsen preparation of sputum.

a cheap, simpler version called the mini peak flow meter which is suitable for use at home by individual patients or for keeping in the doctor's bag. These machines measure the maximal rate of flow which is achieved during a forced expiration and most healthy people will achieve values of greater than 400 litres/min. Patients with lung fibrosis and restrictive changes on the spirogram may also have normal expiratory flow rates so the meter is not suitable for assessment of their disability. Patients with airflow obstruction will have reduced flow rates, with values below 200 litres/min being very significant, and those below 100 litres/min extremely severe.

Gas exchange function of the lungs

Normal gas exchange consists of the uptake of oxygen into the pulmonary capillary blood and the release of carbon dioxide into the alveoli. For this to be achieved, pulmonary ventilation and perfusion need to be reasonably anatomically matched and ventilation needs to be adequate. An approximation of the efficiency of the process of gas exchange may be obtained by measuring the pulmonary transfer

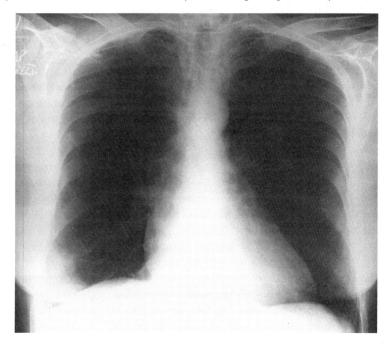

Fig. 7.15 Antero-posterior erect X-ray of chest. There is a wedge-shaped area of opacification in the right costophrenic angle in association with a pleural reaction. The patient had a large pulmonary infarct.

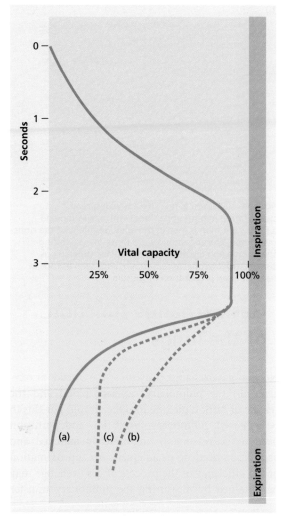

Fig. 7.16   The expiratory spirogram: (a) normal; (b) airway obstruction; (c) restriction (see text for explanation).

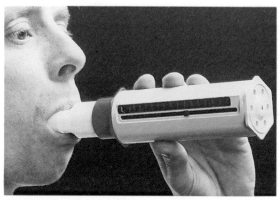

Fig. 7.17   A peak flow meter.

factor for carbon monoxide. A relatively simple single-breath technique can be used. Reduced values are found in patients with interstitial pulmonary fibrosis and pulmonary infiltrative diseases, such as sarcoidosis.

Blood gases

Arterial blood sampling is now widely performed and the advent of automated machines has made the technique routine in most hospitals. The partial pressures of oxygen (P_{O_2}) and of carbon dioxide (P_{CO_2}), and the pH, are measured in arterial blood. The P_{CO_2} is a measure of the effective ventilation of alveoli which are adequately perfused with blood so that efficient gas exchange can take place. This is called *alveolar ventilation* and, provided the rate of

production of carbon dioxide by the body remains constant, the arterial P_{CO_2} (P_{aCO_2}) will be directly related to the level of alveolar ventilation. The normal range is 4.7–6.0 kPa (34–45 mmHg). When alveolar ventilation is reduced, as may occur because of the effects of a sedative drug overdose or severe chronic obstructive bronchitis, then the P_{aCO_2} will rise. Conversely, a low P_{aCO_2} indicates an unusually high alveolar ventilation and may occur as a response to metabolic acidosis, in patients with pulmonary emboli, or in those who are very anxious.

Arterial P_{O_2} (P_{aO_2}) is normally in the range 11.3–14.0 kPa (80–100 mmHg). Breathing an atmosphere in which the partial pressure of oxygen is low, such as occurs at altitude, will cause hypoxia even in the presence of entirely normal lung function. Any lung disease which interferes with gas exchange may reduce arterial P_{O_2} and hypoxia also occurs in arteriovenous or cardiac abnormalities where venous blood is shunted through to the arterial circulation.

Since the advent of Système International (SI) units, it is easier to interpret blood gas measurements, provided that the percentage of oxygen in the inhaled air is known. The barometric pressure at sea level (P_B) is approximately 100 kPa and in atmospheric air which contains approximately 21% oxygen, the inspired P_{O_2} (P_{IO_2}) will be 21 kPa. Alveolar P_{O_2} (P_{AO_2}) will approximate to this value, reduced by the amount of CO_2 present in the alveoli. Thus, if the P_{IO_2} is 21 kPa and the P_{ACO_2} is 5 kPa then the P_{AO_2} will be approximately 16 kPa. The lung cannot be completely 100% efficient and there will always be a difference between the arterial P_{O_2} (P_{aO_2}) and the alveolar P_{O_2} (P_{AO_2}). This is known as the alveolar–arterial difference for oxygen—$(A\text{-}a)D_{O_2}$—and is usually less than 3.5 kPa. If there is significant disturbance of gas exchange function of the lung, then the $(A\text{-}a)Do_2$ will be increased and this can be approximately calculated at the bedside if blood gas results are available. Some examples will illustrate the principle.

EXAMPLE 1

A 24-year-old woman with severe myasthenia gravis, breathing room air (21% O_2), $PIo_2 = 21.0\,kPa$; $P_B = 100\,kPa$; $PAco_2 = 9.0\,kPa$: $Pao_2 = 9.0\,kPa$. Thus $(A\text{-}a)Do_2$ approximately equals $3.0\,kPa$.

Conclusions. $PAco_2$ is increased, so there is inadequate alveolar ventilation because of the muscle disease. Gas exchange function of the lung is normal (alveolar–arterial difference is less than $3.5\,kPa$) even though the patient is hypoxic. The hypoxia is associated with CO_2 retention.

EXAMPLE 2

A 50-year-old man with fibrosing alveolitis, breathing room air. $PIo_2 = 21.0\,kPa$; $PAco_2 = 5.0\,kPa$; $Pao_2 = 8.0\,kPa$. Thus $(A\text{-}a)Do_2$ approximately equals $8.0\,kPa$.

Conclusions. Alveolar ventilation is normal (normal $PAco_2$) but the patient is hypoxic because of abnormal gas exchange function of the lung (increased $(A\text{-}a)Do_2$).

EXAMPLE 3

A 30-year-old man with lobar pneumonia, inspired gas not known, $PAco_2 = 3.0\,kPa$; $Pao_2 = 15.0\,kPa$.

Conclusions. The patient is not hypoxic but has increased alveolar ventilation as shown by the low $PAco_2$. Gas exchange function cannot be assessed. In fact the patient was breathing 28% oxygen so PIo_2 was $28.0\,kPa$ and thus $(A\text{-}a)Do_2$ was $10.0\,kPa$, showing severe disturbance of gas exchange.

The pH of arterial blood is normally kept within the tight limits of 7.38–7.42 but may be altered by renal failure or ketoacidosis. A detailed discussion of acid–base balance is beyond the scope of this chapter.

Additional tests and overall assessment of cardiopulmonary function may be obtained by *exercise testing*. This is usually only carried out in specialized laboratories but a simple assessment of respiratory disability may be obtained by measuring the distance walked by the patient in 6 minutes. This '6-minute walk' is very reproducible when performed according to standardized procedures and has proved useful in assessing the success of rehabilitation programmes and other treatment.

Imaging techniques

Chest X-ray

The chest X-ray is an important extension of the clinical examination (Box 7.8). This is particularly so in patients with respiratory symptoms, and a normal X-ray taken some time before the development of symptoms should not be accepted as a reason for not performing an up-to-date film. In many instances it is of great value to have previous X-rays for the purposes of comparison but if these are lacking then careful follow-up with subsequent films may provide the necessary information.

BOX 7.8 Points to note when assessing the chest X-ray.

- Bony skeleton
- Position of the patient
- Position of the trachea
- Outline of heart
- Outline of mediastinum
- Diaphragm
- Lung fields

POSTEROANTERIOR VIEW

The standard chest X-ray is a posteroanterior view (PA) which is taken with the film against the front of the patient's chest and the X-ray tube 2 m behind the patient (Fig. 7.18). The X-ray is examined systematically on a viewing box according to the following plan:

The bony skeleton. Is the chest symmetrical? Is scoliosis present? Are the ribs unduly crowded or widely spaced in any area? Are cervical ribs present? Are any ribs eroded or absent?

The position of the patient. Is the patient straight or rotated? If straight, the inner ends of the clavicles will be disposed symmetrically with reference to the vertebral column. Any rotation will tend particularly to alter the appearance of the mediastinum and the hilar shadows.

The position of the trachea. This is seen as a dark col-

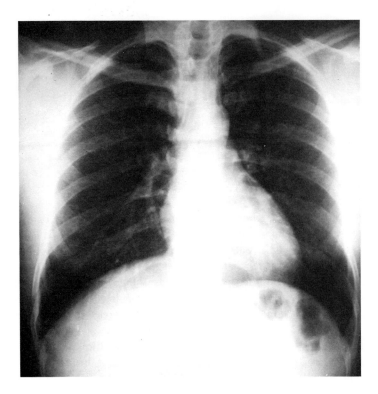

Fig. 7.18 Posteroanterior chest X-ray in a normal person. Note the position of the trachea, the size and shape of the heart and the relatively uniform appearance of the lung fields. The bony skeleton and diaphragm can be clearly seen. There is a little air in the stomach.

umn representing the air within the trachea. The cartilaginous rings are not visible. Is the trachea centrally placed or deviated to either side?

The outline of the heart and the mediastinum. Is this normal in size, shape and position?

The diaphragm. Can the diaphragm be seen on each side and is it normal in shape and position? Normally, the anterior end of the sixth or seventh rib crosses the mid-part of the diaphragm on each side, although the diaphragm on the right may be a little higher than on the left. Are the cardiophrenic angles clearly seen?

The lung fields. For radiological purposes, the lung fields are divided into three zones. The *upper zone* extends from the apex to a line drawn through the lower borders of the anterior ends of the second costal cartilages. The *mid-zone* extends from this line to one drawn through the lower borders of the fourth costal cartilages. The *lower zone* extends from this line to the bases of the lungs. Each zone is systematically examined on both sides and any area which appears abnormal is carefully compared with the corresponding area on the opposite side. The minor interlobar fissure, which separates the right, upper and middle lobes, may sometimes be seen running horizontally in the third and fourth interspace on the right side.

LATERAL VIEWS

Lateral views are most valuable in the localization of lung lesions and again it is useful to follow a plan of examination:

- first, the bone skeleton;
- secondly, the position of the trachea;
- thirdly, the diaphragm (as the level of the diaphragm differs on the two sides a double outline may be seen); and
- fourthly, the lung fields, which are obscured by two relatively opaque areas, one above and behind due to the shoulder joint, and one below and in front due to the heart which rests on the anterior part of the diaphragm. There are thus two relatively clear areas, one above and in front behind the upper part of the sternum and one below and behind including the angle between the diaphragm and the spine. In the lateral views the interlobar fissures are usually seen and their recognition is useful in localizing lesions and detecting shrinkage of a lobe from fibrosis or collapse.

SOME ABNORMALITIES
Pleural effusion

This appears as an opacity on the chest X-ray (Fig. 7.7) with a rising edge on the lateral chest wall. If fluid is not loculated, it can be demonstrated to move freely in the pleural cavity if a PA chest X-ray

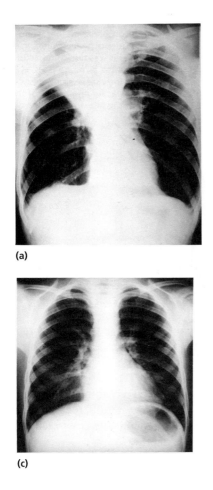

(a)

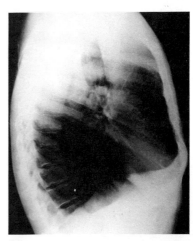

(b)

(c)

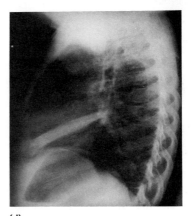

(d)

Fig. 7.19 Consolidation: (a) and (b) right upper lobe; (c) and (d) right middle lobe

is taken with the patient lying on the appropriate side.

Pneumothorax
The presence of air in the pleural cavity means that a clear lung edge can be seen (Fig. 7.6). Sometimes, as shown in Fig. 7.6, associated pleural fluid produces a horizontal air–fluid level at the base of the pleural cavity (*hydropneumothorax*).

Pneumonia
Consolidation may be in a lobe or segment (Fig. 7.19) or more diffuse throughout the lung, as in Fig. 7.20.

Sarcoidosis
The typical appearances of pulmonary sarcoidosis, with hilar lymph node enlargement and a nodular

appearance in the lung fields are shown in Fig. 7.21. In this disease a diffusion defect may occur as a result of the infiltration and fibrosis of lung tissue.

X-ray screening
This investigation is used to demonstrate paralysis of the diaphragm, which is usually caused by malignant involvement of the phrenic nerve. If a patient sniffs, the diaphragm should move downwards but in the case of diaphragmatic paralysis, the affected side moves upwards. Sometimes an indication can be obtained if screening is not practical by taking inspiratory and expiratory plain PA chest X-rays. At the bedside, if the patient cannot sniff, strongly suspect severe diaphragmatic weakness.

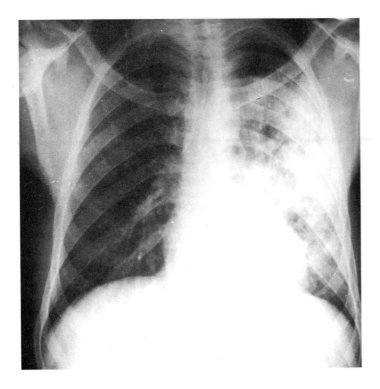

Fig. 7.20 Posteroanterior chest X-ray showing bronchopneumonia. There is patchy consolidation in the mid and lower zones of the left lung. In this patient this was due to tuberculosis. Note that the left lung is less well-expanded than the right, as shown by the more acute angulation of the rib cage on the left side.

Computerized tomographic imaging (CT)

The routine chest X-ray consists of shadows at all depths in the chest superimposed on one another. It has the disadvantage that not more than some 40% of the lung tissue is shown unobscured by shadows of the bony thorax or mediastinum. In CT scanning, X-rays are passed through the body at different angles and a computer is used to build up cross-sectional images at any chosen depth.

The particular value of CT imaging in chest disease is in revealing the presence of small malignant deposits within the lung which are not visible on the chest X-ray, showing pleura in much

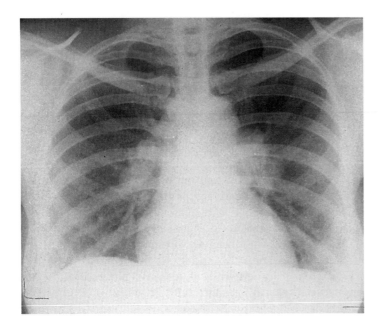

Fig. 7.21 There is a widespread bilateral perihilar bronchial wall thickening in association with faint reticular nodular shadowing and increased density in the mid zones in both bases. The diagnosis is sarcoidosis with widespread mediastinal and hilar lymphadenopathy and some interstitial changes affecting the lungs.

greater detail, and in enabling mediastinal structures to be more accurately demonstrated and delineated (Fig. 7.22).

Radioisotope imaging

Within the lung, the most widely used radioisotope techniques are *perfusion scanning* or combined *ventilation and perfusion scanning*. Radioisotope imaging is important in aiding the diagnosis of pulmonary embolism although the results must be interpreted in conjunction with the clinical situation. The typical symptoms of pulmonary embolism are breathlessness, pleuritic chest pain and haemoptysis, but these are not always all present. There may be no abnormal physical signs and, especially in the early stages, the chest X-ray may be normal. It is in this situation that lung perfusion scanning may be most useful.

A lung perfusion scan is performed by injecting intravenously a small dose of macroaggregated human albumin particles intravenously labelled with technetium-99m and subsequently taking a gamma-camera picture of the impacted particles in the lung (Fig. 7.23). When the distribution of perfusion is abnormal, additional information can be obtained by studying the distribution of ventilation; this can be shown using an inhalation of a radioactive gas, such as krypton-81m. Comparison of the pictures enables matching or mismatching of ventilation and perfusion defects to be observed.

If a patient has a normal chest X-ray and a normal lung perfusion scan within 24 hours of the suspected event, it is unlikely that pulmonary embolism has occurred. Sometimes there is difficulty in interpreting abnormal scans, since perfusion defects may arise not only from emboli but also due to regional abnormalities in ventilation, as is found in patients with asthma or chronic airflow obstruction. In these cases, however, the defect in ventilation and perfusion is often matched, although this may also occur when pulmonary embolism is present. Lung perfusion and ventilation scanning gives a probability estimate of pulmonary embolism having occurred, taking into account the clinical likelihood of the diagnosis being correct.

(a)

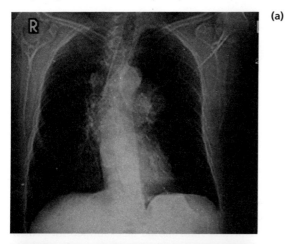

(b)

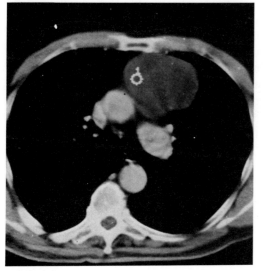

Fig. 7.22 (a) Mediastinal mass shown by CT reconstruction; posteroanterior view. (b) Dense anterior mediastinal mass shown on CT scan.

Ultrasound

Ultrasound is a valuable non-invasive method of assessing pleural fluid and tumours. Sometimes it is not clear from a chest X-ray whether basal shadowing consists of pleural fluid, pleural thickening or tumour, consolidation of the lung, or a combination of all three. A lateral decubitus X-ray may resolve the problem by demonstrating the presence of free fluid, but if this is insufficient then ultrasound examination in a number of positions can show the extent of fluid, whether or not it is loculated, and the locations of associated pleural and pulmonary changes.

Magnetic resonance imaging (MRI)

MRI is useful in demonstrating mediastinal abnormalities but it has few advantages over CT imaging in the evaluation of pulmonary disease.

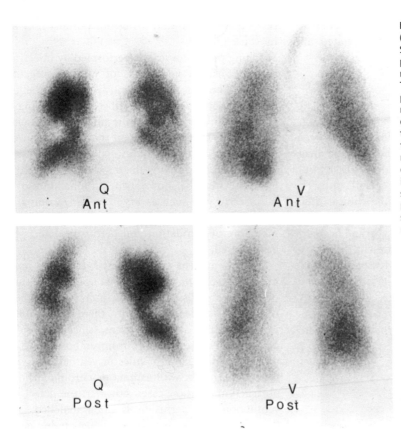

Fig. 7.23 Ventilation (V)/perfusion (Q) isotope scan of the lungs. Segmental and subsegmental loss of perfusion (left) can be seen with relatively normal ventilation (right). The clear punched-out areas in the perfusion (Q) scans indicate areas of reduced isotope concentration during the perfusion scan. Thus these are areas of reduced blood flow. The ventilation scans show normal aeration of the lungs as depicted by the isotope distribution in the pulmonary airways. These sequences of scans are suggestive of pulmonary embolism because they show impaired perfusion with normal ventilation.

Pleural aspiration and biopsy

A pleural effusion can give rise to diagnostic problems and sometimes management problems when the amount of fluid causes respiratory embarrassment. When a pleural effusion is seen as a presenting feature in a middle-aged or older patient, the most likely cause is carcinoma. Less commonly, particularly in younger patients, it may be due to tuberculosis. In either case the diagnosis is best obtained by aspiration and pleural biopsy. Aspiration alone has a lower incidence of accuracy.

A useful technique of pleural biopsy is to use an *Abram's pleural biopsy needle.* This can be inserted under local anaesthesia posteriorly or laterally whilst the patient is in a comfortable sitting position, resting their arms and head on an over-bed tray. The needle should be inserted a little below the upper edge of maximum dullness using local anaesthesia and a small sharp-pointed scalpel incision to aid passage of the needle through the skin and muscle. This needle can be used to aspirate up to 1 litre of fluid in order to obtain samples and relieve symptoms. Before all the pleural fluid present has been aspirated, samples of the pleura can be taken and sent for histological examination.

The pleural fluid should be examined for protein content. A transudate resulting from cardiac or renal failure can be distinguished from an exudate, usually resulting from pleural inflammation, by its lower protein content (less than 30 g/litre). Frankly blood-stained effusions occur with carcinoma, pulmonary infarction, trauma and sometimes tuberculosis. More commonly, however, in tuberculous effusions the fluid is straw-coloured and has a high protein content. The fluid should also be examined for cell content. Many polymorphs may be seen if fluid is secondary to an underlying pneumonic infection. With tuberculosis the fluid usually contains many lymphocytes. Tubercle bacilli are rarely seen, and even in biopsy-proven cases of tuberculous pleural effusion they may only be cultured in less than 20% of cases. Cytological examination of pleural fluid may demonstrate the presence of malignant cells.

In empyema pus is present in the pleural cavity; this pus has a characteristic appearance and will be full of white cells and organisms.

Thoracoscopy

This technique enables the pleural cavity to be directly examined and biopsies to be taken under direct vision. The procedure is commonly performed under a general anaesthetic by a surgeon who uses a rigid thoracoscope after the lung has been deflated. More recently flexible thoracoscopes have been developed which can sometimes be used under local anaesthetic but this technique is only available in specialized centres.

Pleurodesis

Where pleural fluid is troublesome and causing breathlessness, as is often the case in patients with large malignant pleural effusions, it may be useful to perform pleurodesis. In some patients with extensive carcinoma the pleural effusion may be a terminal event but in patients with breast carcinoma there is commonly prolonged survival after treatment of malignant pleural effusion and effective pleurodesis is very worth while.

The best technique is to insert a size 16 plastic catheter into the chest under local anaesthesia and either slowly or intermittently drain the pleural fluid over 24 hours or longer. When the pleural cavity is dry, an agent such as tetracycline (500 mg) can be instilled through the tube and, after a period of clamping, the pleural cavity can again be drained and sucked completely dry, using a suitable vacuum pump. The tube can subsequently be removed; this technique usually produces an 85% success rate in preventing the recurrence of the pleural fluid.

Pneumothorax

When air leaks into the pleural space spontaneously, as commonly occurs in otherwise fit young people, or as a result of an injury with puncture of the lung, a pneumothorax develops. This may require treatment. It is often worth while in the first instance aspirating up to 1 litre of air from the pneumothorax using a small plastic cannula and a 50-ml syringe with the three-way tap connected to an underwater seal. The best position for aspiration of an uncomplicated pneumothorax is with the patient sitting back at an angle of about 45 degrees; the needle is inserted in the second intercostal space in the mid-clavicular line. This technique is successful in many patients and avoids the need for an intercostal drain. If it does not work, however, an intercostal drain must be inserted in the same position and connected to an underwater seal until there has been complete re-expansion.

Bronchoscopy

When an abnormal shadow is detected on the chest X-ray or if the patient has haemoptysis with a normal X-ray, bronchoscopy may be indicated. Normally this is done by the technique of fibre-optic bronchoscopy. The flexible bronchoscope can be passed transnasally in the conscious patient with the help of local anaesthesia. Any endobronchial abnormality can be visualized and biopsies taken using small flexible forceps. In addition, cytological brushing techniques can be performed and specimens of bronchial secretions obtained for microbiological and cytological examination.

The forceps can also be used for obtaining small samples of lung by the technique of transbronchial biopsy. This is particularly useful in diagnosing patients with sarcoidosis.

Useful information about the nature of lung infiltrates can be obtained by broncho-alveolar lavage. For this procedure the bronchoscope is wedged in a bronchus supplying one segment of the lung and a quantity of saline instilled and then removed via the bronchoscope suction channel. The subsequent handling and interpretation of these specimens requires histological examination by a cytopathologist (Fig. 7.24).

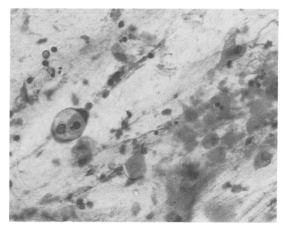

Fig. 7.24 Sputum cytology. A squamous pearl and numerous anucleate abnormal keratinized squamous cells in sputum from a patient with squamous cell carcinoma of the lung. Haematoxylin and eosin. × 160.

Lung biopsy

In addition to obtaining small samples of lung, the technique of transbronchial biopsy can, in conjunction with X-ray screening, be used to biopsy small lesions not in direct vision through the bronchoscope. Solid lesions or cavitating lesions of this type may more usefully be biopsied using a fine aspiration needle. This is inserted percutaneously under X-ray or computerized tomography control.

Rarely it may be necessary to perform a thoracotomy in order to elicit the exact nature of an abnormality but this decision should only be taken after weighing up all the relative risks and benefits.

Immunological tests

Sometimes asthma is related to the development of type I hypersensitivity to certain allergens and part of the assessment of such patients may include skin prick tests. Bronchial provocation tests are used in certain circumstances by specialized laboratories.

The delayed type of hypersensitivity (type IV) is shown by the Mantoux and Tine tests used to detect the presence of sensitivity to tubercular protein.

Precipitating antibodies are present in patients with some fungal diseases, such as bronchopulmonary aspergillosis or aspergilloma. In patients suspected of having an allergic alveolitis antibodies may be demonstrated to the relevant antigens. Immunoglobulin E levels are often raised in patients with asthma.

Typical clinical patterns

Some examples of typical patterns of clinical presentation should help to pull together the symptoms discussed at the beginning of this chapter.

Intermittent breathlessness with wheeze. Asthma may present at any age but is commoner in children. A history of breathlessness on exertion with or without wheezing, or attacks at night should suggest asthma. Exposure to dust or fumes and exertion in cold air will all provoke an attack and asthma is often troublesome at night and disturbs sleep. In older patients this needs to be distinguished from orthopnoea associated with heart disease.

Long-standing breathlessness. A middle-aged patient may come to the doctor complaining of breathlessness on exertion, often associated with a long history of a productive cough, particularly in the winter. On pressing for more history one can often discover that breathlessness has been present for several years, but has only recently become intrusive on the patient's lifestyle. Chronic obstructive bronchitis has this type of insidious onset and can usually be confirmed on clinical examination. If the history genuinely is only for a few weeks or a few months and there is little past history of any respiratory problem, then late-onset asthma needs to be considered.

Haemoptysis in the middle-aged or elderly patient. This should always be considered as suggesting carcinoma of the lung. If the patient is a smoker this is a very likely diagnosis, although full investigations have to be undertaken. A normal chest X-ray does not exclude a carcinoma and bronchoscopy is usually needed as well to rule out this diagnosis.

Haemoptysis in a younger patient. Particularly if associated with pleuritic pain and breathlessness, this should suggest pulmonary embolism. A detailed history will usually reveal the appropriate risk factors, and although the diagnosis can be elusive clinically, it can often be confirmed by special investigations.

A persistent dry cough. A dry cough persisting for many weeks after an apparently simple cold or influenza usually indicates the development of bronchial hyperreactivity. This is common in people with a history of hay fever or those with a family history of asthma.

Increasing breathlessness. Gradually increasing breathlessness over several months, sometimes associated with a dry cough, suggests an interstitial lung disease. Physical signs will vary with the cause and full investigation is usually required.

Snoring or sleep apnoea. Sometimes patients present with a history of snoring or stopping breathing at night. The history is usually given by their sleeping partner, rather than themselves, although they may complain of daytime drowsiness caused by poor sleep quality. Over-weight, middle-aged patients can develop upper airway obstruction during sleep which, in extreme cases, can cause profound hypoxia with cerebral and cardiac damage. The more extreme cases of sleep disordered breathing are unusual, but milder versions may occur and investigation is indicated if daytime drowsiness is a problem.

CHAPTER 8

The cardiovascular system

Introduction

Clinical assessment of the cardiovascular system requires a rational approach in order to analyse the available information in a coherent manner. In each patient the clinician must integrate:
- the facts available from the history;
- the examination and investigations

to reach a conclusion about:
  —the structure and function of the heart, and —the pulmonary and systemic vascular trees.

In this respect, the clinical approach to the cardiovascular system has many similarities with the approach to the nervous system.

General considerations

Careful assessment of the arterial and venous pulses and of the precordial impulse should always precede auscultation of the heart. Many students give insufficient time and attention to these features of the cardiovascular examination. The detection of abnormalities in these areas not only provides valuable evidence about the nature of any cardiac abnormality, but often provides valuable information on the functional severity of any lesion which may be present. Thus, by the time the examiner has reached the stage of auscultation, the salient points of the history and examination frequently suggest findings which may then be detected by stethoscope. By contrast, the beginner's mind may be so filled with anxiety at the thought of failing to hear some unspecified sound that no logical analysis of the auscultatory abnormalities is made. When auscultating the heart it is important to have some idea what abnormalities you expect to hear.

For these reasons it is best to examine the cardiovascular system in the following order:
- Arterial pulses
- Blood pressure
- Venous pulses
- Precordium
- Auscultation.

However, before proceeding to this examination certain general points should be noted.
- *Anaemia*, often recognized by pale mucous membranes, is an important cause of angina.
- Right ventricular failure or other causes of a raised right atrial pressure, such as constrictive pericarditis or tricuspid stenosis, may lead to an *enlargement of the liver* and *ascites*.
- The location of *oedema* depends on the patient's posture. It is always more apparent in dependent parts so that, in a relatively mobile patient, it is most easily detected by pressure over the distal end of the tibia. However, in the patient confined to bed, oedema will tend to collect over the sacrum and the dorsal spine. If the patient is lying in the supine position, oedema can be easily overlooked if it is not specifically sought.
- The presence of *finger-clubbing* in association with *central cyanosis* suggests there is a right-to-left shunt at the intracardiac or intrapulmonary levels.
- In patients with infective endocarditis, finger-clubbing and *splenomegaly* may be present.
- Microvascular embolic phenomena, probably due to antigen–antibody reactions, are manifest by *splinter haemorrhages* in the nailbeds of the fingers and toes, and small petechial haemorrhages in the conjunctivae.
- Larger emboli, probably fragments of vegetations from an infected valve, may present as painful erythematous lumps in the pulps of the fingers and toes,

palms of the hands and soles of the feet (*Osler's nodes*).
- The equivalent phenomena in the retinal circulation, seen on examination of the optic fundi, are called *Roth's spots*.
- Patients with left ventricular failure may be *breathless* at rest to the extent that they cannot complete a sentence without pausing for breath. In these patients *crepitations* (page 151) can often be detected at the lung bases.

Anatomical landmarks

The *precordium* is the term used to indicate the anterior aspect of the chest wall which overlies the heart. It is often convenient to refer to a point on the chest wall, and certain landmarks, some natural and some artificial, are commonly used for this purpose.

The ribs form convenient horizontal landmarks. In order to count them, feel for the ridge which marks the junction of the manubrium with the body of the sternum, known as the angle of Louis, or sternal angle. When this has been found, run the finger outwards until it reaches the second costal cartilage, which articulates with the sternum at this level. The space immediately above this is the first intercostal space. The spaces should then be counted downwards, well away from the sternum, as they are more easily felt here.

The distance of any given point from the midline of the body may be defined in relation to a series of vertical lines. These are the *mid-clavicular* line, defined as the vertical line dropped from the centre of the clavicle or, what amounts to the same thing, the line midway between the middle of the suprasternal notch and the tip of the acromion; and the *anterior*, *mid-*, and *posterior axillary lines*, descending respectively from the anterior border, the centre and the posterior border of the axilla.

Arterial pulses

The presence or absence of the main peripheral arterial pulses (Box 8.1) should be noted and the volume of each pulse compared with the other side.

The arterial pulses are detected by gently compressing the vessel against some firm underlying structure, usually bones.

- The *radial* pulse is felt with the tips of the fingers compressing the vessel against the head of the radius. The patient's forearm should be slightly pronated and the wrist slightly flexed.
- The *brachial* artery is compressed against the humerus just above the antecubital fossa. The examiner should use either the left thumb or right fingertips when examining the patient's right brachial artery.
- The *carotid* may be gently compressed against the transverse processes of the cervical vertebrae. This should always be done carefully in case there is underlying atheroma or hypersensitivity of the carotid sinuses which may cause bradycardia or even syncope. The volumes of peripheral pulses may be compared by simultaneous palpation, but the two carotid pulses should never be examined together because of the danger of critically reducing the cerebral arterial supply. The patient's right carotid is best examined with the left thumb and the left carotid with the right thumb.
- The *femoral* arteries lie midway between the iliac crest and the pubic ramus. In the absence of disease these pulses are relatively easily palpated against the underlying femur.
- The *popliteals* are the most difficult pulses to detect. They are best examined with the patient's knees flexed at an angle of 120 degrees. The fingertips of both hands are placed in the popliteal fossae with the thumbs resting on the patient's patallae.
- The *posterior tibial* pulse is found 1 cm behind the medial malleolus of the tibia. The patient's foot should be relaxed between plantar and dorsi-flexion.
- The *dorsalis pedis* pulse is compressed against the tarsal bones; the patient's left dorsalis pedis is most easily examined with the fingers of the right hand. If the right dorsalis pedis is of diminished volume it is often easiest to detect it by examining the patient from the left side, with the examiner using the fingertips of the right hand.

The following observations should then be made with regard to cardiac function:

- Rate of pulse
- Rhythm of pulse
- Character of pulse
- Volume of pulse
- Presence or absence of delay of the femoral pulses compared with the radials
- The peripheral vessels and circulation.

To assess the rate and rhythm, the radial pulse is generally used. When the character and volume of the arterial pulse are being analysed, one should examine the *carotid* artery, which is the closest pulse to the ascending aorta; here, modifications to the waveform by the vessels of the peripheral arterial system are kept to the minimum.

The blood pressure cannot be measured accurately without a sphygmomanometer (page 169). The terms 'good', 'strong' and 'weak' in relation to the pulse lack precision and should be avoided.

Rate

The rate of the pulse is noted in beats per minute. It should be counted, not when the fingers are first laid upon the pulse, but when any tachycardia due to nervousness in the patient has subsided and the pulse has resumed its normal rate. It is therefore good practice to feel the radial pulse gently, while eliciting the routine parts of the history. Count the beats for not less than half a minute.

In atrial fibrillation, the pulse rate counted at the wrist will not indicate the true rate of ventricular contraction and in such cases, the rate of the heart beat should be counted by auscultation at the apex, and the difference between this rate and the pulse rate at the wrist recorded. This difference is referred to as the *pulse deficit* and is explained as follows. Atrial fibrillation is characterized by a varying length of diastole. When diastole is short, filling of the left ventricle may be so poor that in the subsequent systole there is insufficient stroke volume to cause opening of the aortic valve. The arterial pulse is therefore non-existent. As diastole becomes longer, the stroke volume gradually increases; a pulse might be recorded in the central aorta, yet not be sufficiently large to reach the periphery at the radial artery. Following a long diastole (a slower heart rate) the strength of the subsequent systolic stroke volume is increased. In patients with arterial fibrillation, the potentially rapid ventricular response is the feature which causes most embarrassment to cardiovascular function. Particular attention should therefore be directed to accurate determination of the ventricular rate by auscultation at the apex. For the reasons

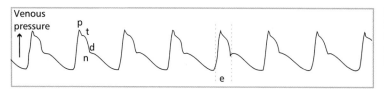

Fig. 8.1 A normal arterial pulse tracing. p = percussion wave; t = tidal wave; d = beginning of diastole; n = dicrotic notch; e = period of ventricular systole (aortic valve open).

given above, the radial pulse will have a variable stroke volume and so cannot be accurately counted, especially at fast rates. The apical rate is therefore a much more useful and accurate clinical observation than the pulse deficit. In atrial fibrillation the pulse deficit inevitably increases in proportion to the ventricular rate because of the consequent shortening of diastole.

The resting heart rate shows considerable variation, ranging between 50 and 120 beats per minute. The parasympathetic and sympathetic components of the autonomic nervous system have a major effect on heart rate. The pulse rate is increased by exercise, fever and in thyrotoxicosis. It is also increased in abnormal tachyarrhythmias. Regular athletic training and myxoedema are the commonest causes of bradycardia. Abnormalities of function of the sinus or atrioventricular nodes may reduce the heart rate to below 50 beats per minute.

Rhythm

Decide next whether the rhythm is regular or irregular. If it is irregular, decide if it is completely irregular, whether the irregularity has a recurring pattern, or whether an otherwise regular rhythm is occasionally interrupted by some slight irregularity. The pulse of *atrial fibrillation* is completely irregular. The irregularity is usually obvious when the rate is rapid, but becomes less easy to recognize when the rate has been slowed by digitalis. If the rhythm has a recurring pattern, or there are occasional irregularities, these are likely to be due to extrasystoles. An *extrasystole* is a beat which occurs prematurely, is therefore of reduced volume and is followed by a lengthened diastole—clinically appreciated as a 'pause'. Disorders of rhythm are described more fully under the section on electrocardiography (page 189).

Character

Study the character or form of the arterial pulse wave (Fig. 8.1) by palpation of the carotid pulse. This is best felt with the thumb, pressing backwards at the medial border of the sternomastoid at the level of the thyroid cartilage. It is not usually possible to detect slight variations from the normal, but in certain diseases the character of the arterial pulse is detectably abnormal. The most important of these are as follows.

Slow rising pulse. The arterial pulse in aortic stenosis (Fig. 8.2) is typically *parvis et tarsus*—of small volume with a large systolic peak. A thrill may be palpable in the carotid pulse and with practice the 'slow rising' characteristic can be appreciated. This slow rising pulse used to be known as an anacrotic pulse.

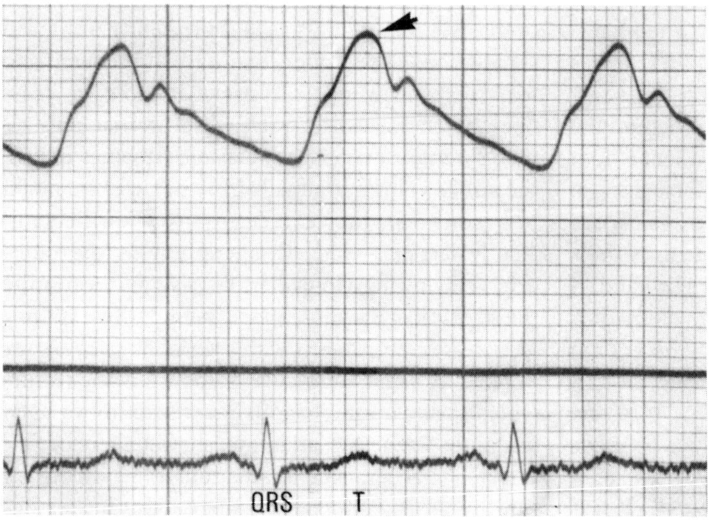

Fig. 8.2 A pressure recording from the aorta in a patient with aortic stenosis. The upstroke of the pressure pulse is slow and its peak (*arrow*) is delayed compared with the normal arterial pulse (Fig. 8.1). The onset of systole is indicated by the QRS complex on the electrocardiogram tracing beneath the pressure pulse.

QRS   T

Collapsing (water-hammer) pulse. A collapsing pulse is characterized by a rapid upstroke and descent of the pulse wave. It characteristically occurs in aortic regurgitation. The abrupt upstroke is due to the greatly increased stroke volume. The collapsing character is caused by two factors: first, the diastolic 'run-off' into the left ventricle; and secondly, the rapid run-off to the periphery because of a low systemic vascular resistance. This type of pulse will also be found with patent ductus arteriosus, ruptured sinus of Valsalva or large arteriovenous communications.

Bisferiens pulse. This is a combination of the low rising and collapsing pulses occurring when aortic stenosis and incompetence are present.

Pulsus paradoxus. When the left ventricle is severely diseased it characteristically develops alternating strong and weak beats. This variation in the strength of the pulse may be detectable clinically, and should not be confused with an arrhythmia.

Volume

Estimate the volume of the pulse. This gives a rough guide to the *pulse pressure*, which depends on the stroke volume and the compliance of the stroke volume. With normal vessels the pulse volume gives an indication of the stroke volume. In older subjects the vessels are more rigid (less compliant), causing a widened pulse pressure for the same stroke volume.

Delay

Delay of the femoral compared with the right radial pulse is found in coarctation of the aorta.

Measurement of the blood pressure

Korotkoff sounds

The Korotkoff sounds may be heard by placing a stethoscope over the brachial artery while the pressure in an occlusion cuff around the upper arm is gradually reduced. The *first* sounds that occur (phase one) indicate the peak systolic pressure. The *second* and *third* phases are due to the turbulent flow of blood through a partially occluded vessel. The *fourth* phase occurs when the sounds become muffled and the *fifth* phase is when they disappear. The fourth phase is 7–10 mmHg above the diastolic pressure recorded directly by an intra-arterial needle, whereas the fifth phase corresponds more accurately to true diastolic pressure. In individual patients, however, the fourth phase may be detected with greater precision than the fifth phase. When recording the diastolic pressure both phases should be noted and recorded if they have been clearly heard.

The sphygmomanometer

Certain details are important in the use of the sphygmomanometer. The patient should be sitting or lying at ease. The manometer is placed so as to be at the same level as the cuff on the patient's arm and the observer's eye. All clothing should be removed from the arm. The cuff should be applied closely to the upper arm, with the lower border not less than 2.5 cm from the cubital fossa.

The radial pulse is palpated while the cuff is inflated to a pressure of 30 mmHg above the level at which radial pulsation can no longer be felt. The stethoscope is then placed lightly over the brachial artery. The pressure in the cuff is lowered, 5 mmHg at a time until the first sounds are heard. This is the systolic pressure. Continue to lower the pressure in the cuff until the sounds suddenly become faint. This is the diastolic pressure (fourth phase). Continue to reduce the pressure and between 1 and 10 mmHg lower the sounds disappear completely (fifth phase).

Occasionally the sounds disappear at a point below 200 mmHg for a period and then reappear, finally disappearing at the point of diastolic pressure. Thus the sounds may first appear when the mercury falls to 210 (systolic pressure), disappear from 180–160 (silent gap), reappear and then finally disappear at 120 mmHg (diastolic pressure). This phenomenon of a silent gap is found in certain patients with hypertension; its significance is unknown, but its occurrence makes it important that at the start of the examination the armlet pressure should always be sufficient to obliterate the radial pulse.

The systemic and arterial pressure is significantly affected by exertion, anxiety, excitement and changes in posture. It should therefore be observed when the patient has been resting quietly. Check that the width of the cuff is correct. For an adult, the standard cuff width is 12 cm. If a narrower cuff is used, the recorded pressures will be falsely high. In obese patients it is essential to use a wider cuff such as a thigh cuff to measure the occlusion pressure in the upper arm. Indeed, it has been recommended that a cuff of 15 cm should be used as the standard adult size. In nervous patients the first reading is often too high; a second reading when the patient has become accustomed to the procedure and is more relaxed may be more representative. It is useful to note the pulse rate at the same time, as circulating catecholamines will affect both measurements. An elevated pulse rate in the presence of an elevated blood pressure suggests that some of the 'hypertension' is due to a temporary increase in circulating adrenaline and noradrenaline levels.

It is essential to work as quickly as is compatible with accuracy, for compression of a limb in itself induces a rise in blood pressure. To reduce this source of error when successive estimations are made, the air pressure in the armlet should always be allowed to fall to zero as soon as each reading has been taken. It is important to measure the blood pressure in patients taking hypotensive drugs or otherwise suspected of postural hypotension in both the recumbent and the standing positions.

For children, there are a variety of cuffs of different widths. Select the size which covers most of the upper arm but leaves a gap of 1 cm below the axilla and above the antecubital fossa. In suspected coarctation of the aorta it may be useful to compare the systolic blood pressure in the arm with that in the leg; the patient lies face downwards and an 18 cm cuff is applied above the knee and auscultation is carried out over the popliteal artery.

NORMAL BLOOD PRESSURE

Average systolic pressure in healthy adults is 100–140 mmHg and average diastolic pressure is 60–90 mmHg. In children it is closer to the lower end of the scale, and in the elderly it reaches or even exceeds the higher figure. The difference between the systolic and diastolic pressures—the blood pressure—is 30–60 mmHg.

ABNORMAL BLOOD PRESSURE

Abnormal blood pressure must be considered in relation to the patient's age. A blood pressure of 140 over 90 would indicate quite severe hypertension in a child while much higher systolic pressures in an elderly patient are inevitable due to loss of elasticity in the peripheral arterial system. The increased rigidity due to degenerative changes (arteriosclerosis) causes the systolic pressure peak to be particularly elevated.

The venous pulse

The neck veins

The importance of studying the level of pressure in the internal jugular veins lies in the fact that these vessels are usually in direct communication with the right atrium. In this way the pressure changes within the heart may be predicted by simple clinical observation. It may be easier to recognize the pulsation in the external jugular veins than in the internal jugular system, but using the former is a less reliable means of predicting pressure changes in the right atrium. There are two reasons for this. First, the presence of venous valves within the external jugular system prevents it being a pure conductor of more central pressure changes. Secondly, the external jugular system passes through more fascial planes than the internal system and so is more likely to be affected by extrinsic compression from other structures in the neck and upper thorax.

The venous pulse (Fig. 8.3) has three positive waves, *a*, *c* and *v*, and two negative waves or descents, *x* and *y*. The *a* wave is due to atrial contraction. This is followed by the *x* descent, which is interrupted by a small *c* wave (rarely visible on inspection of the neck veins). The *c* wave coincides with the onset of ventricular systole and results from the movement of the tricuspid valve ring into the right atrium as the right ventricular pressure rises. The *v*

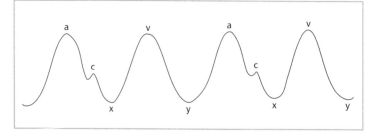

Fig. 8.3   The normal venous pulse (see text for explanation).

wave indicates a passive rise in pressure as venous return to the atrium continues during ventricular systole while the tricuspid valve is closed. When the tricuspid valve opens, blood enters the right ventricle rapidly and there is consequently a lowering of the right atrial pressure—the *y* descent.

Examination

Examine the neck veins with the patient in a good light, and reclining at an angle of about 45 degrees (Fig. 8.4). The neck should be supported so that the neck muscles, especially the sternomastoids, are relaxed. In younger patients it is often possible to detect the normal atrial pulsations—*a*, *c* and *v* waves—transmitted to the neck veins. There is, however, a mean level, and the perpendicular height of this level above the mid right atrium indicates the mean hydrostatic pressure within the right atrium (6–8 cmH$_2$O). In health this level is the same as that of the sternal angle, whatever the position of the patient. The sternal angle is therefore a convenient reference point for measuring or estimating the right atrial pressure. This means that in a healthy person reclining at an angle of 45 degrees, the mean level will be invisible, because it is just below the clavicle, but the *a*, *c* and *v* waves may appear above the clavicle.

Arterial pulsation may be visible in the neck and has to be distinguished from venous pulsation. The venous pulse has a definite upper level, though it may be necessary to sit the patient up higher or lay them lower to find it. This level falls during inspiration when blood is drawn into the heart. When the patient's neck is viewed from the end of the bed the venous pulse is seen to have a dominant inward motion, towards the midline (the *y* descent), whereas the arterial pulse exhibits a dominant outward wave. In addition it is usually impossible to palpate any impulse from the venous waves, whereas the much higher pressure arterial pulses are readily felt by very slight pressure of the examiner's finger.

A raised jugular venous pressure is usually indicative of right heart failure. Occasionally it is due to obstruction of the superior vena cava, in which case the normal pulsations of the venous pulse are absent. A slight rise in venous pressure also occurs with an increase in the circulating blood volume, as in pregnancy, acute nephritis or overenthusiastic treatment with intravenous fluids.

The venous pulse is usually seen quite easily by the methods described, but occasionally difficulties occur. The mean venous pressure may be so high, for instance in patients with constrictive pericarditis, that the pulsation is obscured within the cranium when the patient is semi-recumbent, and is visible only high in the neck when he sits upright. In patients with a very low right atrial pressure the pulsation may be visible only when the patient lies completely flat.

The *a* wave is prominent when right ventricular hypertrophy leads to increased resistance to filling. This is found in pulmonary stenosis or pulmonary

Fig. 8.4 In the normal subject lying with the upper part of the body at an angle of 45 degrees to the horizontal, the peaks of the right atrial pressure waves are just visible in the internal jugular vein. As indicated in the upper diagram, the distance between the right atrium and the sternal angle remains relatively constant regardless of the position of the thorax. However, when the upright position is assumed, the tops of the right atrial pressure waves, while reaching the sternal angle, are hidden from the observer's view by the part of the thoracic cage which is now situated above the sternal angle.

When the venous pressure is grossly elevated (*lower diagram*) the top of the right atrial pressure waves lies above the angle of the jaw. This may make it difficult to observe their pulsatile nature when the patient is positioned at 45 degrees. When the patient is upright the top of the right atrial pressure wave becomes visible in the mid or lower portion of the neck.

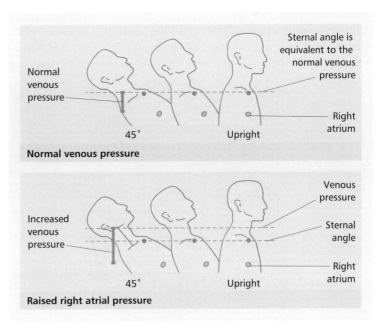

hypertension as a result of increased ventricular work associated with pressure overload. In theory, a large *a* wave is present in tricuspid stenosis but most patients with this condition are in atrial fibrillation and therefore there is no *a* wave. Atrial flutter, however, does cause sufficient atrial activity for rapid waves to be noted.

In tricuspid regurgitation, the *v* wave is replaced by a large systolic wave due to regurgitation of blood in the right atrium during right ventricular systole. The systolic *v* wave is followed by a particularly prominent *y* descent (Fig. 8.5).

In complete heart block (complete atrioventricular dissociation) regular *a* waves can be seen in the neck while carotid pulsation occurs at a slower independent rate. From time to time atrial contraction occurs when the atrioventricular valves are closed during ventricular systole. All the force of right atrial contraction is transmitted backwards into the veins, to give a 'cannon wave'. If the arterial pulse is slow, the neck veins should be carefully examined for more rapid, regular *a* waves and cannon waves. Cannon waves are also seen in atrioventricular junctional rhythm when the atrium and ventricle are activated simultaneously, and the atrium contracts on a closed atrioventricular valve.

The precordium

Inspection and palpation

Deformities of the chest wall can affect the physical signs found in the examination of the heart. The commonest finding associated with these deformi-

ties is an *ejection systolic murmur*, which may be wrongly attributed to organic heart disease. The presence of kyphosis, scoliosis or sternal depression should therefore be noted. Sternal depression is also associated with a loud tricuspid component to the first heart sound, and appearance of cardiac enlargement on the chest X-ray and slight broadening of the QRS complex, with a right bundle branch block pattern. The clinical observation of a depressed sternum in such patients is important since it indicates the absence of cardiac abnormality.

Next identify the apex beat, and assess the cardiac impulse. It should be emphasized that the term 'cardiac impulse' not only refers to the character of the apex beat but also includes other pulsations and palpable murmurs (thrills) and heart sounds.

The cardiac impulse

It is customary to locate the apex beat, which is the lowest and outermost point of definite cardiac pulsation, and to delineate its position in terms of the particular intercostal space and distance from the midline in which it is felt. The normal position of the apex beat is 9 cm from the midline, or 1 cm internal to the mid-clavicular line in the fifth intercostal space.

The position of the apex beat is a valuable physical sign, if its limitations are understood. First, it must be felt with the patient sitting or lying quite straight. The apex beat of a normal person may be felt in the anterior axillary line, if the person is lying on their left side. Secondly, it must be realized that a possible cause of displacement of the apex beat is a deformity

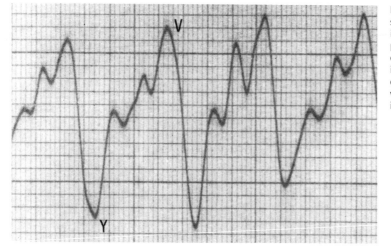

Fig. 8.5 Right atrial pressure trace showing the typical waveform found in patients with an elevated right atrial pressure. Notice that the most dramatic abnormality is the abrupt fall in pressure associated with the *y* descent. On examination of the neck veins this would be observed as a rapid impulse inwards towards the midline.

of the thoracic cage, for instance scoliosis. Pathology in the lungs or pleura may also alter the position of the apex beat. Pneumothorax or pleural effusion will tend to displace the apex beat away from the lungs and pleura whilst loss of lung volume due to collapse or fibrosis will tend to pull the apex beat towards the pulmonary pathology.

If these conditions are absent then displacement of the apex beat may be attributed to disease of the heart itself. The left ventricle normally produces the apex beat. When it is hypertrophied the impulse is more forceful and extends towards the axilla. If the right ventricle is extremely dilated it may form the apex of the heart. A combination of careful inspection and palpation may allow the left and right ventricular impulses to be distinguished. An attempt should be made to differentiate between the impulse resulting from obstruction to outflow (*pressure overload*) and that associated with excess filling of the ventricle (*volume overload*). Pressure overload, due to aortic stenosis or systemic hypertension, causes a forceful sustained heave, whereas volume overload occurring in aortic or mitral regurgitation is followed by easy and rapid (hyperkinetic) ejection of blood from the ventricles, producing an equally forceful but less sustained impulse.

The area immediately to the left of the sternum should be carefully palpated. The finding of a parasternal impulse indicates enlargement or hypertrophy of either the left atrium or the right ventricle. The left atrium lies in a posterior position in the heart; the support of the structures behind it—oesophagus, descending aorta and thoracic spine—causes systolic expansion which is usually transmitted anteriorly as found in severe mitral regurgitation.

Failure to detect an apex beat is usually due to obesity or obstructive airways disease, but may be a feature in patients with pleural or pericardial effusions. Dextrocardia is a very rare reason for failure to detect the apex beat in the left chest.

Other pulsations

In addition to the arterial and venous pulses already described, pulsations may also be noted at the root of the neck, at the front of the chest and in the epigastrium.

- In the *suprasternal notch* any pulsation is usually arterial, an indication of unfolding or aneurysm of the arch of the aorta.

- In the *neck* arterial pulsations may be observed. The carotid pulsation may be visible in anxious patients, in diseases which cause a hyperdynamic circulation, such as thyrotoxicosis, and in aortic regurgitation, hypertension or aneurysm of the aorta. In hypertension or in patients with large-calibre arterial vessels, the right carotid and subclavian pulses may be particularly prominent because of dilation or tortuosity of the great arteries.

- In the *chest wall*, a rare source of pulsation is aneurysm of the aorta. The position of the impulse varies according to the part of the aorta which is involved. If the *ascending aorta* is affected, the pulsation is chiefly to the right of the sternum, whilst the *aortic arch* gives rise to less distinct pulsation under the manubrium sterni, and the *descending aorta* still more to the left.

- In coarctation of the aorta a collateral arterial circulation develops, and pulsation may be detected in the *anastomotic channels overlying the scapulae*. These are palpable over the posterior chest wall and may even be visible on inspection.

- Pulsation in the *epigastrium* is most commonly due to aortic pulsation accentuated by nervousness or excitement in a thin person. Occasionally it is due to hepatic pulsation from tricuspid regurgitation. Aneurysm of the abdominal aorta may present as an expansile swelling in the epigastrium.

Thrills and palpable sounds

The physical energy of a sound or murmur which makes it loud will also allow it to be detected by palpation. A palpable murmur is called a thrill and transmits to the hand a sensation like the purring of a cat. The palpable impulse from a loud, high-pitched sound will be brief with a sharp quality. The loud first sound of mitral stenosis is often palpable and is responsible for the 'tapping' apex beat in this condition. The sounds of aortic and pulmonary valve closure are palpable in systemic and pulmonary hypertension respectively. A third or fourth sound may be easier to feel than to hear.

Percussion

Percussion of the heart is now seldom carried out, adds little to the clinical assessment and has been superseded by the chest X-ray and echocardiogram.

Auscultation

Auscultation of the heart often presents difficulties for the beginner. As with other clinical skills, it requires a great deal of practice and constant repetition. The skilled examiner listens for specific findings, focusing attention on particular parts of the cardiac cycle. An understanding of the events of the cardiac cycle (Fig. 8.6) is a useful basis for ausculta-

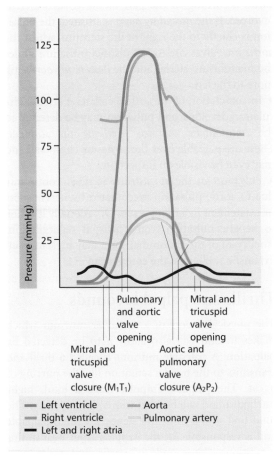

Fig. 8.6   The cardiac cycle. Normally the onset of left ventricular systole precedes the onset of pressure rise in the right ventricle. The mitral valve therefore closes before the tricuspid valve. Because the pulmonary artery diastolic pressure is lower than aortic diastolic pressure, the pulmonary valve opens before the aortic valve. It follows that pulmonary ejection sounds occur closer to the first heart sound than do aortic ejection sounds. During systole the pressure in the ventricles slightly exceeds the pressure in the corresponding great arteries. Towards the end of systole the ventricular pressure falls below the pressure in the great arteries and when diastolic pressure is reached the semilunar valves close. Normally aortic valve closure precedes pulmonary valve closure. The mitral and tricuspid valves begin to open at the point at which the ventricular pressures fall beneath the corresponding atrial pressures.

tion. It is important to identify systole and diastole correctly; intuition is an unreliable guide. Palpation of the carotid artery provides a systolic time reference and it is always wise to feel the carotid artery while auscultating; the delay in the radial pulse may cause confusion.

The stethoscope used for auscultation of the heart should combine both a bell-type chest piece and a diaphragm. High-pitched sounds such as aortic diastolic murmurs, systolic murmurs, the first and second heart sounds and opening snaps are heard better with the diaphragm, and low-pitched sounds such as the third or fourth heart sound or mitral diastolic murmurs with the bell.

Auscultatory areas

Certain areas of the precordium are customarily named according to the valve from which murmurs and sounds arise.
- The *mitral* area corresponds to the apex beat
- The *tricuspid* area lies just to the left of the lower sternum
- The *aortic* area is to the right of the sternum in the second intercostal space
- The *pulmonary* area is to the left of the sternum in the second intercostal space.

Auscultation should not necessarily be confined to these areas, and sounds heard in a particular area do not necessarily come from that particular valve; for example, systolic murmurs originating at the aortic valve are frequently best heard at the mitral area.

Heart sounds

The events of the cardiac cycle are illustrated in Fig. 8.6. At the onset of ventricular systole, the mitral and tricuspid valves close consecutively to give the first heart sound, M_1T_1. Opening of the pulmonary and aortic valves occurs next and is normally inaudible. The closure of the aortic and pulmonary valves gives rise to the two components of the second sound, A_2P_2. It will be seen that because of the lower pressure in the right ventricle compared with the left, closure of the pulmonary valve follows that of the aortic valve. After a brief period the mitral and tricuspid valves open inaudibly in the normal heart.

ABNORMAL HEART SOUNDS

In disease the following deviations from the normal may occur.

- The sounds may have a different intensity, either increased or decreased
- The sounds may be abnormally split
- Low-frequency sounds in diastole—third or fourth sounds—may be heard
- Additional high-pitched sounds, originating from abnormal valves, may be heard.

ALTERATIONS IN INTENSITY

In patients with thick chest walls, and in those with a serious degree of emphysema, the heart sounds may scarcely be audible, though there is no heart disease. Conversely, in the presence of serious heart disease the sounds may be quite normal. Thus alterations in the intensity of the heart sounds are significant only when considered in relation to all other features of the case. For example, in pericardial effusion, the heart sounds are distant or inaudible.

Accentuation of the mitral component of the first sound (M_1) is often noted in mitral stenosis, and in tachycardia from any cause. The tricuspid component of the first sound (T_1) is often loud in atrial septal defect. In *Ebstein's anomaly*, where there is a large leaflet of the tricuspid valve, T_1 is greatly accentuated and there may be an associated opening snap. The intensity of the first sound varies strikingly in complete atrioventricular block.

Accentuation of the sound of aortic or pulmonary valve closure is found where there is systemic or pulmonary hypertension. In calcific aortic stenosis the aortic component of the second sound (A_2) is soft, and in severe pulmonary stenosis the pulmonary component (P_2) is soft.

SPLITTING

The mitral valve closes slightly before the tricuspid valve, and this gives rise to splitting of the first sound. This splitting is often difficult to detect by auscultation because the two sounds are separated by a short interval. When it is heard, splitting of the first sound is not a sign of heart disease and is of importance only because its two components may be confused with an atrial sound followed by a first sound, or with a first sound followed by an ejection click.

Splitting of the second sound is much easier to appreciate because the aortic and pulmonary valve closure sounds (A_2 and P_2) are more widely separated. Aortic valve closure (A_2) is audible in all areas. Pulmonary valve closure (P_2) is normally audible only in the pulmonary area and for a short distance down the left sternal edge. When P_2 is loud it is also audible over a wider area of the precordium. It follows that splitting of the second sound is best sought at and close to the pulmonary area. Splitting is most easily heard in children, and may not be audible in older adults, when muscle noise, a thick chest wall, and emphysema make P_2 inaudible. Normally P_2 follows A_2, and the splitting is widest during inspiration and narrowest in expiration (physiological splitting). Splitting of 0.06 s during inspiration and 0.02 s (a very close split or single sound) in expiration would be average for a child or young adult.

The mechanism of splitting of the second sound is as follows. During inspiration blood is drawn into the thorax and the right ventricular stroke volume increases. The duration of right ventricular systole therefore lengthens, and P_2 is slightly delayed. Conversely the left ventricular stroke volume falls during inspiration, because the greater negative pressure within the thorax enlarges the capacity of the left atrium and pulmonary veins and reduces left atrial pressure and hence left ventricular filling and stroke volume. Thus left ventricular systole is shortened and A_2 occurs earlier and P_2 later, so that the splitting of the second sound widens. During expiration the changes are exactly opposite and the splitting narrows. Movement of P_2 is considerably greater than that of A_2.

THIRD AND FOURTH HEART SOUNDS

In addition to the first and second heart sounds which are both of a high frequency, lower frequency sounds may be heard in diastole. These additional sounds are known as the third and fourth (or atrial) sounds. When either of these additional sounds is present they give a cadence containing three beats rather than the normal two beats—'lub' and 'dub'. When the heart rate is rapid, diastole is shortened and the third and fourth heart sounds coincide. When this occurs the amplitude of the sound increases and is more easily detected, giving rise to a summation gallop rhythm, so called because it gives the auditory impression of a galloping horse.

All these low-frequency sounds are caused by abnormal filling patterns in the ventricles. The third heart sound occurs in early diastole at the time of maximal ventricular filling. This occurs about 0.15 s after the second heart sound. The fourth heart sound occurs when the bolus of blood is delivered into the ventricle from atrial contraction. It follows that this sound is heard only in patients in sinus rhythm.

The third heart sound may occur in healthy young adults, and is also a particular feature of pregnancy. In any other clinical setting, however, the presence of a third heart sound indicates abnormal left ventricular filling. The most important causes of this are left ventricular failure and mitral regurgitation.

Fourth heart sounds are caused by an increased stiffness or non-compliance of the ventricles. Atrial contraction, as a consequence, produces a sudden increase in pressure in the ventricle, rather than the ventricle increasing its volume to accommodate the extra blood delivered by atrial systole. Third or fourth heart sounds may originate from either right or left ventricles. These diastolic sounds are always best heard with the bell of the stethoscope and auscultation should routinely include a search for these sounds with the patient turned slightly on to the left side.

In constrictive pericarditis a very loud low-frequency diastolic sound is characteristically audible. This is known as a pericardial 'knock'. The presence of this sound always coincides with the very abrupt halt to early diastolic filling which is the distinctive haemodynamic abnormality of pericardial constriction.

ADDITIONAL SOUNDS

Ejection systolic clicks arise from the opening of the semilunar valves, either aortic or pulmonary (see Fig. 8.6). These sounds therefore occur in early systole, mimicking splitting of the first heart sound. Aortic ejection sounds are well heard throughout the precordium, but are best appreciated at the apex, where they are preceded by the first heart sound at its loudest intensity. The presence of an aortic ejection sound indicates that the aortic valve cusps are abnormal. In congenital aortic valve stenosis an ejection sound is always associated with the systolic murmur. This physical sign is absent in both subvalvular and supravalvular stenosis. The finding of an aortic ejection sound without an associated systolic murmur indicates the presence of a non-stenotic, bicuspid aortic valve. The pulmonary ejection sounds associated with congenital pulmonary valve stenosis become much softer on inspiration but are loud and sharp on expiration.

When one of the great arteries is dilated, for example the pulmonary artery in pulmonary hypertension, a systolic ejection sound can frequently be heard. A similar sound occurs in long-standing untreated systemic hypertension. These hypersensitive ejection sounds may be due to secondary changes in the corresponding semilunar valves.

Opening of the mitral and tricuspid valves occurs in early diastole shortly after the second heart sound (see Fig. 8.6). Normally these valves open silently but when the valve leaflets are abnormal, as in rheumatic, mitral or tricuspid stenosis, a sound is associated with the opening movement. This sound is analogous to the systolic clicks of the aortic or pulmonary valve opening but, by tradition, the sounds are known as opening snaps when they are related to the mitral or tricuspid valves. The presence of an opening snap is indicative of a thickened but mobile valve leaflet.

Loud extra sounds or clicks occur in mid-systole in association with prolapse of the mitral valve. These mid-systolic clicks may or may not be associated with a late systolic murmur. The presence of a mid-systolic click leads to a cadence which resembles that of a third heart sound. The two can be distinguished by the high frequency of the mid-systolic click and the low frequency of the third heart sound. Mid-systolic clicks arise from the halting of the mitral leaflet as it prolapses into the left atrium during systole.

Murmurs

Murmurs are due to turbulence in the blood flow at or near a valve or an abnormal communication within the heart. It follows that a loud murmur may originate from a rather small orifice such as a ventricular septal defect. Equally a soft murmur may originate from a large abnormal orifice as in very severe aortic regurgitation. Thus, while it is important to note the intensity of a murmur, one should not make deductions about its importance from its loudness. Not all murmurs are produced by a structural disorder of the heart; they may be due to abnormally rapid flow of blood through a normal valve. Such murmurs are called *flow murmurs* and it should be remembered that they do not indicate valvular disease. Flow murmurs have the following characteristics.

- They are always part of an ejection pattern.
- They may have either a grunting or a musical component.
- Their timing is generally earlier in systole than murmurs due to an organic obstruction to outflow.
- They may arise from either the left or right ventricular outflow tracts.
- They are never associated with any abnormality of the thoracic wall, such as a depressed sternum.
- Their intensity may be increased by physiological manoeuvres that increase the cardiac output.

Flow murmurs are most commonly encountered

in children and young adults or in the elderly. They also occur whenever there is an increased stroke volume, such as anaemia, thyrotoxicosis, hypertension, or in chronic anxiety. In pregnancy a flow murmur in the pulmonary area is an invariable finding and does not indicate the presence of a cardiac abnormality.

Murmurs also occur at the site of arterial stenoses, when they are traditionally called *bruits*. In examining a murmur the following points must be noted.

TIMING

Murmurs may be systolic, diastolic or continuous throughout systole and diastole, and can only be timed reliably if the carotid arterial pulse is palpated during auscultation so that systole can be determined. *Systolic murmurs* are either *pansystolic*, as in mitral or tricuspid regurgitation and ventricular septal defects, or *ejection*, when they arise either from the pulmonary or aortic outflow tracts. Pansystolic murmurs start immediately with the first heart sound and continue through to the second heart sound (Fig. 8.7). Typically they have uniform intensity. By contrast, ejection systolic murmurs have a diamond-shaped configuration building to a peak in mid-systole (Fig. 8.8). Ejection murmurs typically diminish before the second heart sound.

Late systolic murmurs are due to mitral valve prolapse, mild ischaemic mitral regurgitation or hypertrophic cardiomyopathy with obstruction. Clinically they are characterized by a clear gap between the first heart sound, which is often loud, and the onset of a murmur in mid- or late systole (Fig. 8.9). The murmur then continues right up to and through the aortic component (A_2) of the second heart sound.

Diastolic murmurs are of two types: *early diastolic murmurs* start at the second heart sound and occur as a result of aortic or pulmonary regurgitation, while *mid-diastolic murmurs*, in which there is a short gap after the second heart sound before the beginning of the murmur, arise from the mitral or tricuspid valve.

THE BEHAVIOUR OF THE MURMUR DURING RESPIRATION

The stroke output of the right heart increases during inspiration, while that of the left heart is reduced. It follows that a murmur originating on the right side of the heart will become louder during inspiration.

POINT OF MAXIMUM INTENSITY AND DIRECTION OF SELECTIVE PROPAGATION

Murmurs due to pulmonary and tricuspid valve lesions are generally well-localized to the areas on the precordium which have been described earlier as overlying the corresponding valves. Aortic and mitral murmurs, however, may radiate extensively. Aortic systolic murmurs, for instance, may be as loud, if not louder, at the cardiac apex than they are in the aortic area. Systolic murmurs that radiate into the carotid arteries are usually aortic in origin. Pansystolic murmurs due to mitral regurgitation may be heard over a wide area of the chest. For example, rupture of an anterior mitral chorda produces a murmur radiating posteriorly to the back, whereas the murmur from

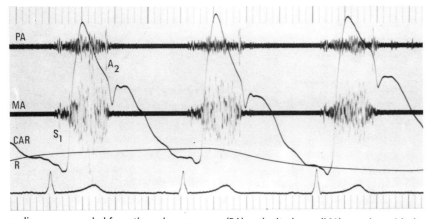

Fig. 8.7 Phonocardiograms recorded from the pulmonary area (PA) and mitral area (MA) together with the carotid pulse (CAR) and the respiration (R) in a patient with mitral regurgitation. The electrocardiogram is shown at the bottom of the tracing. A systolic murmur can be seen in the phonocardiogram recorded at the mitral area. The murmur starts immediately after the first heart sound (S_1) and continues right up to and including the second heart sound (A_2). In this example the presence of the pansystolic murmur at the mitral area obliterates A_2, which would have been audible only in the pulmonary area.

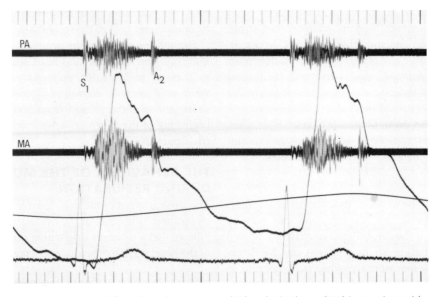

Fig. 8.8 Phonocardiograms recorded from the pulmonary area (PA) and mitral area (MA) in a patient with an ejection systolic murmur. The carotid pulse and respiration are recorded in a manner similar to that in Fig. 8.7. The diamond shape of an ejection systolic murmur can easily be seen. A clear gap is visible between the end of the murmur and the beginning of A_2.

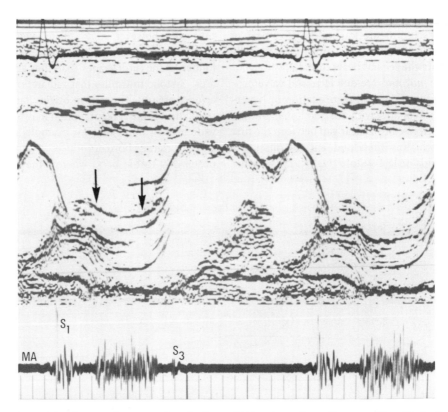

Fig. 8.9 Recording of the phonocardiogram in the mitral area (MA) and an echocardiogram of the mitral valve. The ECG is at the top of the tracing. The phonocardiogram shows a late systolic murmur which starts following a clear gap after the loud first heart sound (S_1). The murmur runs through A_2 and there is another gap before the third heart sound (S_3), which occurs in diastole. The cause of this late systolic murmur is prolapse of the mitral valve. This is indicated by the movement of the mitral leaflets in a downwards direction on the echocardiogram tracing (seen between two arrows).

rupture of a posterior chorda radiates anteriorly, so that it is heard across the precordium and in the pulmonary and aortic areas. It follows that the point of maximal intensity should not be regarded as one of the cardinal diagnostic features of aortic stenosis and mitral regurgitation.

THE CHARACTER OF A MURMUR

Although formerly stressed, the character of a murmur is now considered an unreliable guide to its origin. Rough murmurs are associated with obstruction to flow through a narrowed valve; blowing murmurs are more typical of an incompetent valve.

In the next paragraphs the haemodynamics in the common forms of valvular disease are presented, and the associated auscultatory signs discussed.

Mitral valve disease

MITRAL STENOSIS

The physical signs found in mitral stenosis are attributed to two separate effects of the rheumatic process on the thin, delicate mitral leaflets. First, the valvulitis causes thickening and fibrosis of the cusps themselves. This process tends to progress throughout adult life and is responsible for the alterations in intensity of the first heart sound and the presence of the opening snap. Secondly, the two leaflets become fused at the commissures so that the orifice available for blood to pass from the left atrium to the left ventricle becomes reduced. The ensuing turbulence of blood flow causes the mid-diastolic murmur associated with mitral stenosis.

Heart sounds

The classical findings in mitral stenosis, before the leaflets become very thickened and calcified, are first, a first heart sound much louder than normal and secondly, an opening snap occurring shortly (0.06–0.014 s) after the second heart sound. These cause a striking alteration in the cadence of the heart sounds and once they have been recognized provide the easiest and most sensitive clinical means of detecting mitral stenosis.

The closeness of the opening snap to the second heart sound is a useful indicator of the severity of the mitral stenosis. The reason for this is that the mitral valve opens only after the left ventricular pressure has fallen below the left atrial pressure (Fig. 8.10); consequently the more severe the mitral stenosis, the higher the left atrial pressure and the closer the

mitral valve opens to the second heart sound (Fig. 8.11).

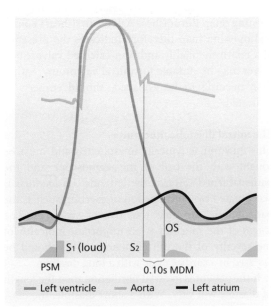

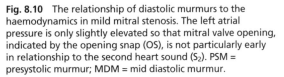

Fig. 8.10 The relationship of diastolic murmurs to the haemodynamics in mild mitral stenosis. The left atrial pressure is only slightly elevated so that mitral valve opening, indicated by the opening snap (OS), is not particularly early in relationship to the second heart sound (S₂). PSM = presystolic murmur; MDM = mid diastolic murmur.

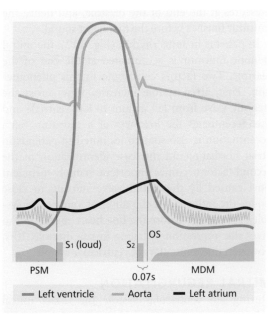

Fig. 8.11 The relationship of murmurs to haemodynamics in severe mitral stenosis. Increasing severity of mitral valve obstruction leads to elevation of the left atrial pressure. Because the left ventricular pressure has less distance to fall to reach this elevated atrial pressure, the time from A₂ to the opening snap is shortened. PSM = presystolic murmur; MDM = mid diastolic murmur.

In later years, as the mitral valve begins to develop calcification and marked fibrotic thickening, the intensity of both the first heart sound and the opening snap diminishes. A loud first heart sound and opening snap therefore indicates the presence of a relatively pliable and non-calcified valve. Such valves may be suitable for mitral valvotomy, rather than needing to be replaced, should surgery be indicated.

The mitral diastolic murmur

This murmur is typically low-pitched and must be sought with the bell of the stethoscope and the patient turned towards the left side. Its *loudness* is accentuated by a brief period of exertion such as the patient touching their toes five or six times. The *length* of the murmur is an important indicator of the severity of the mitral stenosis. This should be assessed in a cardiac cycle with a long diastole.

If the patient is in atrial fibrillation then the length of diastole will vary. With a short diastole, the diastolic murmur may appear to be full length, but the examiner should wait for a long diastole to assess the length of the murmur. In mild to moderate mitral stenosis a length of diastole equivalent to a heart rate of about 70 beats/min is often sufficiently long to allow equilibration of left atrial and left ventricular pressures at the end of the diastole, and hence the murmur finishes before the first heart sound.

In patients in sinus rhythm (Fig. 8.12), the mitral stenotic murmur is accentuated at the end of the diastole. Two factors contribute to this phenomenon. First, atrial systole increases flow across the stenotic valve from left atrium to left ventricle and this accentuates the loudness of a murmur. Such accentuation is also sometimes noted in patients in atrial fibrillation. In this case identification of the second factor becomes important, namely turbulent flow caused by the mitral valve starting to close under the influence of the onset of ventricular systole. This occurs before the first heart sound and so gives the impression of falling in late diastole. It is, however, due to the start of ventricular systole.

MITRAL REGURGITATION

During left ventricular systole the intact mitral valve apparatus prevents blood entering the left atrium. There are a number of different pathologies which may affect the mitral valve, leading to mitral regurgitation.
- The cusps may be affected by rheumatic disease or mitral valve prolapse.

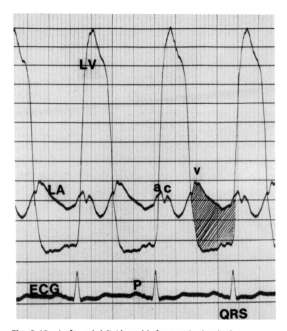

Fig. 8.12 Left atrial (LA) and left ventricular (LV) pressure tracings in a patient with mitral stenosis and sinus rhythm. The *a* and *c* waves together with the *v* wave can be seen in the left atrial tracing. The shaded area between the atrial and ventricular pressures during diastole indicates the size of the gradient across this patient's mitral valve. Each of the horizontal lines represents 10 mmHg; thus the end-diastolic gradient is 20 mmHg, although the gradient in early diastole is closer to 35 mmHg.

- The cusps may be congenitally abnormal.
- The chordae tendinae may rupture, with the result that part of a cusp is unsupported.
- There may be ischaemic damage to a papillary muscle.

Irrespective of its cause, the characteristic auscultatory findings in mitral regurgitation are either a pansystolic or a late systolic murmur.

The mitral pansystolic murmur

The regurgitant jet of blood (Fig. 8.13) starts as soon as left ventricular pressure exceeds left atrial pressure, that is, immediately after the first heart sound, and continues up to and through the second heart sound until left ventricular pressure falls below left atrial pressure. These events account for the characteristics of the pansystolic murmur. The murmur is best heard at the mitral area, and it radiates to the axilla and to the back when the anterior leaflet is normal. When the posterior leaflet is abnormal, for instance due to a ruptured chorda, the murmur usually radiates anteriorly across the precordium, mimicking aortic stenosis.

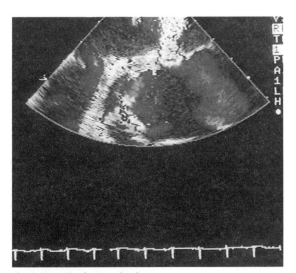

Fig. 8.13 Mitral regurgitation.

The mitral late systolic murmur

A late systolic murmur heard at the mitral area is indicative of mild mitral regurgitation and is usually associated with mitral valve prolapse. A late mitral systolic murmur may also be heard in patients with mitral regurgitation due to ischaemic damage to a papillary muscle or to hypertrophic cardiomyopathy.

The various combinations of murmurs associated with mitral valve disease are summarized in Fig. 8.14.

Aortic valve disease

AORTIC STENOSIS

The haemodynamics in aortic stenosis are shown diagrammatically in Fig. 8.15. There is a pressure gradient between the left ventricle and aorta during systole, and the size of this pressure difference is an indication of the severity of the stenosis. The gradi-

ent is greatest in the middle of systole, and is relatively small early and late in systole. The murmur therefore has a diamond shape, starting soft, building to a peak in mid-systole then becoming quieter in late systole immediately before the second sound. All murmurs due to the ejection of blood through abnormal semilunar valves, or to abnormally high blood flow through normal semilunar valves, have this pattern and are called ejection systolic murmurs.

The *aortic ejection murmur* is heard in the aortic area and radiates into the carotids although frequently it is also heard at the mitral area.

The *aortic ejection click* is produced on opening of the aortic valve in aortic valve stenosis. It is therefore heard just after the first heart sound at the beginning of the ejection murmur. Its presence indicates that stenosis is at the valvular rather than the supravalvular or subvalvular level. In aortic stenosis A_2 is delayed because of prolonged ventricular systole. This causes single S_2 and reversed splitting. Frequently this sign is difficult to detect because A_2, like the ejection click, becomes soft or inaudible when the cusps are heavily calcified. When the valve is rigid from fibrosis or calcification, no click is heard.

Aortic regurgitation

In aortic regurgitation, because of the reversed flow back across the aortic valve during diastole, the systolic stroke volume of the left ventricle is substantially increased (Fig. 8.16). This increased flow across the valve invariably gives rise to an aortic ejection murmur. Thus an aortic ejection murmur in a patient with aortic regurgitation does not necessarily indicate the presence of additional aortic stenosis.

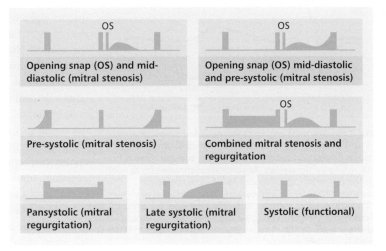

Fig. 8.14 Mitral murmurs; a systolic, functional murmur is shown for comparison.

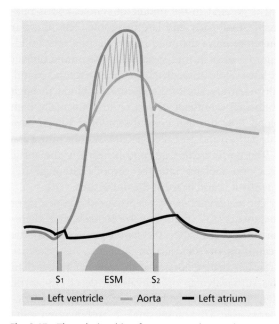

S_1 ESM S_2

— Left ventricle   — Aorta   — Left atrium

Fig. 8.15 The relationship of murmurs to haemodynamics in aortic stenosis. The slow ejection of blood into the aorta causes a slow rise in aortic pressure. The murmur follows the flow pattern, rising to a peak in mid-systole then declining. ESM = ejection systolic murmur.

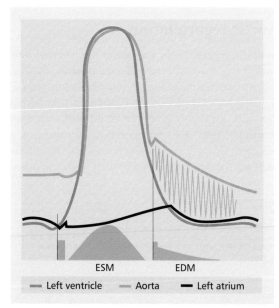

ESM   EDM

— Left ventricle   — Aorta   — Left atrium

Fig. 8.16 The relationship of murmurs to haemodynamics in aortic regurgitation. The increased systolic stroke volume causes an ejection systolic murmur even though there is no coexisting aortic stenosis. Regurgitation commences as soon as the left ventricular pressure falls below the aortic diastolic pressure, i.e. immediately after aortic valve closure. The early diastolic murmur tails off as the diastolic pressure (and hence the gradient across the valve) diminishes and the left ventricle fills. ESM = ejection systolic murmur; EDM = early diastolic murmur.

The latter is best recognized by the contour of the carotid pulse.

The *early* or *immediate diastolic murmur* of aortic regurgitation starts with the second heart sound and continues for a variable time in diastole. It is a high-pitched murmur, often soft, and usually requires intent auscultation for its recognition. It is best heard down the left sternal edge when the patient sits forward and breathes out; the examiner must listen with the diaphragm of the stethoscope.

THE AUSTIN FLINT MURMUR

In severe aortic regurgitation a low-pitched diastolic murmur may be audible at the mitral area. This murmur originates from the anterior leaflet of the mitral valve and is due to the confluence of two streams of blood. On one side there is antegrade flow from the left atrium to the left ventricle, and on the other side there is the regurgitant jet of blood through the incompetent aortic valve impinging on the anterior mitral leaflet. The resulting murmur closely resembles the murmur of mitral stenosis, but since the mitral leaflets are normal, the first heart sound is not loud and there is no opening snap.

Tricuspid valve disease

Although the tricuspid valve may be affected by rheumatic disease, the most common cause of tricuspid regurgitation is stretching of the annulus secondary to dilatation of the right ventricular cavity. In drug addicts who inject themselves intravenously with non-sterile needles and syringes, infective endocarditis of the tricuspid valve may also be a cause of tricuspid regurgitation.

The pansystolic murmur of tricuspid regurgitation is high-pitched and is louder with inspiration. When due to right ventricular failure a third heart sound may be heard at the left sternal edge. In establishing the clinical diagnosis of tricuspid regurgitation, a pansystolic murmur is of less importance than the observation of a giant systolic *v* wave followed by a large *y* descent in the jugular venous pulse.

Rheumatic tricuspid valve disease invariably occurs in association with aortic and mitral valve disease. The murmurs are of a similar timing and quality to rheumatic mitral disease, but typically the opening snap associated with tricuspid stenosis occurs later than the opening snap of mitral stenosis.

In *Ebstein's anomaly*, the main abnormality is a great increase in the size of the anterior leaflet of the tricuspid valve. This is associated with a very loud first heart sound followed by a short systolic murmur. There is usually a tricuspid opening snap.

Myxoma

Myxomas are benign tumours of the atria usually arising from the interatrial septum. They most commonly occur in the left atrium but are also encountered in the right. The condition is of importance since it may cause emboli to the systemic circulation in the case of left-sided tumour and to the pulmonary circulation in right-sided tumour. Both clinically and haemodynamically a left atrial myxoma mimics mitral stenosis. This is because the tumour mass drops down between the mitral leaflets during diastole causing obstruction of flow from the left atrium to the left ventricle.

Hypertrophic cardiomyopathy

Hypertrophic cardiomyopathy is a condition of unknown aetiology in which the muscle fibres of the ventricles become inappropriately hypertrophied and distorted. The commonest site for the process to occur is the intraventricular septum and only in the later stages of the condition or in particularly severe cases are the free walls of the left and right ventricles involved. Two main functional abnormalities occur as a consequence of the abnormal anatomy. First, the hypertrophied ventricle becomes much stiffer than normal and this is manifest by the presence of a loud fourth heart sound. Secondly, the intraventricular septum, when it contracts, bulges into the outflow tract of the left ventricle thus causing an intraventricular gradient. Such gradients do not always occur in hypertrophic cardiomyopathy but when they do they are generally associated with the presence of a systolic murmur. This murmur is essentially ejection systolic in nature but in some patients it may be prolonged until the second heart sound. A degree of mitral regurgitation may be associated with hypertrophic cardiomyopathy due to involvement of the papillary muscles. When present this tends to cause the systolic murmur to extend to the second heart sound.

The pattern of blood flow from the left ventricle is invariably abnormal whether obstruction is present or not. This leads to a typically jerky or sharp carotid arterial pulse. Even when there is severe obstruction the carotid upstroke does not become slow and delayed and this is an important distinguishing feature between hypertrophic cardiomyopathy and aortic valve stenosis.

Pulmonary stenosis

In mild pulmonary valve stenosis the only abnormal signs are found on auscultation (Fig. 8.17). The

Fig. 8.17 Pressure tracings from a patient with pulmonary stenosis. A catheter has been withdrawn from the pulmonary artery (PA) into the right ventricle (RV). The severity of the stenosis is measured by the difference between the peak systolic pressure in the right ventricle and the peak systolic pressure in the pulmonary artery. Each dense horizontal line represents 25 mmHg. The pressure difference in this patient is therefore between 55 and 60 mmHg. Similar principles apply in aortic stenosis; the severity of the stenosis is assessed by the pressure difference between the left ventricle and the aorta.

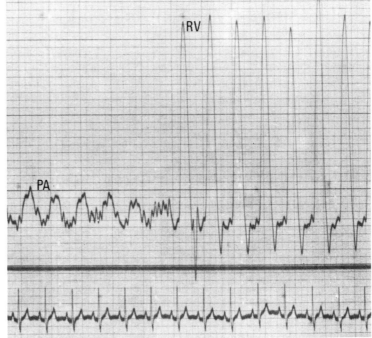

ejection systolic murmur is loudest in inspiration and best heard in the pulmonary area. It is preceded by an ejection click which is loudest in expiration and may be inaudible during inspiration. This distinguishes it from an aortic ejection click, which is of constant intensity. The second sound behaves normally on inspiration, but the width of splitting is wider than normal because of a delay in pulmonary valve closure.

The pulmonary component of the second sound is delayed in proportion to the severity of the stenosis. If the stenosis is severe, the closure of the pulmonary valve becomes soft or inaudible. Pressure overload on the right ventricle leads to a palpable right ventricular impulse at the left sternal edge.

Right ventricular outflow may be obstructed by inappropriate hypertrophy of the muscle which comprises the outflow tract; *infundibular stenosis*. In this case an ejection systolic murmur and delay in P_2 will also be heard but there is no pulmonary ejection sound.

Left-to-right shunts

When there is an abnormal communication between the left and right sides of the circulation, blood will flow from left to right provided the pulmonary vascular resistance is not grossly increased. Such communications occur anatomically at the *atrial level* (i.e. atrial septal defect), the *ventricular level* (i.e. ventricular septal defect), and between the *aorta and the pulmonary artery* (i.e. patent ductus arteriosus) (Fig. 8.18).

ATRIAL SEPTAL DEFECT

The volume of blood flowing from left to right atrium depends on the size of the defect in the atrial septum. The blood flow from the left atrium through the defect is often more than twice the flow entering the left ventricle (i.e. the systemic blood flow). The blood entering the right atrium will then be the systemic flow plus the flow, i.e. the venous return from the superior and inferior vena cavae, from the left atrium, i.e. three times the systemic flow. This increased flow passes from the right atrium to the right ventricle, pulmonary artery, lung vessels and so back to the left atrium.

Because the defect is relatively large and the pressure gradient relatively small (about 1 mmHg) there is little turbulence and no audible murmur from blood flowing through the defect itself. The characteristic auscultatory signs are due to the increased

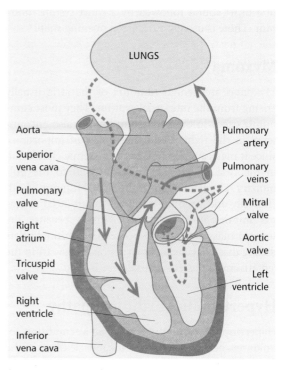

Fig. 8.18 Diagram of the heart to show blood flow through the left and right circulations.

volume of flow in the right ventricle and pulmonary artery. There is *fixed* splitting of the second heart sound, since the increased right ventricular stroke volume does not vary with respiration. The increased blood flow through the pulmonary valve produces a functional ejection pulmonary systolic murmur which is moderately loud. A functional tricuspid flow murmur is often present. It is mid-diastolic, of low frequency and best heard at the lower end of the sternum.

VENTRICULAR SEPTAL DEFECT

Ventricular septal defects are rarely as large as atrial septal defects and usually less than 1 cm in diameter. Defects in the ventricular septum may occur in the upper or membraneous part of the septum immediately below the aortic valve or in the muscular septum. Small muscular defects may, over the years, close spontaneously. The right ventricular systolic pressure is normally about one-fifth of that in the left ventricle, so there is a pressure gradient from left ventricle to right throughout systole.

In mild cases, in which the defect has the cross-sectional area of a pencil lead, the only abnormal sign is a loud pansystolic murmur, best heard at the lower end of the sternum. The murmur is usually accompanied by a thrill.

In more severe cases there is evidence of increased blood flow through the pulmonary vasculature and the left heart. In addition to the pansystolic murmur and thrill there may be a short, soft mid-diastolic murmur due to the increased flow of blood through the mitral valve. Splitting of the second sound is normal, though A_2 may be difficult to hear as it tends to be obscured by the pansystolic murmur which extends to P_2. When there is pulmonary hypertension the second sound becomes single and loud.

PATENT DUCTUS ARTERIOSUS

The ductus arteriosus links the aorta with the main pulmonary artery at a point close to the origin of the left subclavian artery. The communication has the same size range as in ventricular septal defects. A pressure gradient between the aorta and the pulmonary artery is present throughout the cardiac cycle and is greatest towards the end of the systole. The increased flow through the patent ductus increases flow through the pulmonary vascular bed and causes left ventricular volume overload. If the communication is small, a murmur is the only abnormal sign. It is best heard at the pulmonary area in expiration, and is continuous through both systole and diastole. The accentuation of the murmur about the time of the second sound gives it a particular character, and it is sometimes described as a machinery murmur. In addition to the continuous murmur, a short, soft functional mitral diastolic murmur may be present.

Patent ductus arteriosus is the most common but not the only cause of a continuous murmur. Pulmonary arteriovenous fistulae, coronary arteriovenous fistulae or communications between the ascending aorta and pulmonary artery will produce similar physical signs. Particular care should always be taken not to confuse the murmurs of patent ductus arteriosus with a venous hum.

Pulmonary hypertension

There are a number of important physical signs in addition to the auscultatory abnormalities which indicate the presence of pulmonary hypertension. A prominent *a* wave is due to the stiff (non-compliant), thickened right ventricular wall which invariably develops in response to the presence of severe pulmonary hypertension. The carotid arterial pulse volume is small. On palpation of the precordium a prominent parasternal impulse due to right ventricular hypertrophy is detected.

Pulmonary hypertension by itself does not lead to any systolic or diastolic murmurs. The most important finding is that pulmonary valve closure (P_2) is accentuated and may be palpable. In a number of cases, a pulmonary ejection click can also be heard immediately after the first heart sound. In severe long-standing pulmonary hypertension the dilation of the pulmonary artery may lead to secondary pulmonary valve regurgitation (the Graham Steel murmur). This presents as a high-pitched early diastolic murmur loudest in the pulmonary area and radiating down the left sternal border. Pulmonary incompetence is very rarely found other than in association with pulmonary hypertension or following pulmonary valvotomy.

Fallot's tetralogy

Fallot's tetralogy consists of pulmonary stenosis, ventricular septal defect, right ventricular hypertrophy and overriding of the aorta, i.e. the aorta arises astride the ventricular septal defect. The essential features are pulmonary stenosis of at least moderate severity and a large ventricular septal defect, so that the resistance to output from the two ventricles is nearly equal in systole. The right ventricular output is ejected partly into the pulmonary artery through the pulmonary stenosis, and partly into the aorta through the ventricular septal defect. The admixture of deoxygenated blood with the left ventricular septal output makes the patient cyanosed, i.e. there is a right-to-left shunt.

The auscultatory signs are a pulmonary ejection murmur and a single second sound. P_2 is inaudible both because of the low blood flow in the pulmonary artery and because of the associated pulmonary stenosis.

Coarctation of the aorta

In coarctation of the aorta there is a narrowing of the descending aorta at or beyond the insertion of the ligamentum arteriosum. The arterial pressure proximal to the coarctation is increased, so that the blood pressure in the arms is greater than that in the legs. The radial and femoral pulses should be palpated simultaneously. The timing of the femoral pulse is delayed and diminished, or absent. The blood supply to the lower limbs is invariably adequate through collaterals and with a much diminished pulsatile nature to the pattern of flow. The raised arterial pressure leads to left ventricular hypertrophy, which can be detected clinically. There is often an ejection click and an aortic ejection systolic murmur because of an associated congenital bicuspid aortic valve. Collateral vessels linking the subclavian arteries, which arise above the aortic stricture, with intercostal arteries arising below the stricture can usually be felt around the scapulae, and are best seen with the patient bending forwards in a good light.

Exocardial sounds and murmurs

VENOUS HUM
Sometimes in children a continuous murmur can be heard in the neck and upper chest. This is due to kinking and partial obstruction of one of the larger veins in the neck, thus preventing the continuous flow of blood through the vein. The origin of the murmur should be suspected because of the youth of the patient and the loudness of the murmur in the neck. The hum can be obliterated by pressure on the neck, which produces complete obstruction of the vein, or by altering the position of the neck so as to relieve the venous obstruction. It is particularly important to exclude a venous hum if a diagnosis of patent ductus is being considered.

PERICARDIAL RUBS
Pericardial rubs have a characteristic high-pitched quality which has been likened to the noise emitted by compression of new leather. They are generally loudest in systole but often have an additional diastolic component. Because part of the pericardium is in contact with the lung there may also be a marked respiratory element. Pericardial rubs are one of the most evanescent of physical signs and vary greatly from hour to hour. The presence of a pericardial rub indicates that two inflamed layers of pericardium are in contact. The development of an effusion will separate the two layers of pericardium and hence lead to the disappearance of the rub.

Ischaemic heart disease

The arteries of the coronary circulation are at risk of developing atherosclerosis, which may partially or completely occlude their lumen; this disease process is a major cause of mortality and morbidity in many countries. Characteristically, coronary artery disease is symptomless for many years. It then presents when the degree of narrowing of the lumen is sufficiently great to limit the increase in flow required during exercise, resulting in the symptom of *angina*. Alternatively it may present acutely as a *myocardial infarction*. This is caused by rupture or fissuring of a plaque, leading to a total occlusion of the artery and death of the muscle supplied by that vessel. Alternatively, a previous shallow atheromatous plaque causing no stenosis may be converted by plaque-fissuring to a severe stenosis, but without total occlusion, causing the clinical syndrome of *unstable angina*.

The diagnosis of coronary artery disease depends greatly on an accurate history. The symptom of angina pectoris may be described by the patient as a pain, tightness, unpleasant sensation or even a feeling of breathlessness. It characteristically occurs in the upper central chest, radiating both to the left and the right side of the sternum, often in a band-like or constricting fashion. The pain may also radiate down the inner aspect of the left arm, into the left elbow and the little finger of the left hand. Less commonly it radiates to a region between the scapulae or up into the lower jaw, especially around the teeth.

The pain is characteristically provoked by exertion or, in some cases, by emotional stress. It occurs during rather than after exercise. Rest alleviates the pain and it may be possible for the patient to walk much further during a subsequent period of exercise after resting—the warm-up effect. The pain is typically more severe or more easily provoked in cold weather, especially if it is windy. Nitroglycerine relieves the pain within 5 minutes of starting to suck a tablet.

When typical cardiac pain lasts for more than 30 minutes the possibility of a diagnosis of myocardial infarction arises. In this instance the characteristics of the pain are similar to that of angina but it is generally more severe, it is not relieved by nitroglycerine and it is often associated with nausea, vomiting and profuse sweating.

The pain of aortic dissection has a similar quality to that of myocardial infarction, but is usually very severe, radiating through the chest to the back, and often accompanied by circulatory collapse (Fig. 8.19).

UNSTABLE ANGINA
Unstable angina describes a clinical pattern in which angina occurs either at rest or with minimal exertion but without progressing to myocardial infarction. Because the major characteristic of angina, namely its relationship to physical exertion, is absent, it is sometimes difficult to distinguish unstable angina

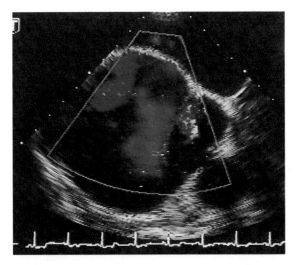

Fig. 8.19 Aortic dissection.

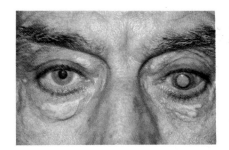

Fig. 8.20 Xanthelasmata palpebrarum and cataract. Yellow xanthelasmata are prominent below both eyes and in the upper lids. There is a mature left cataract (not directly related to the xanthelasmata).

from pain which is not in fact of cardiac origin. Severe or unstable angina is often worse first thing on waking in the morning or after a heavy meal; it may also occur during sleep with or without accompanying nightmares.

Physical signs in coronary disease

Physical examination in patients with angina due to coronary artery disease is generally unrewarding, but it is always important to exclude the diagnoses of aortic stenosis, hypertrophic cardiomyopathy or severe pulmonary hypertension in patients who give this history. There may be signs of associated generalized arterial disease (see section on peripheral vascular system, page 188).

Important general considerations which may precipitate angina are anaemia and myxoedema. The physical signs associated with these conditions should be sought in every patient with angina. There may be clinical evidence to indicate hyperlipidaemia. Lipid deposits may occur as xanthelasmata in the upper or lower eyelids (Fig. 8.20) or they may be found on palpation of tendons, particularly the Achilles or triceps, and the extensor tendons of the hand. Lipid may be deposited in the cornea at its margin with the conjunctiva—the *arcus*. There is a slight gap between the lipid deposit and the conjunctiva itself.

On auscultation the only abnormality in coronary disease is the presence of a fourth heart sound, which is due to an increase in diastolic stiffness of the left ventricular muscle when it has an adequate blood supply. This may be a chronic finding but it occurs typically during the acute phase of myocardial infarction.

Mitral regurgitation may occur as a complication of ischaemia, or infarction, of the papillary muscles. Usually the degree of regurgitation is not severe and the typical finding is of a soft late systolic murmur. Occasionally, ischaemic rupture of a papillary muscle leads to a very severe mitral regurgitation with a loud pansystolic murmur. A similar physical finding presents in association with a ventricular septal defect due to rupture of the intraventricular septum, and on clinical grounds alone it may be difficult to distinguish these two diagnoses. In general, mitral regurgitation is more commonly associated with disease of the right or left circumflex coronary arteries, whereas an acquired ventricular septal defect is often associated with disease of the left anterior descending coronary artery.

The right ventricle is largely supplied by the right coronary artery and there is often a mild degree of right ventricular dysfunction associated with inferior myocardial infarction. This is manifest clinically as a 2–3 cm elevation of the jugular venous pressure, but this is usually a transitory phenomenon.

The peripheral vascular system

Examination of the peripheral vascular system, including both the arterial and venous systems, is often carried out as part of the general examination. It is of particular importance in patients with symptoms of arterial or venous disease of the limbs, and in those with cerebral or coronary disease. Further, many patients with hypertension or diabetes mellitus have associated arterial disease, and degenerative

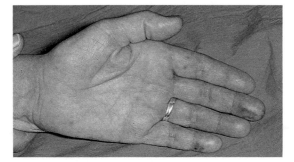

Fig. 8.21 Bacterial endocarditis. The lesions in the fingertips are due to embolic occlusion of branches of the digital arteries.

vascular disease is common in the elderly. Special attention must therefore be paid to the arterial system in these patients. In bacterial endocarditis embolic lesions may be seen in the skin of the digits (Fig. 8.21).

Peripheral arterial system

Intermittent claudication is the term used to describe the cramp-like aching pain felt in the calf muscles during exercise. The pain occurs only during exercise, often walking a certain distance, and it gradually ceases when the patient stops working. It is ischaemic pain due to failure of the peripheral arterial system to allow a sufficiently increased blood flow to the legs to match the metabolic demands of muscular work. In certain forms of inflammatory arterial disease, e.g. polyarteritis nodosa or temporal arteritis, similar ischaemic pain may occur in other muscles. Intermittent claudication of the legs is not associated with numbness or tingling in the feet or legs unless the blood supply of the cauda equina is also affected.

Impaired blood supply to a limb can be assessed by its lowered skin temperature and by its impaired nutritional status. Temperature differences can be reliably assessed only when the limbs have been exposed to a constant room temperature for 10–20 minutes. In an ischaemic leg the skin of the foot is cold and pale or cyanosed, and capillary filling after blanching with light finger pressure is delayed. Reactive hyperaemia is also delayed. This can be demonstrated with the patient lying down. The leg is elevated for several minutes to allow the venous pool of blood in the leg to drain into the circulation, and then the patient sits up and allows the leg to hang over the edge of the bed. Normally the foot will flush pink in about 10 seconds; the flush takes a longer time to appear if blood flow is inadequate.

When there has been *chronic arterial insufficiency* the skin becomes thin and shiny, often losing its hair, and the nails become brittle. Late manifestations of severe arterial insufficiency are chronic ulceration and even gangrene, especially of the distal parts of the toes or feet; the dead area becomes shrivelled, blackened and often demarcated from neighbouring healthy tissue by a thin red zone of inflamed tissue. In *acute interruption of arterial flow* to a limb, as in embolic or thrombotic occlusion of a femoral artery, the affected leg becomes colder than the normal limb, the peripheral pulses below the level of obstruction disappear, and the skin, which is at first white, becomes blue and later gangrenous.

Diminished or absent pulsation of vessels is of great value in localizing arterial lesions, both acute and chronic. In the legs the femoral, popliteal, posterior tibial and dorsalis pedis pulses should be carefully palpated with slightly flexible fingers, and their pulsation compared with that in the contralateral vessels. Using the bell of the stethoscope a careful search for the hissing systolic sound (*arterial bruit*) associated with partial obstruction should be made in both femoral arteries, in the abdomen (*aortic bruits*) and in the loins (*renal artery bruits*).

In patients with claudication, the distal pulses should also be examined after exercise since the diversion of blood flow to exercised muscle may cause previously detectable pulses to disappear, indicating restriction of flow in the affected limb.

In the arms the brachial and radial pulses should be similarly assessed and bruits listened for over the subclavian vessels. The carotid arteries should be carefully examined; it is particularly common to find systolic bruits in these vessels. Carotid stenosis is important in cardiological practice because it is a risk factor for stroke in patients undergoing coronary artery bypass graft surgery for the treatment of angina and ischaemic heart disease. Arterial pulsation in the limbs and the carotids can be assessed quantitatively with a Doppler ultrasonic flowmeter.

Spasm of arterioles may occur in the presence of normal peripheral pulses. This is usually seen in the hands; the digital arteries go into spasm in response to cold or emotional stimuli so that the fingers become white and then cyanosed. When the spasm passes off, the fingers become hyperaemic and pink. This sequence of changes is termed *Raynaud's phenomenon*. Very rarely it may lead to superficial necrosis of the skin of the fingers.

In patients with arterial disease it is important to remember that the arterioles, capillary bed and small veins can be inspected directly in the retina by ophthalmoscopy (page 231). Some patients with hyperlipidaemia show an 'arcus' and xanthelasmata (Fig. 8.20). Lipid deposits within tendons may be detected in the Achilles, triceps and extensor tendons to the fingers.

Peripheral venous system

Varicose veins should be looked for with the patient standing. Superficial varicosities are then obvious. The efficiency of the valves of the long saphenous vein should be assessed by Trendleburg's test. With the patient lying, the saphenous vein is emptied by elevating the leg. The upper end of the vein is then occluded by finger pressure on the saphenous opening. While the examiner maintains this pressure, the patient stands. If the valves are incompetent the veins will fill rapidly from above when the pressure is released.

Venous thrombosis is rare in healthy mobile subjects but may sometimes occur in women taking oral contraceptives. However, it is a frequent complication of enforced bed rest, particularly after surgery. Cardiac failure also leads to venous stasis and thrombosis. The affected limb is swollen, tender and warmer than normal. Dilated superficial veins may be seen which do not collapse when the leg is elevated. Forceful dorsiflexion of the foot will cause pain in the calf (*Homan's sign*). Sometimes extension of deep venous thrombosis upwards to the thigh may lead to a tender, hard palpable femoral vein.

Studies with radioactive fibrinogen, which is taken up by the forming thrombus, and venography, have shown that quite extensive venous thrombosis can occur without significant physical findings. Pulmonary embolism may be the first clinical manifestation of a deep vein thrombosis in the leg.

Routine cardiovascular examination

A record of a normal examination of the cardiovascular system may be constructed along the following lines. The arterial pulse is of regular rate and rhythm and the carotid upstroke is normal. The blood pressure in the right arm with the patient lying is 120/80 mmHg.

The venous pressure is not elevated and there are no abnormal pulsations on palpation of the precordium. On auscultation the first heart sound is normal and splitting of the second sound can be identified. There are no murmurs and no additional heart sounds.

The peripheral pulses in the upper and lower limbs are all present and equal, as are the carotid pulses. There are no bruits.

Electrocardiography

The electrocardiogram (ECG) is a recording from the body surface of the electrical changes that occur within the heart during the cardiac cycle. The main areas in which the ECG can prove useful are:
- analysis of abnormal rhythms;
- detection and localization of changes in the myocardium due to coronary artery disease;
- detection of hypertrophy of the walls of the atria and ventricles;
- detection of changes in electrical activity due to pericardial disease; and
- detection of changes in electrical activity of the heart consequent on general metabolic changes.

Additional valuable information may be obtained by recording the ECG during physical exercise (see section on exercise tests, p. 197)

Definitions

The points of electrical contact—electrode positions —are the four limbs together with specific positions on the thorax. The limb leads are arranged so as to provide an analysis of the vector of the electrical forces arising in the heart. The standard limb leads are shown in Table 8.1.

Leads	Connections
Bipolar	
Lead I	Right arm–left arm
Lead II	Right arm–left leg
Lead III	Left arm–right leg
Unipolar	
aVR	Right arm
aVL	Left arm
aVF	Left foot

Table 8.1 Standard limb leads.

The standard placements of the chest leads are shown in Fig. 8.22. Leads II, III and aVF record changes from the lateral border of the heart, and the

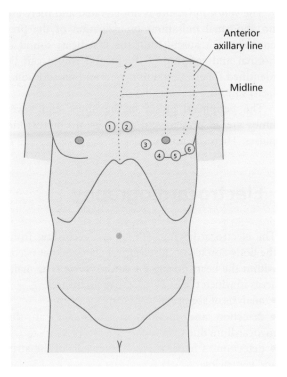

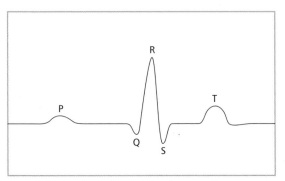

Fig. 8.22 The positions of the electrodes in chest lead recordings.
V_1 Fourth intercostal space at right sternal edge.
V_2 Fourth intercostal space at left sternal edge.
V_3 Halfway between V_2 and V_4.
V_4 Mid-clavicular line in the fifth intercostal space.
V_5 Anterior axillary line nearly horizontal to V_4.
V_6 Mid-axillary line horizontal to V_4.
V, ventricular.

Fig. 8.23   The terminology of the electrocardiogram.

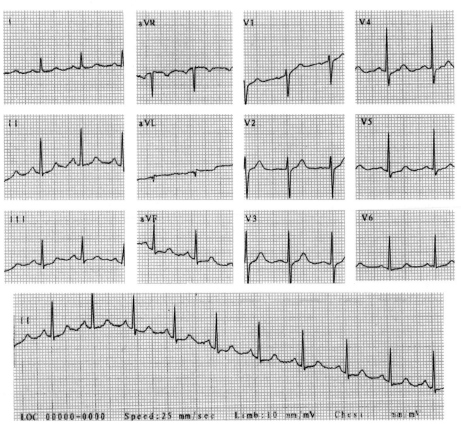

Fig. 8.24 The normal electrocardiogram. Standard leads (I, II, III), aVR, aVL, aVF (unipolar) limb leads, V (unipolar) chest leads $V_1 - V_6$. Note the recording speed of 25 mm/sec. The heart rate can be derived by dividing 300 by the number of large squares (5 small squares) between adjacent P, or QRS complexes. The ECGs in this chapter are taken from original traces and therefore the background colour varies.

Fig. 8.25   Sinus arrhythmia.

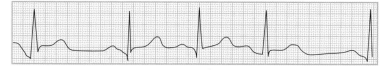

chest leads overlie the interventricular septum and the anterior wall of the left ventricle.

Atrial depolarization is the source of the changes in electrical potentials which cause the P wave. The QRS complex is due to ventricular depolarization and the T wave is due to ventricular depolarization (Fig. 8.23). Atrial depolarization is associated with the very small electrical charges which are not recorded on the conventional surface ECG. The Q wave is an initial negative deflection in the QRS complex.

The P–R interval (measured from the beginning of the P wave to the beginning of the QRS complex) is normally less than 0.2 s. The duration of the normal QRS complex is less than 0.12 s (Fig. 8.24).

Reading and interpreting the ECG

The ECG must be examined systematically. A convenient method is as follows:
● Determine the cardiac rate and rhythm
● Assess the P–R interval and the width of the QRS complex
● Examine the P wave and the QRS complex
● Examine the S–T segment and T wave.

The ECG in disorders of cardiac rhythm

Because it provides a record of both atrial excitation (P waves) and ventricular excitation (QRS complex) the ECG is useful in analysing cardiac dysrhythmias. P waves are usually best seen in lead II or in the right-sided chest leads (V_1) and these leads should therefore be studied particularly carefully when there

is a disorder of cardiac rhythm.

In health the heart beat is initiated in the sinoatrial node (pacemaker), which lies near the junction of the superior vena cava and the right atrium. The impulse spreads through both atria and thence to the atrioventricular (AV) node. From the AV node the impulse is conducted down the bundle of His and from there to the Purkinje fibres in the left and right bundle branches.

SINUS TACHYCARDIA

The cardiac impulse arises normally from the sinus node in sinus tachycardia, and the ECG is normal in form. The pulse rate is increased above 100 beats/min (adults). Sinus tachycardia may result from emotion, exercise, fever, hyperthyroidism and anaemia.

SINUS BRADYCARDIA

Again the ECG is normal in form, but the heart rate is less than 60 beats/min. Sinus bradycardia occurs in trained athletes and in patients with increased intracranial pressure, myxoedema and jaundice. It may also be an indication of fibrosis or ischaemia of the sinus node—sinoatrial disease.

SINUS ARRHYTHMIA

The cardiac impulse arises normally in the sinoatrial node, the rhythmicity of which varies; the heart rate increases with inspiration and diminishes with expiration (Fig. 8.25). The ECG is normal apart from variation in the R–R intervals. This arrhythmia is a normal finding in young people; it is increased by deep breathing and abolished by exercise.

Fig. 8.26   Atrial extrasystoles. Note the abnormal (inverted) P wave. The R–R interval is longer after the extrasystole than in the normal cycle.

Fig. 8.27   Lead II. Atrial fibrillation. The R waves are irregular. The last QRS complex is a ventricular extrasystole.

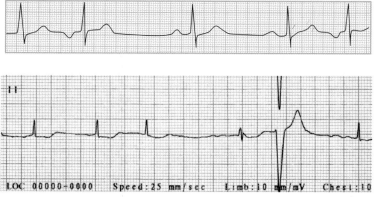

LOC 00000-0000   Speed:25 mm/sec   Limb:10 mm/mV   Chest:10

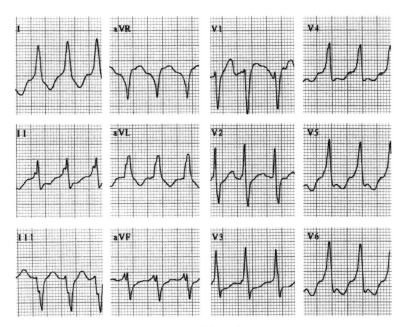

Fig. 8.28   Supraventricular tachycardia. The pulse rate was 150 beats/min.

EXTRASYSTOLES OR ECTOPIC BEATS

Ectopic beats arise from foci in the atria or ventricles which stimulate the heart before the next sinus beat is due. In ventricular extrasystoles P waves are absent and the QRS complexes are broad, the T wave pointing in the opposite direction to the major deflection of the QRS. The extrasystole comes prematurely and is followed by a pause (the compensatory pause).

The ECG of an atrial extrasystole shows the P wave to be abnormal in form, but the QRS which follows it is normal. The pause which follows the extrasystole is longer than normal (Fig. 8.26).

Extrasystoles are thus premature beats followed by an abnormally long pause and can be recognized by auscultation or palpation. Extrasystoles occur both in health and in patients with heart disease (Fig. 8.27). If an extrasystole follows each normal beat the pulse is said to be coupled (*bigeminy*). If the patient is being treated with digoxin the possibility of toxicity should be considered.

ATRIAL TACHYCARDIA AND ATRIAL FLUTTER

Atrial or supraventricular tachycardia (Fig. 8.28) and atrial flutter (Fig. 8.29) are due to the presence of an ectopic focus in the atrium which beats regularly at a rapid rate. The P waves are abnormal in shape, but the QRS complexes are usually normal; however, at faster rates a bundle branch block pattern (page 195) may develop. As a rule not all atrial impulses are

conducted to the ventricles. Often alternate beats are conducted, when 2:1 atrioventricular block is said to be present. Occasionally 3:1 or 4:1 block is present and sometimes the degree of block varies.

Atrial flutter and tachycardia may occur in the absence of other cardiac abnormalities, or in thyrotoxicosis and rheumatic or ischaemic heart disease.

ATRIAL FIBRILLATION

There is no co-ordinate atrial activity (either electrical or mechanical) in atrial fibrillation. The ECG (Fig. 8.30) shows *f* (fibrillation) waves representing the atrial activity instead of P waves, especially in lead V_1. The QRS complexes are normal but occur irregularly.

Atrial fibrillation is recognized clinically by complete irregularity of the pulse rate. Mitral valve disease, ischaemic heart disease and thyrotoxicosis are the commonest causes of atrial fibrillation.

In Wolff–Parkinson–White syndrome (Fig. 8.31) there is an abnormally rapid atrioventricular condition, due to abnormal connection (the bundle of Kent), causing a short P–R interval, an abnormal QRS complex and paroxysmal tachycardia or atrial fibrillation.

ATRIOVENTRICULAR BLOCK (HEART BLOCK)

In *first-degree atrioventricular block* the P–R interval exceeds 0.2 s and all atrial impulses reach the

Fig. 8.29 Atrial flutter. Atrial rate about 300 beats/min. Note the two to four flutter waves to each ventricular complex.

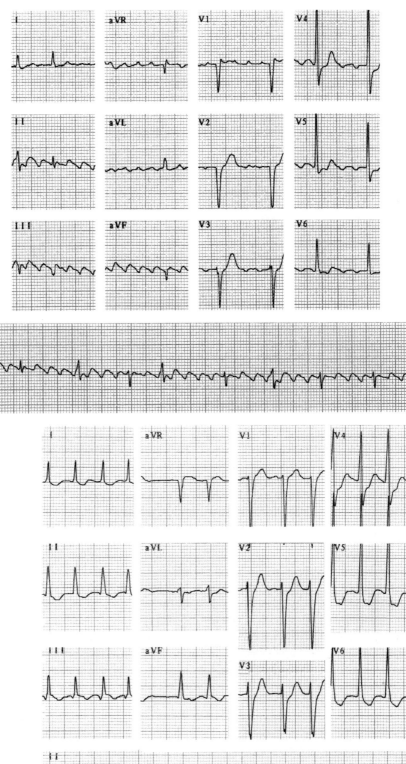

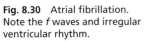

Fig. 8.30 Atrial fibrillation. Note the *f* waves and irregular ventricular rhythm.

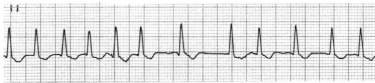

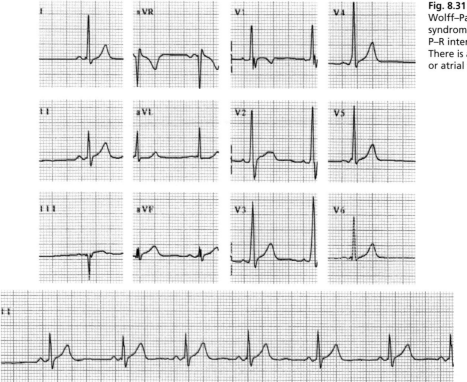

Fig. 8.31
Wolff–Parkinson–White syndrome. There is a short P–R interval and wide QRS. There is a risk of tachycardia or atrial fibrillation.

ventricles. When some impulses fail to reach the ventricles but others do reach it, then there is *second-degree atrioventricular block*. In *third-degree atrioventricular block (complete)* the atria and ventricles beat independently, i.e. they are dissociated (Fig 8.32). The ventricular rate is usually slow, 20–40 beats/min, and often erratic and may fail completely—ventricular standstill.

VENTRICULAR FIBRILLATION

A similar mechanism operates in the ventricles as in the atria with atrial fibrillation. There are no distinct QRS complexes, but bizarre undulations of irregular height and rate. There is no effective cardiac output; loss of consciousness rapidly develops and this rhythm is fatal unless treated promptly.

The ECG in some other conditions

VENTRICULAR HYPERTROPHY

Ventricular hypertrophy is diagnosed principally from the chest leads and in particular V_1 and V_6. Figure 8.33 shows the appearance of the QRS complexes in V_1 (over the right ventricle) and V_6 (over the left ventricle). It must be appreciated that the QRS complex from any lead represents the algebraic sum of the electrical activity of both ventricles (compare this with the normal ECG in Fig. 8.24). At any point in time the ECG will show an R wave (positive deflection) if the resultant current vector is going away from the electrode. Ventricular hypertrophy is associated with an increase in the electrical activity of depolarization. As a result there is an increase in the

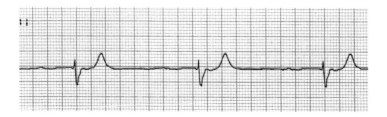

Fig. 8.32 Complete heart block. Atrial rate about 80 beats/min; ventricular rate 35 beats/min.

Fig. 8.33 Left ventricular hypertrophy. Note the deep S wave in V_1; the tall R wave in V_6, and S–T depression and T wave inversion in lead I and V_6,

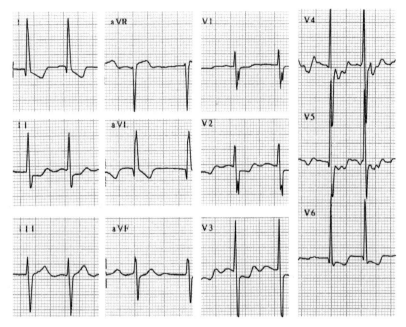

magnitude of the QRS deflections which is best seen in the chest leads. The size of the QRS complex deflections is also affected by the thickness of the anterior chest wall. The QRS complex is larger in thin patients and smaller in obese subjects. Voltage criteria for the diagnosis of ventricular hypertrophy cannot be precise.

Left ventricular hypertrophy

As the left ventricle lies to the left and posteriorly there is an increase in the size of the R wave in the left chest leads (V_5 and V_6) and an increase in the S wave in the right chest leads (V_1–V_2; see Fig. 8.33).

Right ventricular hypertrophy

The R wave in the right chest leads is increased and there is a deeper S wave in the left chest leads, as the increased electrical activity is associated with the anteriorly placed right ventricle.

In addition, both types of ventricular hypertrophy may show a ventricular strain pattern. There is an abnormality of ventricular repolarization associated with hypertrophy. It causes the T wave to point away from the affected ventricle, giving S–T depression and T wave inversion in leads I, aVL and the left chest leads in *left* ventricular hypertrophy, and in leads V_1, V_2, II and III in *right* ventricular hypertrophy. Other causes of T wave abnormalities are mentioned on page 197.

BUNDLE BRANCH BLOCK

In bundle branch block (Fig. 8.34), owing to an interruption of one of the bundle branches, conduction to one ventricle is delayed. The QRS duration is greater than 0.12 s. For example, if the left bundle is interrupted, conduction to the left ventricle is delayed and it becomes activated at a time when it is no longer opposed by the right ventricle, and therefore produces large deflections (Fig. 8.34(a)), as in hypertrophy of the left ventricle.

MYOCARDIAL INFARCTION

Myocardial infarction alters the ECG by the successive production of abnormalities in the S–T segments, the development of Q waves and T wave inversion (Fig. 8.35).

It should be noted that within the first 2 hours of infarction the ECG may be virtually normal. Subsequently the S–T segments become raised. (Fig. 8.35(b)). In a few days the T waves become inverted (Fig. 8.35(c)). The S–T segment gradually returns to the baseline, taking several weeks to do so. T wave inversion may eventually return to normal (Fig. 8.35(d)) but some inversion usually persists. As the S–T segments return to normal the R wave is diminished in height, being replaced by a negative initial deflection—a Q wave. The timing of the appearance of Q waves varies from 1 to 48 hours and they usually indicate permanent loss of viable ventricular muscle.

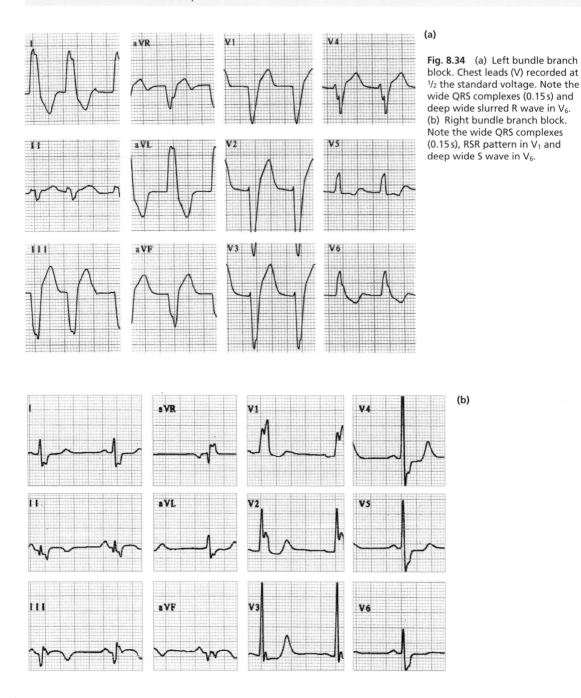

(a)

Fig. 8.34   (a) Left bundle branch block. Chest leads (V) recorded at ½ the standard voltage. Note the wide QRS complexes (0.15 s) and deep wide slurred R wave in V_6. (b) Right bundle branch block. Note the wide QRS complexes (0.15 s), RSR pattern in V_1 and deep wide S wave in V_6.

(b)

The presence of Q waves indicates a full thickness infarct and is usually associated with complete occlusion of a coronary vessel. If only T wave changes occur then this is described as a subendocardial or partial-thickness infarction. The leads showing Q waves or S–T and T wave changes are determined by the site of the infarct. The ECGs illustrating classical anterior and inferior infarction are shown in Fig. 8.36.

In *anterior infarction* the changes are seen in leads I and V_1 to V_5. In *inferior infarction* the changes are seen in leads II and III and aVF. In *lateral infarction* the changes occur in leads I, aVL, V_5 and V_6 (Table 8.2).

P WAVE CHANGES

Because the sinoatrial node is located in the right atrium, right atrial depolarization precedes

Table 8.2 The relationship between the myocardial regions, coronary vessels and the ECG.

Myocardial region	Coronary vessel	ECG leads
Anteroseptal	Left anterior descending	V_1–V_5
Lateral	Left circumflex	I, aVL
Inferior	Right coronary 90% (circumflex 10%)*	II, III, aVF

V_6† (bracketing I, aVL and II, III, aVF)

* In a heavily dominant system with a small or insignificant right coronary circulation, the inferior wall of the left ventricle may be supplied by the left circumflex vessel.

† V_6 (apex) may be supplied by any of three vessels, depending on the anatomy of the coronary tree.

left atrial depolarization. Left atrial hypertrophy therefore causes a broadening of the P wave. This is best seen in standard lead II, where the delayed left atrial depolarization. This gives an M-shaped configuration to the P wave and is often called a *P mitral*, since it is found in patients with severe mitral stenosis and sinus rhythm. Left atrial hypertrophy appears as a terminal negative deflection of the P wave.

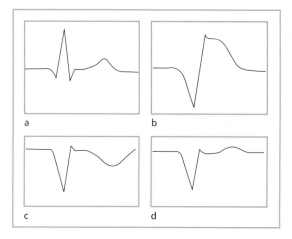

Fig. 8.35 The evolution of the changes in the QRS complex, S–T segment and T wave after cardiac infarction. (a) Normal pattern. (b) A few hours after infarction; a Q wave is present and the S–T segment is elevated (Pardee's sign). (c) After a time the S–T segment returns to the baseline and the T wave becomes steeply inverted. (d) After a further period the T wave becomes inverted, flat and finally upright. Note that the Q wave persists.

In contrast, right atrial hypertrophy leads to a peaked appearance of the P wave in both leads II and V_1. This appearance is sometimes known as a *P pulmonale* since pulmonary hypertension is one of the important causes of right atrial hypertrophy.

Exercise tests

Because the major physiological disorder associated with coronary artery disease is a failure of adequate blood supply in response to increased demand, it follows that an ECG recorded at rest has limited value in predicting a disorder which has its maximum effect during exertion. The objective of an exercise test is, therefore, to stress the patient on either a treadmill or a bicycle ergometer, and to record the ECG during and immediately after the period of exercise. The protocol calls for an increasing level of work to be done until either angina develops or a heart rate of between 140 and 175 beats/min is reached, depending on the patient's age and sex. In the presence of coronary artery disease the S–T segment is often depressed when the myocardium is ischaemic (Fig. 8.37). The presence of S–T segment depression with either a horizontal or downward sloping configuration is then very suggestive of myocardial ischaemia.

Exercise testing cannot at present definitively deny the presence of coronary artery disease (Fig. 8.37) nor is it absolutely specific in predicting its presence. In attempts to increase the clinical usefulness of exercise testing in detecting coronary artery disease the technique has been combined with methods for imaging the heart with radioactive tracer elements. In this way the myocardial perfusion during exercise and subsequently at rest is compared and it is possible to detect areas which were underperfused during exercise. Further refinements of the non-invasive investigation of ischaemic heart disease are currently under investigation. At present coronary angiography (Fig. 8.38(a) and (b)) may be regarded as demonstrating abnormal anatomy and the investigations described above in this section as demonstrating altered physiology.

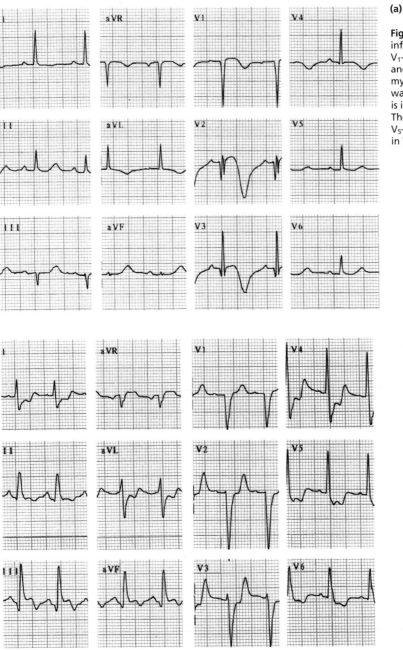

(a)

Fig. 8.36 (a) Anterior myocardial infarction. Note the Q wave in V_1–V_3, with inverted T wave in V_4, I and aVL. (b) Acute inferior myocardial infarction. Note the Q waves in leads II and III. The T wave is inverted in lead II and in lead III. There is T wave inversion in leads V_5–V_6 with S–T segment depression in V_3–V_6.

(b)

Radiographic examination

In addition to the standard posteroanterior X-ray of the chest much information may be gained by taking more penetrated films of the posteroanterior and right lateral views.

Screening of the heart is primarily of value in visualizing calcification of valves; it is occasionally useful in detecting the presence of a left ventricular aneurysm.

The normal cardiac outline

In a standard PA X-ray of the chest the heart (Fig. 8.39) is seen as a flask-shaped shadow, lying between the translucent lungs, about one-third of its area to the right of the midline and two-thirds to the left.

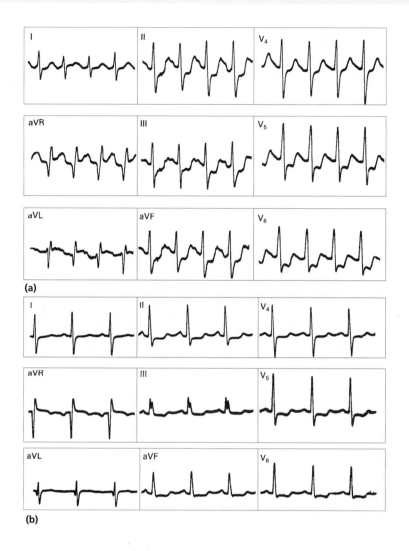

(a)

(b)

(c)

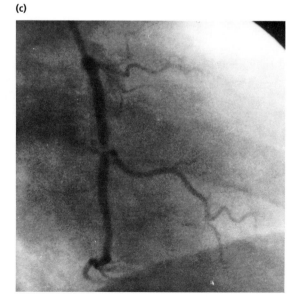

Fig. 8.37 (a) A positive exercise test in a patient who was subsequently shown to have a severe stenosis in the left main coronary vessel. The tracing recorded immediately after exercise shows a heart rate of 160 beats/min with marked depression of S–T segments in the inferior (II, III and aVF) and anterior (V_5 and V_6) leads. (b) Ten minutes after cessation of exercise the S–T segment has returned towards normal although some slight depression still remains. (c) Coronary angiography of the same patient. There is a stenosis in the right coronary artery at a major branch. The illustration is taken from a cineradiograph made as part of the investigation. The patient presented with angina but cardiac infarction had not occurred.

(a)

(b)

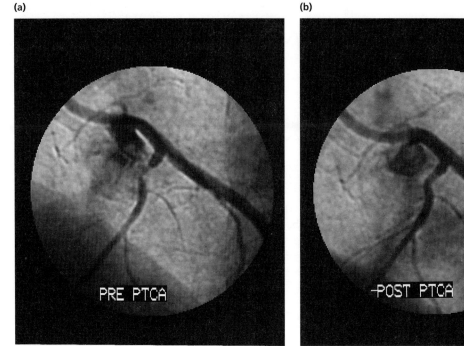

Fig. 8.38   (a) and (b) Stenosis of the branch of the coronary artery before (a) and after (b) percutaneous transluminal coronary angioplasty (PTCA). The patient presented with angina which was relieved after the procedure.

The apex of the heart is internal to the mid-clavicular line.

The right border of the normal cardiac shadow is formed, from above downwards, by two curves:
- a slightly curved portion—the outer edge of the superior vena cava with the ascending aorta; and
- a more convex portion—the outer border of the

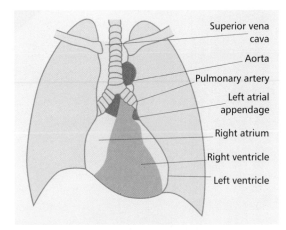

Superior vena cava

Aorta

Pulmonary artery

Left atrial appendage

Right atrium

Right ventricle

Left ventricle

Fig. 8.39   The cardiac silhouette in the anteroposterior position. This is particularly useful in studying the outflow from the left atrium, the pulmonary artery and the aortic knuckle.

right atrium, the lower margin of which lies at the diaphragm.

The left border comprises from above downwards:
- the prominent knuckle produced by the arch of the aorta as it passes backwards, slightly to the left, then downwards;
- the straighter line of the pulmonary artery;
- the left atrial appendage; and
- the wide sweep of the left ventricle, ending at the apex where it rests on the diaphragm.

In the overpenetrated PA film the left atrium can be seen, especially if enlarged, and the aorta is particularly well-shown. Calcification in the pericardium or valves may be apparent. The right lateral film is of value in localizing valve calcification and in addition is helpful in right ventricular hypertrophy when the anteriorly placed right ventricle lies closer to the sternum than normal.

Common alterations in disease

POSITION OF THE HEART IN THE CHEST

Displacement of the heart as a whole is seen in pleural effusion, pneumothorax and fibrosis of the lung. In distension of the stomach and obesity, the heart is raised with the diaphragm and the apex tilted upwards. The common type of scoliosis (convexity of the curve to the right) is a frequent cause of dis-

(a)

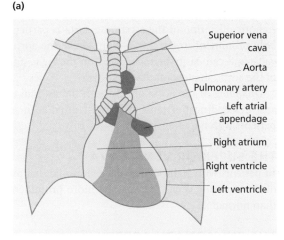

Superior vena cava

Aorta

Pulmonary artery

Left atrial appendage

Right atrium

Right ventricle

Left ventricle

(b)

Fig. 8.40 (a) Diagram of cardiac outline in left ventricular enlargement. (b) Radiograph showing the characteristic shape of left ventricle enlargement in this patient with aortic regurgitation. Thin egg-shell calcification is seen in the aortic wall.

placement of the heart to the left. In narrow chests the heart often lies centrally and seems small and slender.

SHAPE AND SIZE OF THE HEART

Examination of the heart shadow indicates the overall heart size but it can be difficult to identify precisely which cardiac chamber is enlarged. In left ventricular enlargement, as found with aortic valve disease or hypertension, there is a prominent convexity below the diaphragm and forming an obtuse angle (Fig. 8.40). In right ventricular enlargement the outline of the apex is turned up and the heart shadow makes an acute angle with the diaphragm. More commonly it is only possible to indicate that there is an increase in ventricular mass without

BOX 8.2 Detection of left atrial enlargement.

- Prominence of the left atrial appendage at the left border of the heart (Fig. 8.41)
- A doubled shadow seen through the right atrium. This is the caudal edge of the enlarged left atrium, which does not extend down to the diaphragm as does the right atrium
- Upward displacement of the left main bronchus so that it runs horizontally
- Extrinsic compression revealed by using a barium swallow to outline the oesophagus

(a)

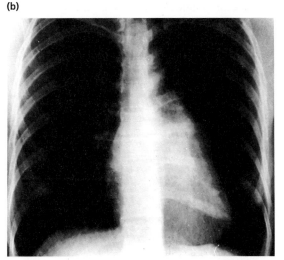

Superior vena cava

Aorta

Pulmonary artery

Left atrial appendage

Right atrium

Right ventricle

Left ventricle

(b)

Fig. 8.41 (a) Diagram of cardiac outline in mitral stenosis showing prominence of left atrial appendage at left heart border. (b) Radiograph of mitral stenosis. Note the characteristic bulging of the left border associated with left atrial enlargement.

being able to predict accurately which chamber is responsible.

There are four ways by which left atrial enlargement may be detected (Box 8.2).

SHAPE AND SIZE OF THE AORTA

Dilatation of the ascending aorta is an important abnormality. It is most usually due to weakening of the media in the aortic wall. In patients with Marfan's syndrome, cystic medial necrosis frequently causes severe aortic dilatation. A less common cause is syphilitic aortitis. Irrespective of the cause of aortic dilatation, if the aortic root is involved the function of the aortic cusps may be disturbed so that aortic incompetence results.

At any site of obstruction in the circulation the phenomenon of *post-stenotic dilatation* is likely to occur. In patients with aortic valve stenosis post-stenotic dilatation of the ascending aorta is particularly prominent in the first 5–8 cm above the aortic valve and can easily be recognized on the right side of the aortic shadow on the chest X-ray.

Unfolding of the aorta affects both the ascending and descending portions. It is most often seen in patients with hypertension.

THE SUPERIOR VENA CAVA

In patients with right ventricular failure the shadow of the superior vena cava may be more prominent than normal.

THE PULMONARY ARTERY

The main pulmonary artery is enlarged in pulmonary hypertension. Pulmonary stenosis leads to

post-stenotic dilatation and this is detected radiologically as enlargement of the main pulmonary artery.

THE PULMONARY VASCULATURE

There are four important indicators of raised left atrial pressure (Box 8.3). It is incorrect to regard these changes as being necessarily due to 'left ventricular failure'. They occur whenever the left atrial pressure is elevated, whether due to mitral valve stenosis or regurgitation, left atrial myxoma, aortic valve disease or primary ventricular disease.

When the pulmonary blood flow is increased, the main branches of the pulmonary artery are increased in size—*pulmonary plethora*. This occurs when there is a left-to-right shunt in the circulation, e.g. atrial septal defect, ventricular septal defect or patent ductus arteriosus. It is especially obvious when some of the

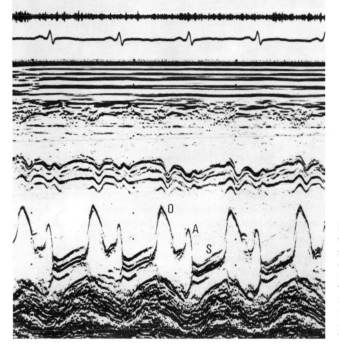

Fig. 8.42 Echocardiogram of a normal mitral valve. The anterior and posterior leaflets are shown moving in opposite directions during diastole. Following the rapid opening of the leaflets in early diastole (O) the leaflets move towards a closed position and then re-open again under the influence of atrial systole (A). During ventricular systole the leaflets are seen as a series of parallel lines moving gradually up the tracing (S).

branches are seen end-on near the hilum. Conversely, in Fallot's tetralogy the vascular markings in the lung field are inconspicuous—*pulmonary oligaemia*.

Special investigations

ECG and chest radiography are essential in the proper assessment of the cardiovascular system and so are

---

BOX 8.4 Abnormality detection using echocardiography.

- On the chest X-ray a pericardial effusion causes non-specific enlargement of the cardiac shadow. On ultrasound the fluid shows up as an echolucent area between the epicardium and endocardium (Fig. 8.43).
- Rheumatic mitral valve disease leads to a characteristically abnormal echocardiographic appearance of the valve (Fig. 8.44): the anterior mitral leaflet, having opened rapidly at the beginning of diastole, moves slowly if at all towards the closed position. If there is any significant fusion of the anterior and posterior leaflets at the commissures, then the ability of the posterior leaflet to move independently from the anterior leaflet is lost. Thus in diastole, instead of the leaflets moving in opposite directions, the posterior leaflet moves anteriorly in parallel with the anterior leaflet. The rheumatic process leads to considerable thickening of the valve structure and this too can be detected echocardiographically.
- Echocardiography makes it possible to study a direct image of the left ventricle. The size of the cavity in end systole and end-diastole can be measured and this permits the quantification of both volume overload of the left ventricle, in which the end-diastolic dimension is increased, and also left ventricular disease, which leads to dilatation of the cavity in both systole and diastole.
- Hypertrophic cardiomyopathy is characterized by thickening of the interventricular septum. Using echocardiography it is possible to measure the thickness of this structure with accuracy. In addition, abnormalities of motion of the mitral and aortic valves found in this condition are well-displayed.
- Calcium in the aortic valve leading to aortic stenosis is recognized on the echocardiogram as an increase of reflected echoes from the abnormal valve structure. Aortic regurgitation leads to a jet of blood impinging on the anterior mitral leaflet and its presence can be predicted from the finding of a fine fluttering motion of the echocardiographic image of this part of the mitral valve.
- The presence of various abnormal masses within the heart can be detected by echocardiography. The commonest of these is a vegetation associated with infective endocarditis and usually attached to one of the valves (Fig. 8.45). Cardiac tumours can also be diagnosed and the most important of these, although rare, is an atrial myxoma.

---

considered as part of the routine examination. The need to establish precisely the diagnosis and functional status of patients, frequently as a preliminary to cardiac surgery, has stimulated the development of special techniques.

External pulse recording and phonocardiography

Using suitable transducers, carotid and venous pulsation can be displayed along with the cardiac impulse (*apex cardiography*) and the recordings of heart sounds and murmurs. This is useful in confirming the time relationships of the physical signs and should be considered an adjunct to the physical examination. However useful in assisting interpretation, these techniques do not elicit new information; phonocardiography will not reveal significant heart murmurs that cannot be heard by auscultation.

Echocardiography

Ultrasound is increasingly used as a diagnostic technique and has become of particular importance in the field of cardiology. The fact that the heart is continually moving and that abnormalities of motion are of diagnostic importance gives echocardiography a particular advantage over other imaging techniques (Fig. 8.42).

Echocardiography is particularly useful in detecting a number of abnormalities (Box 8.4).

Cardiac catheterization

Cardiac catheterization is carried out when it is necessary to obtain detailed information about the heart, aorta and coronary vessels which cannot be obtained from clinical and other non-invasive methods. The technique carries a small risk of both morbidity and mortality and therefore should only be undertaken following a full assessment which defines the objectives of the procedure.

Cardiac catheterization provides information about the pressures in the different cardiac chambers and also allows angiography to be carried out. There are two peripheral sites at which the circulation may be conveniently entered—the femoral artery and femoral vein, and the brachial artery and antecubital vein. This is an important method of determining the need for surgical valve replacement.

Measurement of the pressure difference in the two chambers on either side of a stenotic valve, e.g. left

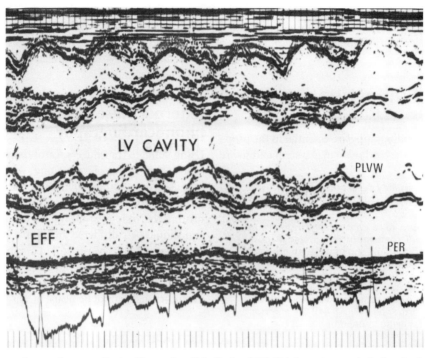

Fig. 8.43 Echocardiogram from a patient with a pericardial effusion (EFF). This is seen as a relatively echo-free space lying above the pericardium (PER). The effusion and pericardium both lie below the left ventricular (LV) cavity and the posterior left ventricular wall (PLVW).

ventricle and aorta in aortic stenosis, indicates the severity of the obstruction to forward flow.

Catheterization of the right heart permits accurate measurement of the pulmonary artery pressure. The left atrial pressure is measured indirectly by 'wedging' the right heart catheter in the peripheral pulmonary arteriolar vessels. Measurement of the right atrial pressure should correlate well with the clinical assessment of the venous pressure. A left ventricular angiogram and an aortogram are the means by which mitral and aortic regurgitation respectively are demonstrated. Radiological contrast may be injected into the cardiac chambers using the same catheter employed for pressure measurements.

Coronary angiography (see Figs 8.37, 8.38 (a) and (b)), in which the ostia of the left and right coronary arteries are selectively cannulated, is at present the only means by which the details of the effects of atheroma on the coronary circulation may be documented. This is an essential investigation prior to coronary artery vein graft surgery (see page 200).

In addition to the above applications, cardiac

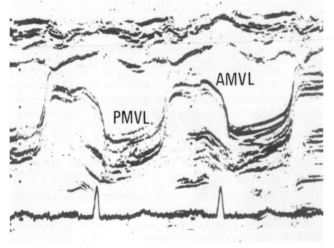

Fig. 8.44 Echocardiogram from a patient with mitral stenosis. In contrast to the normal mitral valve (see Fig. 8.42) the anterior and posterior leaflets both move in the same direction during diastole. Both leaflets are thickened and this is shown by an increased number of lines running parallel to each other. The rate of closure of the leaflets in diastole is much slower than normal. AMVL = anterior mitral valve leaflet; PMVL = posterior mitral valve leaflet.

Fig. 8.45 Echocardiogram of the mitral valve in a patient with a vegetation (VEG) attached to the anterior mitral leaflet.

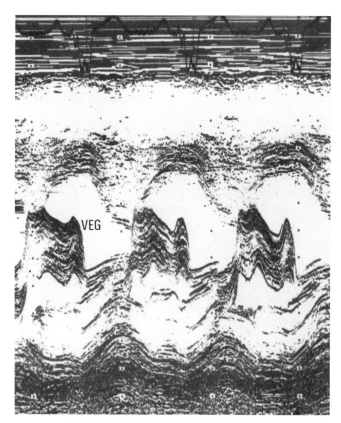

catheterization plays an important role in congenital heart disease. By sampling the oxygen saturation at different points in the circulation the anatomical site of intracardiac shunts can be defined and the size of the shunt may be quantified.

In recent years the technique of *angioplasty* has been used in patients with stenosis in the coronary arteries. A balloon mounted on a catheter is inflated at the site of the atheromatous lesion and the narrowing of the lumen is thereby reduced. In patients in whom this technique seems inappropriate, usually because there is more extensive disease of smaller branches of the coronary arteries, saphenous vein or internal mammary artery grafts are used to bypass the diseased coronary arteries (*coronary artery bypass surgery: CABG*).

CHAPTER 9

The ear, nose and throat

Introduction

The ear, nose and throat are functionally interrelated and should be examined together. For example, a patient with sinus disease, who has pus dripping backwards over the opening of the eustachian tube, may present with acute suppurative otitis media or acute pharyngo-tonsillitis.

Thus, although each region is necessarily described separately, appreciation of the close association of the ear, nose and throat is necessary to ensure a comprehensive examination of this region.

The ear

The main symptoms of ear disease are:
- aural pain (*otalgia*);
- discharge (*otorrhoea*);
- *hearing loss*;
- the sensation of sound in the absence of an appropriate auditory stimulus (*tinnitus*);
- sensation of abnormal movement (*vertigo*).

OTALGIA
The sensory innervation of the external ear canal, tympanic membrane and middle ear arises from the fifth, ninth and tenth cranial nerves, together with branches of the great auricular nerve and lesser occipital nerve (second and third cervical divisions). Since divisions of these cranial nerves also supply the larynx, pharynx (including the tongue base), and the temporomandibular joint and teeth, primary pathology in any of these areas may give rise to referred otalgia. Therefore in any patient with otalgia and normal findings on otoscopy inspection of the nasopharynx is indicated.

Severe pain in the region of the pinna may be secondary to infection of the skin or auricular cartilage (*perichondritis*). As the skin is closely applied to the periosteum of the ear canal, generalized or localized infection (e.g. a furuncle) may also cause severe pain. There is frequently a history of swimming, trauma or dermatitis, especially eczema. Infection may also be caused by trauma from cottonbuds used to remove wax from the ear canal.

An acute onset of a deep, severe, throbbing otalgia may also indicate an acute infection in the middle ear. *Acute suppurative otitis media* is most common in children and is usually secondary to an upper respiratory tract or sinus infection. It is also common in very young children who are teething and should be suspected in a distressed, fretful, crying child with a high fever. Otalgia in a patient with chronic otorrhoea may be due to dural infection or malignant change within the middle ear.

Less severe ear pain follows blunt trauma to the pinna, causing a *subperichondrial haematoma*. Extravasation of blood between the perichondrium and cartilage causes a dough-like swelling which may obliterate the normal contours of the pinna.

Tender nodules on the rim of the helix may be due to *polychondritis helicis*, a chronic, low-grade inflammation of the helical cartilage of unknown aetiology, or to *gouty tophi*. A *squamous or basal cell carcinoma* may present as a slowly growing, painful ulcer on any portion of the external ear, but most commonly affects the helix.

OTORRHOEA

A discharge from the ear may be:
- purulent;
- sanguineous; or
- serous.

An acute onset of otalgia with a prominent discharge indicates either an otitis externa or an acute suppurative otitis media which has caused perforation of the tympanic membrane. If the pus contains mucus (*mucopus*) it must have arisen from glands in the middle ear cleft. Intermittent, profuse, inoffensive otorrhoea suggests that there is a perforation of the pars tensa of the tympanic membrane. This infection passes from the nasopharynx into the eustachian tube (tubo-tympanic disease): such a discharge is unlikely to involve the meninges. By contrast, a chronic, offensive, scanty discharge may be the first symptom of serious underlying disease, which may result in meningeal or intracerebral infection, facial nerve palsy or erosion of the inner ear, causing vertigo or total deafness. Scanty, foul-smelling otorrhoea discharging from a retraction pocket or through a tiny attic perforation may be the only sign of this potentially life-threatening condition. In a chronically discharging ear the onset of bleeding sometimes indicates malignant change within the middle ear.

Trauma is a frequent cause of a blood-stained discharge. A blow to the ear may cause perforation of the tympanic membrane, nearly always associated with otalgia, bleeding and hearing loss. More severe trauma may cause a dural tear, and fracture of the tegmen tympani, which separates the middle ear from the meninges covering the temporal lobe. There will be a history of bleeding from the external ear canal and it may only be when blood has clotted that a watery discharge indicating a cerebrospinal fluid leak is noted.

HEARING LOSS

In patients with hearing loss it is important to establish the cause of the impairment, while also assessing the extent of hearing loss and the handicap that the deafness is liable to produce.

The degree of disability depends on the extent of deafness, on the ability of the patient to compensate by lip-reading and, in unilateral deafness on the retained hearing in the better ear. The overall handicap will depend on the patient's lifestyle and the efficacy of a hearing aid. The cause of the deafness is also important. In *conductive hearing loss*, e.g. a disorder in the external ear canal, tympanic membrane or middle ear, the patient will retain normal auditory acuity and normal speech discrimination provided there is adequate amplification. By contrast, in *sensorineural hearing loss*, due either to cochlear (sensory) or retrocochlear (neural) pathology, speech discrimination is markedly impaired. In particular, patients with a sensory hearing loss may find that a small increase in the intensity of the auditory stimulus above threshold leads to intense discomfort due to perceptual distortion caused by damaged cochlear hair cells. This is known as *recruitment* and may lead the patient to complain of discomfort when well-meaning people raise their voices in an attempt to engage in conversation.

The history may reveal other important clues. Thus a patient may notice an apparent difference in the pitch or frequency of a tone between the two ears (*diplacusis*), and this may lead to a complaint that sound is different in one ear: it is especially associated with endolymphatic hydrops. In such cases the auditory acuity fluctuates. Conversely, if the patient reports that hearing is better in a noisy environment, this may indicate a conductive deafness due to otosclerosis.

Is the hearing loss sudden or progressive? In the majority of patients with *sudden deafness* spontaneous recovery will occur and the aetiology will remain unknown. Identifiable causes (Box 9.1) of

---

BOX 9.1 Causes of deafness.

Sudden deafness
- Viral infections
- Fractured petrous bone
- Acoustic neuroma

Noise-induced deafness

Drugs, e.g. glutamine, quinine

Infection
- Otitis media
- 'Glue ear'

Genetic causes
- Otosclerosis
- Sensorineural deafness

sudden deafness include viral infections, in particular, mumps causing sudden unilateral deafness, and meningitis. Head injuries with a fracture of the petrous temporal bone, and previous surgery in the region of the oval window resulting in perilymphatic fistula, may also result in sudden deafness. Sudden deafness is the presenting feature in a small proportion of patients with an acoustic neuroma.

Deafness in adults may be genetic in origin: a careful family history is therefore important. Conductive deafness caused by fixation of the stapedial footplate in otosclerosis, inherited as an autosomal dominant trait with varying penetrance, is a common cause of hereditary deafness. Dominantly inherited sensorineural deafness due to degeneration of the stria vascularis of the cochlea is also common, and *congenital deafness*, affecting one per thousand live births, is often inherited. There are associations with several neurological, renal and other systemic disorders.

A history of *noise exposure* is also relevant. This is commonly occupational and in many countries legislation has been introduced to compensate certain groups of workers. Social exposure to noise, such as overloud music in discotheques and from personal stereos, can also cause hearing impairment. Occasionally permanent damage may result from a brief exposure to very loud noise such as gun fire or the blast of a bomb. Many drugs are ototoxic, e.g. the aminoglycoside antibiotics, such as *gentamicin*, diuretics such as *frusemide*, cytotoxic drugs such as *cisplatin*, beta-blocker drugs such as *propranolol*, and non-steroid, anti-inflammatory drugs such as *aspirin*. *Quinine* is also ototoxic.

In a child with hearing loss it is important to ascertain the degree of speech impairment and educational delay and to inquire whether the child has appeared withdrawn, or inattentive. Serous otitis media (*glue ear*) is by far the most common hearing impairment in such cases: the deafness varies in severity and may be associated with episodic pain in the ear and clumsiness.

TINNITUS

Tinnitus, defined as a sensation of sound in the absence of an appropriate auditory stimulus, can be caused by any conductive or sensorineural hearing loss.

Most cases are characterized by a ringing, rushing or hissing sound in the ear. Tinnitus must be distinguished from *autophony*, an abnormal perception of the patient's own voice and breath sounds.

Autophony is often likened to the sensation experienced when holding a sea shell to the ear. The commonest cause is a patulous eustachian tube.

Occasionally, simple treatment such as the removal of wax may cure tinnitus. Successful treatment of a conductive hearing loss, e.g. stapedectomy in a patient with otosclerosis, may alleviate or reduce tinnitus. However, in the majority of cases such cures are impossible. Some patients find their tinnitus prevents sleep. Treatment with the use of a hearing aid, or a tinnitus masker (an external source of continuous soft sound), may make life more tolerable.

VERTIGO

Vertigo (Box 9.2) is an hallucination of movement such that the patient has a sensation of movement of self with respect to the world, or of the environment with respect to self.

BOX 9.2 Causes of vertigo.

Of sudden onset
- Acute viral labyrinthitis (vestibular neuronitis)

With focal features
- Brainstem ischaemia (TIA)
- Multiple sclerosis
- Migraine
- Temporal lobe epilepsy

With deafness and tinnitus
- Ménière's syndrome
- Acoustic neuroma

With particular head posture
- Benign positional vertigo

After trauma
- Post-traumatic vertigo
- Perilymphatic fistula

With motion
Motion sickness

Drug induced
- Vestibulotoxic drugs, e.g. gentamicin, salicylates, quinine, antihypertensives

With aural discharge
- Middle ear disease

With systemic disorders
- Postural hypotension
- Syncope
- Cardiac dysrhythmia
- Carotid sinus hypersensitivity
- Anxiety and panic attacks
- Hyperventilation syndrome

Vertigo may be *peripheral*, i.e. labyrinthine, or *central* in origin. Acute peripheral lesions cause vertigo of sudden onset, lasting a few seconds or a few days: movement tends to make the vertigo worse. A more persistent or slowly progressive loss of peripheral vestibular function produces vague symptoms such as dizziness or instability. Although central pathology may occasionally present with a hallucination of rotary movement, a swaying or tilting sensation is more common. Vertigo must be distinguished from gait abnormalities due to cerebellar disease, or disorders of proprioceptive sensory input. Occasionally there is a history of oscillopsia, an inability to stabilize a visual image, a feature of the nystagmus associated with both peripheral and central lesions. Dizziness is a rare feature of temporal lobe epilepsy.

It is important to ascertain the severity, frequency and length of each attack and of any associated otological symptoms. Recurrence of vertiginous attacks and an association with fluctuating hearing loss, fullness in the ear and tinnitus are features of *Ménière's syndrome*. An abrupt onset of transient vertigo with certain head movements occurs in patients with *benign paroxysmal positional vertigo*. In patients with a perilymphatic fistula coughing or sneezing will induce vertigo. In patients with a fistula in the lateral semicircular canal vertigo may be experienced in response to loud sounds (*Tullio's phenomenon*).

Anxiety states in which the patient hyperventilates, has blurring of consciousness and light-headedness may be mistaken for true vertigo.

Examination

The instruments used for examination of the ear, nose and throat are shown in Fig. 9.1.

PINNA

Look first at the pinna and the surrounding skin. Congenital absence of the pinna is termed *anotia*. *Microtia* is incomplete development of the auricle and is commonly seen in conjunction with atresia of the external auditory meatus and with anomalies of the mandibular arch. *Melotia* is displacement of the auricle from its normal position and *macrotia* is enlargement of the pinna. In the common 'bat ear' deformity, this is associated with accessory skin tags and cartilaginous fragments in the skin surrounding the ear. Look also for pre-auricular pits and sinuses. Pre-auricular lymphadenopathy has to be differentiated from cysts or infection in a pre-auricular sinus.

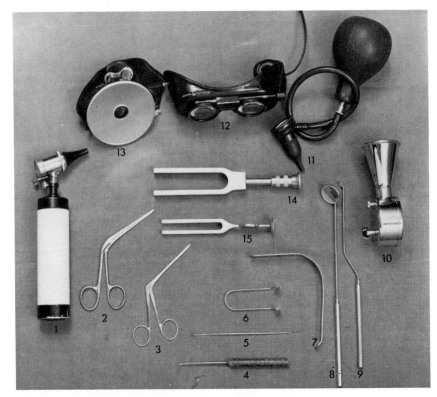

Fig. 9.1 Instruments used in examination of the ear, nose and throat. 1=Auriscope; 2=dressing forceps; 3=crocodile forceps; 4=cerumen hook; 5=Jobson Horne probe; 6=Thudichum's nasal speculum; 7=Lack's tongue depressor; 8=laryngeal mirror; 9=St Clair Thomson postnasal mirror; 10=Bárány noise box; 11=Siegel's speculum; 12=Frenzel's glasses; 13=head mirror; 14, 15=tuning forks.

POSTAURICULAR REGION

Take particular care to examine the postauricular region for signs of a scar indicating previous surgery. Erythema, with a hot, tender swelling in this region indicates that a mastoid abscess may be present. Pus may track from this site along the sternocleidomastoid muscle to the neck or along the posterior belly of the digastric muscle to the submandibular region. In such cases the pinna is pushed forwards and outwards. Occasionally, otitis externa is associated with a tender postauricular lymph node. The latter is distinguished from an abscess by its mobility, its discrete shape and by the absence of fluctuation. If the external meatus is clear the scalp should also be examined as a site of primary infection.

EXTERNAL EAR CANAL

The external auditory canal is examined either with a hand-held auriscope (Fig. 9.1) or with a head mirror, using reflected light and an aural speculum fitted with a magnifying lens (Siegel's speculum). To attain a good view bring the cartilaginous meatus into line with the bony meatus. In a child this is best achieved by retracting the pinna backwards and, in the adult, by retracting the pinna upwards and backwards. In all cases the largest speculum which comfortably fits the ear canal should be used, although a smaller speculum may be necessary to negotiate a particularly difficult meatus. An auriscope should be held like a pen between thumb and index finger with the ulnar order of the hand resting gently against the side of the patient's head (Fig. 9.2). In this way any head movement during examination can be accommodated by appropriate movement of the auriscope, limiting any risk of direct trauma to the ear canal if the patient moves unexpectedly.

Otoscopy may reveal wax, keratin debris, pus or mucopus. This should be removed to visualize the tympanic membrane. If a hard bolus of wax is blocking but not totally occluding the ear canal this may be removed with a probe or a wax hook. Softer wax may be removed by syringing the ear canal with water at body temperature. A stream of water is aimed along the superior meatel wall so that it is deflected by the tympanic membrane. The water accumulates behind the wax and forces it out of the meatus. It is important to ensure the water is at body temperature, otherwise a caloric-induced, vertiginous episode will result. Syringing is contraindicated if there is a history of a painful or discharging ear, since a perforated or thinned tympanic membrane could be further damaged or infected.

In cases of *purulent or mucopurulent* otorrhoea a swab is taken for microbiological studies. The lumen of the ear canal may be *congenitally constricted* or may be narrowed from recurrent bouts of otitis externa, or following surgery. *Bony osteomata*, are associated with repeated swimming in cold water. They may arise from and partially obstruct any portion of the bony ear canal. Occasionally they grow to totally occlude the meatus.

Foreign bodies in the ear canal are found in the external ear mainly in children and in patients with psychological illness. Removal should be preceded by examination of the other ear and the nose. Foreign bodies in the external ear may be difficult to remove, and a general anaesthetic is often necessary.

TYMPANIC MEMBRANE

After examination of the external ear canal look carefully at the tympanic membrane. The lower two-thirds is called the pars tensa and the upper third, the pars flaccida. The whole membrane is surrounded by a fibrous ring (the annulus) which fixes the drum firmly to the surrounding bone (Fig. 9.3). The pars tensa consists of three layers: an outer layer of squamous epithelium, a middle fibrous layer, and an inner layer of mucous membrane which adjoins the

Fig. 9.2 Examination of the right ear using the auriscope. Note the left hand applying gentle traction to the pinna. The fingers of the right hand rest on the patient's cheek.

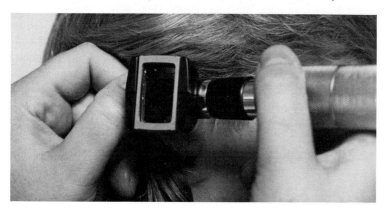

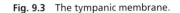

Fig. 9.3 The tympanic membrane.

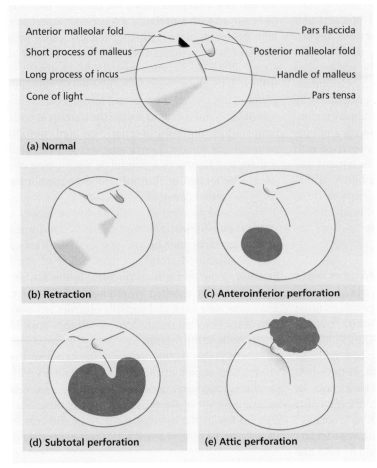

respiratory epithelium of the middle ear cleft. The pars flaccida lacks a middle fibrous layer; it is liable to develop retraction pockets with long-standing negative middle ear pressure. Normally the tympanic membrane is semitranslucent and grey. Within the fibrous layer of the pars tensa lies the handle of the malleus, which has a short process at its upper end and a flattened lower end (the umbo) from which the cone of light from the auriscope beam passes down to the annulus anteroinferiorly (Fig. 9.3). Through the drum, the incus and the chorda tympani nerve, which passes medial to the malleus and lateral to the long process of the incus and which carries taste fibres from the posterior one-third of the tongue, can occasionally be seen.

Any of the three layers of the pars tensa may become thickened. Repeated bouts of otitis externa will lead to the deposition of keratin on the squamous layer of the tympanic drum, and repeated middle ear infection will increase the thickness of the inner layer. Disruption of the integrity of the middle layer due to infection or surgery may lead either to hyaline degeneration, seen as white plaques in the drum (tympanosclerosis) or atrophy, with a resulting thinning of the drum. These two abnormalities often coexist.

In serous otitis media there is often increased vascularity of the drum, causing leashes of vessels travelling radially along the handle of the malleus and a dullness of the drum with either a complete loss or a break in the cone of light. An enhanced vascularity is also seen in the early stages of an acute suppurative otitis media and, as infection progresses, the drum becomes a confluent red colour. If untreated at this stage, pus may form, causing bulging of the tympanic membrane, which may subsequently rupture.

Eustachian tube dysfunction allows air in the middle ear cleft to become absorbed with the development of negative pressure in the middle ear. As a consequence, the tympanic membrane becomes retracted or indrawn. This appears on otoscopy as foreshortening of the handle of the malleus and undue prominence of the short process. If a negative middle ear pressure persists, atrophy of the fibrous layer of the drum occurs with thinning and either hypermobility or adherence of the tympanic membrane to the medial wall of the middle ear; this appearance resembles a large perforation. Negative middle ear pressure also causes exudation of serous fluid into the middle ear so that a fluid level may be visible. A *retraction pocket* may occur in the pars flaccida. This is always secondary to chronic negative middle ear pressure. Retraction into the attic region of the middle ear and antrum may result in the formation of a cholesteatoma.

Perforations of the pars tensa are classified as marginal or central. Marginal defects extend to the annulus whereas with central perforations there is a rim of membrane between the defect and the annulus. Both are described by their position in relation to the handle of the malleus (anterior, posterior or inferior) and by their size; if the perforation involves most of the tympanic membrane it is described as being subtotal.

Assessment of hearing

During clinical testing, due to the interposition of the mass of the head, sounds will be attenuated or masked in the ear furthest from the sound source by an amount that varies according to the frequency of the sound and the proximity of the sound to the test ear. Furthermore, attenuation of sound transmission in tests involving air conduction sound is considerable, whereas it is effectively zero during tests involving bone conduction. Thus a vibrating tuning fork held next to the test ear will, for practical purposes, be heard only in that ear. However, if the same tuning fork is placed on the mastoid process of the test ear it will be heard at the same intensity in the non-test ear—provided that both ears have normal hearing. For these reasons bone conduction thresholds (which are used in audiology to measure inner ear function) should always be masked. In a clinical situation such masking can be achieved by intermittent rubbing of the tragal cartilage at the meatal opening. This produces mixed frequency sound (white noise) of approximately 50 dB intensity. If masking of more than 50 dB is required a Bárány box will be necessary (Fig. 9.1).

It is possible to make a preliminary assessment of the severity of a hearing impairment from the clinical history. Ask whether the patient can hear the doorbell or telephone (sound outputs around 60 dB), and ask if conversation in a quiet environment can be heard (normal levels about 40 dB). If the patient prefers a raised voice in quiet surroundings this implies a hearing loss of 70–80 dB in the speech frequencies.

Clinical testing can also be performed by asking the patient to repeat words spoken at varying intensities. Such free-field voice testing uses phonetically balanced words (e.g. 'dustbin'), number combinations (e.g. '6–3–4') or combinations of numbers and letters (e.g. '7–M–5'). For these tests the examiner stands to the side of the ear to be tested and masks the non-test ear using tragal movement. The test starts with a whispered voice at 60 cm (2 feet) (approximate intensity 15 dB) and proceeds with a whispered voice at 15 cm (6 inches) (intensity about 35 dB). If there is no response a conventional voice at 60 cm (2 feet) (50 dB) is used and this is then repeated, if necessary, at 15 cm (6 inches) (55–60 dB) from the test ear. However, responses in this simple test are often difficult to quantify and may be interpreted erroneously in patients with poor English comprehension. Formal audiometry, therefore, is usually necessary.

Further information about hearing may be obtained at the bedside by using a vibrating tuning fork. For these tests tuning forks of 512 Hz are used since higher frequencies are less accurate at identifying differences between air and bone conduction, and lower frequency forks produce vibrations which may be misinterpreted by the patient as sound. In general, tuning forks as heavy as possible should be used as with these the sound levels decay less rapidly.

In clinical practice two tests are employed. The *Rinne test* compares hearing by air and bone conduction. It is performed by striking the tuning fork and holding it in line with the external ear canal (air conduction) and then against the postauricular skin (bone conduction). The patient is asked in which test position the sound is heard louder. In normal subjects air conduction is better than bone conduction (Rinne positive) and this response is also found in patients with sensorineural deafness. In conductive deafness the converse is true (Rinne negative). In the *Weber test* the base of the vibrating tuning fork is placed anywhere on the midline of the skull and the patient asked whether the sound is heard in the midline or whether it is lateralized. The normal response is to localize the sound to the midline; this is also true if the hearing is symmetrically reduced. However, if there is normal hearing on one side and a pure sensorineural loss on the other the tuning fork will be heard louder in the normal ear. Conversely, if there is a purely conductive hearing loss in one ear and normal hearing in the other the tuning fork will be heard louder on the side with the conductive deficit.

Two fallacies exist with the Rinne test. The first is that up to one-third of patients with an air–bone gap of 30 dB will be Rinne positive and it is only when the difference between air and bone conduction exceeds 40 dB that the Rinne test is negative on 90% of occasions. This lack of specificity is often important clinically. Secondly patients with a profound unilateral sensorineural hearing loss or a dead ear will report a Rinne-negative response when this ear is tested if the better ear has normal or reasonable hearing. This is because of the lack of attenuation of bone-conducted sound which is heard in the non-test ear. This problem is alluded to above and, for this reason, a Bárány box (Fig. 9.1) should be used to mask the non-test ear when a negative response is obtained.

AUDIOMETRY

Formal audiometry is used to assess the degree of hearing loss and in assessing the likely site of pathology in the auditory pathways (see page 223).

Assessment of vestibular function

Balance and orientation is dependent on sensory input from the vestibular system, from the eyes, and from muscle, joint and skin receptors. This information is integrated and modulated by centres within the central nervous system. Examination of the unsteady patient therefore requires not only evaluation of the vestibular apparatus but also of the eyes, the central nervous system and the cardiovascular system. Vestibular input is composed of information from the utricular maculae and the cristae of the semicircular canals. The utricular maculae respond to changes in gravity and to linear acceleration whereas the semicircular canals are responsive to angular acceleration. This information is then integrated to allow compensatory eye movements through central pathways. These include the vestibulo-ocular reflex and postural adjustments.

The assessment of the vertiginous patient starts with an examination of the ears (page 210) followed by an examination of the eye movements (page 291).

NYSTAGMUS

Nystagmus is either induced or spontaneous. It is defined by the direction of the fast movement (page 295).

In general, spontaneous vestibular nystagmus is enhanced by movement of the eyes in the direction of the fast phase and diminished by movement in the opposite direction. Thus, in destructive vestibular lesions, the activity of the contralateral vestibular system predominates and drives the eyes in the direction of the damaged side. This movement, the slow phase, is then interrupted by a fast saccadic compensatory movement in the opposite direction. This nystagmus will be maximal when looking in the direction opposite to the lesion.

Since vestibular nystagmus is enhanced without fixation, and central nystagmus tends to show a reduction of the slow phase velocity with absent fixation, the nystagmus should also be assessed using Frenzel's glasses (Fig. 9.1). These have a 20 dioptre lens and therefore abolish fixation. They contain internal illumination which allows the examiner to adequately visualize the patient's eyes during testing. Eye closure or darkness can also be used to abolish fixation. In such tests, measurements of eye movement are made by *electronystagmography (ENG)*. This monitors changes in electrical potentials recorded from two electrodes close to the eyes. As the eye is a dipole (the cornea is positive with respect to the retina) eye movement results in an altered potential difference between the two electrodes which can be measured and recorded on a moving paper strip. In this way the velocity, amplitude and frequency of eye movements can be measured and a permanent record of the test made.

POSITIONAL VERTIGO

Positional vertigo is elicited by asking the patient to sit on a couch and then with fixation on the centre of the examiner's forehead, the patient's head is turned 45 degrees to the right or left and is rapidly lowered 30 degrees below the horizontal. The patient is instructed not to shut their eyes and the examiner carefully observes the patient for nystagmus. The patient is asked to report sensations of vertigo or dizziness. If none occur the test is repeated with the head turned in the opposite direction.

This procedure, *Hallpike's manoeuvre*, may induce nystagmus in several different disorders. In the classical peripheral disorder, *benign paroxysmal positional nystagmus*, there is a latent period of 5–10 seconds before the onset of severe vertigo and rotatory nystagmus (characterized with the fast component directed towards the lowermost ear). Fatigue of the response then occurs with resolution of subjective symptoms, and immediate repetition of the test will produce little abnormality (adaptation).

The pathophysiology of this disorder is not fully understood but it has been suggested that it is due to disturbance of the utricular otoconia (part of the utricular end-organ) with bias of the response of the ampulla of the posterior semicircular canal when the head is positioned in a particular way. Whatever the cause, the benign nature of this syndrome is characteristic, and the symptoms disappear with time in most cases. Alcohol abuse and psychotropic drugs may also cause transient positional nystagmus.

Persistent positional nystagmus occurring with fixation implies central pathology. In this syndrome the nystagmus appears immediately, is not necessarily associated with vertiginous symptoms and shows no adaptation with repeated testing. This form of positional nystagmus is a feature of cerebellar brainstem disease and lesions in the region of the fourth ventricle.

ROMBERG'S TEST

The patient stands with the feet together and with the arms outstretched, first with eyes open, then closed. Patients with disorders of the posterior columns of the spinal cord will sway and even fall when their eyes are closed but will stand normally with eyes open. Patients with uncompensated unilateral labyrinthine dysfunction show instability to the side of the lesion with their eyes closed rather more markedly than with their eyes open. Patients with central dysfunction sway to both sides, with eyes open or shut. Classically, however, this is a test of proprioception; patients with gross disturbance of position sense in the feet fall with their eyes closed, and are severely disabled when attempting to walk in the dark.

GAIT ASSESSMENT

The patient is asked to walk with the eyes open. Patients with uncompensated peripheral vestibular pathology will tend to veer towards the affected side, whereas those affected with a central pathology may stagger a few steps in one direction before veering to the other side.

CALORIC TESTING

This is the most commonly performed test in assessing the performance of the vestibular end-organ. It is described on page 226.

Radiological examination

Plain views of the temporal bone show the site of the sigmoid sinus and the tegmen tympani, i.e. the roof of the middle ear, and the floor of the middle cranial fossa.

The degree of mastoid aeration can also be assessed. Hazy mastoid air cells or opaque air cells are features of acute suppurative mastoiditis. In chronic mastoid disease with cholesteatoma, erosion with a poorly pneumatized mastoid cortex may be noted. Computerized axial tomograms (CT scanning), or transorbital anteroposterior tomography will demonstrate the internal auditory canal. Enlargement of the internal auditory meatus suggests an acoustic neurinoma. However, normal tomograms do not rule out small acoustic nerve tumours. MR scanning is the investigation of choice in investigating this problem (Fig. 9.4).

CT scanning is also useful in defining the state of the middle ear cleft and the extent of any soft tissue mass in chronic mastoid disease. Congenital abnormalities of the ossicular chain and atresia of the external ear canal can be more precisely defined by CT scanning, as can the position of the facial nerve. CT examination is also the investigation of choice for defining fractures of the temporal bone.

The nose and paranasal sinuses

Sinus infection and nasal disease are interrelated. Thus, severe nasal obstruction may cause breathing through the mouth, leading to dryness in the mouth, persistent sore throat or snoring. Similarly, recurrent sinus infections causing a chronic purulent postnasal drip may present as recurrent tonsillitis or suppurative otitis media. An apical tooth abscess of the upper jaw may drain into the maxillary sinus causing acute sinusitis.

The important symptoms of nasal disease are
- nasal obstruction
- discharge
- sinus pain
- sneezing
- disturbance of smell.

Orbital pain, proptosis, diplopia, periorbital swelling and conjunctival chemosis may develop if

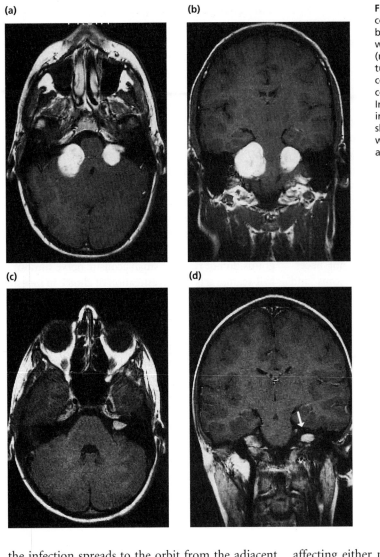

Fig. 9.4 (a) and (b) Transverse and coronal images of the brain to show bilateral acoustic neurinomas in a patient with von Recklinghausen's disease (neurofibromatosis type 1; NF1). The tumours are located in the cerebellopontine angles and are compressing the brainstem. (c) and (d) In these images there is a small tumour in the left internal auditory meatus shown as a bright signal. The tumour was a neurofibroma (as indicated by arrow).

the infection spreads to the orbit from the adjacent paranasal sinuses.

NASAL OBSTRUCTION

Obstruction of the nasal passages causes difficulty in breathing through the nose, is often associated with local discomfort, and with nasal discharge. Acute nasal obstruction following trauma is particularly important as it may be secondary to the formation of a subperichondrial haematoma, or to a fractured, deviated nasal septum. Subperichondrial haematoma may lead to absorption of cartilage and deformity of the nose. Nasal blockage may be unilateral or bilateral, and seasonal or perennial. Long-standing nasal obstruction suggests either a deviated nasal septum or nasal polyposis. Vasomotor rhinitis or seasonal allergic rhinitis with swollen intranasal mucosa cause nasal blockage of varying severity and

affecting either nostril. The alternating laterality of the nasal blockage is due to enhancement of the nasal cycle, a normal, centrally mediated cyclical variation in patency.

RHINORRHOEA

Nasal discharge (*rhinorrhoea*) may be bloody, purulent, watery or mucoid. The amount and duration of the discharge should be noted, and whether the discharge is unilateral or bilateral. A unilateral nasal obstruction with a blood-stained discharge may be the presenting symptom of nasal or sinus malignancy.

Epistaxis (a nose bleed) varies in severity from an insignificant intermittent problem to a life-threatening major haemorrhage. The arterial supply of the nose is from branches of the sphenopalatine (external carotid), and from the anterior and posterior ethmoidal arteries (internal carotid). These vessels anastomose on the anterior nasal septum (Little's area). Nasal bleeding is most common in children; the site of blood loss is either from the anterior nasal septum or from a vessel running on the mucocutaneous junction just inside the nose. Elderly patients tend to have more severe epistaxis than young adults. The epistaxis often originates from the posterior nasal septum, or the lateral nasal wall. Epistaxis is associated with hypertension, nasal trauma and clotting disorders. The patient should be asked about anticoagulant and non-steroidal anti-inflammatory drug ingestion.

Bilateral *watery* or *mucoid discharge* suggests a vasomotor or an allergic rhinitis. A *purulent discharge* may be secondary to a foreign body in the nose, especially in children, or may be a sign of sinus infection. Pus drains into the nose, causing both anterior and postnasal rhinorrhoea.

PAIN

Nasal pain without other symptoms is uncommon. It may be a symptom of infection of the vestibule (tip) of the nose, usually associated with anterior nasal crusting, or it may be secondary to malignant infiltration of the anterior maxillary nerves as they pass along the nasal floor and lateral nasal wall.

Pain centred over a sinus indicates infection, when there is usually a purulent nasal discharge with nasal obstruction, or malignancy, when there may be swelling of the cheek and a bloody nasal discharge. Such pain may also be due to trigeminal neuralgia, or to migraine.

SNEEZING

Sneezing is a protective expulsive reflex which helps clear the nasal airway of irritants. Thus excessive secretion following irritation in the nose as, for example, that which follows an allergic stimulus and histamine release in the nose may provoke paroxysmal sneezing.

Examination of the nose

The external nose should be examined in good light by observation and palpation. Virtually any skin disease can affect the nose. Infective processes, such as erysipelas (streptococcal cellulitis of the skin) may involve the nose and may resemble acute frontal sinusitis or orbital cellulitis. The skin of the external nose is also particularly exposed to ultraviolet light; thus the common skin malignancies are by no means infrequent at this site. The shape of the nose should

be noted. There is some reduction in the elasticity of the soft tissues of the nose with age, resulting in drooping of the nasal tip, and there may be deformities of the nasal bony and cartilaginous dorsum following a nasal fracture. Saddle deformity of the nose may follow destruction of the bony septum from syphilis and of the cartilaginous septum from tuberculosis or leprosy or, following trauma, septal haematoma or septal abscess. Other destructive midline diseases of the nose such as T-cell lymphoma (lethal midline granuloma) or Wegener's granulomatosis may present in the same way, but saddling is most commonly iatrogenic following cosmetic surgery, or due to trauma.

Palpation of nasal bones helps to distinguish cartilaginous from bony distortion. Also palpate the facial skeleton, paying particular attention to the orbital margins. Note any tenderness, swelling, expansion or depression of bone, e.g. after injury or when malignancy is suspected. Facial swelling is unusual in maxillary sinusitis but occurs with dental root infections and in carcinoma of the maxillary antrum. Finally, the palate and alveoli should be inspected and then palpated from inside the mouth, using a gloved finger.

The *patency* of the nasal airway is then assessed. The technique for examination is different in the neonate, child or adult. In a neonate the patency of the nasal airway is best estimated by observing any movement of a wisp of cottonwool held in front of each nostril. Congenital choanal atresia, causing nasal obstruction, may be fatal in the neonate. In children the nasal airway may be assessed either by occluding the front of each nostril in turn and asking the child to sniff, or by holding a Lack's tongue depressor (Fig. 9.1) beneath each nostril: moist expired air will cause surface misting allowing comparison between the two sides. Similar methods can be used in adults; in the latter, collapse of the rim of the nares may occur during inspiration when the nostril is obstructed.

A preliminary examination of the nasal vestibule and intranasal contents can usually be made by exerting gentle upward pressure on the tip of the nose with the finger, using reflected illumination from a head mirror. The nasal vestibule is lined by skin and therefore contains sebaceous glands, sweat glands and hair follicles. These hairs become prominent in later life, particularly in men. The junction of the skin of the vestibule with the respiratory mucosa lining the upper part of the airway is marked by the moist, pink appearance of the mucosa.

All diseases involving the external skin of the nose can also affect the nasal vestibule. The most common disorders are furunculosis and vestibulitis. In the latter condition the vestibule becomes crusted and excoriated as a result of infection, usually secondary to repeated trauma from rubbing or cleaning the nose. Purulent sinusitis and eczema can cause nasal vestibulitis. In a child, unilateral nasal vestibulitis and rhinorrhoea is almost always due to a foreign body in the nose. The nasal cavity is examined with Thudichum's nasal speculum (Fig. 9.5). The nasal septum should lie in the midline, but may be deviated or thickened. When the patency of the nasal airway is reduced, hypertrophy of the contralateral inferior turbinate may develop, causing bilateral nasal blockage. Look for any area of granulation on the nasal septum and for a septal perforation. Perforations may be secondary to nose-picking or to inhalation of industrial dusts, notably nickel and chrome.

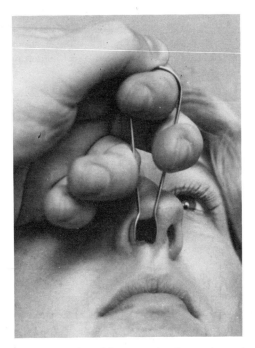

Fig. 9.5 Examination of the nose using the nasal speculum.

Other than the nasal septum the most obvious intranasal structure is the inferior turbinate, situated on the lower portion of the lateral nasal wall. The submucosal vascular bed shows considerable alteration in size with changes in ambient humidity and temperature. When the airway is large the inferior turbinate may undergo hypertrophy. In allergic rhinitis the inferior turbinate may be hypertrophied and its mucosa pallid. Occasionally drying of the nasal mucosa occurs, causing nasal crusting, especially in the aged, and when the air is very dry.

Probing may allow distinction to be made between a nasal polyp and a hypertrophied inferior turbinate. The former will be soft and mobile and, because simple nasal polyps lack pain fibres, the patient will experience no discomfort. By contrast, probing of the inferior turbinate will cause transient mild discomfort. In a child a polyp may be seen seemingly arising from the roof of the nose. This should *not* be probed as it may be the intranasal presentation of a meningocele.

The middle turbinate is also subject to variations in size and shape. Beneath the middle turbinate lies the middle meatus. Here the maxillary, frontal and anterior ethmoidal sinuses drain into the nose. Ethmoidal nasal polyps also present in the nose at this site.

Postnasal space

The posterior choanae and the postnasal space can be inspected by means of a small mirror inserted into the mouth and oriented so that it lies just behind the soft palate. This manoeuvre is difficult and best performed with the patient leaning forward, with mouth opened and the tongue firmly depressed with a Lack's tongue depressor (Fig. 9.1). A postnasal mirror is warmed with the flame of a spirit lamp and passed into the mouth over the upper surface of the tongue until it lies in the space between the uvula, the tongue and the faucial pillars. Inspection should be made rapidly since even the most co-operative patient cannot long resist the desire to swallow. Using this method the posterior end of the nasal septum will be seen as a sharp white dividing line in the middle of the field. On either side of the septum the posterior end of the inferior turbinates can be seen, and directly behind the turbinates are the openings of the eustachian tubes. The fossae of Rosenmuller, which are the sites of origin of postnasal space carcinomas, lie directly above and behind the eustachian tube opening. An antrochoanal polyp, a benign nasal polyp arising from the nasal septum and protruding through the middle meatus to present in the posterior choanae, may be visible using this method. Hypertrophy of the posterior end of the inferior turbinate (mulberry turbinate) can be seen.

Endoscopic examination of the nose

More detailed examinations of the nose may be

made with a flexible fibre-optic endoscope, after preparation of the nose with a suitable anaesthetic.

Radiological examination

Radiological examination has little to offer in the management of nasal fractures. Manipulation of the nasal septum is only required when a fracture has resulted in displacement, and this is best assessed by clinical inspection.

X-Rays are often used in the investigation of sinus disease, but are not required in routine management. In children the maxillary antra are poorly pneumatized and the frontal sinuses have not yet developed. However, the ethmoidal sinuses are well-pneumatized, and the most common sinus infection in children up to the age of 3 or 4 years is therefore ethmoiditis. This is best shown on an occipito-frontal radiograph. With increasing age, the maxillary sinuses enlarge below the nasal floor and the frontal sinuses enlarge into the frontal bone. However, the latter are usually asymmetrical and sometimes fail to develop altogether. Maxillary sinusitis is best demonstrated in posterior–anterior radiographs in the occipito-mental plane; with head tilt any fluid level in the antrum will be seen. In chronic infections the mucosa becomes thickened, but the X-ray appearances are indistinguishable from the mucosal thickening secondary to an allergic or vasomotor rhinitis. A lateral X-ray may demonstrate mucosal thickening or a fluid level in the sphenoid sinus. It is also useful in estimating the degree of adenoidal hypertrophy.

CT scanning of the sinuses with sections taken in the coronal and axial planes, using bone window settings has considerable advantages over conventional X-rays and is useful in the investigation of chronic infection, trauma and neoplasia (Figs 9.6 and 9.7).

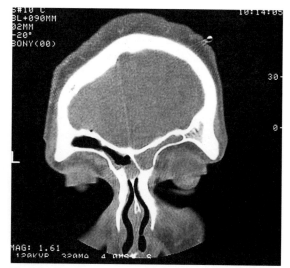

Fig. 9.6 This CT scan of the nasal sinuses in the coronal plane shows fluid levels in ethmoid and frontal sinuses.

laryngopharynx opens anteriorly into the laryngeal inlet. It is bounded above by the posterior surface of the epiglottis and below by the lower border of the cricoid cartilage. The third, fourth, fifth and sixth cervical vertebrae form the posterior wall. The pyriform fossae are small recesses which lie on each side of the laryngeal inlet and form the lateral wall of the laryngopharynx.

Patients with pharyngeal disease may present with

- pain
- stridor (noisy breathing)
- dysphonia (hoarseness)
- dysphagia (difficulty in swallowing) or
- a lump in the neck.

Occasionally lesions in the upper airway may present with symptoms such as overspill of food and ingested fluids into the upper trachea or nose, or with weight loss. However such symptoms are rare in isolation.

Throat

The throat comprises the mouth, the oropharynx (page 222), the nasopharynx (page 218) and the laryngopharynx. The *oropharynx* opens anteriorly into the mouth. It is bounded above by the soft palate and below by the upper surface of the epiglottis. The anterior surface of the second and third cervical vertebrae lie behind it and the palatine tonsils are situated in its lateral wall between the anterior and posterior pillars of the fauces, which enclose the palatoglossus and palatopharyngeus muscles. The

SORE THROAT

A sore throat is one of the commonest symptoms in clinical medicine. Patients with tonsillitis may not only complain of sore throat but, if the attack is severe or is associated with a *quinsy* (peritonsillar abscess), they may also note difficult and painful swallowing, and pain on opening the mouth.

Acute follicular tonsillitis due to *Streptococcus* presents with a punctate, yellow exudate due to pus filling the tonsillar crypts. In glandular fever the tonsils are covered with a white pseudomembrane. A grey membrane may be the result of infection with *Corynebacterium diphtheriae*. With these alternatives

(a)

(b)

(c)

(d)

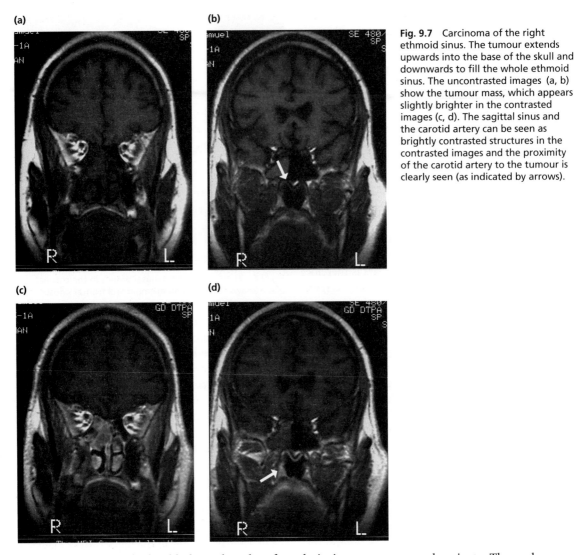

Fig. 9.7 Carcinoma of the right ethmoid sinus. The tumour extends upwards into the base of the skull and downwards to fill the whole ethmoid sinus. The uncontrasted images (a, b) show the tumour mass, which appears slightly brighter in the contrasted images (c, d). The sagittal sinus and the carotid artery can be seen as brightly contrasted structures in the contrasted images and the proximity of the carotid artery to the tumour is clearly seen (as indicated by arrows).

in mind a throat swab should always be taken for culture and sensitivity in these patients. An acute painful peritonsillar swelling results from cellulitis or abscess (*quinsy*) occurring secondary to tonsillitis. The frequency and severity of attacks of tonsillitis as estimated by the amount of time lost from schooling or work and the necessity for antibiotics should be noted: such considerations help to decide whether tonsillectomy is merited.

Tonsillitis may be complicated by a *retropharyngeal abscess*, which forms a smooth, tense, tender swelling bulging from the posterior oropharyngeal wall, or a *parapharyngeal abscess*, which pushes the tonsil medially and presents as a swelling around the angle of the mandible.

Painful vesicles, which break down to create small ulcers on the palate occur with *herpes zoster*. *Aphthous ulcers* may also affect the soft palate, particular-

ly in immunosuppressed patients. These ulcers are tender, and movement causes pain which is also exacerbated by ingestion of acidic fluids. Ulceration in the oropharynx is also seen in glandular fever, rubella and streptococcal tonsillitis, as well as from trauma due to ill-fitting dentures or broken teeth.

STRIDOR

Acute infections within the laryngopharynx and upper respiratory tract are common in children and young adults and usually cause no threat to the airway. However, the narrow diameter of the laryngeal airway in children means that slight oedema may cause stridor, and sometimes rapidly progressive difficulty in breathing.

Acute epiglottitis (due to infection with *Haemophilus influenzae* type B) may present with a rapidly progressive airway obstruction and dyspnoea, fever, pharyngeal pain, and drooling from the corner of the mouth. Examining the throat in such a patient can induce laryngospasm and should be avoided. Instead, blood culture and immediate treatment with antibiotics should be started, and the airway secured by intubation or even by tracheostomy.

Acute laryngotracheobronchitis presents with a longer history (24–48 hours) and the airway obstruction tends to be less severe. However, the patient will have a hoarse voice and the secretions formed tend to be thick and tenacious.

DYSPHONIA

Acute irritation of the vocal cords can follow vocal abuse. It also follows smoke inhalation or exposure to dust. In most cases the symptoms are self-limiting.

Dysphonia may also result from chronic misuse of the voice. There may be oedema of the larynx (Reincke's oedema), a vocal cord nodule (hyperkeratosis), papilloma or polyp. Any abnormality must always be biopsied, as it may be due to carcinoma. If only benign changes are present, speech therapy is necessary.

Hoarseness followed by increasing airway obstruction is the typical presentation of laryngeal neoplasia. There is usually a history of heavy smoking. Dysphonia lasting more than 6 weeks suggests a diagnosis of carcinoma of the vocal cords.

Dysphonia may also be due to a paralysed vocal cord, due to damage to the recurrent laryngeal nerve or the main trunk of the vagus. The recurrent laryngeal nerve may be damaged behind the thyroid, due to malignancy or during thyroid surgery. Disease, especially neoplasia, in the cervical oesophagus, the apex of the lung, and the structures related to the undersurface of the aorta on the left and the subclavian artery on the right may also cause damage to this nerve. The main trunk of the vagus nerve on either side may be involved in the posterior fossa of the skull or in the region of the jugular bulb. The most common cause is infiltrative bronchial carcinoma. Even if no cause has been established the patient must be observed for at least a year with regular examinations before the paralysis is considered idiopathic.

DYSPHAGIA

Squamous cell carcinoma of the distal oropharynx may present as an ulcer or exophytic mass, and direct spread may cause dysphagic local pain and referred pain in the ipsilateral ear. Progressive supraglottic swelling may be due to subepithelial spread of a small carcinoma hidden by subsequent oedema. A *pharyngeal pouch* is a pulsion diverticulum consisting of mucosa pushed out between the two parts of the inferior constrictor muscle of the pharynx, the thyro- and cricopharyngeus muscles. This area is called *Killian's dehiscence*. The pouch tends to present more frequently on the left side of the neck. It causes obstruction of swallowing with regurgitation of partially digested food.

The three primary sites for malignancy in the hypopharynx are the *pyriform fossa, post-cricoid region* and *posterior pharyngeal wall*. Pooling of saliva in the pyriform fossae or at the upper oesophagus in the post-cricoid region is a sign of obstruction in the cervical oesophagus or in the post-cricoid space. Malignancy in the post-cricoid area is more common in women than in men; this is the only primary site in the head and neck where this is true. Tumours in the pyriform fossa present with a muffled voice rather than dysphonia. The voice is said to be like that of someone eating a hot potato. All tumours in this area have a poor prognosis due to their relatively late presentation (compared to laryngeal tumours), and to the rich lymphatic drainage from this site.

LUMP IN THE NECK

Certain deep cervical lymph nodes are described by name due to their frequent enlargement in certain pathologies. The most common of these is the *jugulo-digastric node*, which lies antero–superior in the jugular chain and which can be palpated just posterior to the angle of the mandible. This is the most commonly enlarged node and is swollen in upper respiratory tract infections, especially following tonsillitis. A neoplasm in the pharynx may also present with a cervical node and, in an adult, such a unilateral, enlarged node in the neck has a 60% chance of being malignant. Features that suggest malignancy are progressive enlargement, hardness, lack of tenderness, fixation to deep structures, and size. A node greater than 2×2 cm in diameter is likely to be malignant.

In such patients, the nose and throat should be examined before a fine needle aspiration biopsy of the node is made and sent for cytological examination. With this technique more than 95% of metastatic squamous cell carcinomas will be diagnosed, obviating the need for an excision biopsy. Fine needle aspiration biopsy is much less reliable for other tumour types and, in these circumstances, an excision biopsy may be necessary to establish the diagnosis.

Examination of the oropharynx

It is preferable to examine the anterior oropharynx with a headlight or with a head mirror. This ensures adequate illumination and keeps both hands free for the manipulation of instruments. First check the lips, dentition and gums, floor of the mouth and opening of the submandibular duct, and the buccal mucosa, including the opening of the parotid duct opposite the second upper molar tooth. Then assess tongue mobility and the gag reflex.

A Lack's tongue depressor (Fig. 9.1) is then introduced so that its tip lies at the junction of the posterior and middle thirds of the dorsum of the tongue. In this way the tonsillar pillars, tonsils, soft palate and uvula can be inspected in turn.

Minor salivary glands are found on the soft palate and malignant tumours of these glands may present with a localized swelling on the palate. The tonsils are usually symmetrical in size. Occasionally one tonsil is affected by a benign lymphoid hypertrophy but asymmetry should always be regarded with suspicion as unilateral tonsillar enlargement may be due to lymphoma. A squamous cell carcinoma of the tonsil presents either as an exophytic mass or as an ulcer.

The more distal portions of the oropharynx can be inspected only with a laryngeal mirror or fibre-optic laryngoscope. For indirect laryngoscopy the patient is asked to remove any dentures and to protrude the tongue. The latter is grasped by a cotton swab held between the examiner's thumb and index finger (Fig. 9.8). The patient is then encouraged to concentrate on taking slow deep breaths and, with the mouth opened wide, a warmed laryngeal mirror is introduced gently but firmly to the soft palate just proximal to the uvula. The soft palate is displaced upwards and backwards and, by instructing the patient to say 'ah' or 'eeee', the larynx is elevated towards the examining mirror.

The posterior oropharynx is then examined before inspecting the larynx. The larynx above the vocal cords (*supraglottis*) and the vocal cords (*glottis*) are inspected before the upper tracheal airway (*subglottis*) is examined (Fig. 9.9). The whole length of each vocal cord should be clearly visible and the mobility of each side noted. Visualization may be improved by anaesthetizing the soft palate and posterior oropharyngeal wall with a 2% lignocaine spray to minimize gagging.

Examination of the neck is an essential part of examination of the oropharynx and nasopharynx. Examination for lymph nodes should follow a well-rehearsed routine so that no groups of nodes are missed. Such an examination starts by inspection of the neck from the front in a good light and with the area well exposed, and continues, with the examiner standing behind the patient, with sympathetic palpation of the important structures.

Start by palpating the nodes in the *posterior auricular region* and then progressively feel for the nodes on the *anterior border of the trapezius muscle* down to the *supraclavicular fossa*. The latter area is palpated from behind forwards. The examining fingers then pass up the jugular vein, where the most important groups of nodes in the head and neck are situated, towards the ear. The *jugular*, *parotid* and *pre-auricular* areas are then examined, followed by *submandibular* and *submental* nodes. Finally the nodes associated with the *anterior jugular chain* are examined. This brings the fingers to the thyroid gland.

The position and size of the *thyroid gland* should be noted. Since the thyroid lies deep to the small strap muscles of the neck, it is often best examined with the patient's neck partially flexed; this relaxes the overlying muscles. Consider whether the gland is

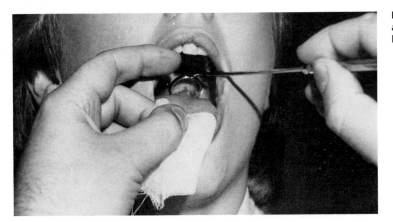

Fig. 9.8 Examination of the larynx and the laryngopharynx by indirect laryngoscopy.

Fig. 9.9 The larynx seen in the laryngeal mirror with the vocal cords in abduction and adduction.

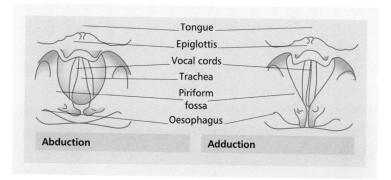

enlarged and, if so, decide whether the enlargement is uniform or lobar. Significance also attaches to whether the gland is smooth or nodular and whether it is possible to get the fingers below the gland on palpation. Irregularity, hardness and fixation of the gland to neighbouring structures are features of neoplasia.

If there is a midline mass, observe it as the patient swallows a little water. The thyroid gland, which is invested with pretracheal fascia, moves as the patient swallows, and such a manoeuvre may draw a small *retrosternal thyroid goitre* above the examining fingers. All other midline lumps should be assessed in this way and also with the patient protruding the tongue. Movement of any mass in these tests suggests attachment to the base of the tongue and implies the presence of a *thyroglossal cyst*.

The larynx should be mobile from side to side and, if the thyroid cartilage is held between thumb and first finger and gently moved against the cervical spine, crepitus should be elicited. Such a grating sensation (*laryngeal crepitus*) is caused by the rubbing of the cricoid and thyroid cartilages against the cervical spine and is a normal phenomenon. If hypopharyngeal pathology such as a *post-cricoid neoplasm* is present, or if there is a mass in the prevertebral space displacing the larynx forward and away from the cervical spine, this crepitus cannot be demonstrated.

Finally, examination should be concluded by auscultation of the carotid arteries and, if indicated, of the thyroid gland.

Radiological examination

A soft tissue lateral neck X-ray is useful in demonstrating the postnasal space. It is not a sensitive investigation in the detection of foreign bodies in the pharynx.

A barium swallow is useful in localizing obstruction in the oesophagus, but is less helpful in evaluating the hypopharynx. Endoscopy is the preferred investigation in such cases.

CT scanning is useful in evaluating any metastases in patients with primary neoplasms of the pharynx.

Special investigations

Pure tone audiometry

In this test the threshold for pure tone sounds introduced into each ear is measured for different frequencies. Standardized sound levels are used, compared to a hearing level of 0 dB. This is the threshold found when testing otologically normal adults in a soundproofed booth using sound attenuation headphones.

The better hearing ear is tested first at frequencies from 250 to 8000 Hz to determine the threshold in decibels at each frequency. Initially an intensity well above threshold is used and the patient is instructed to respond when sound is heard. The sound level is then first reduced in 10-dB steps—until there is no response—and is then increased in 5-dB steps until the threshold is reached. Initial testing is at 1000 Hz and is repeated at 2000, 4000, 8000, 500 and 250 Hz. The other ear is then tested. Bone conduction is assessed in an identical way, but using a bone vibrating earphone. Different symbols are used for right and left ears and for recording responses with air and bone conduction (Fig. 9.10).

In pure sensorineural hearing loss the bone conduction thresholds mirror the air-conducted thresholds, but in a conductive hearing loss the bone conduction thresholds exceed those for air. In these circumstances the difference between these thresholds is known as the *air–bone gap* and gives a measure of the degree of conductive hearing loss. The bone conduction thresholds are also often referred

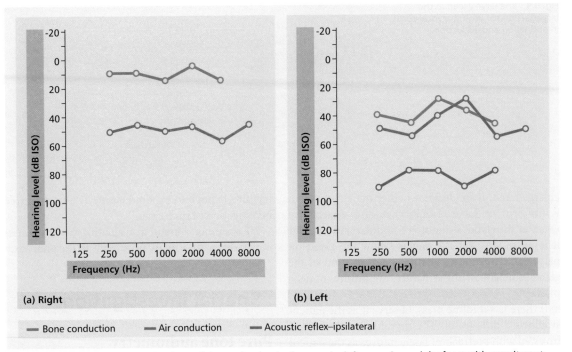

(a) Right

(b) Left

— Bone conduction   — Air conduction   — Acoustic reflex–ipsilateral

Fig. 9.10 Pure tone audiogram showing a right conductive deafness and a left sensorineural deafness with recruitment. The right ear was masked with narrow band noise while testing the left ear for both air and bone conduction.

to as the *cochlear reserve*. They are an indication of the best air conduction thresholds which could theoretically be obtained after surgery to correct a conductive hearing loss.

Speech audiometry

A pure tone audiogram does not test speech discrimination at suprathreshold levels, and it is this that defines hearing disability. For this reason a speech audiogram is often required.

The speech audiogram measures the patient's ability to recognize and repeat lists of phonetically balanced words arranged in groups of 12, delivered at different intensities to the test ear from a tape recording. The percentage of words correctly repeat-

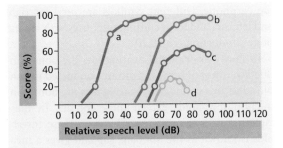

Fig. 9.11 Speech audiogram: (a) normal; (b) conductive deafness; (c) sensory loss; (d) neural lesion.

ed by the subject is noted at each intensity. With normal hearing a score of 100% discrimination is achieved at a sound intensity of 45–55 dB. Patients with pure conductive deafness will also achieve 100% discrimination, but only at a much higher intensity. Patients with sensorineural deafness are unable to achieve 100% discrimination at any intensity (Fig. 9.11).

In subjects with sensory deficit there is often an improvement in discrimination with an increase in intensity until, at a word discrimination of 50–70%, the ability to discriminate either plateaus with increased input, or falls due to recruitment (Fig. 9.11). Neural deafness causes an even more severe impairment of discrimination and the maximum obtained may be as low as 20%, even in the face of reasonably good pure tone thresholds. This is the pattern of abnormality found in acoustic neuroma.

Impedance audiology

An impedance bridge has an earpiece which is inserted into the external meatus. Through this pass three channels. The first delivers a continuous tone into the ear canal during the test (probe tone); the second has a microphone to record the sound intensity level within the ear canal; and the third channel is con-

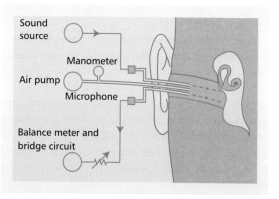

Fig. 9.12 Components of the acoustic impedance bridge. (After S. R. Mawson and H. Ludman in *Diseases of the Ear*, 4th edn (1979), published by Edward Arnold, London.)

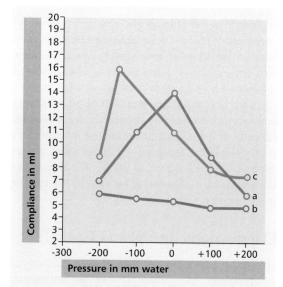

Fig. 9.13 Three types of tympanometry curve: (a) normal; (b) tympanic effusion or adhesive otitis; (c) negative middle ear pressure (eustachian tube dysfunction).

nected to a manometer so that the ear canal pressure can be altered (Fig. 9.12).

In a normal ear the external meatus acts as a rigid tube with a compliant end (the drum). Sound introduced into the ear will be absorbed according to the ability of the tympanic membrane and ossicular chain to conduct the tone into the inner ear.

This impedance to the passage of sound energy is most noticeably increased when the tympanic membrane is thickened and is decreased when it is hypermobile or atrophic. It is also dependent on the state of the ossicular chain and on the pressure difference between the middle and external ears.

The tympanic membrane is at its most compliant when the middle ear and ear canal pressures are equal; in such circumstances the majority of the sound introduced into the system is transmitted into the ear and the amount of sound energy reflected back—and measured by the microphone—is at a minimum.

However, when the pressure difference between the external and middle ear is increased or decreased to 200 mmH$_2$O by changes in the pressure within the meatus from the manometer, the tympanic membrane becomes rigid. In other words such manoeuvres reduce the compliance and increase the impedance to transmitted sound. In these circumstances most of the sound presented to the ear is then reflected from the drum head.

These changes can be plotted graphically on a *tympanogram*. This is a measure of movement of the ear drum and compliance in the middle ear (Fig. 9.13).

The impedance probe can also be used to record changes in the middle ear compliance secondary to contraction of the stapedius muscle. This phenomenon, the *stapedial reflex*, can be measured on an ear

which is ipsi- or contralateral to the probe. It is a bilateral consensual reflex, mediated via brainstem nuclei with input from the normal auditory pathways and output from the facial nerve which innervates the stapedius muscle. Suprathreshold sound is needed to elicit this reflex which is measured as a change in compliance by the impedance probe.

Evoked response audiometry

This is one form of a group of tests in which evoked responses in the brain are recorded following a sound applied to the ear. As with impedance audiology these tests are objective (in that they require no response from the patient) and the responses are displayed by averaging, and thus subtracting the background EEG.

For this test two active electrodes are used, placed on the vertex and on the mastoid. Sound is introduced through earphones and either tone pips or filtered or broad-tone clicks are used. The averaged response is displayed on an oscilloscope as a waveform with 7 peaks:

- first peak—cochlear hair cells
- second peak—cochlear nucleus
- third peak—superior olivary nucleus
- fourth and fifth peak—synapses at the inferior colliculus
- sixth peak—medial geniculate body
- seventh peak—auditory cortex.

It is usual to measure the time taken for the impulse to travel from peaks 1 to 5 (I–V latency). Compressive lesions of the acoustic nerve will cause delay of the impulse as it travels along the nerve with increased I–V latency. Delay also occurs in patients with brain stem tumours or with multiple sclerosis. This technique can also be used to measure hearing threshold by altering the frequency and intensity of the clicks and noting the intensity, at a given frequency, at which the brain stem evoked response (BSER) ceases to have definable peaks. This can be a useful test of hearing in the unborn and in infancy.

Electrocochleography (ECochG)

This test requires the insertion of a needle through the tympanic membrane. It can be undertaken under local anaesthetic in adults. Most of the information comes from the basal turn of the cochlear and is therefore only related to high frequencies.

Broad-band clicks are used and the action potential from the cochlear nerve, the summating potential (related to movement of the cochlear membrane) and the cochlear microphonic recorded. This technique can also be used to assess threshold but is mostly used to assess the presence of endolymphatic hydrops such as occurs in *Ménière's disease*.

Caloric testing

This simple, reliable test is performed with the patient lying on a couch with the head at 30 degrees, in order to bring the lateral semicircular canals into the vertical plane. The patient is instructed to fix upon a point in central gaze and the external ear canal is irrigated with water at 30°C and then at 44°C for 30–40 seconds respectively. This causes a thermal gradient across the temporal bone which is thought to produce convection currents within the endolymph. Cold water induces nystagmus away from the ear being irrigated and the warm water will induce nystagmus towards the ear under test. Each ear is irrigated with water at both temperatures, with a suitable delay of several minutes between each test, and the induced nystagmus is timed for each of the four tests. The evoked

nystagmus may be recorded and analysed using electronystagmography.

As with spontaneous nystagmus of peripheral origin, caloric-induced nystagmus can be significantly enhanced by the abolition of optic fixation. Peripheral lesions tend to cause a diminished response on one side (a canal paresis), although a directional preponderance (where nystagmus in one direction is more prominent than the other) may also be observed (Fig. 9.14). This latter finding is most likely to occur with central disorders, especially in the brainstem.

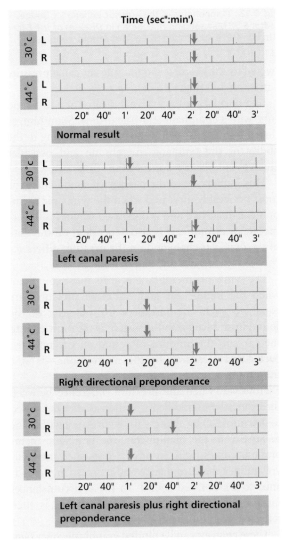

Fig. 9.14 Bithermal caloric tests.

CHAPTER 10

The eye

Before examining the patient with an ocular problem a detailed history of the presenting complaint and associated visual symptoms must be obtained.

History

Disturbances of vision may be sudden or gradual, and involve one or both eyes. The patient may complain of haloes around bright lights, floaters, flashes, or experience visual hallucinations (formed and unformed). Objects may appear smaller (*micropsia*) or larger (*macropsia*). Disorders of ocular movement may manifest themselves as diplopia or just blurring.

Pain in the eye may be described as a foreign body sensation, often exacerbated by eye movement, or as a heavy deep pain within the eye, or sometimes associated with photophobia, as in iritis. Severe ocular pain with vomiting may indicate an acute glaucoma. Migraine may present with visual symptoms and headache and pain may be referred to the eye from neighbouring disease.

There may be abnormal secretions from the eye such as mucus or pus. In tear insufficiency the eye feels dry. Excessive tear production (*lacrimation*) may indicate local ocular disease, whilst overflow of tears (*epiphora*) indicates a defect of the lacrimal drainage system.

Lastly, the patient may complain of physical signs such as red eye, abnormal position of the lids, protrusion of the globe or pupillary abnormality.

In addition to the ocular history a routine general medical and surgical history is necessary. Particular note should be made of the past ophthalmic history such as the presence of a squint in childhood, a previous injury, or the wearing of glasses at any time. The family history may reveal a history of glaucoma, conditions affecting visual acuity, colour vision or squint, or the presence of neurological disease associated with visual loss.

Visual acuity

Tests for distant vision

Visual acuity is measured with *Snellen's test types*, a series of letters of varying sizes constructed so that the top letter is visible to the normal eye at 60 m, and the subsequent lines at 36, 24, 18, 12, 9, 6 and 5 m respectively. Visual acuity (V) is recorded according to the ratio

$$d/D,$$

where d is the distance at which the letters are read, and D the distance at which they should be read. The patient is normally placed at a distance of 6 m from the test types ($d = 6$) and each eye is tested separately. The patient reads down the chart as far as he or she can. If only the top letter is visible, the visual acuity is 6/60. A normal person should read at least the seventh line, i.e. have a visual acuity of 6/6. If the visual acuity is less than 6/60, the patient is moved toward the test types until they can read the top letter. If the top letter is visible at 2 m, the visual acuity is 2/60. Visual acuities of less than 1/60 are recorded as *counting fingers* (CF), *hand movements* (HM), *perception of light* (PL) or *no perception of light* (no PL). A person with an uncorrected refractive error may have reduced visual acuity, and a rough estimate of their corrected visual acuity may be obtained by asking them to view the chart through a pin-hole aperture.

If the patient wears glasses, the type of lens being worn should be determined. Hold the lens up and look at an object through it. Then move the lens from side to side and watch the object. If the object seems to move in the opposite direction to the lens, the lens is convex; if in the same direction, it is concave. Patients with *myopia*, or short sight, use concave (diverging) lenses and those with *hypermetropia* (hyperopia), or long sight, have convex (converging lenses).

In order to tell whether a lens is spherical or cylindrical, look at a straight object through it and then slowly twist the lens round. If the lens is cylindrical, the object will appear to take up an oblique position. Patients who are *astigmatic* need cylindrical lenses.

Tests for near vision

Visual acuity at the ordinary reading distance is assessed by using reading test types of varying sizes, the notation being based on the printers' point system. The smallest print is N5. The near vision is recorded as the smallest type which the patient can read comfortably.

Colour sense

Colour sense is most easily tested by the use of pseudo-isochromatic plates consisting of multi-coloured dots outlining certain digits, the best known being those of Ishihara. People with defective colour vision confuse certain colours. Ishihara pseudo-isochromatic plates are so constructed that a person with abnormal colour vision will read a different number from a normal person on the same colour plate.

The most common anomalies of colour vision are various types of red–green deficiency, inherited as sex-linked recessive conditions, which occur in about 8% of males and 0.5% of females in the UK. People with congenital blue–yellow deficiencies and with total colour-blindness are rare. Acquired defects of colour vision occur in macular and optic nerve disease.

Visual fields

The methods for testing the visual fields are described in Chapter 12.

Examination

After the vision has been tested, the eyes should be examined systematically.

The eyelids

The shape and position of the eyelids should be noted. People of Asiatic origin have a long narrow palpebral aperture with an upward and outward obliquity and a characteristic fold of skin along the upper lid. The highest point of the aperture is at the junction of its middle and inner thirds. In Down's syndrome the palpebral fissure is also oblique. However, in addition, it is short and wide with its highest point at the centre of the lid.

Conditions associated with the eyelids include the following:

Ptosis (drooping of the upper lid). This may be congenital or acquired and examination of old photographs may indicate which it is. A congenital ptosis may be unilateral if due to paralysis of the oculomotor nerve or of the cervical sympathetic, and usually bilateral if due to ocular myopathy.

Lid retraction (Fig. 10.1). If the upper lid is abnormally retracted, a band of white sclera is visible

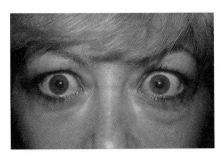

Fig. 10.1 Dysthyroid lid retraction. There is slight exophthalmos (bilateral proptosis).

above the iris when the eyes are looking straight ahead. Lid retraction, which is usually due to thyrotoxicosis, is often associated with infrequent blinking and with *lid lag*, in which the upper lid seems to lag behind the eyeball when the patient looks downwards. Patients with thyrotoxicosis frequently also have a degree of forward displacement of the eyeball (*proptosis* (Fig. 10.2) when unilateral, or *exophthalmos* when bilateral). Some patients with thyrotoxicosis may develop a severe and progressive form of exophthalmos leading to cornal ulceration; optic nerve compression may also occur. Both these complications of hyperthyroidism require urgent medical or surgical orbital decompression. Proptosis also results from space-occupying lesions in the orbit, and apparent proptosis may be a feature of myopia, when the eye is

longer than normal.

Blepharitis. Inflammation of the lids or blepharitis presents as redness and scaling of the lid margins around the base of the lashes.

Entropion. This is inversion of the lid margin with associated malposition of the lashes which may rub on the cornea.

Xanthelasma palpebrarum. Fatty deposits develop below and above the eye, in the eyelids, in patients with long-standing hypercholesterolaemia (Fig. 8.20).

Ectropion. This is eversion of the lid margin, often associated with watering (*epiphora*).

The lacrimal gland

The lacrimal gland is examined by pulling up the outer part of the upper lid while asking the patient to look downwards and inwards. Acute inflammation (*dacroadenitis*) results in a tender swollen gland, with oedema of the upper lid and localized conjunctival injection. Chronic dacroadenitis, a painless enlargement of the lacrimal gland which is frequently bilateral, occurs in sarcoidosis and the reticuloses. Tumours of the lacrimal gland produce a hard swelling of the gland associated with proptosis.

Involvement of the lacrimal gland by any disease process may produce symptoms of a dry eye.

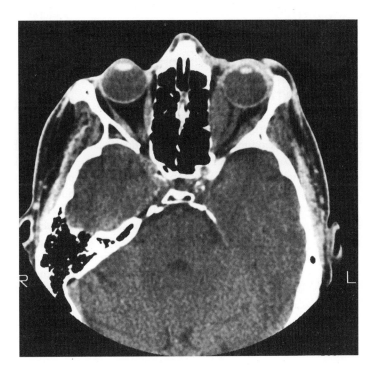

Fig. 10.2 Left-sided thyroid eye disease with exophthalmos and marked hypertrophy (inflammation) of the medial and lateral rectus muscles on that side. These muscles in the other eye are also slightly enlarged. The optic nerve can be seen clearly between the enlarged muscles on the left hand side.

The conjunctiva

The conjunctiva lining the eyeball (bulbar conjunctiva) and that lining the inner surface of the eyelids (palpebral conjunctiva) should be examined. To examine the palpebral conjunctiva of the lower lid, the lower lid should be pulled down and the patient asked to look upwards. To expose the palpebral conjunctiva of the upper lid, ask the patient to look downwards, then place the right thumb at the upper part of the upper lid and pull it up so as to evert the eyelashes. Grasp the lashes between the forefinger and thumb of the left hand and evert the lid by rotating it round the right thumb.

The conjunctiva may be pale in anaemia, jaundiced, or injected in conjunctivitis.

CONJUNCTIVITIS

Marked injection of the bulbar conjunctiva with a mucopurulent discharge suggests a bacterial infection; marked injection with a serous discharge and tender pre-auricular lymphadenopathy is indicative of a viral infection; slight oedema of the conjunctiva with a milky hue suggests an allergic condition. Follicles in the upper palpebral conjunctiva occur in trachoma, whereas their presence in the lower palpebral conjunctiva suggests an allergic condition or a conjunctivitis of viral origin.

Distinction must be made between other causes of red eye such as keratitis, iritis and acute glaucoma (see page 237).

The cornea

INFLAMMATION OF THE CORNEA (KERATITIS)

This may be superficial or deep (interstitial); it is accompanied by circumcorneal injection. Superficial keratitis and corneal ulcers result in breaches in the corneal epithelium; these lesions can be shown with fluorescein. A drop of fluorescein is instilled into the conjunctival sac and the excess dye is then washed out with normal saline. Corneal ulcers are stained green.

Interstitial keratitis causes a hazy cornea, often with an intact epithelium; it is usually caused by a viral infection but can also occur in syphilis. There is growth of capillaries into the cornea. Both keratitis and trauma to the cornea may result in corneal opacities; small opacities are described as *nebulae*, larger ones as *leucomata*.

Severe corneal infections, particularly bacterial, may result in a massive inflammatory response, with pus in the anterior chamber (*hypopyon*). This will progress to a sight-threatening *endophthalmitis* if not treated.

ARCUS SENILIS

Arcus senilis is a crescentic opacity near the periphery of the cornea. It usually starts at the lower part of the cornea, extending to form a complete circle. It is common in old people, but may occur in the young (arcus juvenilis). It is sometimes associated with type IV hypolipoproteinaemia but frequently is of no significance.

The iris

Note should be made of any difference in the colour of the two irides (*heterochromia*), abnormality in the shape of the pupil, or signs of iritis.

IRITIS (ANTERIOR UVEITIS, IRIDOCYCLITIS)

In iritis circumcorneal injection occurs (but also in keratitis and acute glaucoma). In addition, there may be white specks visible on the posterior surface of the cornea (*keratitic precipitates*), or an exudate in the anterior chamber. The pupil may be constricted and irregular due to the formation of adhesions (*posterior synechiae*) between the edge of the pupil and the anterior surface of the lens. Other abnormalities of the pupils are described on pages 238 and in Chapter 12.

Ocular tension

The ocular tension may be roughly assessed by palpating the eyeball, although only gross variations from normal can be appreciated. The sclera is palpated with the two forefingers through the upper lid with the patient looking downwards and the other fingers resting on the patient's forehead. The degree of fluctuation gives an indication of the ocular tension. More accurate measurements of ocular tension can be made with Schiøtz or applanation tonometers. A diminished tension occurs in diabetic coma and in severe dehydration from any cause. A myopic eye frequently feels softer than a normal one. An increased ocular tension is a characteristic feature of glaucoma.

The lens

Lens opacities (*cataract*) develop with ageing, especially after exposure to bright sunlight in fair-skinned people, in diabetes mellitus, after injury, and with hypercholesterolaemia. They are also a feature of certain hereditary diseases, e.g. myotonic dystrophy.

The fundus (Fig. 10.3)

Examination of the fundus of the eye with an ophthalmoscope is an essential part of all complete medical examinations. Valuable information may be obtained about the state of the optic nerve head and of the arteries and veins of the retina, in addition to the detection of local ophthalmic disorders.

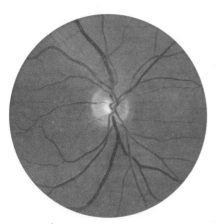

Fig. 10.3 Normal fundus. Note the yellowish colour of the optic disc and the retinal veins (the larger, darker vessels) and arteries leaving the centre of the disc superiorly and inferiorly. A single arterial branch passes laterally to supply the macular part of the retina.

In routine medical examinations it is usually possible, with practice, to examine the optic disc and surrounding retina without dilating the pupil but for a complete examination of the fundus the pupils should be dilated by instilling a few drops of 1% cyclopentolate (Mydrilate) or 1% tropicamide (Mydriacyl) into the conjunctival sacs. In patients with a predisposition to closed-angle glaucoma an acute attack of glaucoma may be precipitated when the pupils are dilated. Before a mydriatic is instilled, the patient should therefore be asked whether they have ever seen haloes (coloured rings) around lights and, if so, this, or the presence of a shallow anterior chamber, is a contraindication to the use of a mydriatic.

The patient should be examined either sitting or lying down in a darkened room. Ask the patient to look straight ahead and to keep their eyes as still as possible. The ophthalmoscope is held a few centimetres from the patient's eyes, and a suitable plus lens is used in the ophthalmoscope so that the iris is in focus. Opacities in the media of the eye (cornea, anterior chamber, lens, vitreous) will appear as black specks or lines against the red reflex of the fundus.

The ophthalmoscope should then be brought as close as possible to the patient's eye and the light directed slightly nasally. In this way the optic disc can be found and, in addition, the light will not shine directly on the macula. If the patient's pupils are not dilated, shining a light on the macula will make the pupils contract and make the examination of the fundus difficult or impossible. If the optic disc is not in focus, the strength of the lenses of the ophthalmoscope should be gradually reduced until the disc becomes sharply focused. If the observer's eye is emmetropic and his or her accommodation is relaxed, the strength of the lens necessary to bring the fundus into focus gives an indication of the refractive error of the patient's eye. Plus lenses indicate hypermetropia (hyperopia), and minus lenses myopia. In astigmatism, the radii of curvature of the cornea in different planes are not regular. The optic disc, the retinal blood vessels, the macular region and the periphery of the fundus should be examined in turn.

The optic disc

SHAPE
The normal disc is round or slightly oval (Fig. 10.3). If astigmatism is present, the disc may appear more oval than normal (Fig. 10.3).

COLOUR
The normal disc is a pale pink colour, distinctly paler than the surrounding fundus. The temporal side of the disc is usually paler than the nasal side.

In atrophy of the optic nerve, the disc becomes pale and white or greyish-white in colour. In oedema of the optic nerve head, resulting from raised intracranial pressure (*papilloedema*) or from inflammation (*papillitis*), the disc is pinker than normal and may approach the colour of the surrounding retina (Fig. 10.4). In *pseudopapilloedema*, a congenital anomaly sometimes associated with hypermetropia, the disc may appear swollen and pinker than normal, but the retinal blood vessels are normal in appearance, corrected vision is normal and the condition is stationary.

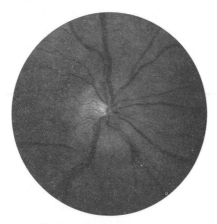

Fig. 10.4 Papilloedema.

PHYSIOLOGICAL CUP

In its central part there is usually a depression in the disc—the physiological cup. The cup is paler than the surrounding disc, and from it the retinal vessels enter and leave the eye. In glaucoma the cup may be greatly increased in size and the retinal vessels will kink as they cross the edge of the disc. When the cup is deep, as in advanced glaucoma, retinal vessels disappear as they climb from the floor to the rim, and reappear as they bend sharply over the cup; in less advanced cases a vertically oval cup extending to the edge of the disc may be seen (Fig. 10.5).

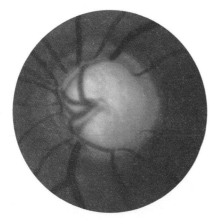

Fig. 10.5 Chronic simple glaucoma. Pathological cupping of the disc. The cup is oval in the vertical plane and appears pale. The retinal vessels are displaced nasally because of the angulation of the optic cup.

EDGE OF THE DISC

This is normally well-defined. In normal eyes there is sometimes a white scleral ring, a dark pigmented ring, or a stippled choroidal ring surrounding the optic disc. These signs are also a feature of highly myopic eyes.

THE RETINAL BLOOD VESSELS

These radiate from the disc, dividing dichotomously into many branches as they pass towards the periphery of the retina. The retinal arteries are narrower than the veins, brighter red in colour, and have a brighter longitudinal streak where light is reflected from their convex walls. *Spontaneous retinal artery pulsation* is an abnormal finding, and occurs in some cases of glaucoma and aortic regurgitation. *Spontaneous venous pulsation* is frequently seen in normal eyes; it is often absent in papilloedema. It is important to study the points where arteries and veins cross. Most frequently it is the artery that crosses the vein, and in normal eyes neither vessel shows any change in colour, diameter or direction.

THE MACULAR REGION

This is defined anatomically as that portion of the posterior retina containing xanthophilic pigment (hence, macula lutea), and two or more layers of ganglion cells. At the centre of the macula (measuring approximately 5.5 mm in diameter) is the fovea. The fovea has a glistening appearance and is devoid of blood vessels. Pathological changes in the macular region are important as they produce a greater reduction in vision than similar changes in any other part of the fundus.

THE PERIPHERY OF THE FUNDUS

This area can be examined only if the pupil is dilated with a mydriatic. Certain disease processes start in this region, for example retinal tears and retinitis pigmentosa.

The abnormal fundus

PAPILLOEDEMA (Fig. 10.4)

This is a passive swelling of the optic nerve head, due to raised intracranial pressure. There is an absence of inflammatory changes and little or no disturbance of visual function. In severe papilloedema the patient may notice transient loss of vision for a second or two (visual obstruction). In the initial stages of papilloedema there is an increased redness of the disc with blurring of its margins; the blurring appears first at the upper and lower margins, particularly in the upper nasal quadrant. The physiological cup becomes filled in and disappears, and the retinal veins are slightly distended. Spontaneous pulsation of the retinal veins is usually absent.

As the condition progresses the disc becomes definitely swollen (Fig. 10.6). In order to measure the

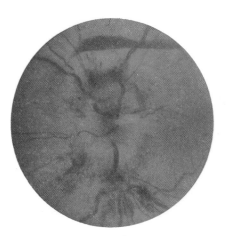

Fig. 10.6   Severe papilloedema with retinal haemorrhages.

degree of swelling of the disc, start with a high plus lens in the ophthalmoscope and reduce the power of the lens until the centre of the disc is just in focus. The retina, a short distance from the disc, is then brought into focus by further reduction of the power of the lens. This further reduction indicates the degree of swelling of the disc (3 dioptres is equivalent to 1 mm of swelling).

If papilloedema develops rapidly, there will be marked engorgement of the retinal veins with haemorrhages and exudates on and around the disc, but with papilloedema of slow onset there may be little or no vascular change, even though the disc may become very swollen (Fig. 10.7). The retinal vessels will, however, bend sharply as they dip down from the swollen disc to the surrounding retina. The oedema may extend to the adjacent retina, producing greyish-white striations near the disc, and a white macular fan between the fovea and disc may develop in some cases. These appearances result from swelling of the nerve axons in the nerve and retina as a result of interference with axoplasmic flow.

Papilloedema occurs frequently in patients with brain tumour, but is particularly liable to occur in children with tumours of cerebellum and fourth ventricle. It is rare in patients with pituitary tumours. An acute form of papilloedema with haemorrhage extending into the vitreous is characteristic of subarachnoid haemorrhage. A subdural haematoma may produce a clinical picture similar to that of a cerebral tumour. Papilloedema is uncommon in acute meningitis, but is a feature in subacute and chronic meningitis and in patients with brain abscess. It may be the only physical sign in benign intracranial hypertension. Papilloedema occurring in malignant hypertension is accompanied by arterial changes characteristic of this condition and the haemorrhages and exudates far beyond the region of the disc.

Pseudopapilloedema (Fig. 10.8) is an anomaly of development of the optic disc that produces an appearance resembling true papilloedema. In this condition there is no oedema of the optic disc.

OPTIC NEURITIS

Inflammatory, demyelinating or vascular disease may affect any part of the optic nerve, producing an optic neuritis, the characteristic symptom of which is loss of vision. There is often pain on moving the eye, and the pupil on the affected side shows an ill-sustained contraction to a bright light (see page 296).

When the disease affects the optic nerve head (papillitis) there is hyperaemia and some swelling of the optic disc. It must not be confused with papilloedema, in spite of their similar ophthalmoscopic appearances. The two conditions can be distinguished by the severe visual impairment that occurs

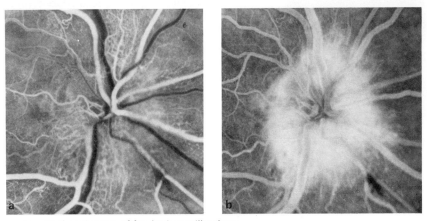

Fig. 10.7   Fluorescein retinal angiogram of fundus in papilloedema.

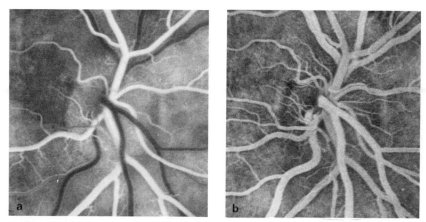

Fig. 10.8 Fluorescein retinal angiogram of fundus in pseudopapilloedema.

with optic neuritis, as compared with the minimal loss in papilloedema. In optic neuritis the swelling of the optic disc is usually slight, the distension of the retinal veins is less marked than in papilloedema, and there may be signs of inflammation, e.g. hazy vitreous and retinal exudates. Optic neuritis is frequently followed by optic atrophy (Fig. 10.9), with residual reduction in visual acuity and central or paracentral scotoma. It may occur alone, bilaterally or during the course of multiple sclerosis.

OPTIC ATROPHY

In this condition the optic disc is paler than normal and may even be white (Fig. 10.9). Because of the wide variation in colour of the normal disc, a useful sign of optic atrophy is the reduction in the number of capillaries on the disc. In optic atrophy the number of capillaries that cross the disc margin is reduced from the normal 10 to 7 or less (*Kestenbaum's sign*). From the appearance of the disc it is customary,

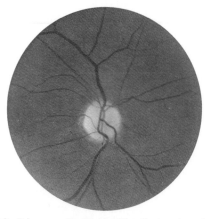

Fig. 10.9 Primary optic atrophy. The disc is pale and whiter than normal, and its edges are unusually sharply demarcated from the retina. The retinal vessels are slightly attenuated.

although not always very useful, to divide optic atrophy into primary and secondary types. In the *primary* type the disc is flat and white with clearcut edges. *Secondary* optic atrophy follows swelling of the optic disc, due to papilloedema. The disc is greyish-white in colour and its edges are indistinct.

Optic atrophy may occur in a number of disorders, of which the following are a few:
● Where there is interference with the blood supply to the optic nerve, as in occlusion of one of the ciliary vessels supplying the optic nerve head (*ischaemic optic neuropathy*).
● Where there is pressure on the nerve, whether in its intraocular, intraorbital, intracanalicular or intracranial portions.
● Following optic neuritis.
● Following trauma, where the optic nerve or its blood supply is involved.
● In toxic conditions due to substances such as tobacco, alcohol, lead, etc.
● In certain congenital disorders, when it is frequently associated with other neurological signs.
● Following widespread chorioretinal inflammation or degeneration.

OPAQUE OR MEDULLATED NERVE FIBRES

These are usually seen as one or more bright white patches radiating for a short distance from the optic disc (Fig. 10.10). The patch has a characteristic feathered edge and retinal vessels may disappear for a short distance within it. This condition is a harmless and non-progressive congenital anomaly.

MYOPIC CRESCENT

This is a crescent of white sclera, usually on the temporal side of the optic disc but in some cases extend-

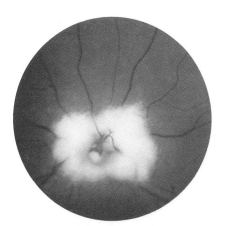

Fig. 10.10 Opaque (myelinated) nerve fibres. The white area obscures the disc, but this is a normal variant.

ing all round it. When marked it may be associated with other degenerative changes in the fundus, which, if they involve the macula, will result in reduction of central vision.

RETINAL HAEMORRHAGES
These occur in a number of different conditions and are due to one or more of the following factors.
- Increased blood pressure within the retinal vessels, as in hypertension.
- Abnormalities in the walls of the retinal vessels, as in arteriosclerosis, diabetes mellitus and occlusion of the retinal veins.
- Abnormalities in the circulating blood, as in severe anaemia, leukaemias, and bleeding diatheses.
- Sudden reduction in intraocular pressure, following a penetrating wound of the eye.

   When *superficial*, within the nerve fibre layer of the retina, the haemorrhages are elongated and flame-shaped, whereas when deep they are round blotches or spots. *Subhyaloid* haemorrhages, situated in front of the retina, are occasionally seen as very large round haemorrhages with a straight, horizontal upper border; they sometimes occur in diabetic retinopathy and after a subarachnoid haemorrhage.

RETINAL ARTERIOSCLEROSIS
This occurs either as an exaggeration of the general ageing process of the body or in association with hypertension. It is characterized by:
- broadening of the arterial light reflex, producing a 'copper wire' or 'silver wire' appearance;
- tortuosity of the vessels;
- nipping, indentation or deflection of the veins where they are crossed by the arteries;

- white plaques on the arteries; and
- in hypertension, flame-shaped haemorrhages and 'cottonwool' spots in the region of the macula.

HYPERTENSIVE RETINOPATHY (Fig. 10.11)
This is characterized by a generalized narrowing of the retinal arteries, particularly in the young patient. In older patients these changes are masked by the accompanying arteriosclerosis. If the hypertension is severe, fullness of the retinal veins and flame-shaped haemorrhages occur around the optic disc, and there is retinal oedema extending towards the macula, sometimes accompanied by a star-shaped collection of white exudates around the macula. In malignant hypertension, papilloedema is also present. The retinopathy seen in some cases of acute and chronic nephritis is due to the associated hypertension.

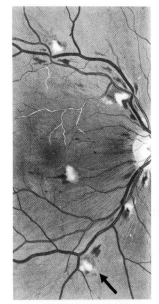

Fig. 10.11 Hypertensive retinopathy. The arteries are irregular in calibre and show 'silver wiring'. Arteriovenous nipping is present. Characteristic 'flame-shaped' haemorrhages and 'cottonwool' spots (arrow) can be seen.

DIABETIC RETINOPATHY (Fig. 10.12)
The fundamental change in this condition is the formation of capillary microaneurysms, seen as tiny red spots around the macula. Microaneurysms are not seen in such abundance in any other condition. Retinal haemorrhages and exudates may occur; the haemorrhages are punctate or round, and the exudates have a waxy yellow-white appearance. In the more severe form of diabetic retinopathy—proliferative retinopathy—new vessels extend into the vitre-

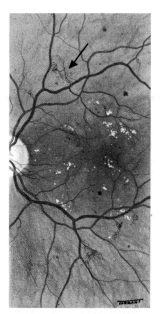

Fig. 10.12 Diabetic retinopathy. Microaneurysms (tiny red dots), blot haemorrhages, hard exudates and areas of new vessel formation (arrow) are characteristic of this condition. In many patients hypertensive retinopathy is also present.

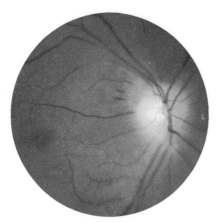

Fig. 10.13 Acute central artery occlusion. The vessels are attenuated, the retina is pale and oedematous and there are a few flame-shaped haemorrhages. The disc is slightly swollen and there is a cherry red spot at the macula indicating preserved choroidal circulation.

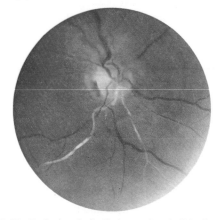

Fig. 10.14 Retinal emboli. Cholesterol emboli in the retinal arteries of a patient with atheromatous disease of the internal carotid artery in the neck.

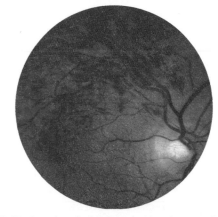

Fig. 10.15 Branch retinal vein occlusion. There are flame-shaped retinal haemorrhages. The disc is normal.

ous and bleed. The resulting glial proliferation may destroy vision by covering the macula or by producing a retinal detachment. Patients with diabetic retinopathy often have associated arteriosclerotic or hypertensive changes in their fundi.

RETINOPATHIES IN DISORDERS OF THE HAEMOPOIETIC SYSTEM

In severe anaemias the fundus may be paler than normal and a few small flame-shaped haemorrhages and small woolly exudates may be present.

In polycythaemia the retinal vessels are dark, tortuous and dilated. There may be oedema of the optic disc, and a few retinal haemorrhages may be observed.

In the leukaemias the retinal veins may be tortuous and dilated. In the later stages of these diseases the arteries and veins may be yellowish in colour, and the fundus may have a generalized pallor. Retinal haemorrhages of various types may occur, the characteristic ones in leukaemia being round with a pale centre.

OCCLUSION OF THE CENTRAL ARTERY OF THE RETINA

The optic disc and surrounding retina are pale, and there is a cherry-red spot at the macula which contrasts with the milky pallor of the adjacent retina. The retinal arteries are narrow or even thread-like

(Fig. 10.13). Embolic occlusion of retinal vessels may occur from atheromatous emboli causing a zone of retinal infarction (Fig. 10.14).

OCCLUSION OF THE CENTRAL VEIN OF THE RETINA

There is intense swelling of the optic disc, gross venous dilatation and numerous retinal haemorrhages which extend in all directions. Branch retinal veins may be affected in isolation, with less resultant abnormality in the retina (Fig. 10.15).

CHOROIDITIS

In acute choroiditis there are one or more round or oval whitish patches in the fundus, lying deep to the retinal vessels. These patches have ill-defined edges and the vitreous may be hazy. When the acute phase subsides, flat white scars with pigment around their edges are left. The numerous causes of choroiditis include tuberculosis, syphilis (which may cause a disseminated choroiditis), and toxoplasmosis (which characteristically produces lesions at the maculae).

Examination of the eye in children

The points made in Chapter 15, on the examination of children in general, also apply to the examination of children's eyes. In particular, children may object strongly to lights and instruments, particularly when they are wielded by white-coated strangers. Allow the child to get used to the surroundings whilst taking a history from the parent. At the same time, constantly observe the child, noting their visual behaviour, the position and movements of the eyes, and the general appearance of each eye.

The assessment of visual acuity should then be made. Babies should rapidly fix a large object and follow it. The examiner's face is the best visual target. In infants, the visual acuity can be assessed by the ability to follow rolling white balls of varying sizes. From the age of $2^{1}/_{2}$ years a more accurate estimate of acuity can be made using the Sheridan–Gardiner test. In this test the child, or the child's mother, holds a card with a number of letters on it. The examiner then shows the child one of the letters on an identical card and asks the child to point to the same letter on his or her own card. When the child has understood the test the examiner moves to a distance of 6 m and shows the child a series of letters of decreasing size, until the child fails to make a match. This test is also useful for assessing visual acuity in patients with whom the examiner has no common language, in illiterate patients, and in patients with dysphasia.

Next, the position and movements of the eyes

should be assessed. The least disturbing method is to observe the corneal light reflex; a light held at about 1 m should produce a reflection in the centre of the pupil of each eye. If the reflection in one eye is at a different location to that in the other, there is probably a squint. If squint is suspected, a cover test should be performed (see page 294). The range of movement of the eyes should then be assessed and the pupillary responses to light, and to accommodation, should be observed. Finally, the media and fundi are examined with the ophthalmoscope. It is best to carry out ophthalmoscopy without touching the child as this can produce resistance and tight closure of the eye. Begin with a relatively dim light and gradually increase the brightness.

Some clinical problems

The red eye

A red eye is usually a sign of ocular inflammation. The dilated vessels giving rise to this appearance produce either *conjunctival* injection (posterior conjunctival vessels) or *ciliary* injection (anterior ciliary vessels). There are essentially four conditions which must be distinguished: conjunctivitis, keratitis, iritis, and acute glaucoma. In assessing these conditions a history of pain and any blurring of vision are important clues to the diagnosis. Examination of the pupil is the most helpful diagnostic sign.

• In *conjunctivitis* pain is of variable severity and vision is unaffected. There is injection particularly involving the palpebral conjunctiva, and often also the bulbar conjunctiva, associated with a sticky discharge. The pupil is normal.

• In *keratitis* there is moderate to severe pain with loss of vision, particularly if the keratitis involves the visual axis. There may or may not be some discharge. The cornea will show signs of inflammation, but the pupil is normal.

• *Iritis* is associated with a dull, boring pain made worse by exposure to bright light (*photophobia*). Vision is reduced to varying degrees depending on the severity of the inflammation (see also page 230). The pupil is small, or irregular if there have been previous attacks.

• *Acute glaucoma* presents suddenly with severe pain, marked loss of vision and often vomiting. There is ciliary injection, the cornea is cloudy and the pupil remains fixed in the mid-dilated position.

• *Subconjunctival haemorrhage*, resulting from rupture of a small conjunctival blood vessel, is an alarming but benign cause of a red eye.

Sudden loss of vision

It is important to decide whether the patient's vision was lost suddenly or if the patient suddenly became aware of relatively long-standing or slowly progressive loss of vision in one eye, for example by inadvertently covering the other eye. Sudden visual loss is usually unilateral and often results from vascular disease. Sudden transient loss of vision, sometimes described as coming on like a curtain falling over the eye, and resolving gradually or like the lifting of a curtain after a few seconds or a minute or so, is usually due to emboli in the retinal vessels. Sudden permanent loss of vision in one eye occurs from central retinal artery occlusion, or from optic nerve ischaemia, due to involvement of the ciliary circulation. The ciliary vessels are often involved in giant cell arteritis. When a retinal detachment involves the macula, it may cause sudden loss of vision.

In all cases of sudden loss of vision, it is essential to test the pupillary light response. When there is disease in the retina or in the optic nerve there will be an afferent pupillary defect (page 296). Sudden blindness with normal pupillary responses to light strongly suggests a functional cause for the loss of vision. Bilateral sudden loss of vision may also be psychogenic in origin, but it can result from acute compression of the optic chiasm and optic nerves, for example in untreated hydrocephalus or in pituitary apoplexy, i.e. infarction of a pituitary tumour. Infarction of both occipital lobes, from vertebrobasilar disease due to embolism from the heart, similarly may produce bilateral loss of vision and in this disorder the pupillary light responses are normal.

Unequal pupils (anisocoria)

Approximately 12% of normal individuals have a slight, but clinically evident, pupillary inequality. Such physiologically unequal pupils react normally. Pathological pupils dilate and constrict abnormally. In the absence of local disease of the eye, a small pupil may be due to paralysis of the dilator pupillae muscle, which is supplied by sympathetic nerve fibres. The sympathetic nerve fibres also supply part of levator palpebrae superioris. Damage to these sympathetic nerve fibres, derived from the stellate cervical sympathetic ganglion, produces slight drooping of the lid on the affected side (*ptosis*). The small pupil, together with slight ptosis, constitutes *Horner's syndrome* (Fig. 10.16). The easiest way to confirm a diagnosis of Horner's syndrome is to put the patient into a semidarkened room for a minute or two. If Horner's syndrome is present, the pupil will dilate very poorly; the normal contralateral pupil dilates much better.

An abnormally dilated pupil suggests a partial *oculomotor palsy*. The internal ophthalmoplegia in partial oculomotor palsy results from damage to the parasympathetic fibres, which arise in the Edinger–Westphal nucleus of the oculomotor nerve. This may be associated with partial or complete weakness of the external ocular muscles supplied by the oculomotor nerve (page 291). In internal ophthalmoplegia due to partial oculomotor nerve palsy, the enlarged pupil reacts very poorly to light and to accommodation. A *tonic pupil* (Holmes–Adie pupil), which is usually smaller than normal, reacts very slowly to light, but better to accommodation. The tonic pupil reacts in a supersensitive manner to weak

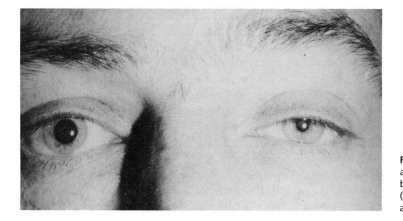

Fig. 10.16 Horner's syndrome. On the affected side there is ptosis, which may be very slight, and a small pupil (miosis), which reacts to both light and accommodation.

cholinergic drugs instilled into the conjunctival sac, e.g. pilocarpine 0.125% solution. After accidental medication with mydriatics, there is no reaction either to light or to accommodation. The pupillary changes in neurosyphilis, the Argyll Robertson phenomenon, are described in Chapter 12.

Trauma

Foreign bodies

In all, 25% of ocular injuries are foreign bodies in the cornea. Symptoms range from mild discomfort to severe pain. Inspection of the cornea with a magnifying glass will aid identification of the foreign body. Further localization may be obtained by instilling sterile 2% fluorescein solution. It is important to search for foreign bodies elsewhere in the conjunctival sac, particularly *subtarsal* foreign bodies (see page 230 on how to evert the upper lid).

Intraocular foreign bodies occur when small pieces of metal, glass, plastic or similar material penetrate the cornea or sclera. Any intraocular foreign body, particularly if it is of vegetable origin, may produce a severe purulent panophthalmitis. Retained iron foreign bodies cause *siderosis*, resulting in gradual loss of vision. It is imperative to X-ray all suspected intraocular and orbital foreign bodies.

Lid lacerations involving the lid margin must be recognized owing to the serious complications, such as ingrowing lashes (*trichiasis*), which may follow inadequate repair. If a laceration of the medial end of the lid also involves the lacrimal drainage system, then *epiphora* may result.

Penetrating injuries

Penetrating or perforating injuries of the eye result in distortion of the ocular anatomy. There may be prolapse of iris, ciliary body, lens, vitreous humour or retina. An X-ray is essential to exclude a foreign body.

Blunt injuries

Mild blunt trauma to the eye and orbit may produce quite marked swelling and bruising of the lids—a 'black eye'. Subconjunctival haemorrhage and corneal epithelial abrasion may also occur; the latter, although painful, heals rapidly.

More severe contusion of the globe may result in bleeding into the anterior chamber (*hyphaemia*). This may vary from a small level of red cells to a large clot. Dislocation of the lens, vitreous haemorrhage and retinal detachment can also occur.

Blunt trauma to the orbit can cause fractures. In particular the orbital contents may prolapse, through a fracture of the floor of the orbit producing a '*blow-out fracture*'. Fracture–dislocation of the zygomatic bone and arch produces the cosmetically unsightly malar fracture.

Chemical injuries

Acid or alkali coming into contact with the cornea and conjunctiva can cause serious complications, including loss of the eye. Severe chemical injuries cause a whitening of the conjunctiva and a marbled appearance to the cornea. There is a danger of corneal perforation in these injuries.

Thermal injuries

The globe is usually spared because of the blink reflex. Contracture of the lids after a burn can result in exposure and subsequent damage to the cornea.

Special techniques in ophthalmology

A refraction test will ascertain the optical power of an eye. This is performed subjectively by placing neutralizing lenses in front of the eye and simultaneously assessing visual acuity. An objective refraction is performed using neutralizing lenses in conjunction with a *retinoscope*.

The intraocular pressure is measured by *tonometry*. It is performed by measuring the force required to flatten a given area of the cornea using an *applanation tonometer*, which is usually attached to a slit lamp.

In addition to standard direct ophthalmoscopy, *binocular indirect ophthalmoscopy*, using a light source supported on the examiner's head and a hand-held lens in front of the patient's eye, allows a much greater area of the fundus to be visualized and permits stereopsis on the part of the examiner.

A *slit lamp* consists of a binocular microscope mounted on a table with an adjustable beam of light.

This can produce a fine slit of light enabling one to examine a magnified optical section of the various structures of the eye.

Fundus photography is a useful adjunct to the diagnosis and management of retinal and choroidal disorders. When used in conjunction with the intravenous injection of sodium fluorescein, detailed assessment of the retinal and choroidal vasculature may be obtained using a blue filter with the fundus camera to excite fluorescence as the dye circulates (*fluorescein angiography*).

Ultrasonography (echography), using sound waves with frequencies of 5000–20 000 Hz is used in the diagnosis of retinal detachments and both intraocular and orbital tumours.

Radiopaque dye may be introduced into the lacrimal drainage system to identify sites of obstruction (*dacrocystography*).

CT and MRI are useful in the diagnosis of orbital disease (see Fig. 10.2).

Visual handicap

The word *blindness* is emotive and for many people implies total loss of vision, but this is rarely the case. In the UK a person can be legally registered blind if they are 'unable to perform any work for which eyesight is essential' (DoH/Dept of Employment regulations). This usually implies a visual acuity less than 6/60. Alternatively, a person can be registered as partially sighted with vision between 6/60 and 6/18, particularly if there is an associated field defect.

Electrophysiological tests

Visual evoked potentials (*VEP*) recorded from the occipital cortex using scalp electrodes while the subject views a powerful alternating stimulus, usually an alternating black and white checker board pattern, are used in the diagnosis of disease of the visual pathway. The principal waveform recorded from the scalp is a positive deflection occurring about 100 ms after the stimulus (the P100 wave). This is attenuated in amplitude and increased in latency in disease, especially disease of the optic nerve, e.g. optic neuritis or optic nerve compression.

Electroretinograms measure the electrical potential across the eye, recorded from a special corneal electrode, with a reference electrode placed on the forehead. Flash or flicker stimuli are used to generate a response, derived from activation of the retina. The waveform is useful in assessing patients with hereditary acquired retinal degenerations.

CHAPTER 11

The locomotor system

Introduction

Musculoskeletal symptoms are common. Although usually due to primary rheumatological disorders, musculoskeletal symptoms may reflect underlying systemic disease; for example, bleeding into a joint, (*haemarthrosis*) may be the presenting manifestation of haemophilia. The first aim of clinical assessment of the locomotor system is to determine whether symptoms are derived from bone, joint, muscle or other soft tissue structures. Pain in a joint may be referred from another organ; for example, pain in the right shoulder may be referred from gall bladder disease, and disease in the hip may present with pain referred from the knee, particularly in children. These examples illustrate the importance of a full clinical assessment rather than examination limited to the apparent site of symptoms. Even in the absence of major musculoskeletal symptoms, basic examination of the joints, muscles and tendons is advisable as part of a general examination. Occult musculoskeletal disease is common. The screening question, 'do you suffer from any pain or stiffness in your arms, legs, neck or back?' is useful.

General assessment: history

The history must include the presenting complaint, i.e. when and how the problem started, and how it has evolved. It is important to define whether the symptoms are causing any *disability* and, if so, the degree of disability must be assessed in terms of the impact on everyday activities and household or work commitments. The impact will vary greatly, depending on the functional requirements of the individual: minor knee pain is a very different problem in an Olympic athlete from that in an elderly patient. Therefore, having established the degree of disability, try to ascertain the patient's expectations of the results of treatment.

Ask simple questions relevant to the individual's disability.

General, for example:
- Do you have difficulty or need any help with dressing, bathing or using the toilet (termed the 'activities of daily living' or ADL)?

Specific to a localized problem, for example:
- *Hip*: Do you have difficulty putting socks/stockings on or cutting toenails?
- *Shoulder*: Do you have difficulty combing your hair?

Specific locomotor history

The history of a fracture is very different from that of a bone tumour. The severe, acute, usually continuous throbbing pain of joint infection is easily distinguished from weight-bearing mechanical pain due to osteoarthritis.

Joint disease

A combination of *pain* and *stiffness*, causing loss of function, is a frequent manifestation of joint disease, but pain and swelling can occasionally occur through overuse of a normal joint. Usually one component predominates, as with stiffness in inflammation, and pain in mechanical joint problems. Therefore, use specific questions to establish whether symptoms are *mechanical* (e.g. degenerative joint disease or meniscal tear) or *inflammatory* (e.g. rheumatoid arthritis or gout).

FEATURES OF MECHANICAL JOINT DISEASE

Pain on activity, usually improving with rest, is typical. In degenerative joint disease there may be a feeling of *inactivity stiffness* in the affected joint after a long period of rest, but this disappears rapidly on activity, unlike the stiffness of inflammatory disease. A clicking sensation in a joint, particularly in the knee, is a common complaint, but it is usually a normal phenomenon (compare with *crepitus*, page 247). *Locking* of a joint may occur. In terms of the knee, this means that the knee becomes jammed in such a way that it will not fully extend, although it may flex. In other joints locking is less well-defined and simply means that at some point through its range of motion the joint becomes jammed, usually associated with pain and often followed by swelling. Locking is due to material within the joint interfering with movement at the articular surfaces. In the knee, this is usually part of one of the menisci, or a cartilaginous loose body.

FEATURES OF INFLAMMATORY JOINT DISEASE

Early morning stiffness

When it persists for more than 30 minutes, early morning joint stiffness is important as a symptom of active inflammatory joint disease. Ask also about *redness* (rubor), *warmth* (calor), t*enderness/pain* (dolor) and *swelling* (tumor), described by Celsius as the classical features of inflammation.

Having recognized that the history suggests inflammation, and if only one joint is involved (monoarticular disease), always exclude infection. Ask if there has been any fever or sweating, and if the joint is hot, red or swollen. If there is inflammation, remember that this could be due to infection and that the joint may well need to be aspirated as part of the clinical examination.

Distribution of joint disease

The pattern of involvement of joints is important in diagnosis. For example, acute inflammation in the 1st metatarsophalangeal joint (*hallux*), suggests a diagnosis of gout, so pay particular attention to family history, previous episodes, usually in small or medium-sized joints, and to the presence of subcutaneous deposits of urate, called *tophi*. Acute attacks of gout are often severe and the patient will not be able to wear a shoe on the affected side or even bear the weight of the bedclothes on the affected joint. The skin overlying the joint is usually dry and often desquamates after the attack. Disease of this joint also occurs, of course, in other disorders.

Recurrent attacks of joint pain

Ask if the same joint is always involved. If not, define the patterns of involvement, the severity and duration of the episodes and any associated clinical symptoms.

Episodic joint pain

Ask if attacks of joint pain are associated with para-articular redness with the attacks lasting about 48 hours (occasionally up to one week) typical of *palindromic rheumatism*.

Flitting joint pains

This term is used to describe joint inflammation, beginning in one joint and then serially involving other joints, usually one at a time for about three days each. Gonococcal arthritis should be considered; it is characterized by typical fleeting skin lesions and urethritis, in addition to joint pain. In rheumatic fever there is associated cardiac involvement and erythema marginatum and subcutaneous nodules may occur.

The other features in the history which should be brought out are best considered under the differential diagnosis of polyarthritis (Boxes 11.1 and 11.2) as all the arthropathies may sometimes have an initial monoarticular presentation.

BOX 11.1 Historical pointers to the differential diagnosis of monoarticular inflammatory joint disease.

First attack
- Exclude infection by aspiration for culture and crystals
- If negative culture, but high risk group, *biopsy*, for example, tuberculosis in Asian immigrants or immunosuppressed patients

Recurrent attacks
- Flitting (gonococcal arthritis; rheumatic fever)
- Episodic (crystal arthritis; palindromic rheumatism)

Persistent synovitis with none of the above features
- Look for systemic features and check serology (e.g. latex fixation test)

BOX 11.2 Importance of distribution of joint involvement in differential diagnosis of oligo- or polyarthritis.

Typically symmetrical
- *Upper and lower limbs*
  - rheumatoid arthritis, SLE, polyarteritis nodosa
- *Especially upper limbs*
  - haemachromatosis (hand, index, middle MCP joints)

Typically asymmetrical
  - psoriatic arthritis

Typically lower limb and asymmetrical
  - spondyloarthritis, e.g. ankylosing spondylitis, Reiter's syndrome

Define any associated features

Soft tissue symptoms

Soft tissue problems are common, usually consisting of pain, dull ache, tenderness or swelling. In the elderly such symptoms often appear spontaneously but, in younger people, there is usually a history of injury or overuse, either through occupation, e.g. tenosynovitis of the long flexor tendons of the hand,

or sport, as with Achilles tendinitis. It is important to define the exact site of the symptoms, factors that usually make them worse, and any factors inducing relief.

The localization of symptoms to specific soft tissue structures can be confirmed by careful anatomical examination (Box 11.3). The possible soft tissues involved are *joint, tendon, ligament, bursa* and *muscle.*

BOX 11.3 Localization of the site of articular and extra-articular features.

Joint
- Diffuse pain and tenderness
- Generalized joint swelling
- Restriction of movement, usually in all directions of movement (specific to each joint)

Tendon
- Localized pain/tenderness at attachment (enthesis) or in the tendon substance
- Swelling, tendon sheath or paratenon
- Pain on resisted action
- Sometimes pain on stretch (e.g. Achilles)

Ligament
- Localized pain/tenderness at attachment or in ligament substance
- Pain on stretch
- Instability, if major tear

Bursa
- Localized tenderness
- Pain on stretching adjacent structures

Muscle
- Localized or diffuse pain and tenderness
- Pain on resisted action
- Pain on stretch (e.g. hamstring)

The bones

Bone pain is characteristically deep-seated and localized, but referred pain may confuse the clinical picture. In the case of fractures, unless pathological, there will almost always be a history of injury. In athletes, however, a fracture may be due to chronic overuse, as in stress fracture, for example, of the tibia in runners. The spontaneous onset of pain may suggest Paget's disease (with bony enlargement, e.g. skull or tibia) or metastatic deposits: infection must also be considered, particularly in younger patients or in immunodeficiency states. Consider also congenital or familial disorders as predisposing factors, e.g. multiple osteochondromata or brittle bone disease (*osteogenesis imperfecta*).

Examination: general principles

Observe the patient entering the room (Box 11.4). Abnormalities of *gait* and *posture* may provide clues that can be pursued in history-taking. Observation of any difficulty in undressing and getting on to the examination couch will further help in assessing the patient. The patient must always be asked to stand and walk, even when it is obvious that this may be difficult. Note how much help the patient requires from others or from sticks, crutches, etc. The locomotor system includes the muscles, bones, joints and soft tissue structures, such as tendons and ligaments. Remember that although muscle wasting may be due to primary muscle disease, e.g. polymyositis, it is more commonly secondary to disuse, perhaps because of a painful joint, or to nerve root compression or peripheral neuropathy (Fig. 11.1). Examination of the muscles is discussed in Chapter 12.

BOX 11.4 Examination of the locomotor system.

General observations
- Gait
- Posture
- Mobility
- Deformity
- Independence
- Muscle wasting
- Long bones

Fractures
- Joints
- Tendons
- Skin

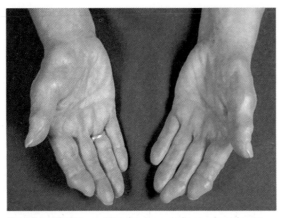

Fig. 11.1 Thenar wasting due to carpal tunnel syndrome. This is often associated with osteoarthritis—note nodal change on the terminal interphalangeal joints of the index fingers.

The bones

The examination of the bones should always be directed by information obtained from the history.

Inspection

Look for any alterations in shape or outline and measure any shortening. In osteitis deformans (*Paget's disease*) bowing of the long bones, particularly the tibia (Fig. 11.2a and b) and femur, is associated with bony enlargement and, usually, increased local temperature. The skull is commonly involved but this may not be apparent clinically until the disease is advanced. Early involvement of the skull bones can be detected on X-rays (Fig. 11.3a and b). Alteration in the shape of bones also occurs in rickets due to epiphyseal enlargement. Deformity of the chest in rickets is due to osteochondral enlargement (*rickety rosary*).

Localized swellings of long bones may be caused by infections, cysts or tumours. Spontaneous fractures may occasionally be the presenting symptom in the diagnosis of secondary carcinoma, multiple myeloma, generalized osteitis fibrosa cystica (*hyperparathyroidism*), or osteogenesis imperfecta.

Palpation

On palpation undue tenderness of the bones is found in local lesions when there is destruction, elevation or irritation of the periosteum, as in generalized osteitis fibrosa cystica, in myelomatosis, in infections of bone, occasionally in carcinomatosis of bones and, rarely, in leukaemia.

FRACTURES

Fractures are common. They are painful, distressing for the patient and expensive for the community (Box 11.5). They may involve any bone. Fractures occurring in healthy bones commonly involve the long bones and are usually due to trauma. Fractures of the ribs, skull and vertebrae are more frequently complications of bone disease. Multiple rib fractures, due to falls, may be found in alcoholics, but may only be seen as healed lesions on chest X-ray. Fractures occur without apparent trauma when a bone is weakened by disease, especially with metastatic malignant deposits in bone (*pathological fractures*). Traumatic fractures invariably present with local pain, swelling and loss of function, but pathological fractures may be relatively silent. The history will reveal the appropriate trauma, whether accidental or due to physical abuse.

(a)

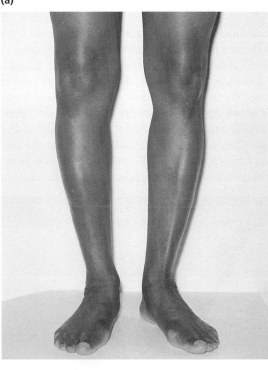

(b)

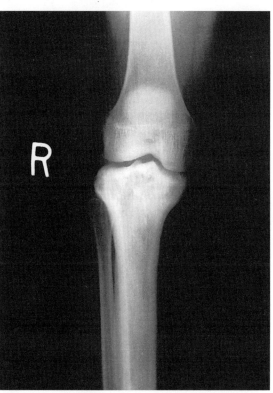

Fig. 11.2 Paget's disease of the right tibia. Note tibial bowing and bony enlargement (a) and bony enlargement sclerosis with some patchy porosis in the X-ray of the upper tibia (b).

(a)

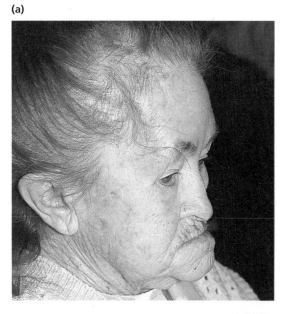

(b)

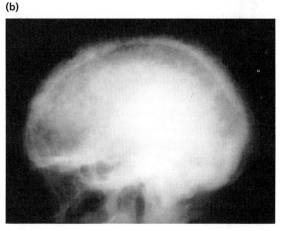

Fig. 11.3 Paget's disease, causing deformity of the skull (a). Note the thickened skull vault with remodelled bone (b).

BOX 11.5 Fractures: clinical features.

Type
- Compound (closed)

Complications
- Accompanying soft tissue injury (indirect)

Features
- Haemorrhage
- Deformity
- Pain
- Crepitus
- Restricted movement

Cause
- Traumatic
- Spontaneous (pathological)

Examination of suspected fracture

On examination, it is essential to establish whether the fracture is open (*compound*), or closed. In *closed fractures* the surrounding soft tissues are intact. In *open fractures* the bone communicates with the surface of the skin, either because the primary injury has broken the overlying skin or because deformation at the fracture site has caused the bone ends to penetrate the skin. There is a major risk of infection when the fracture site communicates with the open air.

Deformity is an obvious feature in the majority of fractures. It may be clinically characteristic, as in Colles' fracture, in which there is a fracture of the distal end of the radius characterized by dorsal displacement and angulation, shortening of the wrist and rotation of the fragment, well-summarized in the description 'dinner fork deformity'. Certain fractures may show little deformity; for example, a fracture of the femoral shaft may be accompanied by only slight deformity, since there is often little separation of the bones at the fracture site and other features are disguised by the thick overlying muscle. A fracture of the neck of the femur causes deformity through external rotation of the foot and shortening of the leg.

Most fractures are characterized by local tenderness and swelling, unless the overlying muscle mass is large. Bony crepitus, due to abnormal motion at the bone ends, is a typical feature of fractures, but this should not be sought for unless necessary for diagnosis since it is very painful and demoralizing to the patient. However, if it is perceived or has been recognized by the patient it is diagnostic.

A fracture of the bone may damage the neighbouring soft tissues directly or, alternatively, a fracture may be a marker of severe injury in which direct damage to the soft tissues, such as the nerves and vessels, may have taken place. It is therefore essential to evaluate the nerve and blood supply to a limb distal to the site of the fracture. Impairment of blood supply distal to a fracture is a surgical emergency.

The presence or absence of *pulses* and *cutaneous sensation* and the colour and perfusion of the limb must always be recorded and any change over time reported. Voluntary movement at joints distal to a fractured long bone, such as ankle movement in a fractured femur, should be noted. If this is absent, nerve injury must be suspected.

The joints

Examination of the joints should proceed from *inspection* to *palpation*, and then tests of the *range of movement*. It is best to proceed in a routine manner, e.g. the jaw, cervical spine, shoulder girdle and upper limb, thoracic and lumbar spine, pelvis and lower limb, so that inconspicuous but important joints, like the temporomandibular, sternoclavicular and sacroiliac, will not be overlooked. Compare the corresponding joints on the two sides of the body. Always take care to avoid causing undue discomfort.

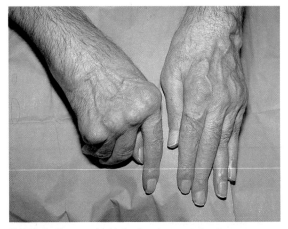

Fig. 11.4   Symmetrical joint involvement due to rheumatoid arthritis.

Inspection

It is important to decide whether joint involvement is inflammatory or not. Look for swelling or deformity of the joint. Inflammation is often associated with *redness* of the joint, and with *tenderness* and *warmth*. The *overall pattern* or joint involvement should be recorded. Note whether the distribution is symmetrical, as is usual in rheumatoid arthritis (Fig. 11.4), or asymmetrical, as in psoriatic arthropathy or gout (Fig. 11.5). The seronegative (non-rheumatoid)

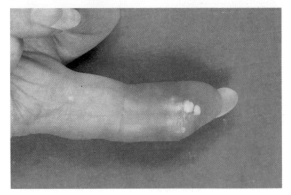

Fig. 11.5   Gouty tophi of the index finger.

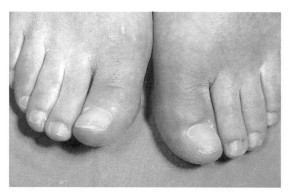

Fig. 11.6 Acute synovitis of the interphalangeal joint, due to Reiter's syndrome of the left hallux. Differential diagnosis includes gout.

spondyloarthropathies (e.g. Reiter's disease, Fig. 11.6) tend predominantly to involve the joints of the lower limb.

Palpation

On palpation of a joint swelling, check first for tenderness. Then determine whether the swelling is due to bony enlargement or to osteophytes (e.g. *Heberden's nodes*: Fig. 11.7), to thickening of synovial tissues such as occurs in inflammatory arthritis, or to effusion into the joint space. Joint effusions usually have a characteristically smooth outline and fluctuation is usually easily demonstrable. Tenderness and enlargement of the ends of the bones, particularly the radius and ulna, can occur in hypertrophic pulmonary osteoarthropathy; a chest X-ray is essential. Gross disorganization of a joint, nearly always foot and ankle joints, associated with absence of deep pain and position sense, occurs in neuropathic (*Charcot's*) joints. Charcot's joints probably arise from recurrent painless injury and overstretching of joints, and are a feature of severe chronic peripheral neuropathy, or, rarely, tabes dorsalis.

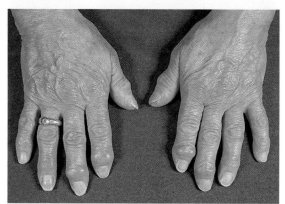

Fig. 11.7 Nodal osteoarthritis (Heberden's nodes).

Joint tenderness may be graded depending on the patient's reaction to firm pressure of the joint between finger and thumb (Box 11.6). Grade 4 tenderness occurs only in septic arthritis, crystal arthritis and rheumatic fever. In gout, the skin overlying the affected joint is dry, whereas in septic arthritis or rheumatic fever it is usually moist.

BOX 11.6 Assessment of joint tenderness.

- Grade 1: The patient says the joint is tender
- Grade 2: The patient winces
- Grade 3: The patient winces and withdraws the affected part
- Grade 4: The patient will not allow the joint to be touched

---

If tenderness is present, localize it as accurately as possible and determine whether it arises in the joint or in neighbouring structures, e.g. in the supraspinatus or bicipital tendon rather than the shoulder joint.

TENDON SHEATH CREPITUS

This is a grating or creaking sensation defined by palpating the tendon, while the patient is asked to contract the muscle tendon complex involved. It is particularly common in the hand. In tenosynovitis of the long flexor tendons in the palm tendon sheath crepitus may be associated with the trigger phenomenon, when the finger becomes caught in flexion and has to be pulled back into extension. Tendon sheath *effusions* can be distinguished from joint swelling by their anatomical location in association with tendons.

JOINT CREPITUS

This can be detected by feeling the joint with one hand while it is moved passively with the other. This may indicate osteoarthritis, or loose bodies (cartilaginous fragments) in the joint space, but should be differentiated from non-specific clicking of joints.

RANGE OF MOVEMENT

In examining joints for range of movement it is usually sufficient to estimate the degree of limitation based on comparison with the normal side, or on the examiner's previous experience. For accurate description the actual range of movement should be measured with a protractor (*goniometer*). Both *active* and *passive* movement should be assessed. Active movement, however, may give a poor estimation of true range of movement because of muscle spasm due to pain. If pain is very severe on attempted active movement, and other findings suggest fracture, neither active nor passive movement should be attempted before X-ray examination. In testing the range of passive movement gentleness must be exercised, particularly in the case of painful joints.

Limitation of movement in a joint may be due to pain, muscle spasm, contracture, inflammation, increased thickness of the capsules or periarticular structures, effusion into the joint space, bony overgrowths, bony ankylosis, mechanical factors such as a torn meniscus, or to painful conditions quite unconnected with the joint.

Extra-articular features of joint disease

Some of the extra-articular features of joint disease are listed in Box 11.7.

> **BOX 11.7 Extra-articular features of joint disease.**
>
> - Cutaneous nodules
> - Cutaneous vasculitic lesions
> - Lymphadenopathy
> - Oedema
> - Tendon sheath effusions
> - Enlarged bursae

SUBCUTANEOUS NODULES
Subcutaneous nodules are associated with various conditions (Box 11.8). If gout is suspected, palpate the helix of the ear for tophi due to subcutaneous deposition of urate, which may also be found overlying joints or in the finger pulps. Subcutaneous nodules in rheumatoid arthritis are firm and nontender; they may be detected by running the examining thumb from the point of the elbow down the proximal portion of the ulna (Fig. 11.8). They can also be found at other pressure and frictional sites, such as bony prominences, including the sacrum. If an olecranon bursa swelling is found, feel also in its wall, as rheumatoid nodules, tophi or occasionally xanthomata may be found at this site. Note that subcutaneous nodules are not specific to rheumatoid arthritis, being found in patients with SLE,

> **BOX 11.8 Types of subcutaneous nodules.**
>
> - Gouty tophi caused by urate deposition
> - Rheumatoid nodules
> - Nodules in SLE
> - Xanthomatous deposits (hypercholesterolaemia)

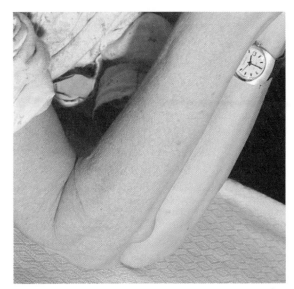

Fig. 11.8 Rheumatoid nodule overlying the olecranon of the right arm.

particularly in the tendons of the hand, and in rheumatic fever.

CUTANEOUS VASCULITIC LESIONS
These may be seen in rheumatoid arthritis, SLE and polyarteritis nodosa. Small vessel involvement is typically seen at the nail fold (cutaneous infarct, Fig. 11.9) but also occurs at pressure sites.

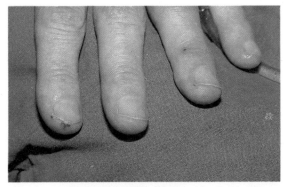

Fig. 11.9 Nail fold vasculitis in rheumatoid arthritis. This also occurs in SLE and polyarteritis nodosa.

LYMPHADENOPATHY
Lymphadenopathy may be found proximal to an inflamed joint, not only in septic arthritis but also in rheumatoid arthritis.

LOCAL OEDEMA
Local oedema is sometimes seen over inflamed joints (Fig. 11.10) but other causes of oedema must be excluded.

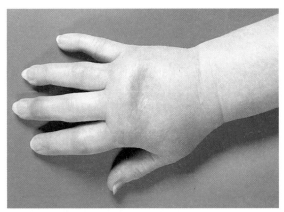

Fig. 11.10 Pitting oedema, right hand.

OTHER SOFT TISSUE SWELLINGS

Tendon sheath effusions are distinguished from joint swellings by their location in association with tendons. Enlarged subcutaneous bursae may be found over pressure areas, particularly at the olecranon surface of the elbow, due to inflammatory joint disease or secondary to friction. Deeper bursae may be defined only by finding local tenderness or by stressing adjacent tissues (e.g. greater trochanter bursitis).

Examination of individual joints

The range of movement of joints is described in the scheme shown in the following pages. All motion should be measured in degrees from a neutral or zero position, which must be defined whenever possible. Some special features seen at individual joints are set out in each section.

The spine

GENERAL EXAMINATION OF THE VERTEBRAL COLUMN

Inspection

Examine the patient standing and sitting in the erect posture. The normal shape of the thoracolumbar spine is an S-shaped curve. If there is an abnormality, note which vertebrae are involved and at what level any vertebral projection is most prominent. Note the presence of any local projections or angular deformity of the spine.

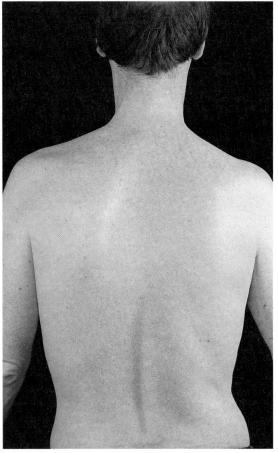

Fig. 11.11 Scoliosis of the lumbar spine, due to prolapsed intervertebral disc.

Palpation

The major landmarks are the spinous processes of C7 (the vertebra prominens) and the last rib, which articulates with the 12th thoracic vertebra. In many patients, however, the last rib cannot be distinctly

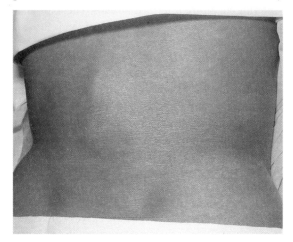

Fig. 11.12 Gibbus of the lumbar spine due to tuberculosis.

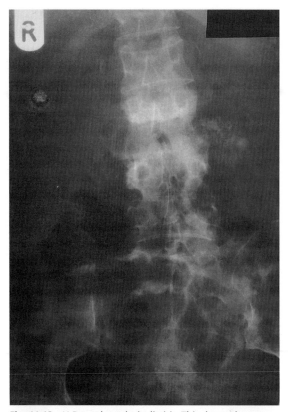

Fig. 11.13 X-Ray tuberculosis discitis. This shows the underlying deformity shown in Fig. 11.12. There is tuberculous infection of the intervertebral disc, causing the spinal deformity.

felt and this is therefore rather untrustworthy as a guide to this level.

The neutral position of the spine is a normal upright stance with head erect and chin drawn in. Note any curvature of the spinal column, whether as a whole or of part of it. The curvature may be in an anterior, posterior or lateral direction (Fig. 11.11). Anterior curvature is termed *lordosis*. There are natural lordotic curves in the cervical and lumbar regions. General posterior curvature is termed *kyphosis*. The thoracic spine usually exhibits a slight smooth kyphosis, which increases in the elderly. It must be distinguished from a localized angular deformity (*gibbus*, Fig. 11.12) caused by a fracture, by Pott's disease (spinal tuberculosis, Fig. 11.13), or by a secondary cancerous deposit.

Lateral curvature is termed *scoliosis* (Fig. 11.11) and may be towards either side. It is always accompanied by rotation of the bodies of the vertebrae in such a way that the posterior spinous processes come to point towards the concavity of the curve. The curvature is always greater than appears from inspection of the posterior spinous processes. In scoliosis due to

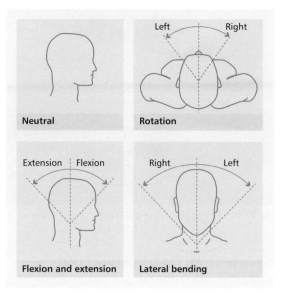

Fig. 11.14 Movements of the neck.

muscle spasm, e.g. with lumbosacral disc protrusion syndromes, the spinal curvature and rotational deformity decrease in flexion. When scoliosis is caused by inequality of leg length it disappears on sitting because the buttocks then become level. Scoliosis

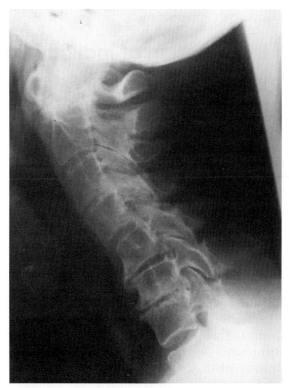

Fig. 11.15 Lateral X-ray of cervical spine showing degenerative spondylosis, with narrowing of the disc spaces and reversed cervical lordosis between C4 and C6.

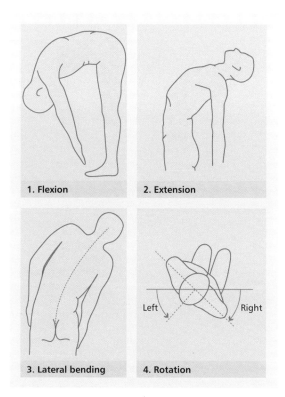

Fig. 11.16   Movements of the lumbar and dorsal spine.

secondary to skeletal anomalies shows in spinal flexion as a 'rib hump' due to the rotation. Kyphosis and scoliosis are often combined, particularly when the cause is an idiopathic spinal curvature, beginning in adolescence.

THE CERVICAL SPINE
The following movements should be tested (Fig. 11.14).
• Rotation (ask the patient to look over one, then the other shoulder)
• Flexion (ask the patient to touch chin to chest)
• Extension (ask the patient to look up to the ceiling)
• Lateral bending (ask the patient to bend the neck sideways and to try to touch the shoulder with the ear without raising the shoulder).

Note any pain or paraesthesiae in the arm reproduced by neck movement, suggesting nerve root involvement. If indicated, check for any associated neurological deficit, particularly of radicular or spinal cord type.

In rheumatoid arthritis particular care is necessary in examining the neck as atlantoaxial instability may lead to damage to the spinal cord when the neck is flexed or extended. If there is any doubt about neck stability in a patient with rheumatoid arthritis

arrange for lateral X-rays of the cervical spine in flexion and extension, together with a view of the odontoid peg through the mouth, and defer clinical examination.

In patients with cervical injury never try to elicit range of motion of the neck. Instead, splint the neck, take a history, look for abnormality of posture, usually in rotation, and check neurological function in the limbs including both arms and both legs. Take X-rays of the neck in the lateral (Fig. 11.15) and anteroposterior planes, *without* moving the neck. Only if the X-rays are normal should neck movements be examined.

THE THORACIC AND LUMBAR SPINE
The thoracic spine permits mainly rotation, while the lumbar spine can flex, extend, and bend laterally. The following movements should be tested (Fig. 11.16).
• Flexion (ask the patient to try to touch toes, without bending at the knees)
• Extension (ask the patient to bend backwards)
• Lateral bending (ask the patient to run the hand

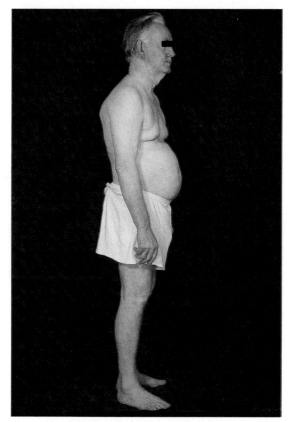

Fig. 11.17   Ankylosing spondylitis. Note dorsal kyphosis and protuberant abdomen due to poor chest expansion with abdominal breathing.

(a)

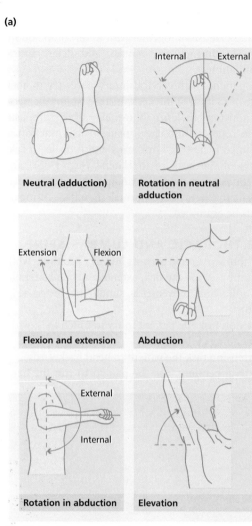

(b)

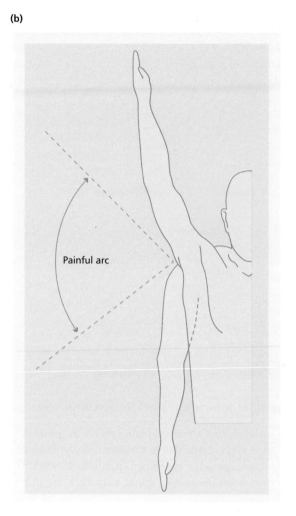

Fig. 11.18 Movements of the shoulder.

down the side of the thigh as far as possible
• Thoracic rotation (ask the seated patient, with arms crossed, to twist round to the left and right as far as possible).

The normal lumbar lordosis should be abolished in flexion. The extent of lumbar flexion can be assessed more accurately by marking a vertical, 10-cm line on the skin overlying the lumbar spinous processes and measuring the increase in the line length on flexion (*modified Shober test*). Painful restriction of spinal movement is an important sign of cervical and lumbar spondylosis, but may also be found in vertebral disc disease or other mechanical disorders of the back or neck. Spinal movements may be virtually absent in ankylosing spondylitis (Fig. 11.17) but, in the early stages of this condition, lateral flexion of the lumbar spine is typically affected first. In mechanical or osteoarthritic back prob-

lems flexion and extension are reduced more than lateral movements.

Chest expansion is a measure of costovertebral movement and should be recorded using a tape measure with the patient's hands behind their head to reduce the possibility of muscular action in the shoulder girdle giving a false reading. Reduced chest expansion is a characteristic early feature in ankylosing spondylitis. It is also found, of course, in primary pulmonary disease, such as emphysema.

Examination of the back is completed by assessing straight leg raising and strength, sensation and reflex activity in the legs. Pain and limitation of *straight leg raising* (SLR) is a feature of prolapsed intervertebral disc when there is irritation or compression of one of the roots of the sciatic nerve. However, tight hamstring muscles may cause a similar picture but, if there is severe pain, it is more considerate to lower the leg to just below the limit of SLR and then to see if gentle passive dorsiflexion of the foot brings back the same pain. If in doubt, dorsiflex the foot once the limit of SLR has been reached. This further stretches the sciatic nerve (the pain increases) but does not affect the hamstrings (*Lasègue's sign*). Sacral sensory loss must always be sought by examination since, if there is a central lumbosacral disc protrusion, bilateral limitation of straight leg raising may be associated with bladder dysfunction. This combination implies the need for immediate investigation and treatment.

The sacroiliac joints

The surface markings of these joints are two dimples low in the lumbar region. Test for *irritability* in three ways:

- direct pressure over each sacroiliac joint;
- firm pressure with the side of the hand over the sacrum;
- inward pressure over both iliac bones in an attempt to distort the pelvis.

In the second and third tests above, a positive test is only indicated by the patient localizing discomfort to the sacroiliac joint.

The shoulder

The neutral position is with the arm to the side, elbow flexed to 90 degrees with forearm pointing forwards. Because the scapula is mobile, true shoulder (*glenohumeral*) movement can be assessed only when the examiner anchors the scapula between finger and thumb on the posterior chest wall. The following movements should be tested (Fig. 11.18a and b).

- Flexion
- Extension
- Abduction
- Rotation in abduction
- Rotation in neutral position
- Elevation (also involving scapular movement).

In practice *internal rotation* can best be compared by recording the height reached by each thumb up the back, representing combined glenohumeral and scapular movement. Similarly, *external rotation* can be assessed by the ability to get the hand to the back of the neck.

Note any pain during the range of movement. In *supraspinatus tendinitis* a full passive range of movement is found, but there is a painful arc on abduction, with pain exacerbated on resisted abduction.

Other tendon involvement should also be defined by pain on resisted action.

Subacromial impingement due to a bursitis or rotator cuff abnormality may produce severe pain at the end of abduction, blocking full elevation. Acute bursitis, however, may be so painful that no abduction is allowed (grade 4 discomfort).

Acromioclavicular joint pain is always very localized and is typically felt in the last 10 degrees of elevation (170–180 degrees arc).

The elbow

The neutral position is with the forearm in extension. The following movements should be tested (Fig. 11.19).

- Flexion
- Hyperextension.

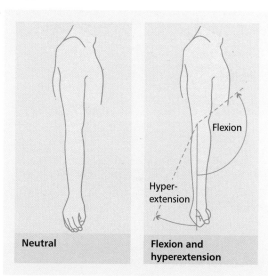

Fig. 11.19 Movements of the elbow.

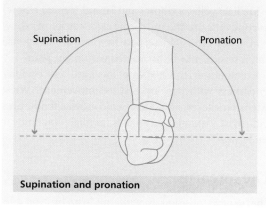

Fig. 11.20 Movements of the forearm.

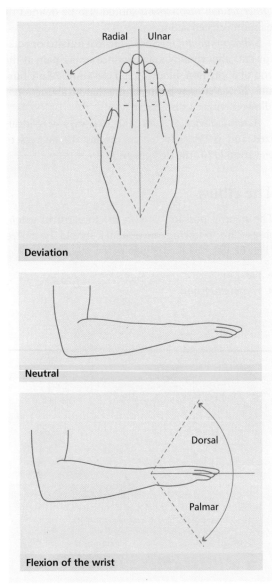

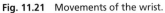

Fig. 11.21 Movements of the wrist.

The following movements should be tested (Fig. 11.20).
- Supination
- Pronation.

The wrist

The neutral position is with the hand in line with the forearm, and palm down. The following movements should be tested (Fig. 11.21).
- Dorsiflexion (extension)
- Palmar flexion
- Ulnar deviation
- Radial deviation.

Even minor limitation of wrist flexion or extension can be detected by comparing movement of both wrists (Fig 11.22). Arthritis of the wrist joints is usually due to inflammatory arthritis. Primary osteoarthritis of the wrist is rare but secondary degenerative change is common.

The fingers

When identifying fingers, use the names *thumb, index, middle, ring* and *little*. Numbering tends to lead to confusion. Digit I is the thumb and digit V is the little finger. The neutral position is with the fingers in extension. Test flexion at the meta-

Medial (golfer's elbow) and lateral (tennis elbow) epicondylitis are the most common causes of elbow pain. They are characterized by pain on active use but, if severe, may be associated with night pain.

Examination must define localized epicondylar tenderness with pain on resisted movement. Wrist extension exacerbates lateral epicondylar tenderness and wrist flexion exacerbates medial epicondylar tenderness.

The forearm

The neutral position is with the arm by the side, elbow flexed to 90 degrees, and thumb uppermost.

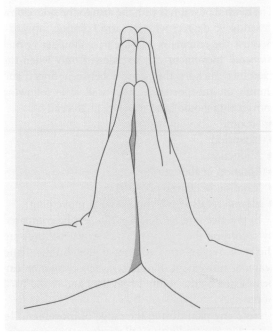

Fig. 11.22 Minor limitation of the left wrist extension compared with the right. Note the slightly different angulation of the left forearm.

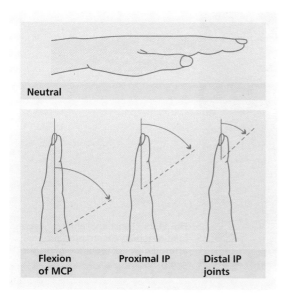

Fig. 11.23 Movements of the fingers

carpophalangeal (MCP), proximal interphalangeal (PIP) and distal interphalangeal (DIP) joints (Fig. 11.23).

In fractures of the fingers the commonest deformity is rotational. If the finger will flex make sure it points to the scaphoid tubercle (all the fingers will point individually in this direction). If it will not flex, look end-on at the nail and make sure it is parallel with its fellows.

The thumb (carpometacarpal joint)

The neutral position is with the thumb alongside the forefinger, and extended. The following movements should be tested (Fig. 11.24).
- Extension
- Flexion (measured as for the fingers)
- Opposition
- Abduction (not illustrated; movement at right angles to plane of palm).

The hand

DEFORMITIES IN JOINT DISEASE

Examination of the individual joints of the hand may be less informative than inspection of the hand as a whole (Fig. 11.25). The combination of Heberden's nodes (see above) and thumb carpometacarpal arthritis occurs in osteoarthritis (see Fig. 11.7). A variety of patterns of deformity are characteristic of rheumatoid arthritis, e.g. metacarpophalangeal joint subluxation, ulnar deviation of

the fingers at the metacarpophalangeal joints, 'swan neck' deformities of the fingers (Fig. 11.26), and 'boutonnière' deformities (flexed proximal and hyperextended distal interphalangeal joints). This is due to the head of the phalanx sliding dorsally between the lateral slips of the extensor tendon, the middle slip having been damaged. In psoriatic arthritis, terminal interphalangeal joint swelling may occur with psoriatic pitting deformity of the nail on that digit.

DEFORMITIES DUE TO NEUROPATHY

The hand may adopt a posture typical of a nerve lesion (see Chapter 12). Slight hyperextension of the medial metacarpophalangeal joints with slight flexion of the interphalangeal joints is the 'ulnar claw hand' of an ulnar nerve lesion. There is wasting of the small muscles of the hypothenar eminence, with loss of sensation of the palmar and dorsal aspects of the little finger and of the ulnar half of the ring finger. In a median nerve lesion the thenar eminence (abductor pollicis brevis) will be flattened (Fig. 11.1) and sensory impairment will be found on the palmar surfaces of the thumb, index, middle and radial half of the ring fingers.

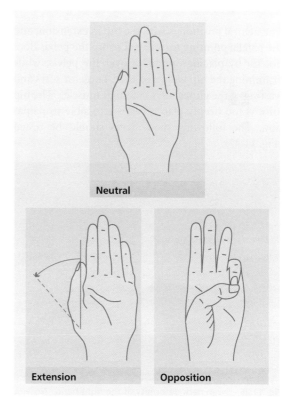

Fig. 11.24 Movements of the thumb.

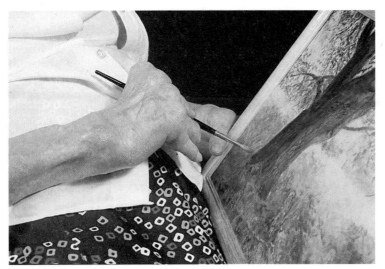

Fig. 11.25 Functional ability. Severe joint deformity due to psoriatic arthropathy, but retention of artistic ability.

ASSESSMENT OF HAND FUNCTION

Assessment of hand function (Fig. 11.25) should include testing hand grip and pinch grip (between index and thumb). The latter may be decreased in lesions in the line of action of the thumb metacarpal, particularly scaphoid fractures.

The hip

The neutral position is with the hip in extension, and the patella pointing forwards. Ensure the pelvis does not tilt by placing one hand over the pelvis, while examining the hip with the other. Look for scars and wasting of the gluteal and the thigh muscles. The hip joint is too deeply placed to be accessible to palpation. The following movements should be tested (Fig. 11.27).

- Flexion: measured with knee bent. Opposite thigh must remain in neutral position. Flex the knee as the hip flexes
- Abduction: measured from a line which forms an angle of 90 degrees with a line joining the anterior superior iliac spines
- Adduction (measured in the same manner)
- Rotation in flexion
- Rotation in extension
- Extension: attempt to extend the hip with the patient lying in the lateral position.

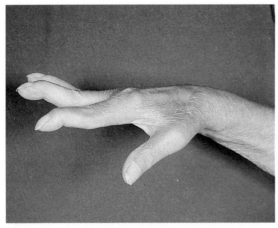

Fig. 11.26 Swan neck deformity of the right hand. Note also wasting of the small muscles of the hand due to disuse in this case of rheumatoid arthritis.

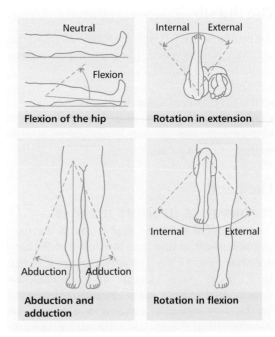

Fig. 11.27 Movements of the hip.

(a)

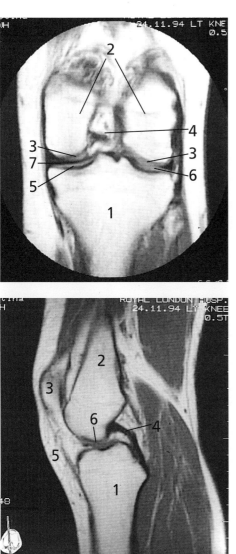

(b)

(c)

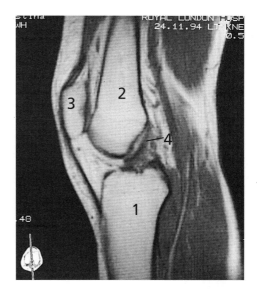

Fig. 11.28 CT scans of the normal knee (MR image, T_1 weighted). (a) Scan to show the medial (5) and lateral (6) menisci, origin of the anterior cruciate ligament (4) and the articular cartilages (3) and synovial fluid (7). Other structures: (1) tibia, (2) articular surfaces of femur. (M) medial, (L) lateral. (b) The anterior cruciate ligament (4). Other structures: (1) tibia, (2) femur, (3) patella, (5) patellar tendon (6) joint space. (c) The posterior cruciate ligament (4). Other structures: (1) tibia, (2) femur, (3) patella.

ADDITIONAL EXAMINATION OF THE HIP JOINT

• Test for *flexion deformity*. With one hand flat between the lumbar spine and the couch, flex the normal hip fully to the point of abolishing the lumbar lordosis. The spine will come down on to the hand, pressing it on to the couch. If there is a flexion deformity on the opposite side, the leg on that side will move into a flexed position.

• *Trendelenburg test*. Observe the patient from behind and ask him or her to stand on one leg. In health, the pelvis tilts upwards on the side with the leg raised. When the weight-bearing hip is abnormal, from pain or subluxation, or when there is muscular weakness on that side, the pelvis sags downwards.

• *Measurement of 'true' and 'apparent' shortening.*

The length of the legs is measured from the anterior superior iliac spine to the medial malleolus on the same side. Any difference is termed '*true*' shortening and may result either from disease of the hip joint or neck of the femur on the shorter side. '*Apparent*' shortening is due to tilting of the pelvis and can be measured by comparing the lengths of the two legs, measured from the umbilicus, provided that there is no true shortening of one leg. Apparent shortening is usually due to an abduction deformity of the hip.

The knee

A CT scan of the normal knee is illustrated in Fig. 11.28. The neutral position is complete extension. Observe any *valgus* (lateral angulation of the tibia) or

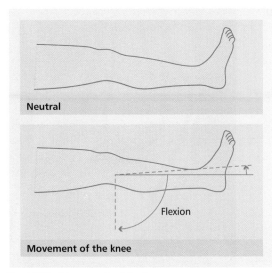

Fig. 11.29 Movements of the knee.

varus (medial angulation) deformity on the couch and on standing. Look for muscle wasting. The quadriceps, especially its medial part near the knee, rapidly wastes in disease of the knee joint. Swelling may be obvious, particularly if it distends the supra-patellar pouch. Check the apparent height of the patella and watch to see if it deviates to one side in flexion or extension of the knee. Feel for tenderness at the joint margins, not forgetting the patello-femoral joint. Palpate the ligaments, remembering that the medial collateral ligament is attached 8 cm below the joint line. Measure the girth of the thigh muscles 10 cm above the upper pole of the patella.

JOINT SWELLING

The presence of swelling in the knee joint may be confirmed by the *patellar tap test* or, for small effusions, by the *bulge test* in which the medial parapatellar fossa is emptied by pressure of the flat of the hand sweeping proximally. It is seen to refill (the bulge) as the supra-patellar area is emptied by pressure from the flat hand. Posterior knee joint cysts, particularly in rheumatoid arthritis, may be palpable in the popliteal fossa and they sometimes rupture, producing calf pain (see below). They may therefore mimic a deep vein thrombosis. When intact, posterior knee cysts can sometimes cause venous obstruction.

The movements of the knee are flexion and extension (Fig. 11.29). Loss of flexion can be documented by loss of the angle of flexion or loss of heel-to-buttock distance in the crouch position, or on the couch. Loss of extension is detected by inability to get the back of the knee on to the flat examining

couch. Hyperextension must be sought by lifting the foot with the knee extended and comparing with the normal side. Lack of full extension by comparison with the normal constitutes fixed flexion deformity. Loose bodies in the joint cause crepitus, interruption of movement (locking) and pain and effusion (Fig. 11.30).

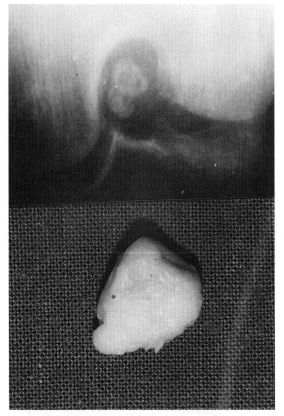

Fig. 11.30 Loose body in tunnel view X-ray of knee, showing the loose body in the intercondylar space.

TESTING FOR STABILITY

Test the stability of the joint by stressing the medial and lateral ligaments, first with the knee in full extension (abnormal motion is due to lax posterior structures), and then in 20 degrees of flexion. Abnormal motion in flexion is due to laxity of the collateral ligaments. With the knee flexed and the foot fixed on the couch by seating your buttock lightly against the patient's toes, check that the hamstrings are relaxed and then try to pull the tibia forward towards you. Abnormal anterior translation implies damage to the anterior cruciate ligament, provided it can be shown that the tibia has not already fallen backwards due to a torn posterior cruciate ligament. Look across both knees similarly flexed to exclude this.

The ankle

The neutral position is with the outer border of the foot at an angle of 90 degrees with the leg, and midway between inversion and eversion. Observe the patient from behind in the standing position. There will be a loss of calf muscle bulk with any longstanding ankle disorder.

Look at the position of the foot with the patient standing. The heel may tilt outwards (*valgus deformity*) in subtalar joint damage. *Varus* (inward) *deformity* is much less common and usually not so painful. Flattening of the longitudinal arch of the foot also produces valgus at the heel but the foot curves laterally as well because the change is in the midtarsal joints in addition to the subtalar joint.

The following movements should be tested (Fig. 11.31).

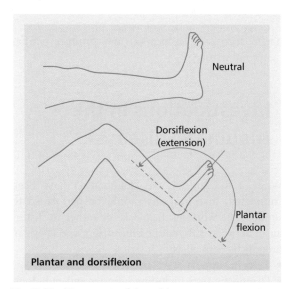

Plantar and dorsiflexion

Fig. 11.31   Movements of the ankle.

• Dorsiflexion: test with the knee in flexion and extension to exclude tight calf muscles
• Plantar flexion: place a finger on the head of the talus to be sure that it is moving. A hypermobile subtalar joint can mimic movement in an arthrodesed ankle.

The foot

Remember that complaints apparently relating to the foot may be features of systemic disease such as gout, or of referred vertebral problems such as a prolapsed intervertebral disc. Look for abnormalities of posture.

Callosities are areas of hard skin under points of abnormal pressure. The most common site is beneath the metatarsal heads because loss of the normal soft tissue pad allows abnormal loads. There may be abnormal spread of two adjacent toes (daylight sign, Fig. 11.32) on weight-bearing if there is a bursa between the metatarsal heads. Check for lateral deviation of the big toe (*hallux valgus*) usually associated with abnormal swelling at its base (*a bunion*). There may be deformities affecting any or all toes with abnormal curvature (*claw toes*), fixed flexion of the terminal joint (*hammer toes*) or over-riding.

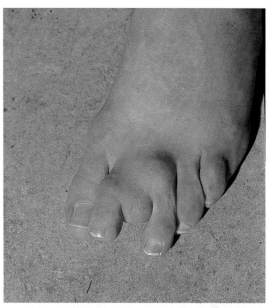

Fig. 11.32   Interphalangeal bursa of left foot. Daylight sign, due to an enlarged bursa, is usually a herald of rheumatoid arthritis.

The following movements should be tested (Fig. 11.33).
• Subtalar inversion and eversion: cup the heel in the hands and move it in relation to the tibia without any up and down movement; this eliminates movement at the ankle or midtarsal joints
• Midtarsal inversion/eversion and adduction/abduction: hold the os calcis in the neutral position in one hand and grasp the forefoot in the other
• Metatarsophalangeal and interphalangeal flexion/extension.
Also look for tenderness at the Achilles tendon insertion on the back of the calcaneum and for plantar tenderness at the site of the plantar fascial insertion. Inflammation of these attachments (*enthesopathy*) is common in ankylosing spondylitis and Reiter's syndrome.

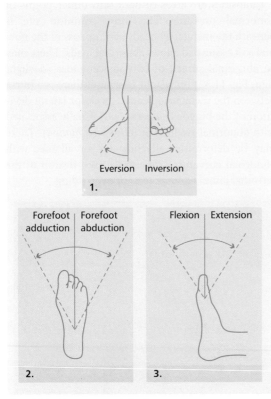

Fig. 11.33   Movements of the foot.

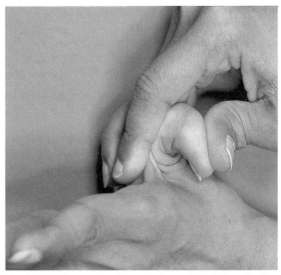

Fig. 11.34   Hyperextensibility of the digits in Ehlers–Danlos syndrome.

The gait

It is best to study gait with the legs and feet fully exposed, and *without* shoes or slippers. Ask the patient to walk away from you, to turn around at a given point and then to walk towards you.

Abnormalities of gait are usually due either to joint problems in the legs or to neurological disorder, although alcohol or drug intoxication, hysteria or malingering may occasionally cause difficulty. A full examination of the legs and feet should reveal any local cause, which may range from a painful corn to osteoarthritis of the hip. Abnormalities due to neurological disorders are described in Chapter 12.

Hypermobility

There is a wide variation in the range of normal joint movement, associated with age, sex and race. Excessive laxity or hypermobility of joints (Fig. 11.34) can be defined in about 10% of healthy subjects and is frequently familial. It is also a feature of two inherited connective tissue disorders—Marfan's syndrome and Ehlers–Danlos syndrome. Repeated trauma,

haemarthrosis or dislocation may produce permanent joint damage.

Investigations in the rheumatic diseases

When a full history and examination have been completed, investigations should be performed to support the working diagnosis, or rather to distinguish between different possible diagnoses. They can broadly be defined as:

• Tests in support of inflammatory disease
• Diagnostic tests including biopsies and radiological investigations.

Tests in support of inflammatory disease

The following acute phase reactant tests are used in the assessment of inflammatory disease activity and in the subsequent monitoring of the patient.

Erythrocyte sedimentation rate (ESR). This is a demanding test in terms of technician time, and is non-specific, as it has poor sensitivity, being affected by the levels of haemoglobin, globulins and fibrinogen. Higher mean values are also seen in elderly patients. Automated centrifuged ESR is much quicker than manual ESR.

C-reactive protein (CRP). This is a more specific indicator of inflammation.

Plasma viscosity. This is much quicker than ESR and a more specific measure of the acute phase response.

Serum complement. Low levels of serum complement reflect activation due to immune complex deposition; this may be a marker of disease activity in autoimmune diseases, such as systemic lupus erythematosus (SLE).

Diagnostic tests

Diagnostic tests differentiate between specific diseases and are relatively specific investigations.

TESTS FOR RHEUMATOID FACTOR

Rheumatoid factors are autoantibodies in the form of immunoglobulin (Ig) directed against other IgG (immunoglobulin G) molecules. IgM rheumatoid factor can be detected by its ability to clump polystyrene particles coated with human IgG (*latex test*). This test is positive in about 80% of patients with rheumatoid arthritis. Results are reported as a titre: 1 in 80 or greater being a positive result. The *Rose–Waaler haemagglutination* test uses sheep erythrocytes coated with rabbit IgG to detect IgM (titres of 1 in 32 or more are positive), but is currently being replaced by other tests. ELISA (enzyme-linked immunosorbent serum assay) techniques are much more sensitive, but produce positive results in many other conditions. Other rheumatoid factors in the IgG or IgA classes can also be detected in the sera of patients with rheumatoid arthritis, but are mainly used in research.

These rheumatoid factor screening tests are useful where a diagnosis of rheumatoid arthritis is suspected, but they are not specific. Rheumatoid factor is frequently found in patients with other connective tissue diseases, for example, systemic lupus erythematosus (SLE), and Sjögren's disease, or other inflammatory disorders, such as, subacute bacterial endocarditis and some viral infections.

ANTINUCLEAR ANTIBODY TESTS

Antinuclear antibody (ANA), often referred to as antinuclear factor (ANF), is a very useful screening test for SLE as it is positive in up to 90% of cases. It is, however, a non-specific test, being positive in many other connective tissue disorders, including about 20% of patients with rheumatoid arthritis. A positive test in children with arthritis may be associ-ated with chronic iridocyclitis, which is frequently asymptomatic. Slit-lamp examination of the eye is mandatory to confirm the diagnosis.

The ANA test is carried out by incubating the patient's serum with frozen sections of normal tissue (usually rat liver). After washing, a fluorescent anti-serum to human IgG is used to detect human antibody adhering to the nuclear antigens. A titre of 1 in 40 or more is significant; adequate standardization is important.

DNA-BINDING TEST

This is a radioisotope immunochemical technique used to detect antibodies to native, double-stranded DNA. The test is usually reserved for patients with a positive ANA test. It is the most specific test for SLE. Occasionally it is positive in patients in whom the clinical suspicion of SLE is very high, but the ANA test is negative.

ANTIBODY TESTS TO EXTRACTABLE NUCLEAR ANTIGENS (ENA)

These tests may be suggested by a particular type of pattern of staining (*speckled*) in the routine ANA test. They can be summarized in terms of their clinical association as follows.

• *Anti-SM* (non-nucleic acid protein), in some cases of SLE.

• *Anti-RNP* (ribonucleoprotein) picks out a group of patients who often have a mixed picture of connective tissue disorder and are therefore often diagnosed as MCTD (*mixed connective tissue disease*). The test can be considered a marker for the combination of clinical features, but the major clinical component of the condition will define management.

• *Anticentromere antibody* is found in 'CREST syndrome' (calcinosis, Raynaud's phenomenon, oesophageal symptoms, sclerodactyly and telangiectasis) and some cases of scleroderma.

Other antibodies used in diagnostic tests include the following.

• *Antineutrophil cytoplasmic antibody* is a marker for vasculitic conditions, especially Wegener's granulomatosis.

• *Antiphospholipid antibodies* in high titre may be associated with a syndrome characterized by thromboses (including cerebral infarction), thrombocytopenia and, in women, recurrent abortion (*antiphospholipid syndrome*). This antibody may be associated with SLE and called *anticardiolipin antibody* or *lupus anticoagulant*, despite the association with thromboses. A false positive VDRL may also be found in these patients.

- *Human leucocyte antigen (HLA) typing:* there is a strong association of the tissue antigen HLA-B27 with ankylosing spondylitis, but it is of limited diagnostic value. Although about 95% of ankylosing spondylitis patients in the UK possess the B27 antigen, it is also found in 8% of the normal population. Ankylosing spondylitis therefore remains a clinical diagnosis, supported by typical X-ray findings. HLA-B27 typing is, however, of some value in the differential diagnosis of seronegative (latex negative) peripheral arthritis, particularly in children.
- *Antistreptolysin-O (ASO) test:* the presence in the serum of this antibody in a titre greater than 1/200, rising on repeat testing after about two weeks, indicates a recent haemolytic streptococcal infection.

URIC ACID

A consistently normal plasma uric acid level (<375 μmol/litre in women, <425 μmol/litre in men) effectively excludes the diagnosis of untreated gout. Raised levels occur in many circumstances and do not establish in themselves the diagnosis of gout (see below). On a low purine diet, the 24-hour urinary urate excretion should not exceed 600 mg. Higher levels indicate 'overproduction' of urate and a risk of renal stone formation.

SYNOVIAL FLUID EXAMINATION

Synovial fluid may be obtained for examination from any joint in which it is clinically detectable. The knee is the most convenient source: after infiltration with a 1% local anaesthetic, a 21-gauge needle is inserted into the joint on its medial aspect between the patella and the femoral condyle. The aspirated fluid should be placed in a plain sterile container; if a cell count is required, some of the fluid should be mixed with ethylenediaminetetraacetic acid (EDTA) anticoagulant.

An injured joint can also be aspirated (Box 11.9). The swollen joint after injury may reveal clear pink fluid suggesting a *meniscal lesion*, or show frank blood. The latter is usually indicative of a *torn*

BOX 11.9 Findings in synovial fluid after aspiration of the knee joint.

- Cloudy fluid or pus: bacterial infection (see text)
- Urate or pyrophosphate crystals: gout or pseudo-gout
- Pink fluid: torn meniscus
- Blood: trauma, haemophilia, villonodular synovitis

(a)

(b)

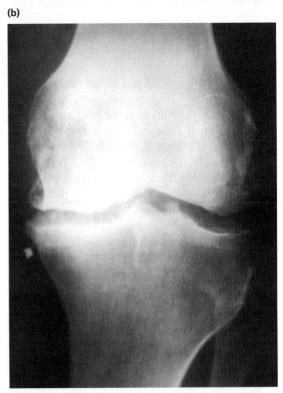

Fig. 11.35 Left and right knee joints. The X-rays show a normal joint (a) and osteoarthritic change (b), on the opposite side. Note the increased bone density and narrowing of the joint space.

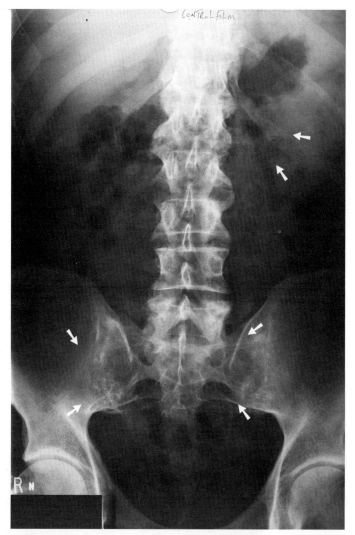

CoNTRoL FILM

Fig. 11.36 X-ray of lumbosacral spine and upper pelvis. There is fusion of several vertebrae, and of the sacroiliac joints (arrows) from ankylosing spondylitis. The renal papillae on the left are calcified, evidence of previous papillary necrosis from analgesic abuse.

anterior cruciate ligament. If blood is aspirated look at its surface for globules of fat. This is derived from the marrow and confirms an intra-articular fracture. Synovial fluid examination is diagnostic in two conditions—*bacterial infections* and *crystal synovitis*—and every effort should be made to obtain fluid when either of these is suspected. Polarized light microscopy can differentiate between the crystals of urate in gout and those of calcium pyrophosphate dihydrate in pseudo-gout. Outside these conditions, synovial fluid examination is unlikely to be diagnostic. Frank blood may point to trauma, haemophilia or villonodular synovitis, while inflammatory (as opposed to degenerative) arthritis is suggested by opaque fluid of low viscosity, with a total white cell count >1000 cells/μl, neutrophils >50%, protein content >35 g/litre, and the presence of a firm clot. Culture of this fluid may produce a bacterial growth,

usually of staphylococci, but occasionally *Mycobacterium tuberculosis* or other organisms.

Biopsies useful in differential diagnosis

The following biopsies may be useful in differential diagnosis of rheumatic diseases.

Synovial biopsy is of little value in the differential diagnosis of inflammatory polyarthritis, but should be considered in any unusual monoarthritis to exclude infection, particularly tuberculous, or rare conditions such as sarcoid or amyloid arthropathy.

Rectal biopsy can be useful in the diagnosis of amyloidosis secondary to chronic inflammatory disease, but renal biopsy may still be necessary if the cause of renal impairment is not clear. Vasculitis may also be confirmed on rectal biopsy but, in

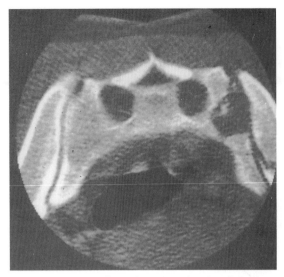

Fig. 11.37 CT scan of sacroiliac joints, showing distinctive lesion on the left side, with a sequestrum due to tuberculosis.

general, tissues found to be abnormal on clinical examination or by further investigation, e.g. skin, muscle, sural nerve or liver, should be considered first for diagnostic biopsy in undifferentiated systemic vasculitis.

Biopsy of the lip may be useful to confirm Sjögren's syndrome.

Temporal artery biopsy is often diagnostic in patients with polymyalgia rheumatica. If there are any clinical features of temporal (giant cell) endarteritis, this is the investigation of choice.

Radiological examination

Only X-rays likely to yield specific information should be ordered. However, in unilateral joint disease it is best to X-ray both sides for comparison (Fig. 11.35a and b). In patients with inflammatory polyarthritis three routine films are helpful in the diagnosis and assessment of progression: both *hands and wrists* on one plate, both *feet* on another, to compare bone density and to look for periosteal reaction or erosive change, and one of the full *pelvis* (Fig. 11.36), to show the sacroiliac and hip joints.

X-Rays taken to confirm or exclude a fracture must be taken in two planes. It is essential that either the whole limb is turned or the X-ray equipment rotated. The limb must not be twisted at the fracture site. When looking for a fracture in a bone, run a pen tip or its equivalent around the cortex of the bone as seen on the film (without leaving marks). Any break in continuity will reveal itself; do not confuse an epiphysis with a fracture. Note soft tissue swelling and distension of joints.

ARTHROGRAPHY

Injection of contrast medium into the knee joint can be used to confirm the diagnosis of a ruptured popliteal cyst. A double-contrast technique is useful

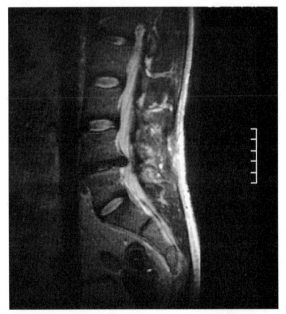

Fig. 11.38 There is a disc protrusion at L4–5, with degeneration of the disc itself, shown by the less bright signal in the intervertebral disc at this level.

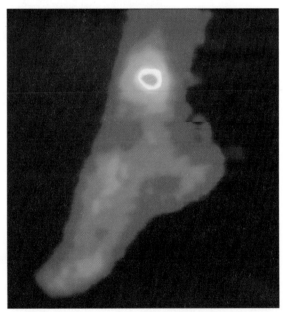

Fig. 11.39 Technetium bone scan in a distance runner, showing focally increased uptake in the lower tibia owing to a stress fracture .

in demonstrating abnormalities of the menisci in the knee (see Fig. 11.28).

SPECIALIZED RADIOLOGY

The following modern imaging techniques can provide precise information about localized pathology but are dependent on the clinician making a clear diagnostic request.

Higher resolution ultrasound is of value in defining soft tissue structures, including muscles and tendons and provides an excellent means for guiding aspiration and biopsy procedures.

Computed tomography (CT). The combination of superior tissue contrast and tomographic technique permits definition of soft tissue structures obscured by overlapping structures, including the intervertebral disc, and other joints normally difficult to visualize, such as sacroiliac (Fig. 11.37), sternoclavicular and subtalar.

MRI provides unique advantages in evaluation of the musculoskeletal system, but it is vital that the clinician defines the pathology suspected, as correct positioning and sequence selection (T weighting) are vital in optimizing image quality. It is of particular value in the non-invasive investigation of disc disease (Fig. 11.38), including spinal infection, and is generally felt to be the most sensitive technique for diagnosis of avascular necrosis. Enhancement by the use of intravenous paramagnetic contrast (e.g. gadolinium) has further improved definition in spinal imaging. MRI is increasingly used in imaging of major joints in the limbs, especially the knee (Fig. 11.28), hip, shoulder and elbow.

Isotopic scanning (scintigraphy) can be used in the diagnosis of acute (e.g. infection or stress fracture) or multiple (e.g. metastases) bone lesions by use of the first 2-minute (dynamic blood flow) phase, second 10-minute (blood pool) and third 3-hour late phase (osteoblastic) (Fig. 11.39) following intravenous injection of diphosphonate compounds. Tomographic scintigraphy can further refine definition of the isotope uptake, e.g. in stress fracture of the pars interarticularis.

CHAPTER 12

The nervous system

Introduction

The aim of the neurological assessment is to delineate the patient's illness in both functional and anatomical terms. A detailed and complete neuro- logical examination is an ordeal for ill patients and a test of concentration and co-operation for those in good general health. Over-long examination may defeat its own ends, especially when sensation is investigated, by leading to variable and incongruous findings. The examination should therefore be planned in relation to the problem posed by the information acquired from the patient's history.

In neurological disorders the history is especially important because it gives information about the course of the disorder. This historical information may in itself be diagnostic, as in the description of attacks of altered function or consciousness in epilepsy, episodes of sudden onset in vascular disease, and of symptoms consistent with disease in multiple sites at different times in multiple sclerosis. The inevitable progression of degenerative disease, and of neoplasms, is also characteristic. The neurological examination in such cases should be planned with the aims of confirming the extent of the disabilities described by the patient, and of assessing the presence or absence of any factors considered to be relevant in the context of the diagnosis suggested by the history. Thus, neck rigidity in a patient with headache and fever is consistent with meningitis, and an extensor plantar response in a patient complaining of a previous episode of hemiparesis is consistent with cerebral infarction.

An abbreviated scheme of examination is often used when screening for occult neurological disease in routine physical examinations (see p. 335) but a careful history is more likely to yield this information.

The order of examination outlined in this chapter should not be adhered to rigidly. For example, if a patient is complaining of sciatic pain, it is appropriate to begin with the examination of the lower limbs and lumbar spine. Observation of the patient's ordinary activity, for example the way they walk into the room and undress for examination, is often helpful in deciding how to begin. Always ask a patient examined in bed to undertake as much activity as possible; it is particularly important to see the patient trying to stand and walk, even if this seems difficult.

Basic concepts

The neurologist looks for patterns of functional abnormality (Box 12.1). These represent features consistent either with *lesions in neuronal systems*, including nuclei and their interconnecting pathways, or with *disease syndromes*. Lower or upper motor neurone syndromes, patterns of sensory disorder or visual dysfunction, are examples of the *negative* expression of dysfunction resulting from lesions in the nervous system.

> **BOX 12.1 Main clinical features of motor disorders.**
>
> **Lower motor neurone syndrome**
> - Weakness
> - Decreased muscle tone
> - Absent tendon reflexes
> - Muscle wasting, often severe
> - Fasciculation in affected muscles
> - Distribution of weakness and wasting consistent with lesion in spinal segments, nerve root or peripheral nerve
>
> **Upper motor neurone syndrome**
> - Weakness in corticospinal distribution, shoulder abduction and finger movements, hip flexion and toe dorsiflexion
> - Spastic increase in muscle tone
> - Increased tendon reflexes
> - Extensor plantar response
> - Little or no atrophy
>
> **Dystonia and extrapyramidal disorders**
> - Plastic or spastic increase in muscle tone
> - Abnormal postures
> - Involuntary movements and tremors
> - Normal or increased tendon reflexes
> - Plantar responses normal or extensor

Positive aspects of these syndromes also develop, for example, seizures in disease of the cerebral cortex, and involuntary movements or tremor in disease of the basal ganglia. This approach is summarized in this section.

The motor system

THE LOWER MOTOR NEURONES

Muscular movement depends ultimately on the integrity of the lower motor neurones. The lower motor neurones consist of the anterior horn cells or homologous cells in the brainstem, their efferent nerve fibres, which pass via the anterior spinal nerve root and peripheral nerves to the muscles, and the muscle fibres innervated by these nerve fibres and their terminal axonal branches.

If the final common pathway is interrupted at any point, *weakness, fasciculation, muscle wasting, loss of tendon reflexes* and *hypotonia* occur. These are the cardinal signs of a *lower motor neurone lesion* (Box 12.1).

Although various reflexes operate at a spinal level, the initiation of voluntary movements and the maintenance of posture and muscle tone depends on neural activity in higher centres, especially the cortex, extrapyramidal system and the cerebellum. These patterns of activity can only reach the muscles if the final common pathway in the lower motor neurone is intact.

THE CORTICOSPINAL SYSTEM

The corticospinal (pyramidal) system consists of the central pathways which directly link the pyramidal cells in the fifth layer of the motor cortex with the motor neurones in the brainstem and spinal cord. The corticospinal tracts contain these fibres and also fibres which arise from the post-central cortex and from subcortical structures. The motor area of the cortex occupies the anterior aspect of the central sulcus (Rolandic fissure) and the adjacent parts of the precentral gyrus. There is localization of function in the motor cortex, with different parts of the opposite side of the body being separately represented. Those parts of the body which carry out the most skilled movements, for example the fingers and thumb, have the largest areas of cortical representation. The areas for tongue, jaw and facial movements lie in the inferior part of the motor cortex, those for the arm, trunk and leg are arranged in sequence in the motor area, which extends to the vertex and on to the medial surface of the cerebral hemisphere (Fig. 12.1).

The fibres of the corticospinal tracts descend from their cells of origin in the motor cortex into the internal capsule, occupying the anterior two-thirds of the posterior limb. Here the order of representation of the body is face, shoulder, elbow, hand, trunk and lower limb from before backwards. The corticospinal fibres then descend through the middle three-fifths of the cerebral peduncles in the midbrain. In the pons, the tract becomes broken into scattered bundles by the transverse pontine fibres and nuclei pontis. In the upper part of the medulla the corticospinal fibres occupy the pyramids, which consist of protuberances on the anterior aspect of the brainstem. In the lower part of the medulla the majority of the corticospinal fibres decussate with those of the opposite side and pass posteriorly into the spinal cord to form the crossed lateral corticospinal tracts. A smaller number of fibres do not decussate, but continue downwards in the anterior columns as the direct corticospinal tracts, which decussate at segmental levels in the anterior commissure. The corticospinal fibres terminate in the grey matter of the brainstem motor nuclei and in the anterior horns of the spinal cord.

The upper motor neurone lesion

The corticospinal system is concerned with the initiation of voluntary and skilled motor acts, particularly of

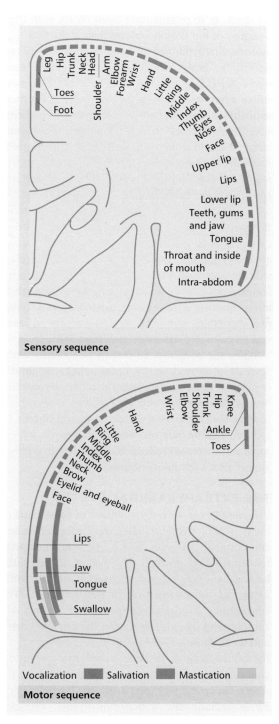

Fig. 12.1 Rasmussen and Penfield's diagram of localization in the sensory (top) and motor (bottom) cortex.

fine distal movements. The syndrome resulting from lesions affecting corticospinal fibres *alone* consists initially of weakness of the contralateral side of the body. Rapid improvement usually occurs, resulting in residual impairment of fine and rapid distal movements of the digits, as in picking up a small object, with mild weakness of hip flexion and shoulder abduction. The more familiar syndrome of widespread paralysis of one side of the body (*hemiplegia*) or of a single limb (*monoplegia*) is usually the result of a more extensive lesion affecting extrapyramidal or other subcortical structures in addition to the corticospinal fibres themselves. Even in cases of dense hemiplegia, movements of the head and trunk (axial movements) are virtually uninvolved. The pathways for such postural movements are predominantly under subcortical control and are represented bilaterally.

In clinical practice, most lesions of the corticospinal system also damage neighbouring extrapyramidal nuclei and pathways. All such cases are loosely grouped as *corticospinal lesions*. The classical signs of such a lesion (an *upper motor neurone lesion*, Box 12.1) are *weakness*, which predominantly affects fine, distal movements, hip flexion and shoulder abduction, *spasticity, increased tendon reflexes*, and an *extensor plantar response* (page 316).

When the corticospinal system is suddenly damaged or destroyed, as by haemorrhage or injury, there is a temporary depressant effect on the anterior horn cells (neuronal shock). Paralysis is accompanied at first by loss of muscle tone and absent or reduced tendon reflexes. The characteristic hypertonia and increased reflexes of a corticospinal lesion appear after a few hours or days.

THE EXTRAPYRAMIDAL SYSTEM

The *extrapyramidal* system consists of those parts of the nervous system, excluding the motor cortex and corticospinal pathways, which are concerned with movement and posture. The system includes the basal ganglia, the subthalamic nuclei; the substantia nigra and other structures in the brainstem. The connections of these extrapyramidal centres are complex and include fibres from the cerebral cortex and the thalamus. There are no direct pathways from the basal ganglia to the spinal cord; extrapyramidal connections with the lower motor neurones are indirect, via several pathways arising in the brainstem. These include the dentatorubrospinal, reticulospinal, vestibulospinal and olivospinal tracts.

The extrapyramidal system is important in the control of posture and in the initiation of movement, especially those movements which affect postural mechanisms, such as sitting, standing, turning over in the lying position, walking and running. Complex volitional movements, such as reaching for an object, require both postural adjustments and fine distal movements, which are under corticospinal control.

Extrapyramidal lesion

Diseases affecting the extrapyramidal system (Box 12.1) are characterized by difficulty in initiating voluntary movement, by impairment of orienting and balancing reflexes, by alterations in muscle tone and by the appearance of involuntary movements. Strength is usually unaffected.

THE CEREBELLUM

The cerebellum receives afferent fibres from the spinal cord, vestibular system, basal ganglia and cerebral cortex. It modulates movement mainly through its connections, via the thalamus, with the basal ganglia and cerebral cortex.

Cerebellar lesions

Lesions of the cerebellum cause incoordination (*ataxia*). Muscle tone may be reduced. Lesions of the cerebellar vermis cause a characteristic ataxia of the trunk, so that the patient has difficulty sitting up or standing. In such patients there may be little or no incoordination of the limbs. Paralysis is not a feature of cerebellar disease. Tendon reflexes are not increased.

The sensory system

Sensory input reaches the nervous system
- from specialized receptors and free nerve endings in the skin and superficial tissues;
- from other receptors, such as muscle spindles, Golgi tendon organs, pacinian corpuscles and free nerve endings in muscles;
- from other specialized receptors in the joints.

Sensory information from internal organs and viscera enters the nervous system via autonomic afferent systems. All afferent fibres enter the central nervous system through the posterior root ganglia and the posterior roots. Disease of these 'first sensory neurones' may thus affect all modalities of sensation. It must be remembered, however, that much sensory input is concerned with the reflex control of posture and movement and, as such, does not reach consciousness or is not consciously perceived. For example, the conscious recognition of posture and position of a limb (*kinaesthesia*) is dependent on input from cutaneous and joint receptors and especially from muscle spindles. However, the major role of muscle spindles and tendon organs is in the control of voluntary and reflex movements. Spindle and

Golgi afferents travel rostrally in the ventral and dorsal spinocerebellar tracts to enter the cerebellum, and cerebral hemispheres.

CUTANEOUS SENSATION

After they have entered the spinal cord, the various cutaneous sensory fibres are ordered, and grouped for projection rostrally to the brain. There are two groups of sensory nerve fibres. One group of fibres projects to cells in the posterior horn of the grey matter at or near the level at which they enter. Second sensory neurone fibres arise from these cells in the posterior horn. Some of these cross immediately, or within a few segments, to the opposite lateral and anterior columns of the cord and so ascend to the brainstem as the *anterior*

and *lateral spinothalamic tracts.* Impulses from which the sensations of pain and temperature are derived ascend in the lateral spinothalamic tract. The fibres from the lower part of the body are arranged in the lateral portion of this pathway, and those from the upper parts of the body more medially.

Other afferent fibres do not synapse in the grey matter of the posterior horns of the spinal cord, but ascend in the ipsilateral posterior columns: these posterior column fibres carry impulses which determine the appreciation of position, movement, size, shape, discrimination and texture, and vibration (which should be regarded only as touch rapidly applied). The medial of the two posterior columns, the *fasciculus gracilis*, contains fibres originating in the lower part of the body, whereas the lateral, the *fasciculus cuneatus*, carries fibres predominantly from the upper limbs. The somatotopic lamination of fibres in the posterior columns, which are uncrossed, is thus the converse of that in the lateral spinothalamic tracts, which are crossed.

At any level of the spinal cord, therefore, there are two major groups of sensory fibres conveying sensory information towards the brain: one in the anterolateral columns carrying pain and temperature from the opposite half of the body, and a second in the posterior columns, conveying the appreciation of posture, weight, size, shape and other qualities of sensation from the same side of the body. A unilateral lesion of the spinal cord, therefore, results in loss of pain and thermal sensibility below the level of the lesion on the opposite side of the body, while on the side of the lesion there is, in addition to spastic paralysis, disturbance of

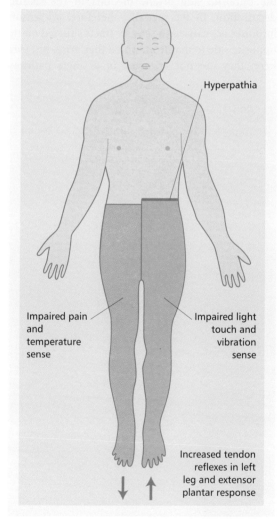

Fig. 12.2   Brown-Séquard syndrome (see Box 12.2). Note the distribution of corticospinal, posterior column and lateral spinothalamic tract signs. The cord lesion is on the left side.

> ### BOX 12.2 Clinical features of the Brown–Séquard syndrome
> This is a clinical syndrome usually due to extrinsic compression of the cord, but it may also arise with intrinsic cord lesions (see Fig. 12.2).
>
> **Below the level of the lesion**
>
> ***Features ipsilateral to the lesion***
> - Impaired light touch
> - Impaired vibration sense
> - Corticospinal tract signs
>
> ***Features contralateral to the lesion***
> - Impaired pain sensation
> - Impaired temperature sensation
>
> **At the level of the lesion**
>
> ***Features ipsilateral to the lesion***
> - Segmental zone of hyperpathia (and spontaneous pain), representing irritation of the compressed segment
> - Sometimes lower motor neurone signs at this level (e.g. in arm)

BOX 12.3 Features of progressive intrinsic and extrinsic spinal cord disease, in their order of development.

This sequence is particularly characteristic of tumours arising within the spinal cord, or compressing it from without.

Intrinsic disease
- Urge incontinence/retention of urine
- Dissociated sensory loss
- Spinothalamic pain
- Bilateral corticospinal tract signs
- Paraplegia and sensory level

Extrinsic disease
- Root pain, worsened by movement
- Progressive asymmetrical paraparesis
- Brown–Séquard syndrome
- Paraplegia with sensory level
- Incontinence/retention of urine and faeces

the sense of position and of movement and loss of recognition of weight, size, shape, touch and vibration. This group of clinical signs is called the *Brown–Séquard syndrome* (see Fig. 12.2 and Box 12.2).

In progressive spinal cord disease a characteristic sequence of clinical events occurs during the course of the untreated illness. The early involvement of sphincter function seen in intrinsic cord syndromes develops because these nerve fibres are situated deeply in the white matter, deep to the corticospinal fibres. Conversely, these fibres are involved relatively late in cord compression (Box 12.3). The sequence of clinical events resulting from intrinsic spinal cord disease, e.g. syringomyelia, is different from that occurring in progressive extrinsic cord disease, e.g. compression of the cord by tumour.

In the upper part of the spinal cord the posterior column fibres terminate in the gracile and cuneate nuclei. The fibres of the second sensory neurone originate in these nuclei and immediately cross to the opposite side of the medulla in the sensory decussation. In the medulla, therefore, *all* sensory impulses are carried in sensory tracts situated on the opposite side to that from which they arise. But even here, they are not arranged in a single pathway:

		Cervical			Dorsal
	5	6	7	8	1
Shoulder Supraspinatus					
Teres minor					
Deltoid					
Infraspinatus					
Subscapularis					
Teres major					
Arm Biceps					
Triceps					
Brachio-radialis					
Supinator					
Extensor carpi radial.					
Pronator teres					
Flexor carpi radial.					
Flexor pollic. long					
Abduct. poll. long.					
Extens. poll. brev.					
Extens. poll. long.					
Extens. digitor.					
Extens. indicis.					
Extens. carpi. uln.					
Extens. digitor. min.					
Flexor digitor. sublimis					
Flexor digitor. profund.					
Forearm Pronator quadratus					
Flex. carpi. uln.					
Palmaris long.					
Abductor poll. brev.					
Flexor poll. brev.					
Opponens poll.					
Flexor digit. min.					
Opponens digit. min.					
Adduct. poll.					
Palmaris brev.					
Abductor digit. min.					
Hand Lumbricales					
Interossei					

Table 12.1 Segmental innervation of the muscles of the upper limbs.

Table 12.1

spinothalamic fibres pass through the lateral part of the medulla, while the posterior columns enter the medial lemniscus. Higher in the brainstem the two sensory pathways are joined by the second sensory neurone fibres from cranial nerve nuclei. The fibres of the medial lemniscus and spinothalamic tract synapse in the thalamus. From this level a third system of sensory fibres conveys sensory input through the internal capsule to the cerebral cortex.

The anatomy and physiology of the sensory system is complex. This complexity is not relevant to ordinary clinical diagnosis, but it is important in understanding certain pain syndromes in patients with lesions in the sensory pathways. The two major pathways themselves are not modality-specific, in the sense that certain fibres 'carry' vibration sense or other forms of sensation; but rather the interaction of different patterns of impulses in different-sized fibres of differing conduction velocity determines the sensation perceived at the highest levels of the nervous system. The importance of spinal mechanisms in the dorsal horn in the control of the flow of afferent information has been emphasized in the 'gate control' theory of sensation. This concept has emphasized, furthermore, the pre-eminent role of the dorsal columns in exploratory, movement-directed behaviour, rather than in the passive reception of sensory input, and the importance of small thinly myelinated or unmyelinated fibres in the generation of the sensation of pain.

The spinal cord

The spinal cord extends from the foramen magnum caudally to the interspace between the 12th thoracic and 1st lumbar spines; the thecal membranes continue down as far as the body of the second sacral vertebra. The cervical enlargement reaches to the 7th cervical spine. Its largest part is at the level of the 5th cervical vertebra. The lumbar segments lie opposite the 10th and 11th thoracic spines and the next interspinous space.

The spinal segments do not correspond exactly with the vertebrae overlying them. This is important in assessing patients with spinal cord compression due to vertebral disease. To determine which spinal

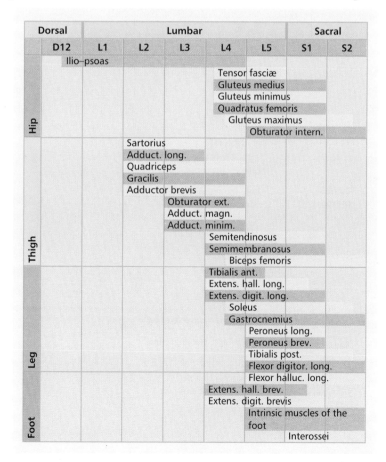

Table 12.2 Segmental innervation of the muscles of the lower limbs.

Table 12.2

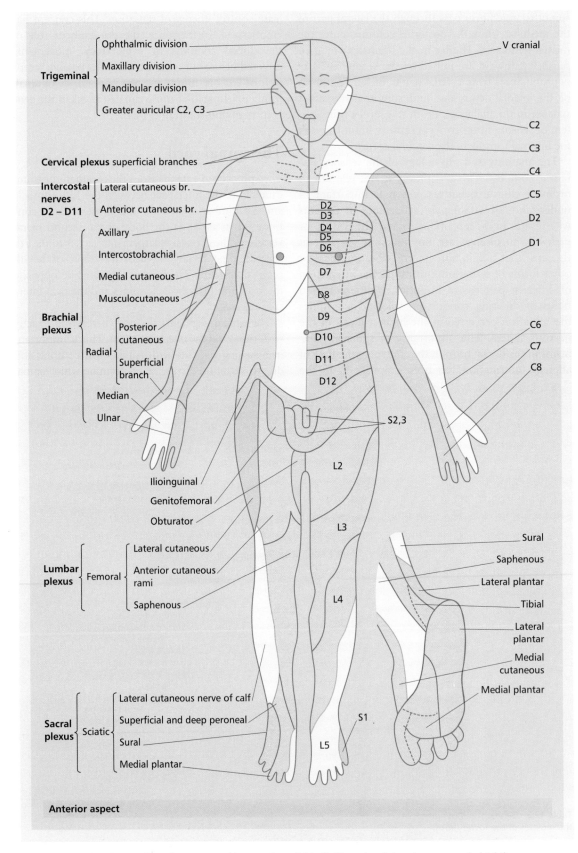

Fig. 12.3   Anterior view to show the segmental innervation of skin (left), and peripheral nerve supply (right).

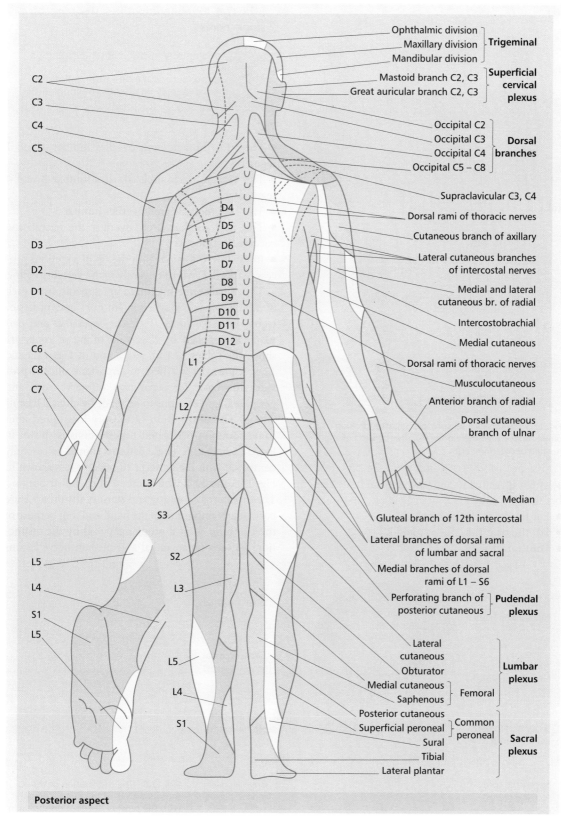

Posterior aspect

Fig. 12.4 Posterior view to show the segmental innervation of skin (left), and peripheral nerve supply (right).

(a)

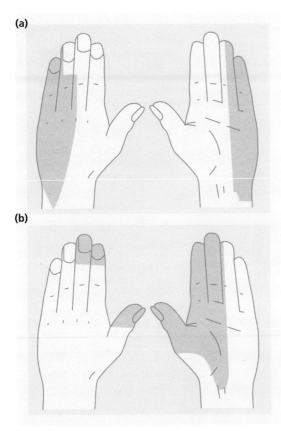

(b)

Fig. 12.5 Cutaneous sensory loss: (a) after division of the ulnar nerve above the elbow; (b) after division of the median nerve in the arm.

segment is related to a given vertebral body remember that:

- For the cervical vertebrae,   add 1
- For thoracic 1–6,   add 2
- For thoracic 7–9,   add 3

BOX 12.4 Mononeuropathies; disorders of single nerves.

- Motor and sensory involvement in distribution of affected nerve
- Acute mononeuropathies are often painful
- Multiple nerves may be affected (mononeuritis multiplex)

- The 10th thoracic arch overlies lumbar 1 and 2 segments
- The 11th thoracic arch overlies lumbar 3 and 4 segments
- The 12th thoracic arch overlies lumbar 5
- The first lumbar arch overlies the sacral and coccygeal segments
- In the lower dorsal region the tip of a spinous process marks the level of the body of the vertebra below.

The spinal cord is organized in segments, from each of which a pair of anterior (motor) and posterior (sensory) nerve roots arise. The *myotomes* and *dermatomes* supplied by the pairs of nerve roots are shown in Tables 12.1 and 12.2 and in Figs 12.3 and 12.4. Knowledge of these is important since it provides the basis for separation of nerve root and peripheral nerve lesions to be made by clinical examination. The distribution of sensory loss found after some common peripheral nerve lesions is shown in Figs 12.5 and 12.6. These patterns should be carefully compared with the patterns of sensory loss shown in Figs 12.3 and 12.4, which represent root distributions. These patterns of motor and sensory disturbance are particularly important in the hand and foot because of the common clinical problems posed by the distinction between ulnar, radial and median nerve lesions

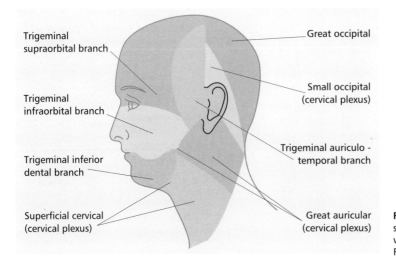

Fig. 12.6 The distribution of the sensory nerves of the head. Compare with the sensory distribution shown in Figs 12.3 and 12.4.

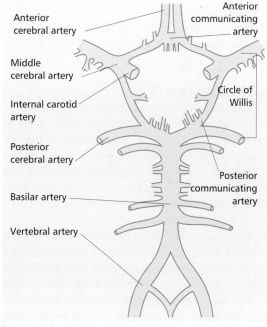

Fig. 12.7 The blood supply to the brain and the circle of Willis.

and lower cervical root problems, and between lumbosacral root disease and common peroneal nerve palsies. The clinical features of mononeuropathies are listed in Box 12.4, and the common causes of brachial plexus lesions in Box 12.5.

Note that C8 and C6 sensory loss extends to the elbow on both ventral and dorsal surfaces of the forearm, but that median nerve sensory loss predominantly affects the palmar surface of the hand. In both ulnar and median nerve lesions sensory loss extends no further proximally than the wrist.

On the body itself there is a line of demarcation between the T2 and C4 segments at the clavicle. The level of the nipple represents T6, the xiphisternum T8, the umbilicus T10 and the inguinal ligament T12. The deltoid area represents C5. The patella and anteromedial shin represent L4. Sensory impairment in an L5/S1 distribution closely resembles that found in a common peroneal nerve lesion, except that the medial borders of the forefoot and large toe are involved in the former but not in the latter.

Vascular supply of the brain and spinal cord

The brain is supplied by the internal carotid and vertebral arteries (Fig. 12.7). Embolic lesions are more frequent in the left than in the right cerebral hemisphere.

The two *vertebral arteries* unite at the lower border of the pons to form the basilar artery, which runs up the anterior surface of the pons in the midline, before dividing into the two posterior cerebral arteries. It gives off paramedian and short and long circumferential branches, which supply the pons and parts of the midbrain and cerebellum.

The *posterior cerebral artery* supplies the occipital lobe, the lower part of the temporal lobe and the uncus, the inner part of the crus and the corpora quadrigemina, and the posterior part of the posterior limb of the internal capsule. Occlusion of this artery at its origin will therefore usually involve the

visual cortex and the sensory fibres but sometimes the calcarine branch, and hence the visual cortex, is affected in isolation.

The *internal carotid artery* gives off the *anterior cerebral artery*, which curves round the anterior end of the corpus callosum, and supplies the inner surface of the cerebral hemisphere as far back as the parieto-occipital fissure. It also supplies the superior frontal gyrus, and gives a branch to the anterior part of the internal capsule and to the basal ganglia.

The *middle cerebral artery*, which lies in the Sylvian fissure, is the main branch of the internal carotid artery. Embolism from the internal carotid artery or from the heart, therefore, often involves the middle cerebral artery. The middle cerebral artery gives off *cortical branches*, which supply the frontal lobes, including the motor cortex, and the superior parts of the parietal and temporal lobes. These branches anastomose freely with those of the adjoining anterior cerebral and posterior cerebral arteries so that occlusion of one of them may sometimes be largely compensated by the establishment of a collateral circulation. The middle cerebral artery also gives off *central branches*, which penetrate into the brain substance and supply the white matter and the basal ganglia. There are two chief groups of these central arteries: an anterior group called the *lenticulostriate*, and a posterior group, the *lenticulo-optic*. The lenticulostriate arteries are particularly associated with hypertensive cerebral haemorrhage. These central arteries also anastomose with one another.

Venous blood leaves the brain in the *venous sinuses*. Blood from the interior of the brain enters the cerebral veins, which end in the straight sinus.

SPINAL ARTERIES

The *anterior* and *posterior spinal arteries* arise from the vertebral arteries and travel caudally in the pia mater, the former in the anteromedian fissure and the two latter alongside the posterior nerve roots. These long vessels receive radicular tributaries from the intercostal and lumbar arteries at each spinal level. In the lumbar region one of these is particularly prominent; this artery of Adamkiewicz is an important tributary. The anterior spinal artery supplies most of the spinal cord; only the posterior parts of the posterior horns and posterior columns are supplied by the posterior spinal arteries. Both anterior and posterior spinal arteries function as anastomotic vessels linking the radicular feeding vessels. Flow does not, therefore, occur in any one direction in these vessels but varies, or may even reverse, in response to local factors such as changes in posture and variations in intra-abdominal and intrathoracic pressure. There are two zones of *watershed flow* in the cord, one in the upper thoracic cord between flow descending from the vertebral circulation and flow derived from thoracic radicular feeding vessels, and another in the lower thoracic region between descending flow derived from thoracic feeding vessels and ascending flow from the artery of Adamkiewicz. These are sites of predilection for infarction of the spinal cord in, for example, aortic dissection.

SPINAL VEINS

The main veins of the spinal cord are situated dorsally and ventrally in the midline. Like the arteries, they communicate by radicular branches with the lumbar and intercostal veins, and empty into the vertebral veins. The blood in them flows upwards; hence in compression of the spinal cord, e.g. by tumour, there is venous engorgement below the level of compression. This may be seen during myelography or magnetic resonance imaging of the spinal cord.

Mental functions

The neurologist is especially interested in the mental state in relation to features suggestive of organic disease of the brain. None the less, the neurological approach to the mental state examination is similar to that taken by the psychiatrist, although with a difference in emphasis that reflects the different symptom complexes of organic and functional brain syndromes.

It is important to analyse the patient's mental state early in the examination, even if the analysis is limited to a subjective assessment of personality, memory, education and abstractional ability formed during the process of history-taking, since this assessment is helpful in the subsequent investigation of symptoms. For example, if the patient's memory is impaired, the patient's description of the illness is necessarily limited. If the patient is comatose, confused, or unable to understand speech, any attempt to investigate sensory functions is likely to be frustrated. If, for any reason, the patient's own history is incomplete, it is essential to obtain a history from relatives or friends. As always in neurology, the history is of cardinal importance. Rapid bedside protocols for mental state testing which can be scored and used to quantify roughly the deficit are available (see Tables 2.1 and 2.2).

Appearance, behaviour and communication

The patient's bearing or actions when lying in bed are important. Note whether there is any disturbance of consciousness, such as confusion, stupor or coma.

• Is the patient unduly disturbed or apathetic, or in a state of agitation or confusion?

• Is attention easily held, or fleeting?

• Does the patient show a reasonable degree of interest in their surroundings?

• What reaction is there to your approach and greeting?

• Is the patient well-groomed or unkempt?

• What is the condition of the hair and hands?

• Any other unusual features in the behaviour (e.g. facial tics or any inappropriate behaviour) should be noted.

Note whether conversation flows easily or not.

• Is the patient silent, monosyllabic or over-talkative?

• Is the content of speech and conversation appropriate and consistent?

• Is there looseness of association?

• Are there features of *flight of ideas* (a rushing stream of ideas with some connection) or *thought disorder*, when one remark follows another without logical connection (see Chapter 2)?

• Does the patient keep on repeating your questions or their own remarks (*perseveration*)?

In patients with a disorder of language (*aphasia*) strange words (*neologisms*) may be used or real words strung together oddly (*word salad*).

Emotional state

It is important to evaluate the patient's mood.

• Is the patient apparently happier than is appropriate (*elation or euphoria*) or filled with despair or dismay (*depression*)?

• Is there a general impression of happiness, distress or depression?

• Does the conversation lead you to feel that there is flattening of emotion, e.g. family or financial success is described without pleasure or in an incongruous manner, as in laughter after relating a misfortune or breaking into tears when given some pleasant news?

• Does the patient enjoy life or, conversely, feel that nothing is worthwhile?

• Does the patient feel fed up with life, even perhaps to the extent that there is a risk of suicide?

• Does the play of facial features suggest preoccupation with a private world?

• Is the patient perplexed at their own mental state?

• Is there insight and understanding of the disorder and its implications?

Find out whether persons or things seem as real as they should, or whether they seem changed in some mysterious way (*depersonalization*). It is, however, unwise to ask leading questions about depersonalization, as anxious patients will often respond affirmatively. Note whether the patient seems irritable or resentful, or whether your words are received with suspicion.

Ask about the patient's sleep.

• Is sleep too long or too brief?

• If too long, is any particular action likely to precipitate this *hypersomnia*?

• If too little, is the difficulty in getting to sleep, waking frequently, or waking early in the morning and being unable to go to sleep again?

Where there is no physical cause for the insomnia, such as pain, cough, asthma or the wearing of an uncomfortable splint or bandage, the insomnia is likely to be due to psychological disorder, e.g. the restlessness of mania, the early waking of depression or, most commonly, the turmoil of the mind found in anxiety states.

Ask about dreams. These are frequent and sleep-disturbing in anxiety states, whether the source of the anxiety is apparent or not. In these conditions, sleep is not refreshing and the patient may complain of waking as tired in the morning as when going to bed at night.

Delusions and hallucinations

Delusions are false beliefs which continue to be held despite evidence to the contrary (page 39). *Hallucinations* are false impressions referred to the special senses (hearing, seeing, smelling, etc.) for which no cause can be found and which the patient knows to be imagined or unreal events (page 41). Hallucinatory experiences are often not volunteered and should be enquired for in patients suspected of suffering degenerative or paroxysmal disorders of the brain.

Hallucinations of taste and smell are especially characteristic of *temporal lobe epilepsy* (*partial seizures*), and may be accompanied by a stereotyped visual hallucination of a half-remembered, unidentified scene perhaps experienced many years previously. Voices may be heard as part of this temporal lobe seizure.

Hallucinations of small animals or insects crawling through the room, or on the walls or bed, are particularly associated with *delirium tremens* during withdrawal from alcohol. They are often accompanied by terror.

In *migraine*, an evolving scintillating patch (*scotoma*) in the visual field, with a hard ragged edge, often precedes the development of headache. In occipital lesions, complex visual hallucinations may occur (page 289).

Orientation in place and time

In order to assess a patient's ability to recognize place or time, the following questions can be asked.

• Does the patient recognize their own surroundings, and know where they are, or are they muddled?

• If he or she offers an inaccurate answer, is this part of *confabulation*, a filling in of forgotten memories by inappropriately recalled material from previous experiences?

• Is the date known approximately, if not correctly?

• Can the patient estimate the approximate time without looking at a watch or clock?

• Is there clear understanding of the reason for, or context of, your consultation?

It is useful to carefully note down the patient's answers to these points.

Clouding of consciousness

States of clouded or altered consciousness are important. They must be described and defined, particularly in patients with head injury or raised intracranial pressure who may gradually deteriorate during a period of clinical observation.

Coma is a state in which the patient makes no psychologically meaningful response to external stimulus or to inner need. In *stupor* the patient, although inaccessible, does show some response, for instance to painful stimuli. Above these levels various degrees of altered consciousness and lethargy can be recognized, which may be accompanied by confusion (see below). The examiner must be alert to observe any minor defects in the patient's capacity to grasp what is required of them and what has happened to them. Such defects will usually be manifest in the responses to tests for orientation, recent memory and appreciation of environment. The assessment of coma and altered consciousness is described in Chapter 13.

CONFUSIONAL STATES

In *dementia* (Box 12.6) the patient is confused in time, place and person, and shows impaired abstractional abilities, but is awake and alert; in *delirium* the patient is similarly confused, but also shows impaired alertness, i.e. is drowsy. Thus, the demented patient may or may not also be delirious, and delirium can occur as an acute abnormality, without underlying dementia.

BOX 12.6 Clinical features of dementia.

Frontal lobe features
- Impaired judgement
- Altered, blunted personality
- Loss of emotional control
- Loss of mental inhibition
- Failure to plan ahead
- Impairment of language production

Temporal lobe features
- Loss of memory for recent events
- Impaired immediate recall
- Language disorder (Wernicke type aphasia)
- Formed visual or auditory hallucinosis

Parietal lobe features
- Impaired sensory integration
- Disorientation in visual space
- Impaired visual recognition
- Receptive aphasia
- Disturbed body image

In the past the term 'dementia' was used to imply an irreversible or progressive brain disorder and, generally, it is still used mainly in this context, although certain causes of dementia are reversible. For example, dementia associated with a frontal lobe tumour may improve after removal of the tumour. Both these abnormal mental states are sometimes termed *organic confusional states* (see Chapter 2). Simple rating scales for assessment of mental state are available for bedside use (see Chapter 2).

MEMORY

Memory consists of the ability to grasp and retain new information. Memory therefore requires adequate processing of input, followed by registration and then appropriate recall. Memory is modality-specific, i.e. can be related to auditory, visual, sensory or olfactory stimuli, or may be related to abstract or internalized experience, e.g. imagined material.

The degree to which *recent memory* is lost is an index of the severity of organic brain disorder (not necessarily permanent). Inquire about the day of the week and of the month and the names of prominent public figures. Ask the patient to recall information recently read in the paper or seen on television. In formulating questions on these lines, attention should be paid to the patient's educational background and their likely personal interests. Bring up a subject discussed a few minutes previously, or give the patient a simple story or address to remember, and note how much is remembered after a short interval or after distraction. *Short-term memory* is memory for events of a few seconds or minutes past. It is characteristically impaired in Wernicke–Korsakoff syndrome, and in many patients with Alzheimer-type dementia. It is usually tested by assessing whether the patient can repeat seven digits backwards, with or without distraction, and by asking the patient to spell 'world' backwards. Working memory, consisting of memory for tasks involving mental manipulations, such as remembering a telephone number while dialling it, is usually spared in patients with disturbances of recent memory, for example in Wernicke–Korsakoff syndrome. *Long-term memory* is relatively resistant to the effects of neurological or psychiatric disease.

Intelligence

It is always necessary to ascertain the patient's general intellectual ability since this is important in assessing the specific effects of brain injury or disease. The educational level reached before leaving school, employment and the work record give a rough-and-ready approximation. Frequent changes of job may indicate mental defect or personality disorder. Frequent changes after an accident or a serious illness in patients with a previously good work record are suggestive of brain damage.

Tests of memory as given above will indicate more serious, specific defects and these can be further explored by tests of *reasoning*, particularly where the tests show that the patient is unable to monitor or correct mental performance. Ask the patient to subtract sevens from 100 (i.e. 100, 93, 86, 79 ...), or to reverse in the mind's eye the hands of a clock. The absurdities test (e.g. 'What would be wrong if I told you I had three brothers, John, Fred and myself?') indicates grosser disability. People of relatively low intelligence can often give the months of the year parrot-fashion but not which month precedes May and which October, etc.

Tests in which the patient is asked the meaning of rare words or to interpret common proverbs or sayings are commonly used as an index of *abstractional abilities*. *Judgement* may similarly be assessed: 'What would you do if you saw a house on fire?' or 'What would you do if you found a stamped addressed envelope lying in the road?' In dementia these questions often provoke *concrete* answers or a confused reply. *Constructional* and *drawing* tests may also be useful. These are described briefly on page 326.

Released reflexes in dementia and confusional states

In the demented patient and in other organic confusional states, certain reflexes, released from the control of higher centres, may be elicited. Some may also be found in patients with large focal lesions; for example, the grasp reflex is characteristically released in patients with contralateral frontal lobe disease. In infancy the presence or absence of these reflexes is used as part of the developmental assessment (page 377). The most important of these higher level reflexes are the *grasping* and *avoiding responses*, the *palmomental reflex*, the *glabellar tap reflex*, and released oral responses such as the *snout response* and tactilely and visually evoked *sucking reflexes*.

Grasping and avoiding responses
Grasping is elicited by stroking the palmar surface of the patient's hand on its radial aspect, preferably using a firm, distally moving stimulus between the patient's thumb and forefinger. The patient's hand grasps the examiner's. This grasp is not easily inhibited even if the patient is distracted, for example, by being asked their address. If traction is applied by lightly pulling against the patient's flexed fingers, the patient tends to oppose with an equivalent force. Grasping is typically associated with contralateral frontal lobe disease.

The *avoiding response* consists of a tendency for the patient's hand to move away from palmar or dorsal contact. It is usually evoked by stimuli on the ulnar side of the hand. It is released in patients with contralateral parietal lobe disease, or lesions in its connections.

The palmomental reflex
This consists of a brief contraction of the ipsilateral mentalis muscle, causing puckering of the chin, in response to scratching the skin near the thenar eminence with a key or pin.

Glabellar tap reflex
A series of sharp finger taps to the glabella normally elicits only two or three blinks before this response is inhibited, but in patients with diffuse degenerative disorders, especially senile dementia, and also in Parkinson's disease, the response is disinhibited and a blink follows each of a rapid train of stimuli.

Snout reflex
Gentle pressure of the examiner's knuckle against the patient's lips causes reflex puckering of the orbiculus oris. This is usually associated with similar contraction of the facial musculature evoked by very light taps to the lips with a tendon hammer or with the fingers.

Sucking reflexes
Anticipatory opening of the mouth as part of released sucking may be elicited by approaching visual stimuli, e.g. the shining metal end of a tuning fork, or by light contact with the cheeks near the corners of the mouth.

Speech and language

In considering speech disorders, it is essential to distinguish between defects of articulation and enunciation of speech, called *dysarthria*, and disturbances of the structure and organization of language itself, *aphasia*.

Dysarthria

Defective *articulation* of speech may seem difficult to distinguish from regional or foreign speech accents but, with practice, this distinction can usually be made quite reliably. Certain constant features of different types of dysarthria can be identified. *Stammering* is a developmental disorder, more common in boys than girls. It is only very rarely due to organic brain disease. In lalling, or 'baby speech', all the difficult consonants are dropped; the patient speaks like a baby. In adults this is usually the result of congenital or infantile deafness. Speech is usually louder than normal in this disorder.

There are four main types of dysarthria: cerebellar, pseudobulbar, bulbar and cortical dysarthria.

Cerebellar dysarthria

The patient speaks slowly and deliberately, syllable-by-syllable, as if scanning a line of poetry. The normal prosodic rhythm of syllable, word and sentence production is lost and in extreme forms each syllable is given equal emphasis. Ask the patient to say 'artillery': it will be pronounced 'ar-til-ler-y'. This scanning or staccato disturbance of speech rhythm is the classical form of severe cerebellar dysarthria. It is important to recognize minor, less obvious forms since its presence indicates bilateral disease of the cerebellum or of its brainstem connections.

Pseudobulbar (spastic) dysarthria

Individual syllables are slurred, and the precision of consonant pronunciation is lost, as in alcoholic intoxication. Thus 'British Constitution' becomes 'Brizh Conshishushon'. This form of dysarthria is due to bilateral lesions in the corticospinal fibres supplying the muscles of the face, larynx, tongue and respiration, i.e. the lesion is *supranuclear* to, or above the level of, these brainstem nuclei. It is therefore a feature of *pseudobulbar palsy*: the jaw jerk is brisk and, in most patients, examination of the limbs reveals evidence of bilateral corticospinal tract lesions, e.g. bilateral extensor plantar responses. *Dysphagia* may be a prominent associated feature, with particular difficulty in swallowing liquids, including saliva.

Sometimes a patient with a profound pseudobulbar palsy may be unable to make a sound, although comprehension is normal. This is called *aphonia*. In hysterical aphonia phonation occurs during spontaneous or voluntary coughing, but in pseudobulbar aphonia coughing is silent.

Bulbar dysarthria

Bulbar palsy, due to lower motor neurone lesions affecting the speech musculature, results in non-specific slurring of speech. This is usually readily separated from other forms of dysarthria. There are usually other features of bulbar palsy, particularly *dysphagia*; fluids tend to be regurgitated through the nose and solid foods are difficult to swallow. Palatal air escape may be audible during phonation.

Cortical dysarthria

This irregular hesitancy in word production, associated with difficulties in abstract, volitional movements of the lips and tongue (*orofacial apraxia*), is commonly associated with aphasia due to left frontal and temporal lesions. It never occurs as an isolated abnormality and the term 'cortical dysarthria' should therefore be used with caution.

Formal tests for dysarthria

Nonsense syllables that test the lips and jaw, e.g. 'papapapa' and 'tatatata', the tip of the tongue 'sasasa' and the body of the tongue 'kakaka' are useful. They can be combined into repetitive tasks as 'patakapataka' and 'fasaxafasaxa' to evaluate rhythm and prosody more objectively. The repetition rate is slowed in patients with dysarthria of any cause.

Aphasia

The word 'aphasia' means a disturbance of the ability to use language, whether in speaking, writing or comprehending. There are several different classifications of aphasia, but, in practice, these are largely of theoretical interest. In assessing an aphasic patient it is important to relate the functional defect in language to the patient's disability as a whole: how does it affect him or her? Formal analysis of the aphasia can then be attempted, and this will enable accurate localization of the lesion to be achieved (Fig. 12.8).

It is especially important to recognize aphasia, even when it is only a very slight deficit, because it implies disease in restricted parts of the dominant hemisphere, almost always the left. A common error is to fail to recognize the language disorder in a patient with fluent aphasia and so to diagnose erroneously a confusional state, which implies diffuse rather than focal brain disease.

Everyday use of language includes the following.
• The ability to *use words* in spoken speech. This includes *articulation*, *fluency* (the ability to put words together into phrases and sentences of varying

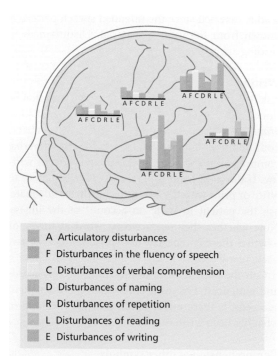

A Articulatory disturbances
F Disturbances in the fluency of speech
C Disturbances of verbal comprehension
D Disturbances of naming
R Disturbances of repetition
L Disturbances of reading
E Disturbances of writing

Fig. 12.8 The average degree of disturbance of various language modalities which occurs when there is an isolated lesion of various lobes (frontal, Rolandic, parietal, temporal and occipital).

complexity, in various grammatical constructions, without hesitations and errors), *naming* and the accurate *repetition* of complex statements and concepts.

• The ability to *comprehend* spoken speech.
• The ability to *read* to oneself (not aloud).
• The ability to *write*.
• The ability to comprehend *other symbols*, e.g. mathematical or musical symbols.

Speech defects can be analysed, therefore, as disturbances of *articulation, fluency, verbal comprehension, naming, repetition, reading and writing*. If a rough score is given to each of these categories (Fig. 12.8), a broad analysis of speech function which has some localizing value can be built up. For example, disturbances of fluency, verbal comprehension, repetition and writing are all prominent in left anterior temporal lobe lesions (amnestic or Wernicke's aphasia). Left frontal lesions affect articulation and fluency more than the other categories of language. Left parieto-occipital lesions impair reading (visual language functions); left parietal lesions impair several other associative functions, but particularly writing. Generally, the lateralization of speech corresponds to handedness, but most left-handed people have left hemisphere dominance rather than right.

Assessment of articulation and fluency, on the one hand, and reading and writing, on the other, enables recognition of lesions in front of and behind the central sulcus (Rolandic fissure). This is a useful clinical concept which may be referred to as the '*anterior*' and '*posterior*' *aphasic syndromes*. The terms '*expressive*' and '*receptive*' *aphasia* are more or less synonymous but they ignore the equally important functions of reading, writing, repetition, articulation and fluency. In the examination of an aphasic patient, spoken and written speech should be assessed separately.

ASSESSMENT OF SPOKEN SPEECH

First be sure whether the patient's hearing is adequate. Begin by assessing speech in the context of an ordinary conversation about everyday things or about the patient's illness itself. Note the presence of hesitations, the searching for a forgotten word, and its compensation by the use of a descriptive phrase (*paraphasia*), *neologisms* (invented or nonsense words), or inappropriately used words or phrases. Note also any articulatory disturbances, particularly clumsiness and difficulty in co-ordinating movements of lips and tongue (*orofacial apraxia*). Orofacial apraxia is a *bilateral* disturbance of these movements that can occur with *unilateral*, left frontal lesions. It is usually very pronounced when the patient is asked to put out their tongue or close their eyes and these movements should not, therefore, be used to establish comprehension of speech or the patient's co-operation. Disturbances of fluency are best addressed in spontaneous conversational speech.

The aphasic patient can often use only a few words. These should be noted, as should words or phrases repeated again and again (*perseveration* or *repetitive utterances*).

If the patient has a considerable vocabulary, first make a note of any examples of slurring etc., as an indication of disturbed *articulation*. Test speech articulation with such words and phrases as 'British Constitution', 'West Register Street', 'biblical criticism', 'artillery'. Then show him common objects—a knife, a pen, a matchbox, etc.—and ask him to *name* them. Sometimes patients with aphasia have a general idea of the word they want to use, but forget exactly how to pronounce it; they may omit some syllables or substitute others for them, so that the listener can hardly make out the word intended. These are signs of *amnestic* or *nominal* aphasia.

In anterior aphasias the patient will often be aware of errors, although unable to correct them. Mistakes in the use of words, e.g. calling a knife a pen, are examples of *word substitution,* a more marked abnormality than *syllabic substitution.* Patients with left posterior lesions, whether in addition to a frontal lesion or occurring alone, show defective ability to monitor their own speech. Their speech not only shows syllabic and word substitutions but it may contain *neologisms.* In extreme examples of this disorder, characteristic of left posterior temporal lesions, speech consists of syllabic neologisms, making no sense at all—*jargon aphasia.* Patients with jargon aphasia tend to talk incessantly, often in relation to inappropriate sounds in their environment, for example, in response to a voice on the radio or in another part of the room. Thus patients with left frontal lesions speak hesitantly, with poor fluency, and those with left temporoparietal lesions speak fluently, but their speech is often devoid of meaning. A further point of difference between these two types of speech defect is that patients with more posteriorly placed lesions show marked difficulties in comprehension of spoken speech. Indeed, this is a marked feature of patients with *fluent aphasia,* since it is an underlying defect in the adequate monitoring of these patients' own spoken speech.

Speech repetition is a useful test. Patients with left frontal lesions can repeat words and simple phrases, although they may introduce syllabic or other errors, but those with more posterior lesions may be unable even to approach the task. The patient should be asked to repeat a simple sentence, clearly stated by the examiner, such as 'Today is Wednesday June 4th, and this is The Royal London Hospital'. Remember never to shout at an aphasic patient: hearing is normal. If the patient is able to repeat what you say, endeavour to find out whether or not what you have said has been heard and understood. Finally, ask the patient to read aloud, note whether they can find their way about the page, and if speech errors appear.

ASSESSMENT OF WRITTEN LANGUAGE
Reading and writing tests are important in the assessment of aphasia.

Reading
Reading aloud tests the visual comprehension of language and spoken speech. Reading silently tests comprehension of language through the visual system; this is best tested by asking the patient to obey simple written commands without reading aloud, e.g. 'Touch your nose with your left hand'. When the patient reads aloud, errors in spoken speech can be readily detected since the intended speech pattern is known from the written material. Disturbances of reading are called *dyslexia.*

Writing
Ask the patient to write their name; this can often be done when the ability to write is otherwise lost (*dysgraphia*). Ask some simple question, such as 'What is your address?' and ask for a written reply. If verbal comprehension is poor, put your question in writing. If the right hand is paralysed, ask the patient to write or print with the left. If the writing is adequate, ask the patient to write an account of the illness. Note whether they use a wrong word at times, or whether there is repeated use (*perseveration*) of any particular word.

Can the patient write to dictation or copy words and sentences? Try, using a newspaper. If the patient succeeds, is there understanding of the meaning of what has been written?

Comprehension of other symbols
Write down some simple calculations, such as:

$$\begin{array}{ccc} 2 & 2 & 2 \\ +2 & +2 & +2 \\ \hline 4 & 5 & 6 \end{array}$$

and ask the patient to point out which is correct. Inability to understand and manipulate mathematical symbols, termed *acalculia,* may occur in posterior parietal lesions affecting the dominant hemisphere.

GESTURE
Many aphasic patients make attempts to use gesture to communicate, but gestural language may be impaired in patients with anterior lesions. Furthermore, many aphasic patients, especially those with Wernicke's (temporal) aphasia, or with posterior fluent aphasias, do not fully understand complex gestural instructions.

Apraxia

The term 'apraxia' is used to describe inability to perform certain acts or movements, even though there is no sensory defect or weakness, or ataxia, and their component movements can be performed easily. Consequently, the apraxic patient is unable to make use of objects, though their use can be recognized and described. Apraxia results from damage to the left parietal cortex or to parietal white matter of the left or of both hemispheres, or from disease of the connections between the two hemispheres through the corpus callosum. When the corpus callosum is damaged, apraxia may affect only the left side, since the dominant left hemisphere is then disconnected from the right hemisphere, but it is more commonly a bilateral disorder.

Apraxia can be formally tested for by asking the patient to use objects or to make or imitate certain movements. For instance, when given a box of matches and asked to strike a match the apractic patient may fail to open the box, or to take a match from it, or to strike the match, or may show an inability to recognize which end to strike against the box. It is, of course, important to be sure that the patient understands the request.

The cranial nerves

Examination of the functions of the cranial nerves is an important part of the clinical assessment. The third to twelfth cranial nerves arise from the brainstem and innervate facial, cranial and cervical tissues. The first and second cranial nerves actually consist of central nervous tissue rather than peripheral nerve. All the cranial nerves may be involved in disease processes in their intracranial and extracranial courses, and at their sites of origin within the brain and brainstem.

The olfactory (first) nerve
ANATOMY
The central processes of the bipolar sensory cells in the olfactory epithelium pass through the cribriform plate to the olfactory bulb, where the cells of the second olfactory neurones lie. Nerve fibres project to the olfactory area of the cerebral cortex: the uncus and the parahippocampal gyrus.

TESTING SMELL
Have three small bottles containing pungent odours, such as oil of cloves, oil of peppermint, or tincture of asafoetida. Common bedside substances such as soap, fruit or scent may also be used. Present these to each nostril separately and ask the patient to name them. Avoid the use of irritating substances such as ammonia, for these partially stimulate the trigeminal nerve. In *anosmia* the sense of smell is absent. Before concluding that this is due to neurological disease exclude local changes in the nose itself, e.g. catarrh. *Parosmia* is a rare abnormality of olfaction in which, for instance, pleasant odours seem offensive.

Inquire also regarding *hallucinations of smell*. These sometimes constitute the aura of an epileptic fit, originating in the temporal lobe.

The optic (second) nerve
ANATOMY
From the retina, the fibres of the optic nerve (Figs 12.9 and 12.10) pass back to the optic chiasm. Here

Fig. 12.9 Computerized tomographic (CT) scan of the head in a normal subject. This CT image is oriented in the plane of the orbits. Both eyes are visible. In the right eye the lens appears as a relatively high-attenuation zone. In the orbits the medial and lateral rectus muscle and the optic nerves can be seen forming a cone with its apex at the posterior margin of the orbits. The temporal lobes are situated on either side of the pituitary fossa and optic chiasm. The two orbits are separated by the nose and ethmoid sinuses.

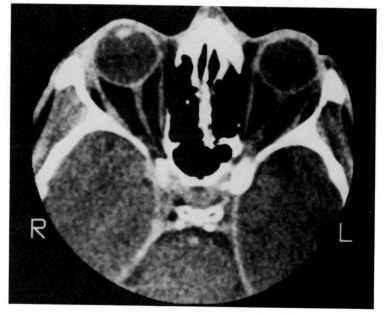

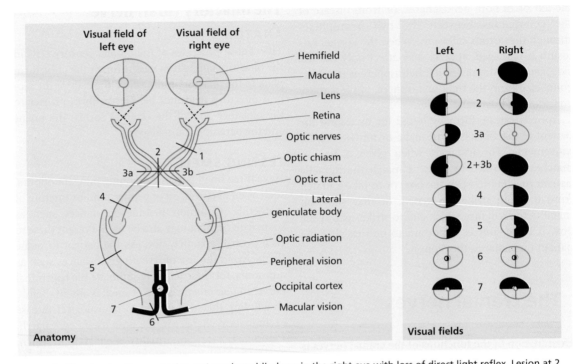

Fig. 12.10 The visual pathways. Lesion at 1 produces blindness in the right eye with loss of direct light reflex. Lesion at 2 produces bitemporal hemianopia often beginning in the central fields as a bitemporal scotomatous defect. Lesions at 3a and 3b produce binasal hemianopia (a rare disorder). Lesions at 2 and 3b produce blindness of the right eye with temporal hemianopia of the left visual field. Lesion at 4 produces right homonymous hemianopia with macular (splitting) involvement. Lesion at 5 produces right homonymous hemianopia with sparing of the macular field. Lesion at 6 produces right homonymous central (macular) hemiscotoma.

the fibres from the inner nasal half of each retina, representing the temporal field, decussate, whilst those from the outer temporal half, representing the nasal field, remain on the same side. Each optic tract, formed after this chiasmal decussation, therefore consists of fibres from the outer half of the retina on the same side and from the inner half of the retina on the opposite side. Each optic tract passes posteriorly to the lateral geniculate body of the same side; some pregeniculate fibres project to the superior colliculi. The optic radiation originates in the lateral geniculate body on each side, passes through the posterior limb of the internal capsule and then projects posteriorly to the calcarine cortex of the occipital lobe. Those fibres subserving the upper visual fields pass through the white matter of the temporal lobe, whilst those mediating impulses from the lower field pass through the parietal lobe. Thus, in the occipital cortex around the calcarine fissure, the left half of the field of vision is represented in the cortex of the right hemisphere and vice versa (Fig. 12.10).

The input from the two homologous fields of the two eyes is represented in adjacent columns of neurones. The most peripheral part of the visual fields is represented anteriorly in the calcarine fissure and the most medial part, the macular field, is represented at the occipital pole (Fig. 12.10).

TESTS

The *visual acuity* and the *visual fields* must always be examined. Other aspects of visual perception, including colour vision, visual localization and visual recognition may also be tested, if clinically appropriate. When testing vision it is important to ensure that any refractive error is corrected and that no other ocular disease is present that might impair the visual acuity or the visual fields. Each eye must be tested separately.

Visual acuity

For technique of testing, see chapter 10.

Visual fields

When we look at an object, we not only see that object but also a number of other objects in the neighbourhood, more or less distinctly. The full extent of this vision is called the visual field. The field of vision is limited both by the area of the retina and by the margins of the orbit, nose and cheek. Hence the position of the eye is important. The extent of the visual field varies with the stimulus used. For example, the field is larger to large than to small objects, or to brightly illuminated than to dimly lit objects. Colour sensitivity is mainly confined to the central or macular field, corresponding to the central part of the retina rich in cone cells. The rod cells, sensitive to white light, are more uniformly distributed across the whole area of the retina. Moving stimuli, on the other hand, are best perceived in the peripheral field since specialized movement-sensitive receptor cells are located mainly in the peripheral parts of the retina. This part of the retina is also particularly responsive to the sudden appearance or disappearance of stationary visual stimuli, but the appreciation of the form of an object is only poorly developed in this part of the field. Form and detail are best perceived in the central field and this aspect of visual function is tested by assessment of the *visual acuity*.

Physiological investigations have disclosed the existence of columns of cells in the visual cortex responsive to precise visual stimuli, for example, dark surrounds, linear dark–light junctions oriented in particular planes, and specialized colour-receptive cells. This cortical organization enables the matrix of cells in the retina to function as a very precise transducer of visual information in terms of position, shape, size, colour and movement. The higher level cortex related to vision contains groups of cells, and even individual cells responsive to environmental recognition, visual memory (modality-specific memory) and facial recognition. Colour vision itself is processed in a particular part of the visual-related cerebral cortex.

The *visual fields* can be assessed by several methods of varying sophistication. The simplest consists of comparing the extent of the patient's visual field with your own: testing the field by *confrontation*. Both eyes should be tested together first (binocular vision), and then each must be tested separately (monocular testing) to exclude a field defect limited to part of the visual field of one eye only.

Confrontation tests. Seat yourself opposite the patient, at a distance of about 1 metre. To test the patient's right eye, ask the patient to cover their left eye with their left hand and look steadily at your left eye. Cover your right eye with your right hand and gaze steadily at the patient's right eye. In this way slight movements of the patient's eye, which would introduce error into the test, can be detected. Hold up your left hand in a plane midway between the patient's face and your own, at first almost a full arm's length to the side. Keep moving the fingers of the hand and bring it nearer until you yourself can just perceive the movements of the fingers 'with the tail of your eye'. Ask the patient whether he or she sees the movements, making sure at the same time that the patient fixes their gaze on your eye. If the patient fails to see the fingers, keep bringing your hand nearer until he or she does see them. Test the field in this fashion in every direction—upwards, downwards, to right and to left—using the extent of your own field for comparison.

Red pin test. This outlines the central field. Since this field may be relatively intact when the fields for other forms of stimulation are markedly abnormal, the field for small objects must also be tested when disease of the visual pathways is suspected. This test can conveniently be done using a red pinhead held up in the patient's field in the manner described above. A central area of impaired vision (*central scotoma*) can also be recognized by this method because the red or white pinhead cannot be perceived in the scotoma or, in less severe examples, because the intensity of the red colour is reduced (desaturated) in this part of the field.

This method allows the patient's field, including the size of the physiological blind spot (see below), to be compared precisely with the examiner's field. A good test in preliminary assessment is to ask the patient to compare the contour and colour of the palm of the examiner's hand held up in the right, left and central fields of each eye separately.

The physiological blind spot is situated to the temporal side of the central point of fixation of the visual field. It corresponds to the point of entry of the optic nerve into the retina; this is the *optic disc*, found slightly to the nasal side of the macula when visualized with the ophthalmoscope. At the optic disc there are no retinal receptor cells and there is thus a small blind spot in the field corresponding to this region. It should always be possible to identify this blind spot when testing the visual field to confrontation with a red pin, and its size should correspond with the examiner's own blind spot when the red pin is held equidistant between the examiner's eye and the patient's eye. The blind spot sometimes appears to be absent in an uncooperative patient, or if the patient is attempting to mislead the examiner. Little reliance can be placed on the visual fields in such patients.

Perimetry. The visual field may be mapped using a perimeter. Several types of perimeter are available but all utilize the same principles. The patient is seated comfortably with the chin resting on a chin rest adjusted so that the eye to be tested is oriented at the centre of a hemispherical, illuminated field, upon which spots of light of various intensities, colours or sizes may be projected, or moved, in order to detect the limits of the field and its sensitivity in various parts. In the more elaborate perimeters, the examiner can observe the patient's eye through a small telescopic eyepiece in the centre of the hemisphere, in order to detect any movement of the patient's eye away from fixation on the central point of the hemispheric field. Simpler, portable versions of the perimeter do not allow this. These consist only of a hemispheric arm along which stimulus may be moved by a simple mechanical system. Stationary, rather than moving, targets can be used for perimetry in the central fields, using special perimeters with targets of variable luminance.

Perimetry surveys the monocular field of vision, from which the limits of perception can be charted (Fig. 12.11). The centre point of the chart corresponds to the point of fixation. Around this point are arranged a series of more or less concentric lines, each of which denotes equal visual acuity—an *isopter*.

Since the fixation point is not exactly central, the outer and inner parts of the field are unequally divided. Further, the field is limited medially and superiorly by the nose and brow. With an object of 5 mm diameter the extent of the average field of vision is 100 degrees laterally, 60 degrees superiorly and medially, and 75 degrees inferiorly. The field charted with a 20-mm object is shown in Fig. 12.11; note the restriction of the lower nasal field by the bridge of the nose.

The binocular field extends 200 degrees in the lateral plane and about 140 degrees vertically. The major area of the visual field is binocular. On each side of this area of binocular vision is a lateral semilunar area which is unpaired (i.e. it is monocular) and which accounts for the remainder of the field. This is called the temporal crescent. Since the visual acuity is much lower at the periphery than at the point of fixation, it is possible, by using a graduated series of objects, to plot out a series of isopters, each of which corresponds to the field for a known size of object, at a known distance from the eye and at a constant illumination.

The area within 30 degrees from fixation is best examined either with a sophisticated perimeter, having first corrected any refractive errors with lenses, or by presenting objects against a 2 m² wall-mounted black screen (*Bjerrum's screen*) at a distance from the patient of 1 or 2 metres. In the latter method the patient is seated comfortably, preferably with the head steadied by a chin and head rest, and a white object 1 cm in diameter is fixed to the screen on a level with the patient's eye. The blind spot is mapped first using a white object 10 mm in diameter. The peripheral field is then mapped with the same 10-mm object: at a distance of 2 metres the field should be circular and extend to about 25 degrees, that is, to the edge of the 2-m² screen. With a smaller white or red object areas of blindness or defective perception should be sought around the blind spot, especially between this area and the macula (the *centrocaecal* area), and in the horizontal meridian on the nasal side of the fixation spot. The findings are marked upon the screen with black pins, and subsequently transferred to a chart for recording in the patient's case notes.

Changes in the field of vision

A zone of loss of vision confined to the centre of the field is called a *central scotoma*. A unilateral central scotoma is a common feature of demyelination in the optic nerve (*retrobulbar neuritis*), which in most cases is a symptom of multiple sclerosis. Paracentral scotomas arise from local disease of the choroid or of the retina in the neighbourhood of the macula, espe-

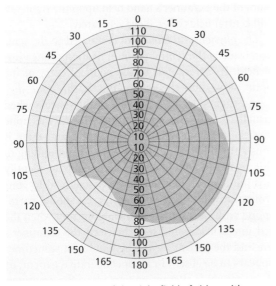

Fig. 12.11 The extent of the right field of vision with a white target of 20 mm diameter mapped on a perimeter at a distance of 330 mm.

cially with vascular disease. In that case it often affects only one eye. Less commonly, they may be due to toxic causes, especially alcoholism or to vitamin B$_{12}$ deficiency, when they are generally bilateral. Untreated glaucoma can cause a paracentral 'arcuate' scotoma, which has a characteristic comma-like shape and which results from damage to a nerve fibre bundle. Pressure on the optic nerve is another cause. A paracentral scotoma may also result from a lesion of the posterior part of the visual cortex and is then bilateral, but this is very rare (see Fig. 12.10).

Hemianopia means loss of sight in one-half of the visual field. When the same half of both fields of vision is lost, the hemianopia is described as *homonymous*, e.g. right homonymous hemianopia when the right half of the field of each eye is affected (see Fig. 12.9). Blindness limited to one quadrant of a field is termed a *quadrantanopia*.

When the outline of the visual loss in the homonymous fields of the two eyes is similar (*congruous hemianopia*) the lesion is likely to be pregeniculate, i.e. in the optic tracts or chiasm, but in central, post-geniculate lesions, because of the relative separation of fibres in the optic radiation, the two field defects are often *incongruous*.

Superior or *inferior altitudinal hemianopia* means loss of the upper or lower halves of the visual field respectively. This may occur with damage to an optic nerve by ischaemia or trauma. Bilateral altitudinal field defects are uncommon; they are usually due to occipital lesions.

Bitemporal hemianopia means loss of vision in the temporal (outer) halves of both fields, and is due, therefore, to loss of function of the nasal half of each retina. It can only be produced by a lesion of the optic chiasm, involving those fibres of the optic nerves, derived from the nasal parts of the retina, which decussate at this site. It is usually due to a tumour of the pituitary gland but is also a feature of inflammatory or traumatic lesions of the optic chiasm (Fig. 12.12).

Binasal hemianopia means loss of the nasal or inner half of each field, indicating loss of function of the temporal half of each retina. It is very rare, but results from bilateral lesions confined to the uncrossed optic fibres on each side of the optic chiasm. It may also occur in open-angle glaucoma.

Concentric constriction of the visual fields sometimes occurs in long-standing papilloedema, in bilateral lesions of the striate (visual) cortex and in some retinal disorders, e.g. retinitis pigmentosa. It is also found in hysteria.

Bitemporal and binasal hemianopias are sometimes described as *heteronymous*, in contradistinction to the homonymous variety.

Colour vision
For methods of testing, see chapter 10.

SUBJECTIVE VISUAL SENSATIONS
Among the commonest subjective visual sensations are floaters (*muscae volitantes*)—little grey specks seen floating before the eyes, especially on looking at a white surface or up to the sky. They are a normal phenomenon due to awareness of parts of the retinal blood vessels seen reflected from the posterior surface of the lens, or to vitreous opacities. In migraine, zigzag lines, known as 'fortification figures' or *teichopsia* are a characteristic feature at the beginning of the attack. *Visual hallucinations* occur in a number of neurological diseases, notably in delirium tremens and in temporal and occipito-parietal disorders; they may also form part of the aura in epilepsy. *Photopsias*, tiny white flashes seen in the visual field may occur in acute retrobulbar neuritis. They often seem to be induced by ocular movement.

VISUAL AGNOSIA AND CORTICAL BLINDNESS
Complex disturbances of visual perception and of visually directed behaviour result from lesions in the parietal connections of the occipital cortex especially inattention to visual stimuli in the abnormal field. In *visual agnosia (Anton's syndrome)*, in which the lesions are in the central connections of the striate cortex, the patient is unaware or uncomprehending of the visual deficit. In *cortical blindness*, in which the lesions are in the striate cortex of both hemispheres, the patient is aware of the visual disorder. The pupillary light reflexes are normal in both these disorders.

Ocular movements and pupils

The external ocular movements, and the pupils, are controlled by the third (oculomotor), fourth (trochlear) and sixth (abducens) nerves. These nerves arise from nuclei in the brainstem, and function as a physiological unit.

ANATOMY
The brainstem nuclei from which these nerves arise are located in the brainstem close to the Sylvian aqueduct at the level of the superior corpora

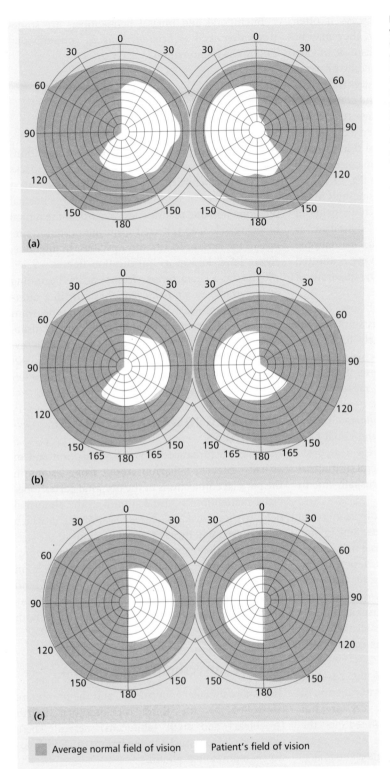

(a)

(b)

(c)

Average normal field of vision   Patient's field of vision

Fig. 12.12   Fields of vision in a patient with a pituitary tumour (chromophobe adenoma) showing the development of bitemporal hemianopia. These fields were plotted many years ago; in the modern era of safe neurosurgery, operative decompression of the optic chiasm by hypophysectomy would have been carried out at the time of initial diagnosis in May.   (a) May: VA (visual acuity) Lt 6/12 Rt 6/18.   (b) August: VA Lt 6/12 Rt 6/12.   (c) October: VA Lt 6/12 Rt 6/12. The fields were plotted on a Bjerrum's screen at a distance of 2 m from the eye to the point of fixation at the centre of the screen, using a 10-mm white object. The coloured areas show the average normal field of vision and the white areas show the patient's field.

quadrigemina, and extend as far caudally as the eminentia teres in the floor of the fourth ventricle. The nucleus of the third nerve is farthest forward; its most rostral nerve cells supply parasympathetic innervation to the ciliary muscle and iris (Edinger–Westphal nucleus), those for the extraocular muscles being located in the more caudal part of the nucleus. Caudal to this is the nucleus of the fourth nerve. The sixth nerve nucleus is situated in the floor of the fourth ventricle at the level of the pons.

The third nerve emerges on the inner aspect of the cerebral peduncles, between the superior cerebellar and posterior cerebral arteries, and passes forward in close relation to the posterior communicating artery before entering the lateral wall of the cavernous sinus. It is thus at risk in certain patients with brain herniation associated with cerebral mass lesions, and in aneurysms of the posterior communicating arteries.

The fourth nerves emerge on the rostral part of the roof of the fourth ventricle. They are unique both in that they are the only cranial nerves which decussate between their nuclei and their point of emergence from the brainstem, and that they emerge dorsally.

The sixth nerve emerges between the medulla and pons. Its long intracranial course renders it particularly vulnerable to the effects of pressure, leading to diplopia on lateral gaze. The sixth nerve innervates the external rectus muscle and the fourth nerve innervates the superior oblique muscle. All the other extraocular muscles, the sphincter pupillae (the muscle that causes pupillary constriction during accommodation) and the levator palpebrae superioris, are supplied by the third nerve.

OCULAR MOVEMENTS

Horizontal movement of an eye outwards (laterally) is termed *abduction;* inwards (medially) *adduction;* vertical movement upwards, *elevation;* and downwards, *depression.* The eye is also capable of *diagonal* movements at any intermediate angle. *Rotary* movements, the eye rolling like a wheel towards the nose (internal rotation) or away from the nose (external rotation), are not possible voluntarily, but occur normally as part of the reflex compensation necessary to adjust for slight degrees of head tilt during tasks involving macular fixation, e.g. when reading. Note that *the superior and inferior recti act as elevators and depressors alone when the eye is in abduction, and the superior and inferior obliques act similarly when the eye is in adduction* (Fig. 12.13). Their function may therefore be assessed by testing the movements of elevation and of depression in both full abduction and full adduction. This method of testing gaze movements is much more informative than simply testing elevation and depression in the mid-position of gaze. Lateral gaze must always be tested separately. Vertical and horizontal ocular movements made from the mid-position of gaze are called

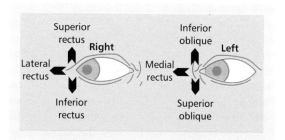

Fig. 12.13 The action of the external ocular muscles with the patient confronting the examiner.

cardinal movements. The medial and lateral recti always act directly in a single plane, but all movements require the co-ordinated activity of the whole group of extraocular muscles. The eyes normally move 50 degrees medially, 30 degrees upwards and 50 degrees downwards.

Normally the movements of the two eyes are symmetrical, so that the visual axes meet at the point at which the eyes are directed. This is referred to as *conjugate* movement of the eyes. Conjugate ocular movements depend on brainstem integration of the third, fourth and sixth nerve nuclei. Thus *infranuclear* (lower motor neurone) lesions of the third, fourth and sixth nerves lead to weakness of individual eye muscles or groups of muscles, and *supranuclear* (upper motor neurone) lesions lead to paralysis of conjugate movements of the eyes. The classification of disorders of ocular movement is shown in Box 12.7.

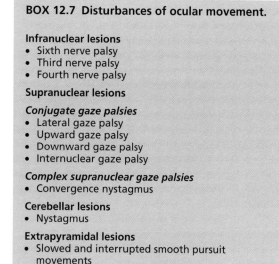

BOX 12.7 Disturbances of ocular movement.

Infranuclear lesions
- Sixth nerve palsy
- Third nerve palsy
- Fourth nerve palsy

Supranuclear lesions

Conjugate gaze palsies
- Lateral gaze palsy
- Upward gaze palsy
- Downward gaze palsy
- Internuclear gaze palsy

Complex supranuclear gaze palsies
- Convergence nystagmus

Cerebellar lesions
- Nystagmus

Extrapyramidal lesions
- Slowed and interrupted smooth pursuit movements

Lower motor neurone (infranuclear) lesions
Infranuclear lesions of the sixth, fourth and third nerves lead to the following abnormalities.

Sixth nerve. Inability to move the eye outwards (laterally) and diplopia (double vision) on looking in that direction. Sometimes convergent squint because of the unopposed action of the medial rectus, innervated by the ipsilateral third nerve.

Fourth nerve. Impaired downward movement; on attempting to look downwards in the mid-position of gaze the eyeball is rotated outwards by the unopposed action of the inferior rectus (Fig. 12.13). Diplopia only below the horizontal plane, with the images uncrossed, but the false one tilted. There is rarely a visible squint.

Third nerve. Ptosis: the eye is displaced downwards and laterally and further movement is only possible laterally and a little downwards. Because the third nerve contains parasympathetic nerve fibres that cause pupillary constriction, the pupil in a third nerve palsy is often dilated, with loss of accommodation and unopposed action of the cervical sympathetic innervation of the dilator pupillae muscle. These are the features of a complete oculomotor nerve palsy (Fig. 12.14). However, third nerve palsy is often partial, and in some cases, particularly diabetic third nerve palsy, the pupil is spared.

In the upper eyelid there is smooth muscle as well as striated muscle. This smooth muscle is innervated by the cervical sympathetic nerves. Slight ptosis therefore occurs after a lesion of the cervical sympathetic but the pupil is then small (Horner's syndrome; see Fig. 10.16, page 238), rather than large as in third nerve palsy.

Thus, the features of a lesion involving one or more of these three nerves may be:

- Defective movement of the eye
- A squint
- Double vision (*diplopia*)
- Pupillary abnormalities.

Of these signs diplopia and pupillary abnormalities are the most consistent.

STRABISMUS

A squint or strabismus is an abnormality of ocular movement such that the visual axes do not meet at the point of fixation. There are two types: *paralytic* and *non-paralytic (concomitant)*.

Paralytic strabismus

Paralytic strabismus is due to weakness of one or more of the extraocular muscles. The following clinical features occur.

Limitation of movement. Since paralytic strabismus is due to weakness of one or more extraocular muscles, a prominent feature is impairment of ocular movement in the direction of action of the muscle(s) affected. Although this weakness is usually obvious it is sometimes so slight, or the unaffected muscles mask it so much, that the defective movement of the eye is hardly apparent.

If an eye fails to move at all, or fails to move through its normal angular excursion, the observed deviation of this eye in a direction opposite to the physiological action of the muscle is called the *primary deviation* or *squint*. It is measured by the angle which a line from the object to the nodal point of the eye makes with the visual axis. If the unaffected eye is covered, so that the patient fixates with the affected eye (cover test; page 294), the covered normal eye will deviate still more than the primary deviation of

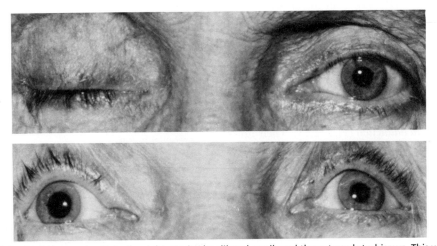

Fig. 12.14 Right third nerve palsy. Note the right ptosis, the dilated pupil, and the external strabismus. This was due to a berry aneurysm of the right posterior communicating artery.

the affected eye. This deviation of the healthy eye is called *secondary deviation* and occurs because of the 'mental effort' made by the patient to move the eye with the weakened muscle. The difference between the primary and secondary deviations in paralytic strabismus is the most important feature differentiating it from concomitant, non-paralytic strabismus.

False orientation of the field of vision. This consists of erroneous judgement by the patient of the position of an object in that portion of the field of vision toward which the paralysed muscle should normally move the eye. For example, if a patient who has paralysis of the right lateral rectus muscle closes the left eye and attempts to touch an object held in the horizontal plane on their right side, they will point wide, to the right side of the object. This results from information reaching the brain from the retina due to the weakness of action of the affected lateral rectus muscle failing to match the position expected to result from the execution of the motor program for that movement. This is a form of sensory mismatch.

Dizziness or instability. This is occasionally a symptom of paralytic strabismus when both eyes are opened. It is due partly to the confusing experience of double vision and partly to false orientation, a symptom also due to sensory mismatch.

Diplopia. Patients with paralytic strabismus complain of double vision. This occurs because defective movement of one eye results in the images from the two eyes arising from different points on the two retinae. Binocular fusion cannot therefore occur in the visual cortex and two separate or overlapping images are perceived. Furthermore, in paralytic strabismus, the image from the macula of the healthy eye is seen distinctly and is called the *true image*, whereas in the affected eye this image is derived from the retina outside the macula. This latter image is indistinct and blurred; it is called the *false image*. Most patients can therefore clearly recognize which of the two images they perceive is the true image and which the false. The false image is projected into that part of the field of vision into which the paralysed muscle should move the eye if it were normal; it is perceived *in the direction of action of the weak muscle*. Doubt as to which is the false image can usually be resolved by covering one eye with a red glass and asking the patient whether the red or the normally coloured image is the real one (*red glass test*).

In order to overcome diplopia the head may be involuntarily turned in the direction of action of the paralysed muscle. This *head tilt* gives information as to which muscle is involved.

Diplopia is of value in the diagnosis of paralytic strabismus. First make certain that the diplopia is *binocular,* since lens opacities and astigmatism may produce monocular diplopia. Diplopia should always be assessed in the nine cardinal directions of gaze (Fig. 12.13 and Box 12.8). The objective of this formal analysis is to decide to which eye the *furthest displaced of the two images, i.e. the false image, belongs*. The test object is therefore moved in the cardinal directions until the position of maximal displacement of the two images is ascertained.

BOX 12.8 Charting diplopia in the nine cardinal directions of gaze in paralytic diplopia (see also Fig. 12.13).

The muscles used in each direction of gaze are listed.

Upwards to the left	*Upwards*	*Upwards to the right*
left SR	left and right SR	right SR
right IO	left and right IO	left IO
To the left	*Straight ahead*	*To the right*
left LR	contraction of all	right LR
right MR	extraocular muscles	left MR
Downwards to the left	*Downwards*	*Downwards to the right*
left IR	left and right IR	right IR
right SO	left and right SO	left SO

SR = superior rectus; IR = inferior rectus;
LR = lateral rectus; MR = medial rectus;
SO = superior oblique; IO = inferior oblique.

In order to find the direction of maximal diplopia, the patient is seated, preferably with their head in a head rest, with a red glass over the right eye and a clear glass over the left. At a distance of about 0.5 m the observer moves a light in the directions indicated in Box 12.8. Each of the lateral squares corresponds to a pair of associated muscles. Thus maximal vertical diplopia produced when the patient looks up and to the right, into the right superior square, shows that either the right superior rectus or the left inferior oblique muscle is the one affected. In this example, the higher of the two images, the false image, indicates the affected eye, and from this it is easy to decide which muscle is affected.

In *paralytic* strabismus the angular deviation of the two visual axes varies with different positions of the two eyes, and the secondary deviation is always greater than the primary deviation.

Non-paralytic strabismus

In non-paralytic (concomitant) strabismus, as its name implies, the angular deviation of the visual axes is the same in whatever position the eyes may be moved; in other words, the primary and secondary deviations are always equal (see page 292). Thus, the ocular axes are misaligned; there is no weakness of the external ocular muscles.

The *cover test* can be used to assess the primary and secondary deviations. Ask the patient to look at an object immediately in front of him or her. Suddenly cover the apparently fixing eye. If the uncovered eye makes any movement in taking up fixation, it must have previously been deviating, indicating that a squint is present. If the eye now behind the cover (which was previously fixing) is now tested by uncovering it, it will deviate in the same relative direction as was the other eye, and *to the same angular amount,* that is, the primary and secondary deviations are equal.

The *clinical features* of non-paralytic strabismus are characteristic.

- It begins in early childhood, usually before the fifth year and almost always before 3 years of age.
- The movements of the eyes, tested individually, are full in all directions.
- Diplopia is almost never a symptom.
- The primary and secondary deviations are equal.
- The deviating eye usually has defective vision (amblyopia ex anopsia).

A squint may be *intermittent* or *constant* and, if constant, *monocular* when only one eye deviates whilst the other usually fixes, or *alternating* when either eye fixes independently.

SUPRANUCLEAR GAZE PALSIES

In addition to abnormalities of ocular movement due to weakness of individual ocular muscles, impairment or paralysis of the movement of *both* eyes in one direction sometimes occurs (*conjugate gaze palsy*). Thus the patient may be unable to look to either side, or upwards or downwards; or convergence alone may be lost. Paralysis of *lateral conjugate gaze* is characteristically found with lesions in the pons. The lesion is in the pontine paramedian reticular formation (PPRF) near the abducens and vestibular nuclei. *Bilateral paralysis of lateral conjugate gaze* may occur with centrally placed pontine lesions above the level of the abducens nuclei. Weakness of lateral conjugate movement also occurs in hemiplegia due to cerebral lesions, especially in the acute stage. Palsies of *conjugate upward gaze* are

always associated with disease of the central parts of the mid-brain or inferior thalamic region, or in the neighbourhood of the oculomotor nuclei. Impaired *downward gaze* is very rare, but occurs with brainstem lesions at a lower level.

Tonic conjugate deviation of the eyes is an abnormality in which both eyes are kept persistently turned in one direction, usually in the lateral plane. It is usually due to a lesion causing weakness of conjugate gaze, as above, but may also occur in irritative cortical lesions. In the former, the eyes (and usually also the head) are turned towards the side of the lesion, if the lesion is in the cerebral hemisphere, as in a patient with acute hemiplegia, i.e. the patient 'looks towards his lesion'. An irritative lesion in a similar situation causes deviation towards the healthy side, usually accompanied by nystagmoid jerks of the eye toward this side. This is a form of *focal epilepsy*. If, however, the lesion is in the pons, these rules are reversed, the deviation being towards the sound side in a paralytic lesion. Irritative lesions in the brainstem, it should be remembered, are exceptional.

Skew deviation of the eyes—in which one eye is directed upwards and the other downwards—occurs in lesions of the labyrinth and in cerebellar disease. Other abnormal ocular movements, such as *ocular bobbing, opsoclonus* and *ocular dysmetria*, also associated with acute cerebellar lesions, are rare.

Assessment of *saccadic* (rapid, programmed, conjugate fixation movements) and *pursuit* (following) gaze movements can be performed separately by asking the patient to move his or her eyes rapidly from fixation on one finger to another held about 30 degrees away in the horizontal plane, and by asking him or her to follow a slowly moving finger across visual space in the same, or in the vertical, plane. In Huntington's chorea, pursuit movements are slowed, or interrupted by slowed saccades, and a similar disturbance may occur in Parkinson's disease. In higher level disturbances of visual perception, e.g. parieto-occipital lesions causing agnosia or misperceptions of visual space to one side, saccadic movements may be impaired toward the midline in the affected field.

Internuclear ophthalmoplegia is due to a lesion in one medial longitudinal fasciculus in the mid-brain or upper pons. On attempted lateral gaze there is pronounced rhythmic nystagmus of the abducting eye and impaired medial deviation of the adducting eye. The latter may cause diplopia. In addition, the adducting eye moves more slowly than the contralat-

(a)

Right   Left

Weak adduction   Nystagmus

(b)

Fig. 12.15   (a) Right internuclear ophthalmoplegia. This abnormality is a frequent clinical feature in patients with multiple sclerosis. (b) Diagrammatic representation of interconnection of oculomotor, trochlear and abducent nerve nuclei with the pontine paramedian reticular formation (PPRF) via the medial longitudinal fasciculus (MLF). A lesion (X) in the right MLF will cause impaired adduction of the right eye with nystagmus of the abducting left eye during attempted lateral gaze to the left. A lesion in or near the PPRF causes impaired conjugate lateral gaze to the same side.

eral abducting eye, especially during attempted saccadic movements. All other gaze movements, and the pupils, are normal. The lesion is on the side of the impaired adduction, not on the side of the nystagmus (Fig. 12.15a and b). This sign is important because it is common in multiple sclerosis, when it is often bilateral.

In the 'one-and-a-half syndrome' a lesion in the parapontine region involves both the PPRF and the medial longitudinal fasciculus (Fig. 12.15a and b) on the same side. There is failure of lateral conjugate gaze to one side (the side of the lesion), together with impairment of adduction of the eye on that side and nystagmus on abduction (lateral movement) of the opposite eye. The latter is the only horizontal movement possible; one eye will not move at all horizontally and the other only in abduction— one-and-a-half lateral movements are paralysed. Vertical gaze movements and the pupillary reactions are normal.

NYSTAGMUS

The term 'nystagmus' is applied to a disturbance of ocular movement characterized by involuntary, conjugate, often rhythmical oscillations of the eyes. These movements may be horizontal, vertical or rotary. In any given direction of gaze the speed of the movement is usually quicker in one direction than the other; the *quicker movement* describes the direction of the nystagmus.

To examine for nystagmus, ask the patient to look straight ahead and note whether the eyes remain steady. Then ask the patient to look to the extreme right, then to the left, and then upwards and downwards. It is best to ask the patient to look at your finger in these positions. Observe the rate, amplitude and rhythm of nystagmus in each direction and whether or not it is sustained.

Nystagmus can be graded, for example:
- Grade 1: Nystagmus with fast phase to left, looking toward the left.
- Grade 2: Nystagmus with fast phase to left, looking straight ahead.
- Grade 3: Nystagmus with fast phase to left, looking toward the right.

Nystagmus occurs with disorders of the vestibular system (either centrally or peripherally); lesions affecting the central pathways concerned in ocular movements, e.g. the vestibulo-cerebellar connections in brainstem or cerebellum or the medial longitudinal fasciculus; or with weakness of the ocular muscles. Nystagmus is often induced by drugs, especially benzodiazepines, phenytoin and other anticonvulsant drugs, and barbiturates. Nystagmus due to long-standing visual impairment (e.g. 'miner's nystagmus') is pendular and often rotary on central fixation of the eyes. *Congenital nystagmus* also shows this pendular quality.

Some forms of nystagmus, particularly that associated with benign epidemic vertigo, and with posterior fossa neoplasms, may be induced only by certain movements of the head (*positional nystagmus*, see chapter 9).

A few irregular jerks of the eyes are often seen in full lateral deviation in normal subjects. The brief duration and irregularity of these movements distinguish them from true nystagmus.

Optokinetic nystagmus is a physiological phenomenon that occurs when the patient follows a rapidly moving scene (*railway track nystagmus*). The eyes fixate and follow the moving stimulus and then refixate by making a rapid saccade back to the primary position of gaze. There is thus a slow component in the direction of the moving stimulus and a fast phase in the opposite direction. This phenomenon may be used as a crude test of visual acuity by utilizing a striped drum or tape, but the test is used mainly to assess patients with hemianopia or brainstem lesions. In *parietal hemianopia* there may be neglect of the visual environment on the hemianopic side, even with a very mild degree of visual impairment and this is accompanied by suppression of the fast phase of optokinetic nystagmus when the stimulus is moved from this abnormal visual field toward the normal field. The fast phase is replaced by a slow tonic deviation of the eyes in the direction of movement of the stimulus. In *brainstem lesions* optokinetic testing is useful in establishing the presence of conjugate gaze palsies, internuclear ophthalmoplegia and abnormalities of the velocity of saccadic eye movements.

EXAMINATION OF THE PUPILS

The following must be noted about the pupils in every patient.

Size

Compare the size of the two pupils, first in a bright light and then in a dim light. Note whether the pupils are large or small and whether any irregularity is present. The size of the pupil in healthy subjects is very variable. As a rule, the pupils are larger in dark eyes than in light eyes. They tend to be small in elderly subjects. Slight inequality of the pupils may be present in perfectly healthy subjects.

If one pupil is larger than the other, which is the abnormal? This is not always easily decided, but the pupil which is less mobile is usually the abnormal one.

Shape

Note whether the pupil is circular in outline, as it should be, or whether its contour is irregular. Irregularities are usually due to adhesion of the iris to the lens, as a result of an old iritis.

Mobility

Reaction to light. The pupillary reaction to light is a reflex. The afferent fibres involved travel in the optic nerve, leaving it before the synapse in the lateral geniculate bodies to enter the brainstem in the pretectal region. These fibres synapse in the oculomotor nuclei; the efferent fibres, which are parasympathetic, reach the pupillary sphincters via the oculomotor nerve after synapsing again in the ciliary ganglion in the orbit.

Use a shady, indirectly illuminated room, and examine each eye separately. Ask the patient to look into the distance, e.g. across the room, to be sure accommodation is relaxed. Shine a bright light into one eye; the pupil should contract almost immediately, then dilate again a little and, after undergoing a few slight oscillations, settle down to a smaller size. When the light is switched off the pupil will rapidly dilate to its previous diameter.

Swinging light test for afferent (optic nerve) pupillary abnormality. Because some of the fibres in the optic nerves decussate in the optic chiasm, light shone into one eye stimulates the brainstem nuclei (oculomotor nerve) concerned with pupillary constriction bilaterally. As a consequence, if bright light is shone into one eye only, both pupils contract; and if light is shut off from one eye, both pupils dilate slightly. The former is the *consensual pupillary reaction*. It should be tested by keeping one eye in the shade while shining a bright light into the other. The effect on the pupil of the unilluminated eye is then observed. The pupillary constriction may be brisk and well-sustained in one eye but, when the light is shone immediately into the other eye, this pupil may slowly dilate a little, indicating that the consensually mediated light reaction of the second eye is more active than its direct reaction. On this second side there must therefore be an *afferent defect* (Gunn's pupil), i.e. a lesion in the optic nerve. This is a particularly useful sign in optic neuritis and in ischaemic or compressive lesions of the optic nerve.

In some patients with post-chiasmal, but pregeniculate hemianopia, the pupillary light reaction is less active when a narrow beam of light is shone from the hemianopic side than when shone from the normal side. However, this hemianopic pupillary reaction sign is difficult to elicit.

Reaction to accommodation. The pupils become smaller on accommodating for a near object (*miosis*). Convergence of the eyes, accommodation and miosis are closely related reflexes.

Hold up one finger close to the patient's nose. Ask the patient to look away at a distant object. Then ask him or her to look quickly at your finger. As the eyes converge to accomplish this the pupils become smaller. The test may be carried out in patients with defective vision by asking them to hold their own finger about 30 cm in front of their face, and then asking them to 'look at the finger'. Accommodation is only rarely lost in brainstem lesions, but may be impaired with lesions of the oculomotor nerve and autonomic neuropathies.

The *Argyll Robertson pupil* is the classical pupillary abnormality of neurosyphilis. The pupil is small and irregular, reacts briskly to accommodation, but does not react to light directly or consensually. The pupil dilates slowly or imperfectly to atropine. The abnormality is typically bilateral but it is usually more marked on one side. The lesion is in the pretectal region of the mesencephalon.

Hippus is a rhythmic dilatation and constriction of the pupil, either in response to light or occurring spontaneously. It is particularly prominent in retrobulbar neuritis, but is often of no clinical significance.

The *Adie pupil* is an abnormality characterized by absent or delayed pupillary constriction to light or to accommodation/convergence. Once constricted the pupil dilates only very slowly, either in response to darkness or to far gaze. The pupil may thus appear small or large and this sometimes leads to confusion with the Argyll Robertson syndrome. The pupil in Adie's syndrome varies in size from day to day but *never* reacts promptly to light. The abnormality is frequently unilateral so that it may cause unequal pupils (*anisocoria*). It is sometimes associated with absent tendon reflexes, often on the same side as the pupillary abnormality (Holmes–Adie syndrome). The distinction between the Argyll Robertson and Adie pupillary abnormalities is important since the latter, probably due to partial parasympathetic denervation, is of little clinical significance. The distinction may be made by instillation of sterile 2% methacholine into the conjunctival sac; the Adie pupil constricts but the Argyll Robertson pupil does not.

Horner's syndrome is due to paralysis of the cervical sympathetic nerve. The sympathetic nerve fibres supplying the pupil originate in the lower cervical and upper thoracic regions of the spinal cord (C8 and T1), from which they emerge in the first thoracic nerve roots and pass to the sympathetic ganglia by the rami communicantes. From the cervical sympathetic chain the sympathetic nerve fibres pass along the internal carotid to the cavernous plexus, and thence via the ophthalmic division of the trigeminal nerve to the eye. Sympathetic nervous activity causes pupillary dilatation and elevation of the upper lid, the latter through contraction of the smooth muscle fibres in the levator palpebrae superioris.

Horner's syndrome consists of:
- slight drooping of the upper lid (ptosis);
- pupillary constriction;
- absence of pupillary dilatation on shading the eye or on instillation of cocaine; and
- abolition of the ciliospinal reflex.

Less commonly, there may be absence of sweating on the corresponding half of the face and neck, both in front and behind, extending as low as the third rib and third thoracic spine, and over the whole of the upper limb on the same side. An apparent enophthalmos is also often present, and is a useful clue to the diagnosis when the patient is first seen (see Fig. 10.16).

Dilatation of the normal pupil when the skin of the neck is pinched (*ciliospinal reflex*) is due to reflex excitation of the pupil-dilating fibres in the cervical sympathetic: it is abolished by lesions of that nerve and, sometimes, by medullary, cervical and upper thoracic cord lesions.

The fifth (trigeminal) nerve

ANATOMY

The *sensory root* takes origin from nerve cells in the trigeminal (Gasserian) ganglion and enters the lateral surface of the pons at about its middle. The fibres which conduct impulses for light touch terminate in a large nucleus in the pons, situated lateral to the motor nucleus near the floor of the fourth ventricle, while the fibres for pain and thermal sensation enter the 'descending' or bulbospinal tract, which extends as low as the second cervical segment of the cord before ascending in the medial lemniscus.

Immediately distal to the trigeminal ganglion the nerve separates into its three divisions (Fig. 12.16).

The *first* or *ophthalmic division* supplies the conjunctiva and the conjunctival surface of the upper but not of the lower lid, the lacrimal gland, the mesial part of the skin of the nose as far as its tip, the upper eyelids, the forehead, and the scalp as far as the vertex. Lesions of the ophthalmic division result in loss of cutaneous and corneal sensibility in the areas described above. Trophic changes in the cornea (*neuropathic keratitis)* may occur. The corneal reflex is abolished: this must be tested with great care when corneal anaesthesia is suspected because of the risk of causing corneal ulceration.

The *second* or *maxillary division* supplies the cheek, the front of the temple, the lower eyelid and its conjunctival surface, the side of the nose, the

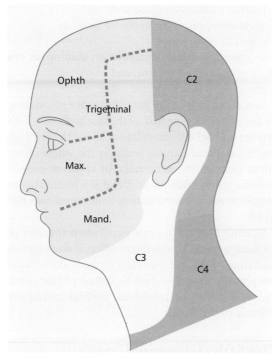

Fig. 12.16 Lateral view of the skin area supplied by the trigeminal (fifth) nerve and the second, third and fourth cervical segments.

upper lip, the upper teeth, the mucous membrane of the nose, the upper part of the pharynx, the roof of the mouth, part of the soft palate, the tonsils, and the medial inferior quadrant of the cornea. Lesions of the maxillary division lead to loss of sensation in the above areas and occasionally to loss of the palatal reflex.

The *third* or *mandibular division* supplies the lower part of the face, the lower lip, the ear, the tongue, and the lower teeth. It also supplies parasympathetic fibres to the salivary glands. The mandibular division is joined by the motor root and this innervates the muscles of mastication. The *motor root* originates from a small nucleus, medial to the main sensory nucleus, and partly also from nerve cells scattered around the cerebral aqueduct. It emerges at the side of the pons, just anterior to the sensory division, passes inferior to the trigeminal ganglion, and joins the mandibular division.

Lesions of the whole trigeminal nerve lead to loss of sensation in the skin and mucous membrane of the face and nasopharynx (see Fig. 12.16). The salivary, buccal and lacrimal secretions may be diminished and trophic ulcers may develop in the mouth, nose and cornea. Taste is spared, but lack of oral secretions may result in its subjective impairment. Weak-

ness of the muscles of mastication is often a prominent feature.

TESTING THE MOTOR FUNCTIONS

Ask the patient to clench their teeth: the temporal and masseter muscles should stand out with equal prominence on each side. This sign is better checked by palpation than by inspection. If there is paralysis on one side, the muscles on that side will fail to become prominent and, on opening the mouth, the jaw will deviate towards the paralysed side, being pushed over by the healthy lateral pterygoid muscles.

TESTING THE SENSORY FUNCTIONS

The sensory acuity of the area supplied (see Fig. 12.16) is tested in the usual way (page 324).

TESTING THE CORNEAL REFLEX

Twist a light wisp of cotton into a fine hair and lightly touch the lateral edge of the cornea at its conjunctival margin with the wisp, having asked the patient to gaze into the distance or at the ceiling. If the reflex is present the patient blinks. It is helpful to steady your hand by gently resting the little finger on the patient's cheek. The two sides should be compared. This can sometimes be done more easily by lightly blowing a puff of air into each cornea in turn. The cornea should *not* be wiped with the cotton and the central part of the cornea should *never* be touched, since to do so in the presence of corneal anaesthesia carries the risk of corneal ulceration and subsequent visual impairment.

The seventh (facial) nerve

ANATOMY

The course of the nerve fibres from the cortex to the nucleus of this nerve has already been described (page 269). The facial nucleus is situated in the pons lateral to the nucleus of the abducens nerve. On leaving the facial nucleus the fibres wind round the abducens nucleus and emerge medial to the vestibulocochlear nerve, between the olive and the restiform bodies.

The facial nerve itself then lies in close contact with the vestibulocochlear nerve and enters the internal auditory meatus with it, so that a lesion of one at this part often also affects the other. During its course through the temporal bone, in close proximity to the aditus of the tympanic antrum, it gives off a branch to the stapedius muscle. It is joined by the chorda tympani, which contains taste fibres from the anterior two-thirds of the tongue, at the geniculate ganglion. In this part of its course the nerve is vulnerable to trauma and oedema, since it is enclosed in a bony tube. It emerges at a point opposite the junction of the anterior border of the mastoid process with the ear, and spreads out on the side of the face to supply the facial muscles.

The facial nerve is almost entirely a motor nerve. It supplies all the muscles of the face and scalp, except the levator palpebrae superioris. It also supplies the platysma. The chorda tympani travels with the facial nerve during part of its course and taste may therefore be lost on the anterior two-thirds of the tongue when the proximal part of the nerve is damaged. There is sometimes a small area of altered cutaneous sensation at the auricle in such cases, representing the somatic afferent component of the facial nerve.

TASTE

The sense of taste should always be examined when a cranial nerve lesion is suspected. The nerve fibres subserving taste from the anterior two-thirds of the tongue pass from the lingual nerve into the chorda tympani and thence through the geniculate ganglion of the facial nerve and the nervus intermedius into the medulla oblongata. These taste fibres sometimes enter the brainstem in the maxillary division of the trigeminal nerve, rather than through the chorda tympani and the facial nerve, but this is rare. The taste fibres from the posterior third of the tongue enter the brainstem in the glossopharyngeal nerve.

All the taste fibres enter the tractus solitarius and relay in the nucleus of this tract. The ascending fibres pass via the thalamus to the temporal part of the post-central gyrus and to the amygdala. *Ageusia* or loss of taste occurs with lesions of the peripheral pathways or with centrally placed pontine lesions, which may involve the gustatory lemnisci. Loss of taste may result from lesions in any part of the peripheral and central course of the taste fibres.

To test the sense of taste, using strong solutions of sugar and common salt, and weak solutions of citric acid and quinine, as tests of 'sweet', 'salt', 'sour' and 'bitter' respectively. These are applied to the surface of the protruded tongue. The patient should be asked to indicate perception of the taste *before* the tongue is withdrawn in order to decide whether taste is disturbed anteriorly or posteriorly. After each test the mouth must be rinsed. The bitter quinine test should be applied last, as its effect is more lasting than that of the others. Both the anterior and posterior parts of the tongue should be tested when rele-

vant. Taste may also be assessed using a weak electrical stimulus.

In addition to loss of taste, one should always ask the patient whether there have been any abnormal taste sensations or hallucinations of taste. These may form the aura of an epileptic fit, especially in temporal lobe epilepsy.

MOTOR EFFECTS OF FACIAL NERVE LESIONS

These are usually obvious. The affected side of the face has lost its expression. The nasolabial fold is less pronounced, the furrows of the brow are smoothed out, the eye is more widely open than on the normal side and, when the patient smiles, the mouth is drawn towards the normal side. The patient is unable to whistle and food fragments collect between teeth and gums. Saliva, and any fluid that has been drunk, may escape from the affected angle of the mouth.

TESTING THE FACIAL NERVE

Five tests can be used to test for facial nerve lesions.

• Ask the patient to shut their eyes as tightly as possible. Note that the affected eye is either not closed at all or, if the eye is closed, the eyelashes are not so deeply buried in the face as on the healthy side. Try to open the eyes while the patient attempts to keep them closed. If the orbicularis oculi is acting normally, it should be almost impossible to open them against the patient's effort. The effect of screwing the eyes tightly shut causes the corners of the mouth to be drawn upwards. In paralysis of the lower part of the face, the corner on the affected side is either not drawn up at all, or not so much as on the healthy side.

• *Bell's phenomenon*, in which the eyeball rolls upwards during attempted forced eye closure, is a normal phenomenon which is preserved in facial palsies of lower motor neurone type. It is thus particularly obvious when eye closure is impossible in a patient with facial nerve palsy.

• Ask the patient to whistle. This is impossible.

• Ask the patient to smile or show the upper teeth. The mouth is then drawn to the healthy side.

• Ask the patient to inflate their mouth with air and blow out the cheeks. Tap with the finger in turn on each inflated cheek. Air can be made to escape from the mouth more easily on the weak or paralysed side.

• T st the sense of taste on the anterior part of the tongue (page 299).

Remember that *bilateral* facial weakness can be surprisingly difficult to recognize.

SIGNS OF PARALYSIS OF THE FACIAL NERVE IN DIFFERENT PARTS OF ITS COURSE

Lesions situated above the facial nucleus, in the nucleus, or distal to it, result in different types of facial weakness. Lesions above the facial nucleus cause *upper motor neurone* or *supranuclear facial palsies*, lesions in the nucleus cause *nuclear facial palsy*, and lesions distal to the nucleus cause *lower motor neurone* or infranuclear paralysis.

In *supranuclear paralysis* the lower part of the face is chiefly affected. This is because the muscles of the upper part of the face are bilaterally innervated. A unilateral lesion, therefore, will cause only partial paralysis of the upper part of the face, including eye closure, on the one side, but movements of the mouth on that side will appear much more severely affected. Sometimes a supranuclear lesion affects only the fibres concerned in emotional movement and this function should be assessed separately from voluntary movement. Taste is not affected in supranuclear lesions. Facial reflexes, elicited by lightly tapping the facial muscles around the mouth, are often increased in supranuclear lesions.

In *infranuclear paralysis* both the upper and lower parts of the face are equally involved. Infranuclear facial paralysis may be produced by a lesion of the nucleus or of the facial nerve itself. A lesion inside the facial canal—unless it is towards the outer end—involves the fibres of the chorda tympani and therefore also causes loss of taste sensation in the anterior two-thirds of the tongue. Because the stapedius muscle is paralysed, sounds on the side of the facial palsy may seem unusually loud (*hyperacusis*).

A lower motor neurone lesion, whether nuclear or infranuclear, causes atrophy of the facial muscles. Supranuclear lesions do not produce atrophy.

ABNORMAL FACIAL MOVEMENTS

The muscles supplied by the facial nerve are frequently affected by spasmodic (*synkinetic*) movements. These may involve all the facial muscles, or only groups of them. They occur most commonly as a result of aberrant regeneration of facial nerve fibres during partial recovery from an infranuclear (e.g. Bell's) lesion. Facial spasms of a different type occur in some patients with dystonia and in other extrapyramidal disorders, especially tardive dyskinesias following phenothiazine medication. They may also occur in multiple sclerosis and without evident cause in the syndrome of hemifacial spasm.

The eighth (vestibulocochlear) nerve

ANATOMY

This nerve consists of two sets of fibres. One supplies the cochlea and subserves hearing; the other supplies the labyrinth and semicircular canals and subserves equilibration, balance and sensations of bodily displacement. The *auditory* fibres, which arise from the cochlear ganglion, enter the brainstem at the lower border of the pons and are distributed to the dorsal and ventral cochlear nuclei.

The secondary auditory tracts, after partial decussation, terminate in the inferior colliculi and the medial geniculate bodies, and another system, that takes origin from these, passes through the internal capsule to the cortical centre for hearing, in the first and second temporosphenoidal gyri. Sounds received in one ear reach the opposite hemisphere of the brain, but owing to the partial decussation of the secondary auditory tracts neither unilateral cerebral nor brainstem lesions produce unilateral deafness.

The *vestibular* fibres originate in the vestibular ganglion, and terminate in a group of nuclei in the pons and medulla. The vestibular nerve is closely connected with the cerebellum. It also has a cerebral projection to the temporal lobe.

TESTS OF HEARING

See Chapter 9.

ABNORMAL AUDITORY SENSATIONS

The patient may complain of 'ringing in the ears' (*tinnitus*). The precise character of the sound varies in different cases. It may be of a humming, buzzing, hammering or whistling character. This symptom, although common, is almost never due to neurological disease.

Hyperacusis, a disorder in which even slight sounds are heard with painful intensity, sometimes occurs when there is paralysis of the stapedius muscle due to a facial nerve palsy. A similar phenomenon, *recruitment*, occurs in patients with sensorineural deafness due to damage to the cochlea, e.g. Ménière's syndrome (chapter 9).

Auditory hallucinations and *delusions* of voices are common in the non-organic psychoses, e.g. schizophrenia, but may also occur in organic psychoses. Hallucinations of voices may also occur in normal people. Other complex auditory hallucinations, e.g. music, sometimes arise as epileptic auras when there is a lesion in the temporal lobe.

VERTIGO

The patient will usually describe this as *giddiness* or *dizziness*. In vertigo, external objects seem to move round the patient. Ask if this is the case and, if so, in what direction the objects seem to move. Ask also whether the vertigo or giddiness causes loss of balance. The distinction between vertigo and giddiness is rarely of great importance. Both may occur in disease of the vestibular system, i.e. the ear, vestibulocochlear nerve, brainstem, or temporal lobe. The method of examination of this problem is described in Chapter 9.

Positional vertigo

In some patients vertigo is induced by certain head postures, or by sudden changes in head posture. The subjective sensation of rotational disequilibrium is accompanied by a rotary nystagmus in the primary position, often enhanced by gaze to one or other side. If this posture is reproduced during examination, for example by suddenly laying the patient in the supine position, the nystagmus and vertigo will develop either after a short delay (*benign positional vertigo,* associated with labyrinthine disease) or immediately (an indication of brainstem disease). It usually continues for only a few seconds. Benign positional vertigo can often be reproduced only once or twice in an examination (page 219).

The ninth (glossopharyngeal), tenth (vagus) and eleventh (accessory) nerves

ANATOMY

The glossopharyngeal, vagus and accessory nerves arise, in order from above downwards, in an elongated nucleus in the floor of the fourth ventricle. They emerge by several roots along the lateral aspect of the medulla, beginning rostrally in the groove between the olive and restiform bodies. The spinal part of the accessory nerve emerges from the lateral column of the cord, perhaps beginning as low as the sixth cervical root. It passes up through the foramen magnum to join its medullary part, and emerges with it through the jugular foramen. After emerging, its two divisions separate, the medullary or accessory portion joining the vagus nerve and supplying motor fibres to the larynx and pharynx. The spinal portion supplies the sternomastoid and the upper part of the trapezius muscle.

THE GLOSSOPHARYNEAL NERVE

The glossopharyngeal nerve is sensory from the posterior third of the tongue and the mucous membrane of the pharynx. It supplies motor fibres to the middle pharyngeal sphincter and the stylopharyngeus muscle. It contains taste fibres from the posterior third of the tongue.

The glossopharyngeal nerve is rarely damaged alone, but damage can best be diagnosed by examining the nerve's sensory and reflex functions. Loss of taste in the posterior part of the tongue may occur with a lesion of the trunk of the glossopharyngeal nerve.

Tickle the back of the pharynx, and note if reflex contraction occurs (*palatal reflex*). This is also a test of the vagus (below).

THE VAGUS NERVE

The vagus is motor for the soft palate (with the exception of the tensor palati), pharynx and larynx. It is sensory and motor for the respiratory passages, the heart and, through the parasympathetic ganglia, for most of the abdominal viscera. The fibres for the soft palate, pharynx and larynx take origin in the nucleus ambiguus, emerge in the upper roots of the accessory nerve, reach the pharyngeal plexus, and innervate the muscles of the palate, pharynx, and larynx. The visceromotor and the cardio-inhibitory fibres are derived from the dorsal nucleus of the vagus in the floor of the fourth ventricle. Damage to the vagus is obvious clinically only through its *palatine* and *laryngeal* branches.

The palate

Ask the patient whether there has been any regurgitation of fluids through the nose during swallowing. This is a common symptom in total paralysis of the soft palate, due to defective elevation of the palate during swallowing. In addition, the patient is unable to pronounce words which require complete closure of the nasopharynx. Thus 'egg' is sounded as 'eng', 'rub' becomes 'rum', and so on. In unilateral paralysis these symptoms are not so severe, or may even not be apparent. Difficulty in swallowing (*dysphagia*) particularly affects fluids in lower motor neurone lesions, but may be more marked for solids in upper motor neurone lesions.

For direct examination of the soft palate, place the patient facing the light with the mouth open and introduce a tongue depressor. The position of the uvula at rest is variable even in health. One must watch the movements of the palate during phonation. Ask the patient to say 'ah' and observe whether both sides of the palate arch upwards. If one side is paralysed, it will remain flat and immobile and the median raphe will be pulled towards the other side. In bilateral paralysis the whole palate remains motionless.

Remember that minor degrees of asymmetry of the palate and of the tongue occur as part of a hemiparesis due to an upper motor neurone lesion. This is not what is meant by palatal palsy since then the lesion is invariably of lower motor neurone type.

The larynx

The *superior laryngeal* branch of the vagus contains sensory nerve fibres from the larynx above the level of the true vocal cords, and motor fibres which innervate the cricothyroid muscle. Unilateral damage to the nerve is usually symptomless. Bilateral paralysis causes the vocal cords to be relaxed. The voice is therefore hoarse and deep and the utterance of high notes is impossible.

The *recurrent laryngeal* branch supplies sensation to the larynx below the level of the vocal cords and motor fibres to all the laryngeal muscles *except* the cricothyroid. Paralysis leads to characteristic laryngoscopic features (see page 223). *The speech is characteristically blurred and ineffectual* and the patient cannot cough clearly ('bovine cough'). Bilateral paralysis may cause serious stridor or even respiratory obstruction because the paralysed cords lie in partial adduction, thus partially blocking the airway.

THE ACCESSORY NERVE

The accessory nerve is purely motor in function, contributing to the innervation of the larynx and pharynx as well as the sternomastoid and trapezius muscles. The spinal part of the nerve dips below the sternomastoid muscle about 2 cm below the tip of the mastoid process and re-emerges from underneath that muscle at about the middle of its posterior border.

Paralysis of the upper part of the *trapezius* is demonstrated by asking the patient to shrug his or her shoulders while the examiner presses downward on them. Paralysis of the *sternomastoid* causes weakness of rotation of the chin towards the opposite side.

The twelfth (hypoglossal) nerve

ANATOMY

The hypoglossal nerve arises from its nucleus in the lower part of the floor of the fourth ventricle, close to the midline. It emerges between the anterior pyra-

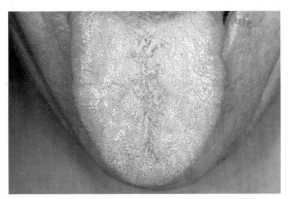

Fig. 12.17 Wasting of the tongue. The atrophy is slightly more marked on the right than the left in this patient with motor neurone disease. The tongue was fasciculating.

mid and the olive. It is a purely motor nerve, supplying the tongue and the depressors of the hyoid bone.

TEST

Ask the patient to put out the tongue as far as possible. If the hypoglossal is paralysed, the tongue is pushed over to the paralysed side instead of being protruded straight. Be careful not to mistake an apparent deviation of the tongue, really due to the mouth being twisted to one side, for a real deviation. Such an apparent deviation occurs in facial paralysis. Ask the patient to move the tongue from side to side, and to lick each cheek with it; observe whether this can be done freely. Strength may also be assessed by pressing against the tongue with a finger as the patient protrudes it into each cheek in turn. Note whether there is any *wasting* of the tongue (Fig. 12.17), and whether there is any tremor or fasciculation of it. The presence of wasting indicates that the lesion is either nuclear or infranuclear (lower motor neurone). *Fasciculation* should be assessed with the tongue relaxed in the mouth, not when protruded. *Tremor* of the tongue is common in Parkinson's disease, either when the tongue is at rest or protruded.

Motor functions

The motor system should be examined with the following aspects of motor function in mind.

- Movement and strength
- Bulk of muscles
- Tone of muscles
- Reflexes
- Gait
- Involuntary movements.

(a)

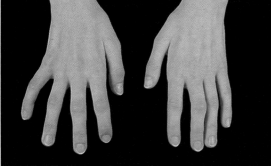

(b)

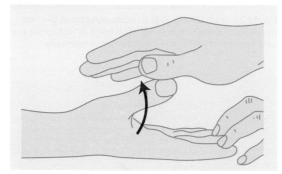

Fig. 12.18 Wasting of the small hand muscles in a chronic neuropathy. (a) There is marked wasting of the abductor pollicis brevis and (b) guttering of the dorsal surface of the hand indicating atrophy of the dorsal interossei.

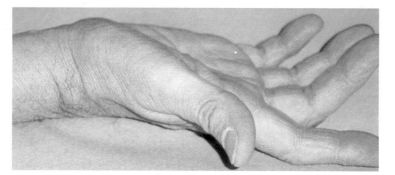

Fig. 12.19 Testing the abductor pollicis brevis.

Fig. 12.20 Atrophy of the thenar eminence.

Strength of muscles

Much the quickest and most reliable method of making a quick or preliminary assessment is to watch the patient walking, standing up from lying and sitting positions, and dressing or undressing, and lightly jumping or hopping. These movements require proximal and distal strength and co-ordination of a considerable degree and much can be learnt by observing them carefully. The strength of individual muscles should then be assessed more formally. Each movement made during this assessment is tested by comparison with the examiner's own strength or by comparison with what the examiner judges to be normal in a person of comparable build to the patient. It therefore requires practice and experience. Very simple requests produce better results than long explanations: a demonstration or gesture is often more effective than any verbal explanation. Remember that most patients have no knowledge of anatomy.

TESTING THE MUSCLES OF THE UPPER LIMB

Abductor pollicis brevis. This muscle (see Fig. 12.18a and b) is supplied by the median nerve, which is commonly damaged by compression in the carpal tunnel at the wrist (*carpal tunnel syndrome*). The patient is asked to abduct the thumb in a plane at right angles to the palmar aspect of the index finger, against the resistance of the examiner's own thumb. The muscle can be seen and felt to contract (see Fig. 12.19). Atrophy of the thenar eminence (Fig. 12.20) is often evident.

Opponens pollicis. Ask the patient to touch the tip of the little finger with the point of the thumb. Oppose the movement with your thumb or index finger (see Fig. 12.21).

First dorsal interosseous (see Figs 12.22, 12.23 and

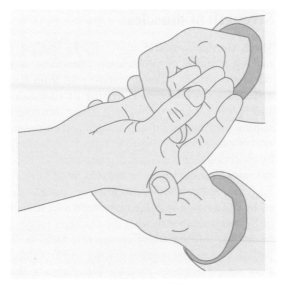

Fig. 12.21   Testing the opponens pollicis.

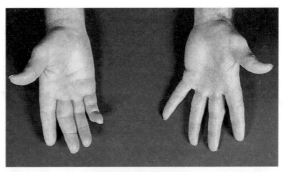

Fig. 12.22   Right ulnar nerve palsy showing marked atrophy of the left first dorsal interosseous muscle and flexion of the little finger. The left hand is normal.

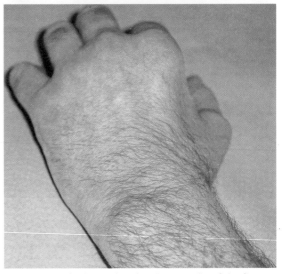

Fig. 12.23   Left ulnar palsy, showing atrophy of the first dorsal interosseous muscle with the hand at rest, often the best posture in which to recognize the abnormality.

12.24). Ask the patient to abduct the index finger against your resistance.

Interossei and lumbricals (see Fig. 12.25). Test the patient's ability to flex their metacarpophalangeal joints and to extend the distal interphalangeal joints. The interossei also adduct and abduct the fingers. When these muscles are paralysed and power is retained in the long flexors and extensors of the two fingers, as in ulnar nerve palsy, a 'claw-hand' deformity is produced. The first phalanges are over-extended and the distal two are flexed. The fingers are slightly separated (Fig. 12.18).

Flexors of the fingers. Ask the patient to squeeze your fingers. Allow the patient to squeeze only your index and middle fingers—this is sufficient to assess strength of grip without them painfully crushing your fingers (see Fig. 12.26a–d).

Extensors of the wrist. Ask the patient to make a fist, a movement which results in firm contraction of both the flexors and extensors of the wrist, and try forcibly to flex the wrist against this effort to maintain the patient's posture. It should be almost impossible to overcome the wrist extensors of a healthy man or woman. The wrist flexors can be similarly tested (see Fig. 12.27).

Slight weakness of the extensors of the wrist may be elicited by asking the patient to grasp something firmly in their hand. If the extensors are weak the wrist becomes flexed as they do so, because the flexor muscles are then stronger than the extensors.

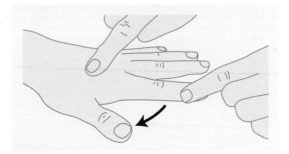

Fig. 12.24   Testing the first dorsal interosseous muscle.

Weakness or paralysis of the extensors of the wrist, as in radial nerve palsy, leads to *wrist-drop*.

Flexors of the wrist. Ask the patient to squeeze your fingers. Allow the patient to make a fist, and try to overcome wrist flexion (see Fig. 12.28).

Brachioradialis. Place the arm midway between the

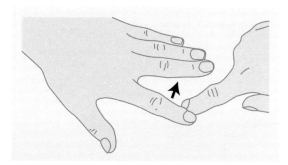

Fig. 12.25   Testing the first palmar interosseous muscle.

(a)

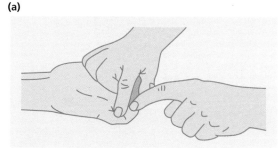

(b)

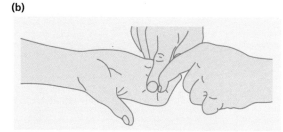

(c)

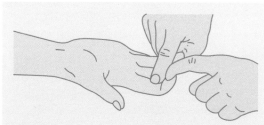

(d)

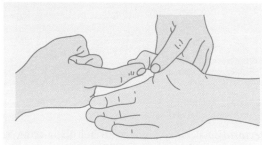

Fig. 12.26   Testing (a) flexor digitorum profundus III and IV; (b) flexor digitorum sublimis; (c) flexor digitorum profundus I and II; (d) flexor pollicis longus.

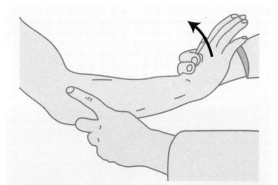

Fig. 12.27   Testing the extensor carpi radialis longus.

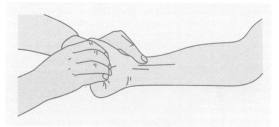

Fig. 12.28   Testing the flexor carpi radialis.

prone and supine positions; then ask the patient to bend up the forearm, whilst you oppose the movement by grasping the hand. The muscle, if healthy, will be seen and felt to stand out prominently at its upper part.

Biceps. Ask the patient to bend up the forearm against resistance, with the forearm in full supination. The muscle will stand out clearly (see Fig. 12.29).

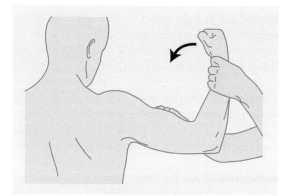

Fig. 12.29   Testing the biceps.

Triceps. Ask the patient to straighten out their forearm against your resistance (see Fig. 12.30a and b).

(a)

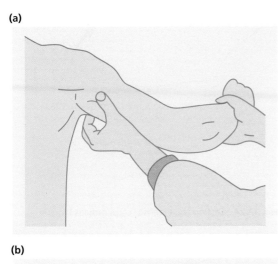

(b)

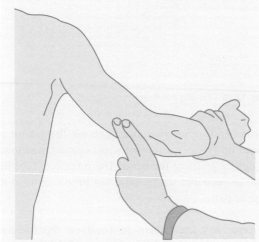

Fig. 12.30   Testing the triceps: (a) long head; (b) whole muscle.

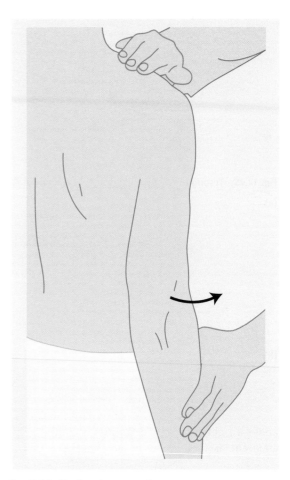

Fig. 12.31   Testing the supraspinatus.

Supraspinatus. Ask the patient to lift their arm straight out at right angles to their side. The first 30 degrees of the movement is carried out by the supraspinatus. The remaining 60 degrees is produced by the *deltoid* (see Fig. 12.31).

Deltoid. The anterior and posterior fibres help to draw the abducted arm forwards and backwards respectively. The middle fibres abduct the shoulder (see supraspinatus, above) (see Fig. 12.32).

Infraspinatus. Ask the patient to tuck the elbow into the side with the forearm flexed to a right angle. Then ask the patient to rotate the limb outwards against your resistance, the elbow being held against the side throughout. The muscle can be seen and felt to contract (see Fig. 12.33).

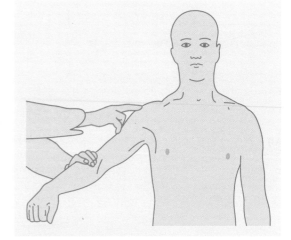

Fig. 12.32   Testing the deltoid.

Pectorals. Ask the patient to stretch their arms out in front, and then to clap their hands together while you endeavour to hold them apart (see Fig. 12.34).

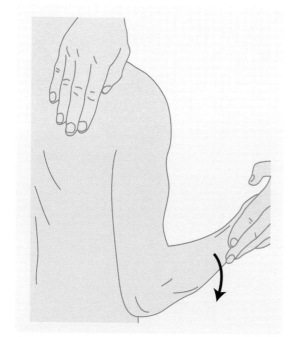

Fig. 12.33 Testing the infraspinatus.

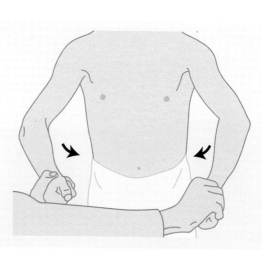

Fig. 12.34 Testing the pectoralis major.

Serratus anterior. When this muscle is paralysed the scapula is 'winged', with the vertebral border projecting. The patient is unable to elevate the arm above a right angle, the deformity becoming more apparent as they try to do so. Pushing forwards with the hands against resistance, such as a wall, also brings out the deformity (see Figs 12.35 and 12.36).

Latissimus dorsi. Ask the patient to clasp their hands behind their back while you, standing behind the patient, offer passive resistance to the downward and backward movement. Alternatively, the two posterior axillary folds can be felt as the patient coughs (see Fig. 12.37).

TESTING THE MUSCLES OF THE TRUNK

Weakness of the muscles of the abdomen is shown by the patient's inability to sit up in bed from the supine position without the aid of the arms. *Babinski's 'rising up sign'* consists in making the patient lie supine with the legs extended and rise up without using their hands. In spastic paralysis of a leg the affected limb will rise first, but in hysterical paralysis this does not occur.

Paralysis of a portion of the anterior abdominal wall can be detected by the displacement of the umbilicus that occurs when the patient attempts to lift up their head from the pillow against resistance.

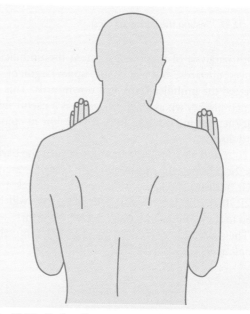

Fig. 12.35 Testing the serratus anterior.

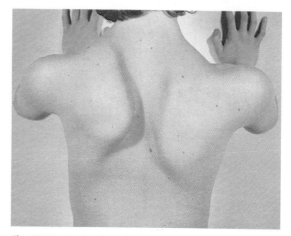

Fig. 12.36 Testing for winging of the scapulae.

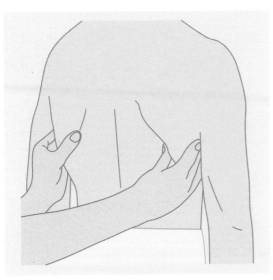

Fig. 12.37 Testing the latissimus dorsi.

With paralysis of the lower segment the umbilicus moves upwards, but when the upper segment is affected the umbilicus is pulled downwards. This is sometimes known as *Beevor's sign*: it is a useful sign since it may indicate the level of a lesion in spinal cord disease.

To test the *erector spinae* and muscles of the back, ask the patient to lie prone, and then to try to extend their head from the bed by extending the neck and back. If the back muscles are healthy, they will be seen to stand out prominently during this effort.

The method of detecting paralysis of the *diaphragm* is described on page 159.

(a)

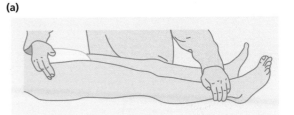

(b)

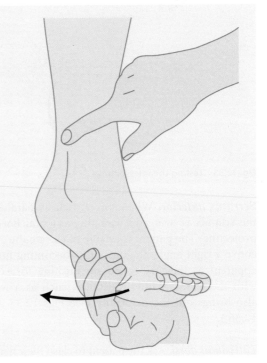

(c)

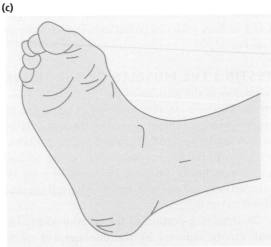

Fig. 12.39 Testing (a) tibialis posterior; (b) peroneus longus and brevis; (c) small muscles of the foot.

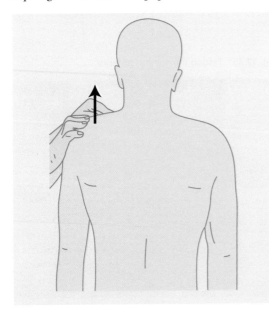

Fig. 12.38 Testing the trapezius.

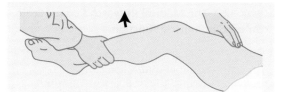

Fig. 12.40   Testing the quadriceps femoris.

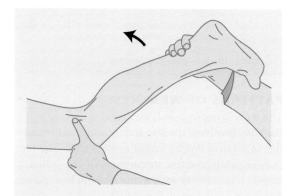

Fig. 12.41   Testing the hamstring muscles.

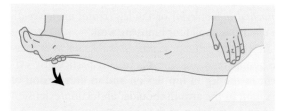

Fig. 12.42   Testing the adductors of the thigh.

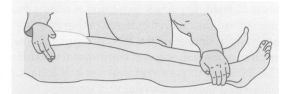

Fig. 12.43   Testing the gluteus medius and minimus, and tensor fasciae latae.

The upper part of the *trapezius* is tested by asking the patient to shrug their shoulders while you try to press them down from behind. Its lower part can be tested by asking the patient to approximate the shoulder blades (see Fig. 12.38).

The cranial musculature is described above.

TESTING THE MUSCLES OF THE LOWER LIMB

The *intrinsic muscles of the foot* are difficult to examine (see Figs 12.39–12.43). When the interossei are

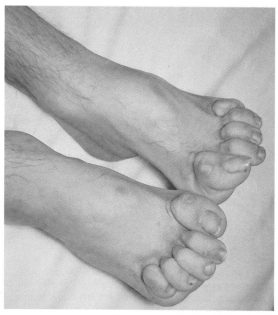

Fig. 12.44   Pes cavus, with clawing of the toes in a patient with familial neuropathy. This patient had Refsum's disease and the peripheral nerves were slightly enlarged.

weakened or paralysed a foot deformity may develop. A similar deformity may develop in patients with spastic hemiparesis of very long duration; this is due to a form of dystonia and not primarily to muscular weakness. In familial peripheral neuropathies a hollow wasted foot deformity '*pes cavus*' is characteristic (Fig. 12.44).

Dorsiflexion and *plantar flexion* of the feet and toes are tested by asking the patient to elevate or depress the part against resistance.

Extensors of the knee. Bend up the knee, and then, pressing with your hand against the shin, ask the patient to try to straighten it out again. This muscle is stronger than your arm. Look for atrophy of the quadriceps compartment musculature (Fig. 12.45).

Flexors of the knee. Raise a leg up from the bed, supporting the thigh with your left hand and holding the ankle with your right. Then ask the patient to bend the knee against your resistance. You should not be able to overcome this muscle.

Extensors of the hip. With the knee extended, lift the patient's foot off the bed, and ask them to push it down against your resistance. This is normally a very strong movement and should be impossible to overcome.

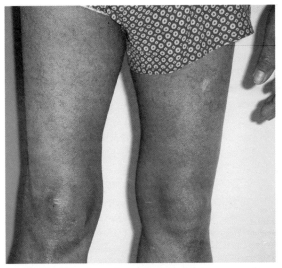

Fig. 12.45 There is wasting of the thigh extensor muscles, particularly evident in the medial component of the quadriceps group. The small scar on the left side is from a muscle biopsy. The patient had limb girdle muscular dystrophy.

Flexors of the thigh. With the leg extended ask the patient to raise the leg off the bed against resistance. Alternatively, the related movement of flexion of the thigh, with the thigh already flexed to a right angle, can be tested.

Adductors of the thigh. Abduct the limb and then ask the patient to bring it back to the midline against resistance.

Abductors of the thigh. Place the patient's legs together and ask them to separate them against resistance.

Rotators of the thigh. With the lower limb extended on the bed, ask the patient to roll it outwards or inwards against resistance.

GRADING OF STRENGTH

The Medical Research Council Scale is used to grade muscle function (see Box 12.9). This scale is clinically based, easy to reproduce, but essentially nonlinear. Grades 1, 2 and 3 are similar, but grades 4 and 5 contain a wide variation in strength. The MRC scale was devised to evaluate muscles during recovery from peripheral nerve palsies in war-time, and therefore emphasizes assessment of very weak muscles. Several quantitative techniques are now available that measure force or torque in contracting muscles, reflecting *isometric* and *isokinetic* strength.

PATTERNS OF WEAKNESS

The term *hemiplegia* indicates paralysis of one side of the body involving the arm and leg, and usually also of the face (*facio-brachio-crural hemiparesis*). The term *crossed paralysis* refers to paralysis of the ipsilateral cranial musculature with a contralateral hemiparesis; it is a sign of brainstem disease. The term *paraplegia* is applied to a paralysis of both legs; the term *monoplegia* to a paralysis of one limb, which may be the arm (*brachial monoplegia*) or the leg (*crural monoplegia*). In *quadriplegia* all four limbs are weak.

In weakness due to a *corticospinal lesion*, as in spastic hemiparesis, weakness is usually particularly evident in the leg in hip flexion and in dorsiflexion of the foot; in the arm in shoulder abduction/extension and in dorsiflexion of the wrist; and in the face, in a supranuclear distribution. The face and arm, or the leg, may be particularly involved. Slowness and clumsiness of rapid, fine finger movement is often a feature. Antagonistic movements, such as hip extension, and plantar flexion of the foot, are strikingly less involved in the early stages of corticospinal weakness. The characteristic pattern of weakness in this clinical syndrome is thus of great value in diagnosis.

The detection of hemiplegia in a patient who is comatose may be difficult. However, if the paralysis is of recent onset, one can usually detect hypotonia in the paralysed limbs. If the arm, for example, is raised from the side and allowed to drop, it falls, if it is paralysed, as if it did not belong to the patient; the sound arm also falls, but not in such an utterly limp fashion. The face is asymmetrical, the angle of the mouth more open on the paralysed side, and the affected cheek moves loosely outwards and inwards with respiration. The abdominal and tendon reflexes may be absent on both sides, but an extensor plantar response can usually be obtained on the hemiplegic side (see section on reflexes, page 315).

MYASTHENIC WEAKNESS

In *myasthenia gravis* (Fig. 12.46), weakness, which commonly affects the external ocular and bulbar muscles more than the rest of the skeletal muscu-lature, is characteristically exacerbated or pro-voked by repeated contraction of the affected muscles. The degree of detectable weakness there-fore varies during the course of the day. This is referred to as myasthenic weakness. In the myas-thenic syndrome (*Lambert–Eaton syndrome*) there is weakness initially, but during contraction of a muscle or movement an increase in strength occurs at first, followed by weakness if exertion is continued. This is often quite difficult to detect and the diagnosis is usually made by electromyog-raphy (EMG). Lambert–Eaton syndrome occurs in association with small cell carcinoma of the bronchus, but may also occur as an idiopathic autoimmune disorder.

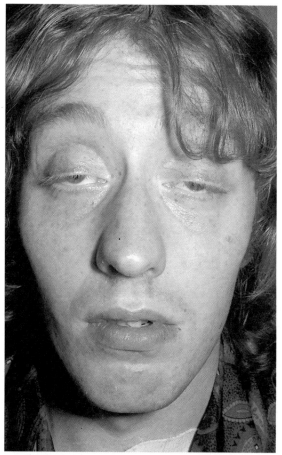

Fig. 12.46 Myasthenia gravis. There is bilateral ptosis with resting divergence of the eyes and lower facial weakness, so that the mouth and jaw hang open. There is compensatory overactivity of the frontalis muscles in an effort to open the eyelids.

NEUROGENIC WEAKNESS

In lower motor neurone lesions weakness is associat-ed with marked muscular atrophy, and with reduced tone and absent tendon reflexes. The distribution of the weakness and atrophy is important in diagnosis (Figs 12.47 and 12.48) since it may be *localized*, as in

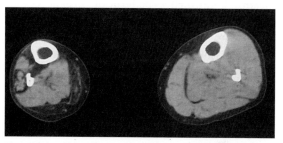

Fig. 12.47 Old poliomyelitis. CT scan. Wasting of the muscles of the right leg (to the left of the picture). Note that all the muscles are wasted compared with the normal left side. Also, the tibia and femur are smaller, indicating that the wasting must have been present since childhood.

Fig. 12.48 Type 3 spinal muscular atrophy. CT scan. There is atrophy, fibrosis, and fat replacement of most of the muscles of the thighs and the abnormality is symmetrical. The patient is immobile and has become obese.

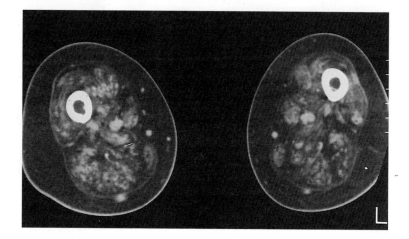

peripheral nerve (see Figs 12.18 and 12.22) or root disease, or *generalized,* as in anterior horn cell disease, e.g. motor neurone disease. In the latter and, to a lesser extent in other types of neurogenic weakness, *fasciculations* may occur. These are spontaneous contractions of groups of muscle fibres, representing enlarged re-innervated motor units or parts of such motor units. They vary in distribution and frequency, and may also occur in fatigued normal subjects. They originate from abnormal generator sites in the peripheral nervous system. In chronic neurogenic weakness *action fasciculation* may be noted. This occurs during initial contraction of a muscle; the muscle is seen to undergo rhythmic fasciculation-like contraction as motor units are recruited into the muscular effort. Fatigue is a common feature of neurogenic weakness, but also occurs in some myopathies.

PERIPHERAL NEUROPATHY

When there is a generalized disease of the peripheral nerves, whether affecting axons or myelin sheaths, a distinctive pattern of weakness and, often, of sensory disturbance is found (Box 12.10). In disease of individual peripheral nerves (*mononeuropathies*) the clinical features are restricted to the distribution of the affected nerve (Box 12.4), and in brachial plexus lesions (Box 12.5) to the wider motor and sensory distribution of the cervical roots.

BOX 12.10 Peripheral neuropathy; major clinical features of polyneuropathies.

- Symmetrical distal weakness and wasting
- Symmetrical distal sensory impairment
- Loss of tendon reflexes
   generalized loss in demyelinating neuropathies
   distal loss in axonal (dying back) neuropathies
- Tremor of outstretched fingers in chronic neuropathies
- Pes cavus in early-onset, familial neuropathies
- Enlargement of peripheral nerves in chronic demyelinating neuropathies, and in leprosy (Hansen's disease)
- Distal burning pain in small fibre neuropathies, e.g. diabetes mellitus

---

MYOPATHIC WEAKNESS

In myopathies (Fig. 12.49), dystrophies (Fig. 12.50) and polymyositis muscle weakness is strikingly proximal, usually symmetrical and often affects the pelvifemoral muscles more severely than the pectoral girdle muscles. Affected muscles are atrophic and may feel firmer than normal. In Duchenne muscular

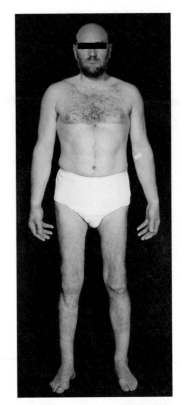

Fig. 12.49 Myopathy due to adult onset acid maltase deficiency (type III glycogenosis). There is atrophy of proximal muscles, usually involving the pelvic femoral and pectoral girdle muscles, e.g. thighs and deltoids. In this disease the diaphragm is particularly affected.

dystrophy pseudohypertrophy of some weak muscles develops (Fig. 12.51). Fasciculations do not occur in myopathic weakness.

MYOTONIA

In certain inherited muscular disorders, of which *myotonic dystrophy* is the commonest, relaxation is

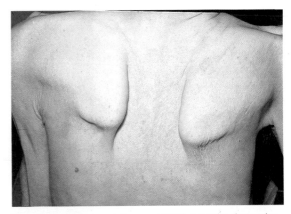

Fig. 12.50 Facioscapulohumeral (FSH) muscular dystrophy. Note the wasted, winged scapulae and the severe wasting of the left upper arm musculature.

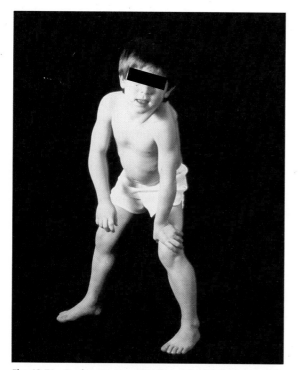

Fig. 12.51 Duchenne muscular dystrophy (Xp21 dystrophy). There is pseudohypertrophy of the weak muscles, e.g. the calves and deltoids. The child is 'climbing up himself' with legs widely placed as he gets up from the sitting position to the standing position. This is Gowers' sign.

impaired following contraction of a muscle. The phenomenon of myotonia is most evident when the muscles are cold and it is therefore often best demonstrated in the hand. Ask the patient to grip your hand firmly and then to let go suddenly. The grasp is maintained for a moment and then is slowly and gradually released. Myotonia can be demonstrated in the tongue and in other muscles, e.g. the thenar eminence, by lightly striking the muscle with a small patellar hammer. A dimple of contraction appears that relaxes only slowly.

Bulk of muscles

Muscle bulk (Fig. 12.52) is best estimated clinically by inspection and palpation. Wasted or atrophic muscles are not only smaller, but also softer and more flabby than normal when they are contracted. When muscular wasting is accompanied by fibrosis, as in muscular dystrophy or polymyositis, the muscles feel hard and inelastic. They may become shortened so that it is difficult to stretch them passively to a normal degree—*contractures*. Contractures may also occur as a result of prolonged hypertonia in a group of muscles.

Muscular atrophy is not only caused by neurological disorders. Generalized muscular wasting is seen in cachexia of any cause. Localized muscle atrophy may be due to injury or disease of a joint; this occurs, for example, in the quadriceps in patients with diseases of the knee. In such instances strength is well-preserved in relation to the degree of muscular wasting. Some patients, especially boys with Duchenne muscular dystrophy (Fig. 12.51), develop large muscles (*pseudohypertrophy*) due to pathological changes in the muscles themselves. The calves, buttocks and infraspinati are particularly affected. These enlarged muscles are weak in spite of their size. True hypertrophy of muscles occurs in response to continued excessive workloads as in certain occupations, or following athletic training. It may also occur in certain myotonic disorders. Hypertrophy and atrophy can be quantitatively assessed by transverse CT or MR imaging of muscles, or by ultrasound studies.

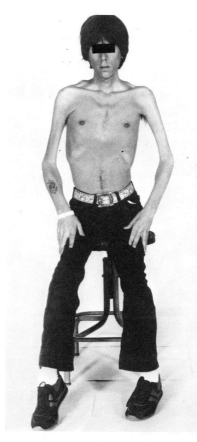

Fig. 12.52 Muscular atrophy due to facioscapulohumeral muscular dystrophy. Note the atrophy of the limb and shoulder muscles, especially the biceps and deltoids. Thinning of the thigh musculature can be recognized even through the trousers.

Tone of muscles

Muscular tone is a state of tension or contraction found in healthy muscles. An increase in tone is called *hypertonia* and a reduction *hypotonia*. The degree of tone is estimated by handling the limbs and moving them passively at their various joints. The maintenance of tone is dependent on a spinal reflex arc. Afferent fibres from the primary and secondary endings of the muscle spindles enter the spinal cord and synapse with the anterior horn cells, from which efferent fibres arise and pass to the muscles. Tone is diminished or lost if this reflex arc is damaged. *Hypotonia* therefore occurs in lower motor neurone lesions, in lesions of the afferent sensory pathways, as in tabes, and in cerebellar disease, in which suprasegmental mechanisms are abnormal. Tone may be reduced in sleep and by certain drugs.

Muscle tone is mainly regulated by corticospinal and extrapyramidal pathways. *Hypertonia* following lesions of the corticospinal system (upper motor neurone lesions) is termed *spasticity*. Spasticity is a term which has a precise meaning. It describes a state of increased tone which is of 'clasp-knife' type when the limb is fairly rapidly flexed or extended. That is, the resistance to stretch increases during the applied stretch, and then suddenly gives way, like opening a pen-knife. These are the lengthening and shortening reactions described by Sherrington. Spasticity is therefore a form of rigidity which is *stretch-sensitive*. Moreover it can usually be shown that the degree of increased tone developed during any given passive stretch is velocity-dependent, i.e. it is proportional to the speed of the applied stretch.

Spasticity due to cerebral or brainstem lesions has a characteristic distribution shown by the typical posture of the limbs in such patients. The upper limbs are held in flexion and the lower limbs in extension with the feet in plantar flexion (physiological extension). Thus in the arms the flexor muscles are mainly involved but, in the legs, the extensor muscles are predominantly affected. This distribution is most evident in the erect posture, and may even be reversed if the patient is placed head down, showing that it is driven by labyrinthine/vestibular afferent activity.

Hypertonia resulting from disease of the basal ganglia is termed *extrapyramidal rigidity*. The resistance to passive movement in this disorder is regularly or irregularly variable and is aptly described as like a lever rubbing on the teeth of a cogwheel (*cogwheel rigidity*). It can usually be enhanced by asking the patient to contract another muscle, e.g. to clench the fist on the opposite side (*Jendrassik's manoeuvre*). In the commonest extrapyramidal disorder, *Parkinson's disease*, the hypertonia is accompanied by a general attitude of flexion of the limbs and trunk. This type of rigidity is often accompanied by *akinesia*, a tendency for the patient not to spontaneously move the affected limb or part of the body. Parkinson himself termed this 'a peculiar disinclination to move' (Fig. 12.53). Sometimes a plastic type of rigidity is found in which the resistance developed to passive movement is uniform during all phases of the applied movement. This is *paratonic rigidity* or *gegenhalten* (literally: 'go-stop'). It is found in catatonic states and in patients with clouded or confused consciousness from any cause, especially dementia. It is not simply evidence of lack of co-operation. Its physiological basis is unknown. In *hysterical rigidity* the resistance to passive movement increases in proportion to the effort applied by the examiner. The increased resistance is usually developed in a characteristically irregular, jerky fashion.

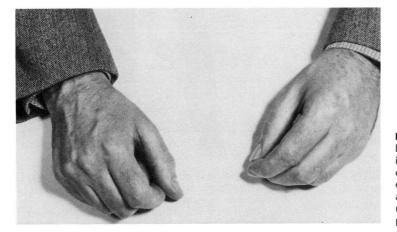

Fig. 12.53 Parkinson's disease. The left hand is held partially flexed and immobile. This has resulted in slight oedema of the skin of the hand causing the joints and tendons to appear indistinct. Since the hand is not used, its venous return is not as prominent as on the other side.

When the muscles are *hypotonic,* there is little or no resistance to passive movement of the limb and when handled or shaken the unsupported part flops about inertly. Hypotonic muscles are abnormally soft to palpation. The outstretched hypotonic upper limb may assume an abnormal posture, as in cerebellar disease or chorea. It is hyperextended at the elbow, the forearm is overpronated, the wrist flexed, and the fingers hyperextended at the metacarpophalangeal joints.

Reflexes

TENDON REFLEXES

If the tendon of a lightly stretched muscle is struck a single sharp blow with a soft rubber hammer (thus suddenly stretching the muscle and exciting a synchronous volley of afferent impulses from the primary sensory endings of the muscle spindles in the stretched muscle), the muscle contracts briefly. This is the *monosynaptic stretch reflex.* It is a test of the integrity of the afferent and efferent pathways, and of the excitability of the anterior horn cells in the spinal segment of the stretched muscle. Properly performed, examination of the tendon reflexes offers a reliable and reproducible method of assessment of this system of neurones and their higher connections. It is therefore very important to become skilled in the technique for eliciting these reflexes.

Always use the same type of hammer; always examine these reflexes in the same manner, standing on the same side of the bed; always make sure the patient is warm and comfortable; and reassure him or her that the hammer is soft and not an offensive weapon. When examining the tendon reflexes in the legs, care taken to allow the patient's genitalia to be properly covered is repaid by more easily elicitable reflexes. The patient should be asked to relax or to 'let the muscles go to sleep'. Some neurologists prefer to assess the tendon reflexes with the patient sitting on the edge of the couch facing the examiner. However, they are more usually tested with the patient supine on a couch.

Knee jerk

The patellar hammer derives its name from its invention as an instrument for eliciting this reflex, the first tendon reflex to become a regular part of the neurological examination. The knee jerk consists of contraction of the quadriceps when the patellar tendon is tapped. The spinal segments concerned are the second, third and fourth lumbar. It is best tested with the patient supine. The examiner's hand is passed under the knee to be tested and placed upon the opposite knee; the knee to be tested rests on the dorsum of the observer's wrist. The patellar tendon is struck midway between its origin and insertion. Following the blow there will be a brief extension of the knee from contraction of the quadriceps. The reflex can sometimes be more easily elicited with the patient sitting up, the legs dangling freely over the edge of the bed.

The briskness of the knee jerk varies greatly in different individuals. In health it is hardly ever entirely absent. Sometimes, as in the case of the other tendon reflexes, it cannot be elicted without applying *reinforcement* (Jendrassik's manoeuvre). This is done by asking the patient to make a strong voluntary muscular effort with the upper limbs; for example, to hook the fingers of the two hands together and then to pull them against one another as hard as possible, or to make a fist with the ipsilateral hand. While the patient is doing this, a further attempt is made to elicit the knee jerk. Reinforcement acts by increasing the excitability of the anterior horn cells and by increasing the sensitivity of the muscle spindle primary sensory endings to stretch (by increased gamma fusimotor drive).

Ankle jerk

Place the lower limb on the bed so that it lies everted and slightly flexed. Then with one hand, slightly dorsiflex the foot so as to stretch the Achilles tendon and, with the other hand, strike the tendon on its posterior surface. A sharp contraction of the calf muscles results. This reflex can also be conveniently elicited when the patient is kneeling on a chair. It depends upon the first and second sacral segments.

Triceps jerk

Flex the elbow and allow the forearm to rest across the patient's chest. Tap the triceps tendon just above the olecranon. The triceps contracts. The reflex depends upon the sixth and seventh cervical segments. Care must be taken to strike the triceps *tendon* and not the belly of the muscle itself. All muscles show a certain amout of irritability to direct mechanical stimuli; but this is a direct response, not a stretch reflex.

Biceps jerk

Flex the elbow to a right angle and place the forearm in a semipronated position; then place your own thumb or index finger on the biceps tendon and strike it with the patellar hammer. The biceps contracts. The fifth and sixth cervical segments of the cord are concerned in this reflex.

Supinator jerk

A blow upon the styloid process of the radius stretches the supinator causing supination of the elbow. This reflex depends on the fifth and six cervical segments.

With lesions at this level the supinator reflex or biceps reflex may be lost but, when it is tested, brisk flexion of the fingers is seen. This phenomenon is known as *inversion* of the reflex and it is evidence of hyperexcitability of the anterior horn cells below the C5/6 level. The responsible lesion is in the C5/6 spinal segments.

Jaw jerk

Ask the patient to open the mouth, but not too widely. Place one finger firmly on the chin and then tap it suddenly with the other hand as in percussion. A contraction of the muscles that close the jaw results. This jerk is sometimes absent in health and is increased in upper motor neurone lesions at a level above the trigeminal nerve nuclei.

Clonus

The phenomenon of clonus is often elicitable, especially at the ankle, when the tendon reflexes are exaggerated as a result of a corticospinal lesion. To test for *ankle clonus* bend the patient's knee slightly and support it with one hand, grasp the forepart of the foot with the other hand and suddenly dorsiflex the foot. The sudden stretch causes a brief reflex contraction of the calf muscles, which then relax; continued stretch causes a regular oscillation of contraction and relaxation which is called *clonus*. *Sustained clonus* is abnormal, and is evidence of an upper motor neurone lesion. It is then always associated with increased tendon reflexes and an extensor plantar response.

Unsustained clonus may occur in healthy persons, particularly in those who are very tense or anxious; in these subjects the plantar responses are flexor.

GRADING THE REFLEXES

The tendon reflexes may be graded:

0 Absent
1 Present (as a normal ankle jerk)
2 Brisk (as a normal knee jerk)
3 Very brisk
4 Clonus.

ABNORMAL TENDON REFLEXES

The tendon reflexes are diminished or absent with lesions affecting the afferent pathways, the anterior horn cells themselves, or the efferent pathways (lesions of the lower motor neurone). For example, in tabes dorsalis the posterior roots are affected; in poliomyelitis the anterior horn cells are diseased; and in most peripheral neuropathies both the efferent (motor) and afferent (sensory) nerve fibres are abnormal. In all these conditions tendon reflexes may be absent.

Hyperreflexia occurs with upper motor neurone lesions at all levels above the anterior horn cells. It may also occur with anxiety or nervousness, in thyrotoxicosis and as a manifestation of tetanus. Hyperreflexia is therefore only of pathological significance if it is asymmetrical or if it is associated with other signs of an upper motor neurone lesion.

In cerebellar disease the reflexes may have a characteristic *pendular* quality. This is clearly evident only when there is a severe cerebellar ataxia and it is not a sign of diagnostic importance. It may be considered a manifestation of hypotonia.

In myxoedema both the contraction and relaxation phases of the tendon reflex may be prolonged. This is sometimes called, somewhat confusingly, a *myotonic reflex*. It is also found in hypothermic patients. The relaxation time of the ankle jerk can be estimated by simple observation with surprising accuracy in relation to the normal, and is a sensitive and reliable clinical index of hypothyroidism.

SUPERFICIAL REFLEXES (Table 12.3)
The plantar reflex

Assessment of the plantar reflex (the Babinski response) is of great clinical importance; it is an objective response which can easily be compared by various observers. To elicit it the muscles of the lower limb should be relaxed. The *outer edge of the sole of the foot* is stimulated by gently scratching a key or a stick along it from the heel towards the little toe and then medially across the metatarsus. In healthy adults even a slight stimulus produces contraction of the tensor fascia lata, often accompanied by a slighter contraction of the adductors of the thigh and of the sartorius. With a slightly stronger stimulus, flexion of the four outer toes appears, which increases with the strength of the stimulus until all the toes are flexed on the metatarsus and drawn together, the ankle being dorsiflexed and inverted. This is called the *flexor plantar response*. With still

Reflex	How excited	Result	Level of cord concerned
Anal	Stroking or scratching the skin near the anus	Contraction of anal sphincter	3rd and 4th sacral segments
Bulbocavernosus	Pinching dorsum of glans penis	Contraction of bulbocavernosus	3rd and 4th sacral segments
Plantar	Stroking sole of foot	Flexion of toes, of foot and toes, or leg	Lower part of lumbar enlargement (5th lumbar and 1st sacral segments)
Cremasteric	Stroking skin at upper and inner part of thigh*	Upwards movements of testicle	1st and 2nd lumbar segments
Abdominal	Stroking abdominal wall below costal margin, at level of umbilicus and in iliac fossa	Contraction of abdominal muscles	7th and 12th thoracic segments
Scapular	Stroking skin in interscapular region	Contraction of scapular muscles	5th cervical to 1st thoracic segment

*The cremasteric reflex can often be more easily elicited by pressing over the sartorius in the lower third of Hunter's canal.

Table 12.3 Chief superficial reflexes of spinal origin.

stronger stimuli withdrawal of the limb occurs. The plantar reflex is never completely absent in healthy subjects.

An abnormality in the plantar response in lesions of the corticospinal system was first described by Babinski. This abnormal response, *Babinski's extensor plantar response,* replaces the normal flexor plantar response; it is found only in patients with corticospinal tract lesions and is thus a pathognomonic feature of an upper motor neurone lesion. In the extensor plantar response dorsiflexion (extension) of the great toe precedes all other movement (Fig. 12.54). It is followed by spreading out and extension of the other toes, by dorsiflexion of the ankle and by flexion of the hip and knee.

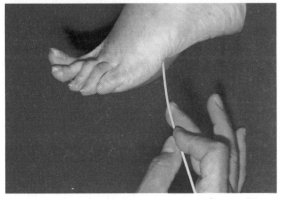

Fig. 12.54 The Babinski plantar response. A firm stroking stimulus to the outer edge of the sole of the foot evokes dorsiflexion (extension) of the large toe and fanning of the other toes.

This abnormal response is called the *extensor plantar response* because the movement of the toes is in extension according to anatomical terminology. None the less it is important to recognize that the extensor plantar response is, in reality, part of the nociceptive flexion withdrawal response described in the decerebrate preparation by Sherrington. Like the normal flexor plantar response, the extensor plantar response is best elicited from the outer edge of the sole of the foot; more medial stimuli usually elicit flexion as part of the *grasp response,* a different phenomenon. In major corticospinal lesions the area from which the extensor plantar reflex can be elicited (receptive field) enlarges, spreading first inwards and over the sole of the foot, and then upwards along the leg to the knee or even higher. For this reason extension of the great toe, generally associated with some dorsiflexion of the foot, can sometimes also be obtained by squeezing the calf or pressing heavily along the inner border of the tibia (*Oppenheim's sign*), or by pinching the calcaneus tendon (*Gordon's reflex*).

In adults, the extensor plantar response occurs with disease involving corticospinal pathways, but in children below the age of 1 year the extensor response is the normal response. The flexor response appears in the subsequent 6–12 months as myelination of the corticospinal pathways is completed.

Flexor spasms may occur during testing of the plantar reflex. These consist of an exaggerated extensor plantar response, the whole limb being suddenly drawn up into flexion and the large toe extended. This is the fully developed human counterpart of Sherrington's nociceptive flexion withdrawal response. It is common in spinal cord disease and in some patients with bilateral upper motor neurone lesions at a higher level. Flexor spasms are often particularly severe in the presence of posterior column disease (as in multiple sclerosis or subacute combined degeneration), or when there is a constant barrage of small unmyelinated fibre input to the spinal cord, as in the presence of bedsores or urinary tract infection in a patient with a cord lesion. *Extensor spasms,* conversely, are more likely to occur in patients with corticospinal tract lesions when posterior column function is normal.

Superficial abdominal reflexes

These are elicited with the patient lying relaxed and in a supine position, with the abdomen uncovered. A light stimulus, such as a key or a thin wooden stick, is passed across the abdominal skin in the plane of the dermatome from the outer aspect towards the midline. A ripple of contraction of the underlying abdominal musculature follows the stimulus. These reflexes are absent in upper motor neurone lesions above their spinal level. In disease of the thoracic spine they may indicate the segmental level of the lesion by their absence below this level.

It is often impossible to elicit abdominal reflexes in anxious patients, in the elderly or obese, and in multiparous women.

Corneal reflex

See page 298.

Palatal reflex

See pages 301–302.

SPHINCTERIC REFLEXES

These are the reflexes concerned with swallowing, micturition and defecation. They depend upon complex muscular movements excited by increased tension in the wall of the viscus concerned, and involve both unstriated and striated muscles.

Swallowing

Ascertain whether there is any difficulty in swallowing (*dysphagia*), noting especially whether there is any regurgitation of food through the nose. Patients with neurological disorders causing dysphagia usually note difficulty in swallowing liquids, whereas those with mechanical obstruction to the oesophagus or pharynx cannot swallow solids.

Defecation

The patient should be questioned as to any difficulty with defecation or continence, both to formed and liquid stool and to flatus. The presence of normal or abnormal anorectal sensation should be noted.

The reflex action of the voluntary anal sphincter may be tested by introducing the lubricated gloved finger into the anus and noting whether contraction of the sphincter occurs with normal force, whether the sphincter is weak or paralysed, or whether any spasm is excited. The activity of the reflex may also be tested by gently pricking the skin on either side near the anus. A brisk contraction of the sphincter should immediately occur—the *anal reflex.* In addition, the anal sphincter normally contracts briskly in reflex response to a sudden cough—the *cough reflex.*

The degree of tension in the anal sphincter during a voluntary sphincter squeeze—'tighten on my finger'—should be noted. In patients with weakness of the pelvic floor, usually due to damage to the innervation of the pelvic floor musculature, coughing is accompanied by descent of the pelvic floor a distance of several centimetres on to the examiner's finger. This is often associated with stress incontinence of faeces or of urine.

Micturition

The patient must always be asked whether there is any difficulty in controlling or initiating micturition and whether bladder and urethral sensation are normal. Retention, incontinence or urgency of micturition should be noted.

Incontinence in neurological disorders may be due to overflow from an atonic distended bladder in which sensation has been lost. In this case the bladder will be enlarged to palpation or percussion and a suprapubic pressure may result in the expulsion of urine from the urethra (*stress incontinence*). Incontinence may also be due to *reflex micturition,* occurring either at regular intervals as the bladder partially fills, or precipitately and unexpectedly in response to a sudden noise, to movement or to exposure to cold (*unstable bladder; urge incontinence*). Urge incontinence is frequently idiopathic but may be an early feature or intrinsic disease of the spinal cord.

Sexual function

When there is incontinence associated with neurological disease, difficulty with penile erection, ejaculation or, in both sexes, orgasm, may be noted.

Co-ordination of movement

By co-ordination is meant the smooth recruitment, interaction and co-operation of separate muscles or groups of muscles in order to accomplish a definite motor act. If such co-ordination is imperfect (*ataxia*), motor performance becomes difficult or even impossible.

The co-ordination of groups of muscles is a function of various factors, among which are the afferent impulses coming from the muscle and joint receptors, cerebellar function and the state of tone of the muscles. When ataxia is present it is not always easy to say which of these factors is at fault. The movements that constitute a motor act can be controlled and directed by vision, but sight itself is not concerned in the co-ordination of most normal movements. When, however, there is loss of the sense of position of a limb or joint, the sensory defect may be compensated for by vision, and the disturbance of movement may become apparent only when the eyes are closed or the patient is in the dark (Fig. 12.55). Such ataxia occurs typically in tabes dorsalis, when position sense is diminished or lost in the legs. Before ataxia can be ascribed solely to cerebellar disease, therefore, it is important to ascertain whether joint position sense is impaired or not. Proximal weakness may mimic cerebellar ataxia, but this can usually be distinguished easily when muscular strength is tested.

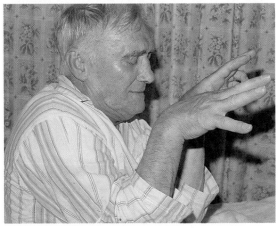

Fig. 12.55 Paraneoplastic sensory neuropathy due to small cell carcinoma of the lung. With the eyes closed the patient's outstretched arms become flexed and abnormal postures develop in the fingers.

HOW TO TEST CO-ORDINATION

In the upper limbs

Ask the patient to touch the point of the nose first with one forefinger and then with the other; or ask them to touch first the nose and then your forefinger with their index finger. If these movements are performed naturally and without making random errors, co-ordination is normal. The patient should then be asked to perform the same actions with the eyes closed; any additional irregularity indicates that there must be impairment of position sense in the limb. Co-ordination of the fingers in rapid movements, e.g. touching each finger in turn with the thumb, should also be tested. In *cerebellar ataxia* the errors of movement tend to occur at right angles to the intended direction of movement. In *anxious subjects* errors tend to occur in the direction of the movement itself.

A special and very useful sign of cerebellar ataxia is *dysdiadochokinesia;* it consists of impaired ability to execute rapidly repeated movements. The patient is asked to flex the elbows to a right angle and then alternately to supinate and pronate the forearms as rapidly as possible 'as though screwing in a light bulb'. All normal persons can do this very rapidly but usually slightly less rapidly with the non-dominant than with the dominant arm. When dysdiadochokinesia is present the movements are slow, awkward and incomplete, and often become impossible after a few attempts. In addition, the rhythm of the movement is characteristically irregular. The sign can also be elicited by asking the patient to tap the examiner's palm with the tips of the fingers as fast as possible. Minor degrees of ataxia can then be both felt and heard.

It is often useful to watch the patient dressing or undressing, handling a book or picking up pins, since these more complex and more practised everyday movements offer a very sensitive way of assessing co-ordination.

In the lower limbs

If the patient is able to walk, a good test of lower limb co-ordination consists of asking them to walk along a straight line. If incoordination is present the patient will soon deviate to one side or the other. Watch particularly for unsteadiness as the patient turns to walk back towards you. The test is made more difficult by asking the patient to 'tandem walk' along a line drawn on the floor, like a tightrope walker, placing the heel of one foot immediately adjacent to the toe of the one behind.

Ask the patient, as they lie in bed, to lift one leg high in the air, to place the heel of this leg on the opposite knee and then to slide the heel down the shin towards the ankle. In cerebellar ataxia a characteristic, irregular, side-to-side series of errors in the speed and direction of movement occurs. The test should be performed *with the eyes open*. A similar test is to ask the patient to draw a large circle in the air with toe or forefinger. The circles should be drawn smoothly and accurately.

Romberg's sign is a test for *loss of position sense* (sensory ataxia) in the legs: it is not a test of cerebellar function. The patient is asked to stand with feet close together and, if this can be done, to stand in this posture but with the eyes closed. If Romberg's sign is present, as soon as the eyes are closed the patient begins to sway about or may even fall. *The essential feature of the sign is therefore that the patient is more unsteady standing with the eyes closed than when they are open.* With defective position sense in the legs, as in tabes dorsalis or sensory neuropathy, the patient is unable to maintain posture without visual fixation. Patients with labyrinthine lesions or with cerebellar ataxia show only a little increase in instability in this test.

Gait

Analysis of a patient's gait is of major importance in diagnosis (Box 12.11). The legs should be adequately exposed and free of constricting clothing such as a dressing gown. The feet should be bare. The patient is asked to walk away from the observer, to turn round at a given point and then to come back again.

The points to be noted are the following.

- Can the patient walk at all?
- How much help is needed?
- Does the patient walk in a straight line or tend to deviate to one side or the other? To assess this point, ask them to walk along a straight line, e.g. a crack in the floor.
- Does the patient tend to fall? In what direction?

The next point to be decided is whether the gait conforms to any of the well-recognized gait disorders. Begin by excluding local causes, e.g. osteoarthritis of the hip, an old knee injury, or local pain in the leg or pelvis.

In a *spastic gait* the patient walks on a narrow base, has difficulty in bending the knees and drags the feet along as if they were glued to the floor. This can be heard as well as seen. The foot is raised from the ground by tilting the pelvis, and the leg is then

---

Box 12.11 Gait disorders.

Upper motor neurone
- Hemiplegia: Circumduction of leg with inability to flex hip and dorsiflex foot against resistance (or gravity). Triple flexion posture of upper limb
- Paraplegia and quadriplegia: Scissoring, stiff-legged gait and flexed posture

Lower motor neurone
- Foot drop: Weakness of dorsiflexion and eversion of the foot leads to excessive hip flexion to compensate; due to common peroneal nerve palsy or L5/S1 root lesion, or to peripheral neuropathy
- Quadriceps weakness: Knee extension weak, leading to sudden falls, difficulty rising from chair or descending stairs
- Proximal weakness: Rolling gait, with difficulty climbing stairs. Arms cannot be lifted above shoulder height. Axial weakness may be present
- Peripheral neuropathy: Distal weakness and sensory loss

Cerebellar syndrome
- Ataxia: Unsteadiness and inability to walk on a narrow base, or to turn quickly

Extrapyramidal syndromes
- Parkinson's disease: Shuffling festinant gait, with flexed posture, tremor of hand and face
- Dystonia: Involuntary movements and rigid postures
- Involuntary movements: Chorea, athetosis, ballismus
- Sensory ataxia: Cerebellar-like ataxia associated with distal loss of position sense
- Apraxic gait: Loss of concept of walking, often associated with tiny rapid steps
- Hysteria: Bizarre, 'functional' gait disorder, miraculously the patient does not fall

---

swung forwards so that the foot tends to describe an arc, the toe scraping along the floor—*circumduction* of the leg. A spastic gait is a characteristic feature of patients with corticospinal lesions, especially in spinal cord disease. The *hemiplegic gait* is essentially a spastic gait in which only one leg is affected.

The gait in *sensory ataxia* may be described as 'stamping'. The patient raises the foot very suddenly, often abnormally high, and then jerks it forward, bringing it to the ground again with a stamp, and often heel first. By using their eyes in place of position sense the patient may succeed in walking fairly steadily, but when walking in the dark, or with the eyes closed, there is severe ataxia. This gait is best seen in tabes dorsalis. Other signs of loss of postural sensibility will be present.

The gait of *cerebellar ataxia* appears 'drunken' or 'reeling'. Patients with this gait disorder walk on a broad base, the feet planted widely apart and placed irregularly. The ataxia is equally severe whether the eyes are open or closed. Other signs of cerebellar disease are usually present (Box 12.12).

> **BOX 12.12 Clinical signs of cerebellar lesions.**
>
> - Cerebellar ataxia
> - Intention tremor
> - Involvement of limbs, trunk and external ocular movement (nystagmus)
> - Past-pointing
> - Rebound
> - Impaired ability to generate alternating rhythmic movements

A *festinant gait* is characteristic of Parkinson's disease (Box 12.13). The patient is bent forwards (flexion dystonia) and advances with rapid, short, shuffling steps, so that the gait appears as though the patient is trying to catch up with the centre of gravity. The arms do not swing. In some cases, if the patient is suddenly pulled backwards, the patient begins to walk backwards, and is unable to stop (*retropulsion*). In bilateral corticospinal lesions in the deep cerebral white matter a rather similar short-stepped but rapid tapping gait occurs, called *marche à Petipas* (the Russian ballet master of 100 years ago), to describe its resemblance to the rapid steps of a ballet dancer on her points. In dystonia and chorea the involuntary movements are usually exaggerated during walking, and unusual foot placement responses may occur so that the toes may extend away from the floor (*avoiding response*) or the feet may appear glued to the floor (*grasping response*).

The *waddling gait* is like the gait of a duck. The body is usually tilted backwards, with an increase of lumbar lordosis; the feet are planted rather widely apart and the body sways from side to side as each step is taken. The heels and toes tend to be brought down simultaneously. This gait disorder is due to difficulty in maintaining truncal and pelvic posture because of proximal muscular weakness. It occurs, therefore, in the myopathies and the muscular dystrophies. A similar gait may occur with bilateral disease of the hip joints (*Trendelenberg's sign*).

A *high-stepping gait* is adopted in order to avoid tripping, from the toes catching the ground. It occurs when there is weakness of the extensor muscles of the feet, for example, in common peroneal nerve palsy.

Involuntary movements

In a number of different diseases of the nervous system, involuntary, unintended movements occur, either at rest or during voluntary movement. The different clinical varieties of involuntary movement are not specific disease entities, but represent clinical patterns of involuntary movement. Most are due to diseases of the basal ganglia and extrapyramidal system.

EPILEPSY

The possibility should always be considered that an involuntary movement limited to one side of the body, or to one limb, might be due to focal epilepsy. Very rarely such an attack may continue for hours or even days (*epilepsia partialis continua*). The movement is usually complex and repetitive, even if brief. It may be exacerbated by arousal or by handling or touching the limb and it will usually be relieved by anticonvulsant drugs. The movement differs from the involuntary movement disorders principally by its stereotyped repetitiveness. A classification of epilepsy is given in Box 12.14, and of the causes of epilepsy in Box 12.15.

MYOCLONUS

Myoclonus is a rapid, irregular jerking movement of a group of muscles in a limb or even of the whole

> **BOX 12.13 Parkinson's disease: main clinical features.**
>
> - Distal pill-rolling tremor (about 5 Hz)
> - Tremor mainly involves hands
> - Often unilateral predominance
> - Cogwheel rigidity
> - Akinesia of face and limbs
> - Impassive facies
> - Drooling
> - Flexed posture
> - Loss of righting reflexes, and impaired balance, with postural instability
> - Autonomic features; e.g. incontinence, postural hypotension

> **BOX 12.14 Seizures; a basic clinical classification.**
>
> **Generalized epilepsy**
> - Major generalized seizures: grand mal epilepsy
> - Minor generalized seizures: petit mal epilepsy, myoclonic seizures
>
> **Partial epilepsy**
> - Simple partial seizures: temporal lobe epilepsy
> - Complex partial seizures: with secondary generalization
> - Focal motor seizures of childhood
> - Myoclonus epilepsy

body, often occurring in response to extraneous stimuli, such as a sudden loud noise. A sudden start when surprised, or bodily jerks on falling asleep or waking, are common varieties of myoclonus experienced by most normal people. In exaggerated form these jerks of *flexion myoclonus* may occur as a manifestation of major epilepsy or with degenerative disorders of the cerebellum. Generalized flexion myoclonus also occurs in certain types of encephalitis, when it often exhibits an obvious periodicity. Less commonly, irregular myoclonic jerks may occur in a single limb, or a ripple of jerky irregular contraction may pass through the muscles of a limb—*segmental myoclonus*. Myoclonus can occur with lesions at many levels in the nervous system and it does not, therefore, have localizing value.

TREMOR

Regular or irregular distal movements having an oscillatory character are classified as tremors (Box 12.16). The tremor of *anxiety* is usually fine and rapid, but it may be coarse and irregular. The tremor found in *thyrotoxicosis* is characteristically rapid. Coarser distal tremor, often exaggerated in awkward postures, as when the outstretched fingers are held pointing at each other in front of the patient's nose and usually relieved to some extent during move-

ment, occurs as a familial disorder—*benign essential tremor*. This tremor is often coarse, but usually irregular, and it is present both at rest and during movement. It must therefore be distinguished from parkinsonian and cerebellar tremor. The latter is present only during movement (*intention tremor*) and the former is accompanied by signs of extrapyramidal disease. *Senile tremor* is similar to benign essential tremor. *Hysterical tremor* tends to involve a limb or the whole body and it is characteristically worsened by the examiner's attempt to control it. Secondary gain (see Chapter 2) is a feature of the psychological disturbance associated with the underlying personality disorder in hysterical symptoms.

The tremor of *parkinsonism* is usually easily recognizable. It consists of a rapid, rhythmic, alternating tremor, predominantly in flexion/extension but often with a prominent rotary component between finger and thumb (*pill-rolling tremor*). Proximal muscles may be involved, and the lips and tongue are frequently affected. The tremor is invariably more severe in the arm than in the leg. It is often asymmetrical and is associated with other symptoms and signs of this extrapyramidal disease, such as hypokinesia, cogwheel rigidity, postural abnormalities, gait disorder and an expressionless, quiet voice.

ATHETOSIS

Athetosis is a writhing movement, usually more pronounced in distal than in proximal muscles, in which the play of movement is very complex. It often seems to consist of an interaction between two postures, those of *grasping* and *avoiding* (see page 281). The fingers are alternately widely extended, the arm following into an extended, abducted and externally rotated posture, and then the fingers clench, often trapping the thumb in the palm, and the limb flexes slightly and rotates internally. In very severe forms of this disorder, as for example in *dystonia musculorum deformans* (torsion dystonia) the trunk and axial musculature is also affected and the patient may scarcely be able to stand. Deformities may develop and become fixed.

Athetosis may be unilateral or generalized. The latter form is usually associated with degenerative disease of the basal ganglia. Very rarely it may occur as a paroxysmal phenomenon.

CHOREA

The word chorea means 'a dance'. The involuntary movements are brief, fluid and often difficult, at first, to discern. Ordinary voluntary movements, such as walking or picking up a cup and saucer, may be embellished with smooth, rapid extra little flourishes of movement. Muscular tone is often decreased. The outstretched upper limbs may assume a hyperpronated posture and little flicks of movement of the digits or wrist may occur. At rest the patient appears 'fidgety' and 'unable to sit still'. The movements often appear less obvious during voluntary movement, and are increased by agitation or nervousness.

Chorea occurs as part of an inherited presenile dementia (*Huntington's chorea*), with rheumatic fever (*Sydenham's chorea*) and rarely in pregnancy and after certain drugs (e.g. phenothiazines). It may also occur with other systemic diseases, e.g. thyrotoxicosis and systemic lupus erythematosus, and in old age (*senile chorea*). Unilateral chorea may occur with deeply placed lesions in one hemisphere, which may be violent, consisting of ballistic, flinging movements of the limbs (*hemiballismus*).

DYSKINESIA

The word 'dyskinesia' is particularly used to describe *phenothiazine-induced* involuntary movements, which predominantly affect the pharyngeal and facial perioral musculature, and *levodopa-induced* axial torsional movements, although similar movements occur in choreo-athetoid and dystonic patients not previously treated with these drugs. Levodopa-induced involuntary movements tend to develop at times of peak plasma levels of dopamine (*peak-dose dyskinesias*).

DYSTONIA

This is an *abnormally maintained posture*, often associated with a plastic rigidity. The dystonias are closely related to choreo-athetosis (dystonic movements), but the term can also be used to describe the flexed posture of Parkinson's disease (*flexion dystonia*) or the hemiplegic posture (*hemiplegic dystonia*). The abnormal posture varies in relation to different circumstances: for example, it is often relieved by lying supine or by standing in contact with a wall. The term dystonia is often used to include all involuntary movements that are accompanied by abnormal postures.

TORTICOLLIS

Spasmodic torticollis consists of a jerky or maintained rotational and abducted posture of the neck. It is a form of dystonia. It can often be partially self-modified by certain postural adjustments, e.g. touching the chin with the index finger.

TICS

These are simple, normal movements which become *repeated* unnecessarily to the point that they become an embarrassment. They may be a source of, or reaction to, psychiatric problems. In contrast to the other involuntary movement disorders, they can be readily imitated. Head-nodding is a common example.

MYOKYMIA

This is a persistent twitchy and often rhythmical movement usually affecting the periorbital muscles. It may occur as a benign phenomenon in fatigued or anxious people. It is sometimes due to lesions in the facial nerve or its nucleus. Myokymia is rarely a generalized disorder (Isaac's syndrome).

ASTERIXIS

An irregular, abrupt, brief loss of posture, especially evident in the outstretched hands or tongue, occurs in decompensated hepatic failure (*hepatic flap*) and in other metabolic disorders, e.g. uraemia, poisoning with hypnotic drugs, and in respiratory failure.

TETANY

In tetany, commonly due to hypocalcaemia or alkalosis, there is a characteristic posture of the affected hand (see page 19). The fingers and thumbs are held stiffly adducted and the hand is partially flexed at the metacarpophalangeal joints; the toes may be similarly affected (*carpopedal spasm*). Ischaemia of the affected limb, produced by a sphygmomanometer cuff inflated above the arterial pressure for 2 or 3 minutes, will augment this sign or produce it if it is not already present (*Trousseau's sign*). Another useful test is to tap lightly with a patellar hammer in the region of exit of the facial nerve from the skull, about 3–5 cm below and in front of the ear. The facial muscles twitch briefly with each tap (*Chvostek's sign*).

CRAMP

This spasm of part or whole of a muscle, especially of the calf muscles, is common in normal people. It is a frequent feature in chronic or progressive neurogenic muscle weakness, and in metabolic disorders, e.g. hyponatraemia (as in *heat stroke*) and hypomagnesaemia. It is due to hypercontraction of muscle fibres, and is relieved by passive stretch of the affected muscle.

Sensation

The following different forms of sensation can be tested at the bedside.
- Tactile sensibility. This includes light touch and pressure, and tactile localization and discrimination.
- Position sense; the appreciation of passive movement.
- Recognition of the size, shape, weight and form of objects.
- Vibration.
- Pain.
- Temperature.

These 'sensory modalities' do not necessarily represent different, discrete sensory functions, but rather are commonly experienced sensations in normal life. Perception depends on a complex physiological interaction of afferent input at many levels in the nervous system. In some instances, as in the recognition and naming of objects, it depends also on the ability to manipulate the object felt. Perception of vibration, for example, does not depend on a special set of nerve fibres responsible only for transmitting vibration sense to the central nervous system, but rather is a form of sensation subjectively similar to rapidly applied light touch which, in clinical practice, is found to be disturbed when there is a lesion of the large-diameter afferent fibres in the peripheral nerves, posterior columns or, more rarely, at a higher level.

Technique of sensory examination

Begin testing sensation with touch and position sense. Use a pin later, when you have gained the patient's confidence. Always apply the sensory stimulus first to an area of impaired sensation and mark out its borders *from the abnormal to the normal.* The patient should readily note the sudden change to normality. Areas of diminished sensation should be carefully, *but quickly,* mapped out so that their distribution in relation to root lesions, peripheral nerve lesions or lesions in the central nervous system can be studied. It is important to do this quickly, accurately and, as far as possible, without repetition. The longer the time spent on this the more confusing will be the result: it requires great concentration and co-operation from the patient and from the examiner.

Inconsistency in the patient's replies may be due to fatigue, poor co-operation, dementia or undue suggestibility. This can be checked by asking the patient to say 'now' whenever the stimulus is felt, with the eyes shut; by examining a related form of sensation such as temperature sense in the case of pinprick, or position or vibration sense in the case of light touch; or by encouraging the patient to be very careful to make the correct response. Never make much of small differences. Remember that many patients will experience changes in the acuteness or sharpness of a pin between the nailbed and the dorsum of the finger, or at about the level of the clavicle when the stimulus ascends the anterior chest wall. The pulp of the fingers is rather insensitive to pain but very sensitive to light touch and to discriminative tests such as two-point discrimination. Vibration sense is best perceived over a bony prominence.

On the whole it is better to test sensation with the patient's eyes open although it is, of course, necessary to prevent the patient seeing their fingers and toes when testing position sense. People are usually more alert and attentive with their eyes open than with them shut, and alertness is crucial in sensory testing. During most sensory testing it should not affect the result to have the patient actually watching the procedure. Remember it can be a frightening experience to be suddenly pricked with a pin when one's eyes are closed. Such surprises, which destroy a patient's confidence in the examiner, should be avoided. Compare the findings with the abnormalities, if any, described by the patient as part of the neurological history. Most people are very aware of sensory abnormality, except perhaps in the case of temperature sense which may be lost without the patient being aware of it, especially if the area affected is around the shoulders, as in syringomelia, rather than involving the hands or feet.

Tactile sensibility (light touch)

Use a wisp of cotton wool or the tip of your index finger. Ask the patient to indicate whether the touch is felt, and if it feels normal. If not, *how* is it abnormal? It may be abolished or reduced (*hypaesthesia*), misperceived as a painful, irritating or tingling sensation (*hyperaesthesia*) or mislocalized. Very rarely there may be a delay between the stimulus and its recognition by the patient. Areas of diminished sensation should be carefully delineated and recorded.

The ability to discriminate between two points is tested by the use of blunt dividers. The patient is asked whether one or both points can be felt. Normally 2 mm of separation of the points can be recognized as two separate stimuli on the fingertips, and slightly wider separation on the pulps of the toes. This is an excellent objective sensory test which is particularly useful in cases of posterior column or parietal cortical lesions and in some peripheral nerve lesions (such as the carpal tunnel syndrome) that involve large afferent fibres and impair discriminate sensation.

Position sense

Ask the patient to look away or shield their eyes. Explain that you will move a finger (or toe or elbow) up or down and ask the patient to tell you which way it has been moved. Normal people can recognize movements of only a few degrees at all joints, including knee, ankle, elbow and wrist, in addition to the more commonly tested fingers and toes. It is sometimes helpful to ask the patient to imitate with the opposite limb or digit the position of the limb or digit being tested. It is essential that the patient should be relaxed sufficiently to allow the limb to be moved *passively*.

When position sense is disturbed in the upper limbs, the outstretched fingers may twist, rise and fall when held out with the eyes closed. These involuntary movements (*pseudoathetosis*) occur unknown to the patient and disappear almost completely when the patient watches the position of their fingers. Patients with defective position sense may be unable to manipulate small objects, fasten buttons and so on without visually observing their movements (*sensory ataxia*).

The *appreciation of movement* is closely related to the sense of position and can be tested at the same time. Gradually move a digit or limb into a new position, with the patient's eyes closed, and ask them to say 'now' as soon as movement is perceived. Note the angle through which the limb was moved. If the appreciation of movement is diminished, this angle is many times greater than that in a normal limb. Movements of less than 10 degrees can be appreciated at all normal joints.

Recognition of size, shape, weight and form

These faculties can be tested most accurately in the hands with the eyes closed. To test size, place in the patient's palm objects of the same shape, but of different sizes, for example small rods or matches of different length. Ask which is the larger. The objects should be applied consecutively.

To test recognition of shape familiar objects such as coins, a pencil, a penknife, scissors, etc., are placed in the hand, and the patient is asked to identify them or to describe their form. Loss of this faculty, called *astereognosis*, may occur, with parietal lesions, when position sense and light touch are normal, although there is usually some associated defect in these modalities. When astereognosis occurs with posterior column lesions, position sense, vibration sense and light touch are invariably profoundly disturbed.

Appreciation of vibration

If the foot of a vibrating tuning-fork is placed on the surface of the body the vibrations can be felt, providing they are sufficiently strong. This is a valuable test, as the ability to appreciate vibration may be lost in various diseases, as in tabes dorsalis, in peripheral neuropathies and in posterior column disorders. A tuning fork of 128 Hz (lower C) should be used. Vibrations of higher frequency are more difficult to perceive. If the patient perceives the vibration, as it gradually fades in intensity, ask them to say when they cease to feel it. If the examiner can then still perceive it, the patient's perception of vibration is impaired. There is often some loss of vibration sense in the feet and legs in old age.

Pain

Pain may be evoked either by a cutaneous stimulus, e.g. the prick of a pin, or by pressure on deeper structures, such as muscles or bones. Superficial and pressure pain should be tested separately.

Superficial pain

The point of a pin should be used as the stimulus. Care must be taken that the patient distinguishes between the *sharpness* of the point (that is, its relative size) and the *pain* which the prick evokes; it often happens that, even when sensibility to pain is abolished, the patient can recognize that the stimulus is pointed, and thus confuse the observer by calling it 'sharp'. The pin used should be an ordinary domestic pin, rather than a hypodermic needle: the latter is designed to cut skin relatively painlessly and is not suitable for sensory testing. Pins used to test sensation should be adequately sterilized before re-use, or destroyed, because of the possibility, however remote, of transmission of hepatitis B or human immunodeficiency virus (HIV) infection. Disposable pins are available for testing, and these should be used whenever possible.

Pressure pain

This is examined by squeezing a distal muscle or the Achilles tendon. This sensation is particularly disturbed in tabes dorsalis.

Absence of sensibility to pain is termed *analgesia;* partial loss of pain sensibility is called *hypalgesia;* an exaggerated sensibility, so that even a mild stimulus causes an unnatural degree of painful sensation, is known as *hyperalgesia.* This occurs in some patients with spinal cord disease, for example in tabes dorsalis, and in certain patients with deep-seated parietal or thalamic lesions (thalamic pain). The pain experienced has a peculiar, ill-localized and persistent character. It often has a burning quality and it may occur as an intractable spontaneous phenomenon or only in response to cutaneus stimuli.

Temperature sense

Temperature sense is conveniently examined by using test tubes containing warm and cold water. The part to be tested is touched with each in turn, and the patient says whether each tube feels hot or cold. At the bedside it is often sufficient to use the cold metallic sensation of the touch of the end of an ophthalmoscope or tuning-fork for rough assessment of temperature sensation.

Other disturbances of sensation

Sensory inattention is an important feature of lesions of the parietal lobe. Ask the patient to close their eyes and stimulate homologous points on opposite sides of the body simultaneously by touch or by pinprick. Then ask the patient to indicate which side, or sides, are touched. In sensory inattention the stimulus on the abnormal side is not perceived even though there is no subjective difference between left and right to conventional comparative testing. This is also called *sensory extinction* or *sensory neglect. Bilateral simultaneous sensory stimuli* can also be used when testing vision and hearing; a similar defect may be found. In the presence of fixed hemisensory loss, of course, the sign is invalid.

Some patients with parietal lesions will also show *spatial summation* in which a stimulus is perceived only if an area of skin larger than a certain critical area is stimulated, or *temporal summation* in which an ill-localized and often perverted or painful sensation is felt after rapidly repeated stimuli applied to the same point. Single stimuli will be missed. These abnormalities are part of a perceptual defect related to *agnosia,* a disorder in which the patient is unaware

of the nature or the severity of a sensory disorder. In its most extreme form there may even be denial of illness (*anosognosia*). In patients with higher perceptual defects of this type a number of other bedside tests may be useful. These include *constructional tests* such as the patient's ability to draw a map of their surroundings, to copy a complex figure (for example, two interlocking irregular pentagons), to draw a clock face or a human face, or to draw more complex figures, for example a house. Visual and tactile memory can be tested by variations of these tests. Constructional ability is particularly impaired with right parietal lesions (*constructional apraxia*). Specific sensory disorders, such as inability to recognize faces, visual and tactile perseveration and synaesthesias (sensations perceived in a different modality than that applied) are some features of parietal cortical lesions.

Autonomic function

The autonomic nervous system consists of afferent and efferent, post-ganglionic, sympathetic and parasympathetic neurones in the periphery, together with the central preganglionic components of these systems in the intermediolateral cell columns in the spinal cord, and rostral connections in the brainstem and cerebral hemispheres. These neuronal systems are autonomous, but not entirely free from voluntary control. They are concerned with modulation of function in the cardiovascular and gastrointestinal systems, with temperature regulation, sexual reflexes, bladder and bowel detrusor and sphincter activity, and pupillary and respiratory reflex control mechanisms. Thus, patients with disturbances of the autonomic nervous system may show complex clinical abnormalities; the clinical presentation will be determined by the distribution of abnormality in the central or peripheral components of this neuronal system (Box 12.17).

BOX 12.17 Features of autonomic disorders.

- Postural hypotension
- Impotence and erectile failure
- Retention or incontinence of urine
- Poor urine stream (detrusor failure)
- Constipation, and faecal incontinence
- Oesophageal and GI dysmotility
- Pupillary immobility
- Impaired sweating
- Snoring and sleep apnoea

In the rare syndrome of progressive autonomic failure there is degeneration of both preganglionic and post-ganglionic neurones, leading to inability to maintain the blood pressure in the erect position (*orthostatic hypotension*), constipation, incontinence of urine, impotence, pupillary areflexia, and disturbances of sweating. Orthostatic hypotension causes syncope in the erect posture. Loss of cardiovascular reflexes causes tachycardia at rest, with absence of the normal slowing of the pulse in response to the Valsalva manoeuvre, of the normal slight increase in the pulse rate and blood pressure on standing, and of increased blood pressure during hand grip, or in stressful tasks, such as mental arithmetic. Some of these clinical features may also develop in patients with peripheral neuropathies, especially in diabetic neuropathy, when the post-ganglionic neurones of the sympathetic and parasympathetic nervous system may be involved.

These features form the basis of a series of simple clinical tests, in which emphasis is placed on measurement of the pulse rate from a continuously running electrocardiographic (ECG) record. The pulse rate can be calculated, in an ECG recorded at conventional paper speed, from the R–R interval using the formula:

$$\text{Heart rate} = \frac{\text{R–R interval}}{60}$$

Bedside assessment of autonomic function

Check the pupillary responses to light and accommodation. Is the skin normal? If dry, suspect absence of sweating. Is there a resting tachycardia? Does the pulse rate slow with deep inspiration?

Standing test for orthostatic hypotension

Ask the patient to lie quietly on a couch for 15 minutes, with sphygmomanometer and cardiac rate meter, or lead 1 ECG attached. Check the resting blood pressure. Then ask the patient to stand. Note the pulse rate from the R–R interval at the 15th and 30th beats after standing, and measure the blood pressure 1 and 3 minutes after standing. In normal subjects the systolic blood pressure should not decrease by more than 10 mmHg. In patients with autonomic dysfunction the systolic blood pressure falls more than 30 mmHg. The 30th:15th pulse ratio is >1.03 in normal subjects, and 1.0 when there is autonomic disturbance.

Deep breaths test

Lay the patient flat. When the pulse has steadied, record the pulse rate during six *maximal* deep breaths. In normal subjects the pulse rate should fall by >15 beats/min; with autonomic disturbances the pulse rate slows <10 beats/min.

Handgrip test

With the patient lying flat measure the maximal handgrip by having the patient grip a sphygmomanometer cuff as hard as possible. Then measure the rise in diastolic blood pressure after a 30% handgrip sustained for 5 minutes. The diastolic pressure should rise >16 mmHg; in autonomic disorders the diastolic pressure will rise <10 mmHg.

Valsalva test

The patient blows into a sphygmomanometer, maintaining a pressure of 40 mmHg for 15 seconds. The ratio of the highest pulse rate in the preliminary rest period to the lowest pulse rate during the test is >1.5 in normal subjects and <1.1 in patients with autonomic disturbances. The test may be repeated up to three times if the initial result is equivocal.

Other tests

Tests of bowel motility and of bladder and urethral function using cystometrography are also useful in evaluating the extent of autonomic dysfunction. Quantitative pupillometry, and the response to conjunctival application of parasympathomimetic and sympathomimetic drugs can also be used (see Chapter 10).

Signs of meningeal irritation

Neck stiffness

Ask the patient to flex the neck as fully as possible to ascertain the degree of movement possible, and then to relax. Then passively flex the neck. The chin should normally touch the chest without pain.

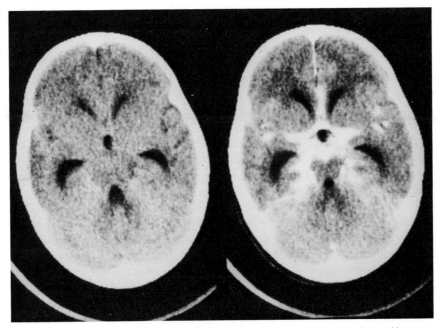

Fig. 12.56   CT scans of tuberculous meningitis. The basal cisterns are obliterated in the unenhanced image on the left. On the right the inflamed meninges and the inflammatory exudate have been visualized (enhanced) following intravenous injection of iodine-based contrast. The white central areas represent the abnormality. The clinical sign of neck stiffness represents reflex spasm in the neck extensors caused by inflammation of the basal meninges.

In meningeal irritation neck flexion causes pain in the posterior part of the neck, sometimes radiating down the back, and the movement is resisted by spasm in the extensor muscles of the neck. Neck rigidity is also caused by diseases of the cervical spine. Head retraction represents a marked degree of neck rigidity.

Kernig's sign

Kernig's sign is tested with the patient supine on the bed by passively extending the patient's knee when the hip is fully flexed. In patients with meningeal irritation affecting the lower part of the spinal subarachnoid space this movement causes pain and spasm of the hamstrings. It is a less sensitive test than neck stiffness.

These two tests depend upon the fact that stretching the spinal nerve roots in meningeal irritation causes reflex muscular spasm in the paraspinal and sacral muscles. They are both positive in meningitis (Fig. 12.56) and subarachnoid haemorrhage, and also in patients with 'meningism', a state of irritation of the meninges seen most commonly in young children with acute fevers. In some patients with raised intracranial pressure in whom herniation of the cerebellar tonsils into the foramen magnum has occurred, neck stiffness may also be present.

Straight leg raising

This test is useful in patients with sciatica. The sciatic nerve and its roots are stretched by passively elevating the patient's extended leg with the hand, which is placed behind the heel. The movement is restricted by sciatic pain when a lumbosacral spinal root is entrapped, as in lumbosacral intervertebral disc protrusion.

Special investigations

The following special methods of investigation are in common use.

Lumbar puncture

This procedure is used for obtaining samples of cerebrospinal fluid (CSF) by puncturing the lumbar meninges with a long hollow needle inserted between the spines of two lumbar vertebrae, below the level of the termination of the conus medullaris. It is performed as follows.

First, always examine the fundi to exclude raised intracranial pressure; lumbar puncture is contraindicated in the presence of raised intracranial pressure because of the risk of consequent transtentorial or tonsillar herniation.

Mark out the 3rd and 4th lumbar spines. The 4th lumbar spine usually lies in the plane of the iliac crests. The puncture may be made through either the 3rd or 4th interspace. The patient should be lying on their side on a firm couch or on the firm edge of a bed, with the knees and chin as nearly approximated as possible; the patient's back should be right at the edge of the couch, and it is *important that its transverse axis,* i.e. a line passing through the posterior superior iliac spines, *should be vertical.* Local anaesthesia may be produced by injecting 2% sterile procaine, first raising a bleb under the skin, and, when this is insensitive, anaesthetizing the whole dermis. It is not necessary to inject procaine into the deep ligaments; this usually causes more pain than it relieves. A special needle containing a withdrawable stylet about 8 cm in length should be used. The stylet should fit accurately and should not protrude through the bevelled cutting edge of the needle.

Push the needle firmly through the skin in the midline or just to one side of it and press it steadily *forwards and slightly towards the head,* with the bevel pointing towards the side on which the patient is lying. When the needle is felt to enter the spinal cavity the stylet is withdrawn and the CSF which escapes is collected in three sterilized stoppered test tubes. If any blood is present, a marked difference in the amount in the first and subsequent tubes indicates that the blood is due to trauma from the puncture. The patient should lie flat for 8–24 hours afterwards, in order to reduce the chance of post-lumbar puncture headache developing.

It is useful to have a manometer, connectable with the needle, so that the pressure of the fluid can be measured at the time of puncture. For this measurement, the patient should be lying with their head on the same level as their sacrum, breathing quietly and with muscles relaxed. The neck and legs should *not* be too intensely flexed. The normal CSF pressure is 60–150 mm of CSF. The pressure rises and falls a centimetre or two with respiration. The pulse is also reflected in pressure fluctuations in the CSF.

Queckenstedt's test was formerly used to detect a block in the circulation of CSF in the spinal canal, for example, in spinal tumours. If spinal tumour is suspected it is nowadays preferable to proceed to magnetic resonance (MR) scanning, or to myelogra-phy without previous lumbar puncture, since the latter may result in deterioration of the patient's signs. With the needle and manometer in position and the patient breathing quietly as described above, an assistant compresses one or other, but not both, jugular veins. This causes a sudden increase in intracranial pressure, which is immediately seen in the manometer as a sudden rise of CSF pressure, followed by an equally rapid fall when the pressure on the vein is released. A similar sudden rise and fall is seen if the patient is asked to cough. This is a useful check that the needle tip is in free communication with the subarachnoid space. With slight degrees of block in the spinal canal there may be a rise of pressure in the manometer followed by a very slow fall when the pressure on the vein is released; and with more severe block no rise of pressure will be seen when the jugular vein is compressed. *This test should never be carried out in the presence of raised CSF pressure* since it may then precipitate transtentorial or tonsillar herniation.

DIFFICULTIES WITH LUMBAR PUNCTURE

The commonest cause of a 'dry-tap', the failure to obtain CSF, is an incorrectly performed puncture, and this is usually due to the patient not being in the correct position. The needle will then not be introduced at right angles to the transverse axis of the back, and will miss the spinal canal.

A common error is to introduce the needle too deeply so that it traverses the spinal canal and wedges against the posterior margin of the intervertebral disc; if the needle is withdrawn slightly CSF will begin to flow. Occasionally, however, a 'dry-tap' is due to a complete block to the flow of CSF through the spinal canal. In this circumstance urgent MRI or myelography is required. For the latter procedure *cisternal puncture* or *lateral cervical puncture* may be required. This should be performed only by an experienced physician or surgeon. It is best undertaken under radiographic control.

ABNORMALITIES OF THE CSF

Normal CSF is clear and colourless like water. Any yellowness is pathological and is due either to old haemorrhage, jaundice or excess of protein. In *Froin's syndrome* a pronounced yellow colour (*xanthochromia*) is associated with great excess of protein and the formation of a coagulum. It is a very rare phenomenon. Even slight increases in CSF protein, however, cause a noticeable increase in viscosity of the fluid and an excessive frothiness of its surface when it is gently shaken.

Turbidity of the fluid may be due to the presence of white blood cells, either as a result of infection or of subarachnoid haemorrhage. If it does not clear on standing it is due to microorganisms.

The presence of *blood* may be due to injury to a vessel by the needle or to subarachnoid haemorrhage. In the latter case the blood is more uniformly mixed with the fluid, and the supernatant fluid remains yellow after centrifugation.

Cytological examination of a turbid fluid is of great importance. A centrifugal deposit should be examined with Leishman's stain in order to obtain an idea of the character of the cells present; and by Gram's and Ziehl–Neelsen's methods for bacteria (Fig. 12.57). Cell counts are performed with a counting chamber and must be done immediately the fluid has been collected. Counts done some hours later give inaccurate results because the leucocytes stick together and to the sides of the tube, and endothelial cells break up in a short time. If any clot has formed, an accurate cell count cannot be obtained but the cells in the clot can be stained and examined. Normal fluid contains 2–5 lymphocytes/μl.

An increased cell count may consist of polymorphonuclear cells or lymphocytes. The increased cell count is termed *polymorphonuclear* if these cells are above 75% of the total, or *lymphocytic* if more than 98% are lymphocytes. Bacterial meningitis is associated with a polymorphonuclear pleocytosis, viral meningitis and syphilis with a lymphocytic one, and tuberculous meningitis with either a lymphocytic or a mixed type. The latter is termed *pleocytosis*. Cytological examination of the centrifugal deposit may reveal malignant cells in patients with secondary neoplastic invasion of the meninges from lymphoma or carcinoma (see Fig. 12.58).

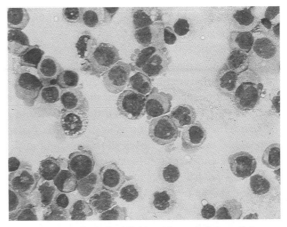

Fig. 12.58   Cerebrospinal fluid cytology. Cell deposit from cerebrospinal fluid almost exclusively comprising carcinoma cells shed from the leptomeninges. Metastasis to meninges from primary carcinoma of the breast. May–Grünwald–Giemsa stain. × 160.

The CSF should also be examined bacteriologically and chemically. Normal CSF contains only a trace of albumin and hardly any globulin, the *total protein* being not more than 40 mg/dl. In some neurological diseases, particularly in multiple sclerosis and in many acute and subacute virus infections, the globulin fractions in the CSF are increased. The *Lange test* takes advantage of this. Varying dilutions of CSF are mixed in 10 tubes with a colloidal gold suspension of constant strength. The degree of precipitation which results is expressed by arbitrary figures 0–5, 0 representing no change and 5 complete precipitation. The *CSF IgG concentration* can also be directly estimated by immunoelectrophoresis, an investigation that has rendered the Lange test obsolete. It is compared with the blood IgG and albumin levels in order to show whether a raised CSF IgG level is due to endogenous IgG synthesis within the central nervous system. Techniques are also available to study the various components of IgG found in the CSF; in multiple sclerosis the abnormal IgG may be oligoclonal.

Glucose is present in normal CSF in a concentration of 2.5–4.2 mmol/l, which is about a half to a third of the blood glucose concentration. In purulent tuberculous or fungal meningitis and rarely in carcinomatous meningitis the CSF sugar is *reduced to less than half of the blood glucose*. It is also low if the patient is hypoglycaemic.

One or more of the tests for syphilis are often performed on the CSF.

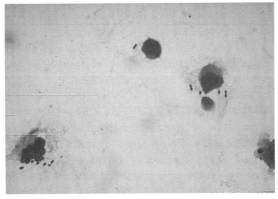

Fig. 12.57   Smear from cellular deposit in CSF from a patient with acute meningitis showing Gram-positive diplococci, many located intracellularly in polymorphonuclear leucocytes.

The typical changes in the CSF in various neurological diseases are summarized in Table 12.4.

The electroencephalogram (EEG)

Electrodes applied to the patient's scalp pick up small changes of electrical potential, which after amplification are recorded on paper or displayed on a video monitor. The EEG is of particular value in the investigation of epilepsy; it is also used in the localization of cerebral tumours, other expanding intracranial lesions and encephalitis, and in the assessment of patients with dementia.

The electromyogram (EMG)

Electrical activity occurring in muscle during voluntary contraction, or in denervated muscles during rest, can be recorded with needle electrodes inserted percutaneously into the belly of the muscle, or with surface electrodes (silver discs attached to the skin overlying the muscle with a salty paste). This electrical activity is amplified and displayed as an auditory signal through a suitable loudspeaker and as a visual signal on an oscilloscope. It may be recorded on magnetic tape or printed out on a paper recorder. Analysis of such electrical activity is useful in the

Disease condition	Physical characteristics	Cytology (cells/μl)	Protein (g/l)	Glucose (mmol/l)	Tests for syphilis	Stained deposit	Culture
Normal	Clear and colourless	Lymphocytes 0–5	0.1–0.4	2.5–4.2	Negative	No organisms	Sterile
Meningitis Bacterial	Yellowish and turbid	Polymorphs 200–2000 Lymphocytes 5–50	0.5–2.0	<2.0	Negative	Bacteria	Positive
Tuberculous	Colourless and sometimes viscous	Polymorphs 0–100 Lymphocytes 100–300	>0.5	<2.0*	Negative	Tubercle bacilli in films in some cases	Positive by special methods
Viral (includes poliomyelitis)	Usually clear	10–100 mixed cells at first, becoming lymphocytic in 36 hours	0.1–0.6; Poliomyelitis 0.3–0.2, remaining high 6–8 weeks	2.5–4.2	Negative	No organisms	Sterile
Multiple sclerosis	Clear and colourless	Rarely 5–15 lymphocytes	0.1–0.6 Rarely higher. IgG level raised with monoclonal bands	2.5–4.2	Negative	No organisms	Sterile
Neoplastic infiltration	Clear or yellowish	5–1000 cells of mixed type	0.5–2.0	<3.0	Negative	Inflammatory and indignant cells	Sterile
Syphilis GPI	Clear and colourless	5–100 lymphocytes	0.4–1.0	2.5–4.2	Positive	No organisms	Sterile
Tabes	Clear and colourless	5–100 lymphocytes	0.3–0.6	2.5–4.2	20% Negative by reagin tests†	No organisms	Sterile
Meningitic	Clear and slightly turbid	10–50 polymorphs 50–500 lymphocytes	0.5–2.0	May be slightly low	Positive	No organisms	Sterile

GPI = general paralysis of the insane.
*CSF glucose is usually about half the blood glucose. Simultaneous blood and CSF glucose estimations should always be performed.
†Nearly all are positive by FTA-ABS (Fluorescent Treponemal Assay) or TPHA (Treponema Pallidum Haemagglutinin Assay).

Table 12.4 Typical changes in the cerebrospinal fluid (CSF) in various diseases.

(a)

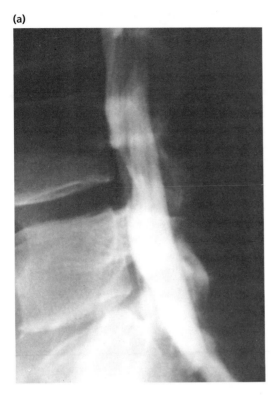

(b)

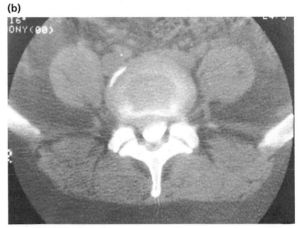

Fig. 12.59 (a) Lateral view of myelogram, or radiculogram, since only the cauda equina nerve roots are displayed in this limited view. There is disc protrusion opposite the L4/5 disc interspace which is indenting the column of water-soluble contrast within the theca. The nerve roots can be seen above this level. (b) CT scan of the contrasted theca shown above. The disc protrusion can be seen a little to the left of the midline, displacing the dense, contrast-filled thecal sac posteriorly. There is also a lateral disc protrusion extending toward the invertebral foramen and thus compromising the nerve root. The scan shows the paraspinal muscles and, anteriorly, the upper parts of the two psoas muscles.

diagnosis of primary diseases of muscle (*myopathies* and *dystrophies*) and of lower motor neurone lesions (*denervation*).

The speed of conduction of afferent impulses (*sensory nerve conduction velocity*) and efferent impulses (*motor nerve conduction velocity*) in peripheral nerves

(a)

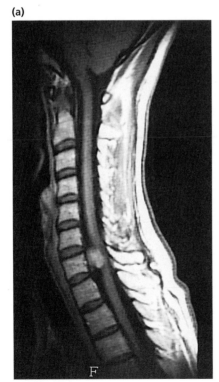

(b)

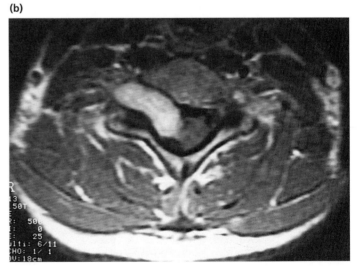

Fig. 12.60 (a) MRI scan with gadolinium enhancement. There is a neurofibroma at the C6 spinal level which is compressing the spinal cord, causing progressive paraparesis. (b) The tumour enhances slightly and can be seen as a sausage-shaped mass arising in the intervertebral foramen and compressing the spinal cord in the axial view.

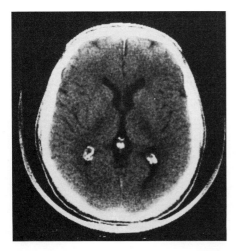

Fig. 12.61 Normal CT scan. The cerebral ventricles, the sulci at the surface of the brain, the central calcified pineal gland and the two calcified parts of the choroid plexus. In the posterior parts of the skull there is a linear an artefact resulting from the computer processing required to produce the image.

can be calculated using an electrical nerve stimulation technique and suitable recording electrodes with amplifying or digital averaging equipment. These measures are useful in the diagnosis of peripheral nerve disorders, particularly those due to local compressive lesions such as, for example, carpal tunnel syndrome. Similar investigations of sensory conduction in the central nervous system can be achieved by averaging signals recorded from the head (*somatosen-*

sory evoked potentials), and *visual* and *auditory evoked potential* measurements can be used to study visual and auditory pathways in the brain.

Neuroimaging

Apart from routine radiographs of the skull and spine a number of special techniques are useful.

MYELOGRAPHY

This is a method for demonstrating the subarachnoid space in the spinal canal (Fig. 12.59a and b). A lumbar or cisternal puncture is performed with the patient on

(a)

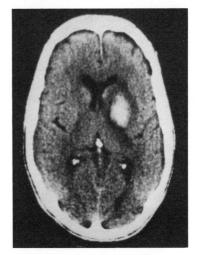

(b)

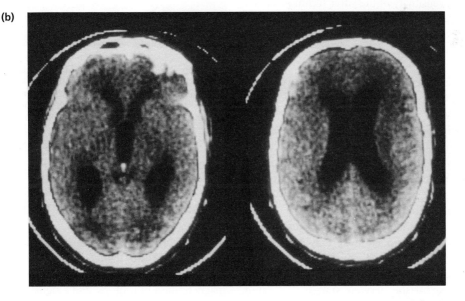

Fig. 12.62 CT scans illustrating lesions in the brain. (a) Left capsular haemorrhage. The haemorrhage appears relatively dense; it is surrounded by a zone of oedema, and has caused displacement of the midline structures to the opposite side. The haemorrhage is in the typical location associated with hypertensive haemorrhage. (b) Hydrocephalus. The ventricular system is enlarged and there are periventricular lucent zones, due to oedema or seepage of CSF into the cerebral white matter in these regions, indicating that the hydrocephalus is progressing (decompensated hydrocephalus).

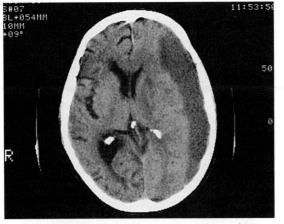

Fig. 12.63 CT scan in a patient presenting with confusion. There is a chronic left subdural haematoma with midline shift. The patient had been involved in a fight a few weeks previously.

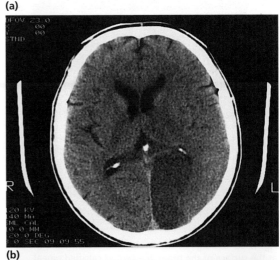

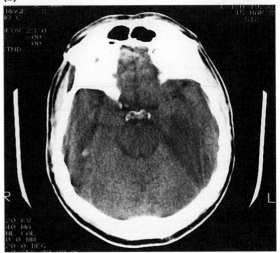

Fig. 12.64 CT scan. (a) Infarction in a left posterior cerebral artery territory involves the occipital lobe and its deep white matter. The infarct extends anteriorly into the posterior part of the temporal lobe (b). There is a slight mass effect with swelling of the left hemisphere causing herniation of the midline to the right. The sagittal sinus is clearly seen in (a).

the myelogram table in the X-ray department and 2–10 ml of a special water-soluble radiopaque contrast medium is injected into the subarachnoid space. By tilting the table the contrast medium can be made to flow up and down the spinal canal under direct vision, preferably using TV amplification; and radiographs can be taken of regions of deformity or obstruction to the flow of contrast. This is a very useful method for accurate localization of tumours in the spinal canal. Transverse axial computerized tomography, combined with contrast myelography, greatly enhances the sensitivity of the latter technique in the detection of small lateral intervertebral disc protrusions (Fig. 12.59b), but is itself giving way to magnetic resonance imaging (Fig. 12.60).

COMPUTERIZED TOMOGRAPHY (CT) SCANNING

CT scanning provides tomographic images of the brain of high resolution, without the need for invasive procedures. A crystallographic X-ray detection device is used instead of conventional X-ray film and a photographic image is produced by computerized averaging techniques. The resulting pictures are displayed as sections of the head in the coronal or basal plane (Figs 12.61 and 12.62). Intravenous or subarachnoid iodine-based contrast may be used to enhance the vascular or CSF compartments respectively (Fig 12.59b).

CT scanning of the nervous system is a rapid, widely available, high-resolution technique that is particularly useful in the assessment of trauma (Fig. 12.63), stroke (Fig. 12.64), suspected haemorrhage or tumours (Fig. 12.65) of the nervous system.

Tuberculomas are well demonstrated by this technique (Fig. 12.66).

MAGNETIC RESONANCE IMAGING (MRI)

In this technique the patient is placed in a uniform high magnetic field. Radiofrequency current is used to interpose brief pulses into the field causing changing magnetization of protons, and a signal recorded from the coil surrounding the magnet. Computerized reconstruction of this pattern of signals allows a water-based image of the tissue, of very high resolution, to be generated. Lesions such as multiple sclerosis (Fig.

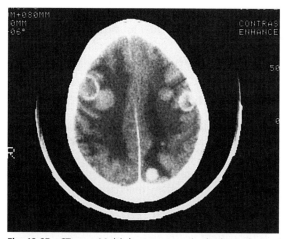

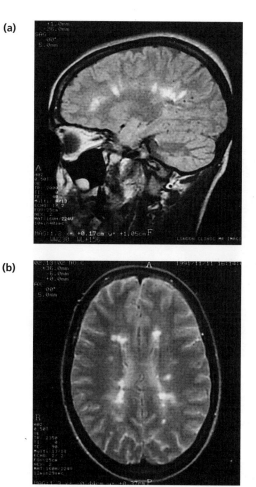

Fig. 12.65 CT scan. Multiple metastases in the brain from primary carcinoma of the breast. There is marked oedema of the white matter.

(a)

(b)

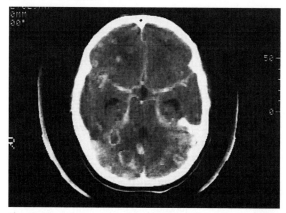

Fig. 12.66 Enhanced CT scan. Multiple tuberculomas in the brain. The lesions show enhancement of their capsules. They vary in size. Note that there is effacement of the cortical pattern suggesting widespread meningeal inflammation.

Fig. 12.67 MRI scan. Multiple sclerosis. T_2-weighted scans of a woman aged 45 showing (a) axial and (b) sagittal images. There are bright lesions in the periventricular white matter. In the sagittal image the abnormal signals have a finger-like form pointing towards the lateral ventricle (Dawson's fingers).

12.67), infections, infarction and infiltrative tumours (Fig. 12.68) can be detected readily (see Fig 12.69).

ANGIOGRAPHY

This is a method for studying the intracranial and extracranial vessels. A water-soluble radio-opaque contrast medium is injected percutaneously into a carotid artery in the neck, or into a vertebral artery either by catheterization of a major vessel, such as the femoral, axillary, brachial or subclavian arteries. Radiographs are taken in various planes in the following few seconds as the contrast medium traverses the cerebral circulation. The arterial, capillary and venous circulations can be studied and abnormalities of the distribution, size, position and lumen of these vessels can be seen.

The technique is particularly useful for diagnosis of aneurysms (Fig. 12.70), arteriovenous malforma-

tions and cerebral tumours. It is also useful in cerebral vascular disease.

The application of digital averaging has enabled angiography to be performed using intravenous contrast injections to visualize circulating contrast in the cerebral and extracranial circulation, thus reducing the risk of the vascular complications of arterial catheterization or puncture.

Routine examination of the nervous system

A detailed examination of the whole nervous system is time-consuming and something of an ordeal for

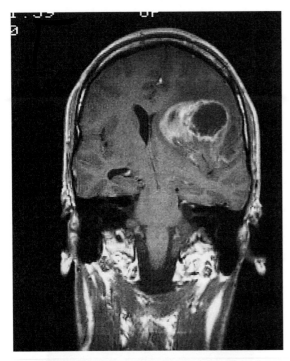

Fig. 12.68   MRI scan. T$_1$-weighted coronal slice. There is a large cystic malignant glioma in the left hemisphere which is causing subfalcine herniation of the brain to the right with compression of the lateral ventricle, and pressure on the mid-brain.

the patient. A scheme for a quick routine examination is therefore useful in the examination of patients *not suspected of neurological disease*, in order to exclude major neurological disability.

Mental state

Much useful information can be obtained during history-taking and physical examination; no specific questions need usually be asked.

- Is the history given *accurately, concisely* and *with insight?* Or is the patient *concrete, circumlocutory* or *vague?*
- Is the patient's *memory* normal?
- Is the patient *neatly dressed* and *well-cared for?*
- Is the patient's *behaviour* normal?
- Is the patient *aphasic* or *dysarthric?*
- Is the patient *confused?*
- Can the patient *find his or her way* in and out of the room?
- Can the patient *dress* and *undress* him or herself?

Gait

- Is it *spastic, hemiparetic, ataxic* or *parkinsonian?*
- Is there a *foot drop?*

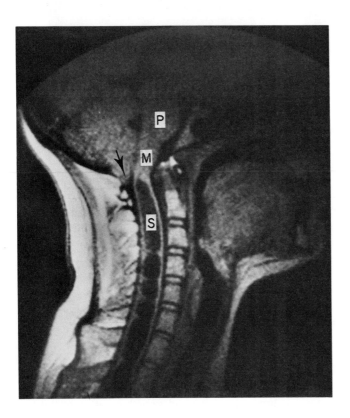

Fig. 12.69   MRI scan of the brain. Sagittal view of the craniocervical junction in a patient with syringomyelia. The neck and chin can be recognized to the left and right in the picture. Note the normal density representing the water content of the central parts of the intervertebral discs. The tongue, pharynx and larynx, and soft tissues of the neck are recognizable. Note the pons (P) and medulla (M). There is tonsillar herniation (arrow) into the foramen magnum and a long irregular cyst (syrinx) has caused enlargement of the cervical spinal cord (S).

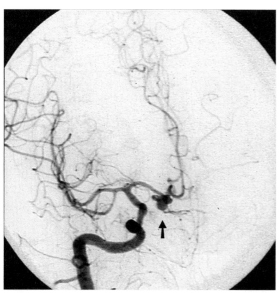

Fig. 12.70 Oblique right carotid angiogram with digital subtraction showing a multioculated anterior communicating artery aneurysm (arrow).

Cranial nerves

- Test *ocular movements* and look for nystagmus.
- Test *facial movements.*
- Test *tongue protrusion* and *palatal movement.*

Visual fields

These, like *aphasia,* may provide absolute evidence of disease above the tentorium cerebelli.
- Is there a *hemianopia?*
- If so, is it *homonymous, bitemporal, unilateral* or something else?
- Is *central vision* normal? This is crudely assessed by testing the visual acuity.

- Can the patient read small print with or without glasses?

Fundi

- Is *papilloedema* present?
- Is *optic atrophy* present?
- Are there *hypertensive, uraemic* or *diabetic* changes present?

Motor

- Is there any *weakness* of the outstretched upper limbs?
- Is there *distal* or *proximal weakness* or *wasting?*
- Is *muscular tone* normal, spastic or extrapyramidal in type?
- Look for *cerebellar ataxia* in the limbs.
- Assess the *tendon reflexes* and *plantar responses.*
- Assess *gait* and the ability to get up from a low chair.

Sensory

- Test *position sense* in the fingers and toes and vibration sense in the feet (posterior columns).
- Test *pinprick* in the four limbs and on the face (lateral spinothalamic tracts).
- *Light touch* need only be tested if the patient complains of numbness.

General

- Examine the *skull, spinal movements* and posture.
- Look for *cutaneous naevi.*
- Listen for *bruits in the neck.*

CHAPTER 13

The unconscious patient

Introduction

Coma is a common medical problem. Diagnosis can usually be achieved at the bedside, provided attention is given both to the history and to the examination. In this chapter clinical methods relevant to diagnosis of the comatose patient will be described.

Consciousness is a state of normal cerebral activity in which the patient is aware both of self and environment and is able to respond to internal changes, for example hunger, and to changes in the external environment. *Sleep*, although a state of altered consciousness, is a normal variation in consciousness. The sleeping patient can be roused, both spontaneously and in response to external stimuli, to a full state of wakefulness. Altered consciousness resulting from brain disease may take the form of a *confusional state*, in which the patient's alertness is clouded; this is associated with agitation, fright and confusion, i.e. disorientation. Such patients usually show evidence of misperception of their environment, and hallucinations and delusions may occur. Confusional states must be carefully distinguished from apha-

sia, in which a specific disorder of language is the characteristic feature, and from continuous temporal lobe epilepsy, a form of focal status epilepticus in which the behavioural disorder is often accompanied by aphasia if the epileptic focus is left-sided. Usually this can be recognized by the occurrence of frequent but slight myoclonic jerks of facial and especially perioral muscles and by variability in the patient's confusion from moment to moment during the examination. The examiner should always pause and observe an unconscious or drowsy patient for a few moments before disturbing them.

A state of abnormal drowsiness is often found in patients with space-occupying intracranial lesions or metabolic disorders before stupor or coma supervenes. The patient appears to be in normal sleep but cannot easily be wakened and, once awake, tends to fall asleep despite attempts to continue conversation or clinical examination. Further, while awake such patients can usually be shown to be disorientated; higher intellectual function, such as the ability to perform abstract tasks or to make judgements, is disturbed. Stupor means a state of disturbed consciousness from which only vigorous external stimuli can produce arousal. Arousal from stupor is invariably

Eye-opening		Best verbal response		Best motor response	
Spontaneous	4	Oriented	5	Obeying	5
To speech	3	Confused	4	Localizing	4
To pain	2	Inappropriate	3	Flexing	3
None	1	Incomprehensible	2	Extending	2
		None	1	None	1

The three categories of information required in the assessment require no special skills and are thus particularly suited for observations to be carried out serially in a patient after a head injury, for example by relatively untrained staff. The best score is 14. This simple non-linear clinical rating scale enables relatively accurate assessment of improvement or deterioration in a patient's conscious state.

Table 13.1 The Glasgow coma scale.

BOX 13.1 Outline of causes of coma.

Metabolic
- Drug overdosage (including alcohol)
- Hypoglycaemia
- Diabetes mellitus
- Renal failure
- Hepatic failure
- Hypothermia
- Hypothyroidism
- Cardiorespiratory failure
- Hypoxic encephalopathy

Structural
Diffuse
- Meningitis
- Encephalitis
- Other infections (e.g. cerebral malaria)
- Subarachnoid haemorrhage
- Epilepsy
- Head injury
- Hypertensive encephalopathy

Focal
  Supratentorial lesions
  —Cerebral haemorrhage
  —Cerebral infarction with oedema
  —Subdural haematoma
  —Extradural haematoma
  —Tumour
  —Cerebral abscess
  —Pituitary apoplexy
  Subtentorial lesions
  —Cerebellar haemorrhage
  —Pontine haemorrhage
  —Brainstem infarction
  —Tumour
  —Cerebellar abscess
  —Secondary effects of transtentorial herniation of brain due to cerebral mass lesions

Causes of coma

The objective of examination of the unconscious patient is to achieve a diagnosis and so to plan management. Coma may be due to *metabolic* or *structural* disease of the brain: it is only very rarely a psychogenic disorder. Coma results from lesions affecting the brain widely, diffusely or multifocally, and from lesions of deep, centrally placed structures in the diencephalon or brainstem (Box 13.1). For example, supratentorial mass lesions, such as tumours, may damage deep diencephalic structures, while subtentorial neoplasms may directly damage the brainstem reticular formation. Metabolic disorders, for example hypoglycaemia, hypnotic drugs or hypoxia, widely depress brain function. It is important to distinguish supratentorial (cerebral) from subtentorial (posterior fossa) space-occupying lesions. An immediate basic assessment will direct the subsequent series of investigations, and management (Box 13.2).

History

The history is of great importance and attempts should always be made to find family or other witnesses of the onset of the coma. Coma occurs suddenly in vascular disorders such as *subarachnoid haemorrhage* or stroke, especially with cerebral or cerebellar haemorrhage. A history of trauma with concussion followed a few days later by fluctuating drowsiness and stupor, suggesting subdural haematoma, should never be regarded lightly. Concussion followed by a brief lucid interval before rapidly deepening coma suggests extradural haematoma. A history of headache before coma supervenes is frequent in patients with intracranial space-occupying lesions of any cause. Seizures of

both brief and incomplete. Stupor is a non-quantitative description of an altered mental state that is difficult to define exactly. In *coma* the patient is less responsive: the term coma was originally used to describe a patient who is unrousable and unresponsive to all external stimuli. The *Glasgow coma scale* (Table 13.1) represents an attempt, now generally used, to replace these ill-defined terms with descriptions of the state of consciousness confined to three categories of performance—*eye-opening to command, verbal responses* and *motor responses*.

BOX 13.2 Immediate assessment of coma: seven questions.

Question	Check	Action
1 Is the airway clear?	Blood gases	Intubate and give oxygen
2 Is the patient fitting?	EEG/blood glucose	IV glucose, oxygen and diazepam
3 Are there signs of cranio-facial trauma?	CT scan	Neurosurgical opinion
4 Is the neck broken?	X-ray	Splint neck
5 Is there major haemorrhage?		Maintain circulation
6 Is there evidence of diabetes mellitus?	Blood/urine glucose	Treat appropriately
7 Is there evidence of drug overdose or misuse?	Pupils/ventilation	Naloxone?

recent onset, whether focal or generalized, strongly suggest cerebral disease, which may be due to tumour, encephalitis, abscess or trauma. Patients with drug-induced coma may be known by neighbours, family, medical attendants or the ambulance driver to have taken drugs by the presence of drug containers or alcohol in their homes. A history of depression might be known. A search of the patient's clothing may reveal hospital out-patient attendance cards, unfilled prescriptions, drugs or even syringes. Diabetic or epileptic patients often carry some form of identification either in their clothing or as a wrist-band or necklace. If there is any suspicion that the patient might be hypoglycaemic, a blood sample should be taken for blood glucose estimation and then 20 g of 50% glucose given intravenously, before the test result is necessarily available. Hypoglycaemia is characterized by stupor or coma from which the patient can be roused to a resentful and aggressive state of partial awareness, with pallor and sweatiness, bounding pulse, and often focal or generalized seizures.

It is important to try to discover whether the coma was of gradual or sudden onset; the latter clearly suggests vascular disease. Before examination commences the doctor must make sure that the patient is breathing adequately, that the pulse and blood pressure are satisfactory and that the patient is not bleeding rapidly. If oxygenation is not satisfactory, whatever the breathing pattern, oxygen should be administered. If the patient is clearly in status epilepticus this must be treated appropriately immediately, and clinical examination continued afterwards (Box 13.2). Remember, also, always to consider whether there may be a fracture of the cervical spine; if this is suspected splinting of the neck and an X-ray in the AP and lateral planes is mandatory (Box 13.3).

Examination

Always proceed to examine the patient in a logical order (Box 13.3). Certain general features of the patient's clinical state are of great importance. Does the patient appear clean, well nourished and generally cared for, or are there signs of social decline such as a dishevelled appearance, lack of personal cleanliness, malnutrition or infestation? Is there evidence of trauma or exposure? A rapid search must be made for fractures and especially for signs of cranial trauma (Box 13.4). Bruises in the scalp are difficult to see

---

BOX 13.3 Basic neurological examination in coma.

- Assess level of consciousness (Glasgow coma scale)
- Signs of head injury: local bruising, fractures and penetrating wounds, bleeding from nose or ears
- Splint the neck: head injury may be associated with fracture of the cervical spine
- If no neck injury (clinically and by X-ray) check for neck stiffness
- Check resting pupillary size, and pupillary responses to light
- Ocular movements: spontaneous, following and to 'doll's head' (if no voluntary response)
- Limbs: posture, tone and movement
- Reflexes and plantar responses
- Fundi

---

but scalp oedema or haematoma can usually be palpated and bruising of the skin behind the pinna, called a 'battle sign', is a useful sign of basal or temporal skull fracture. Likewise, bleeding from the external auditory meati is a reliable sign of cranial trauma, with basal skull fracture. Pallor, circulatory failure and other evidence of shock must be recognized and a search made for external or internal haemorrhage, especially if trauma is suspected.

BOX 13.4 Head injury: basic management.

- Exclude intracranial haemorrhage by CT scan
- Control circulation
- Control intracranial pressure
- Control ventilation
- Obtain neurological/neurosurgical opinion

Metabolic coma is common, and has many causes (Box 13.1). It is characterized by altered consciousness without focal neurological signs or neck stiffness, and with preservation of vestibulogenic ocular movements (doll's head responses) (Box 13.5). In certain drug-induced coma states there may be signs of repeated intravenous injections under conditions of imperfect sterility, causing venous thrombosis in

---

BOX 13.5 Causes of coma without focal neurological signs, or neck stiffness.

Metabolic coma
- Hypoglycaemia
- Hyperglycaemia
- Liver failure
- Renal failure
- Respiratory failure with CO_2 retention
- Endocrine/electrolyte imbalance

Drug poisoning (consider gastric lavage)

forearm or antebrachial veins. The odours of alcohol, uraemia, diabetic acidosis and hepatic coma may be recognizable in some instances. The stertorous, rapid respiration of acidotic coma (air hunger), usually due to diabetes, can be quickly recognized (see below). The presence of jaundice, liver palms, or spider naevi, even in the absence of hepatic enlargement, raise the suspicion of hepatic coma.

Meningitis can usually be recognized by the presence of drowsiness, lethargy or stupor with fever and signs of meningeal irritation (see Chapter 12). The pulse may be unexpectedly slow in relation to the fever in pyogenic meningitis, although the respirations are usually rapid. Seizures and focal neurological signs may develop and there is usually a history of headache and neck stiffness, perhaps with vomiting. Further, there may be a skin rash (Fig. 13.1), or a primary site of infection such as otitis media or sinusitis may be apparent. The ocular fundi must always be examined by ophthalmoscopy for signs of papilloedema, retinal haemorrhages or exudates, or intraarterial emboli, which appear as luminescent, highly refractile yellow or white plaque-like material occluding vessels (see Fig. 10.14) Coma with neck stiffness (Box 13.6) implies meningeal irritation and infection must be excluded.

Consciousness

Define the state of consciousness by using the Glasgow coma scale (Box 13.1), as described above, particularly noting any variation or tendency to improve or deteriorate during the period of observa-

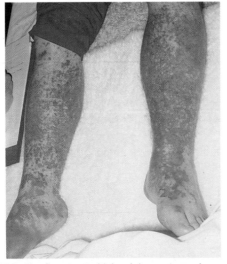

Fig. 13.1 Confluent petechial rash in an unconscious patient with overwhelming meningococcal septicaemia and meningitis.

> **BOX 13.6 Causes of coma with neck stiffness.** The stiffness may be relatively inapparent in deeply comatose patients.
>
> - Subarachnoid haemorrhage
> - Meningitis
>   —Bacterial
>   —Viral (aseptic)
> - Encephalitis
> - Intracerebral haemorrhage
> - Cerebral malaria

tion. *Change in level of consciousness* is the single most important piece of information which will indicate the need for a change of management. The scoring system applied to the Glasgow coma scale is useful in warning of this change, and this can readily be done by nursing as well as by medical staff. It is important to note exactly the *degree of responsiveness to external stimuli*, including conversation, calling the patient's first name, a sudden loud noise, a flash of light, contactual or painful stimulation, passive movement of the limbs and deep noxious stimuli such as squeezing the Achilles tendon, sternal pressure applied with a hard blunt object or supraorbital pressure from the examiner's thumb. Special attention must also be directed to *pupillary reactions and ocular movements*, both volitional and reflex, *to the pattern of breathing* and to *motor responses*, either spontaneous or reflexly evoked. Localizing responses to painful contractual stimuli are meaningful and imply stupor or a state of light coma, with preservation of sensation and associated motor responses. If localized responses are absent, there may be hemiparesis, or deep coma. Substituted flexion or extension responses of an upper limb signify decortication or decerebration, respectively (see below). In the leg, extension to a painful stimulus applied to the sternum suggests decerebration or decortication.

PUPILS

Pupillary size and responsiveness to light should be noted (Fig. 13.2). If the pupils are unequal a decision as to which is abnormal must be made. Usually the larger pupil indicates the presence of an oculomotor nerve palsy, whether from damage to the oculomotor nerve by pressure and displacement or from a lesion in the mesencephalon itself, but occasionally the smaller pupil may be the abnormal pupil, as in *Horner's syndrome*. If the larger pupil does not react to light it is likely that there is a *partial oculomotor nerve palsy* on that side. If the smaller pupil also fails to react to light this may be the *mid-position pupil* of complete sympathetic and parasympathetic lesions, indicating extensive brainstem damage. Pupillary dilatation in response to neck flexion or to pinching the skin of the neck is not a reliable phenomenon.

In drug-induced coma and in most patients with metabolic coma the pupillary responses to light are normal. Exceptions to this rule are glutethimide poisoning and very deep metabolic coma, in which the pupils may become dilated and, rarely, may become unreactive to light. In pontine and in thalamic haemorrhage the pupils may be very small (*pinpoint pupils*), and unreactive to light.

OCULAR MOVEMENTS

In comatose patients the eyes become slightly divergent at rest. If there is a pre-existent strabismus, deviation of the ocular axes may be pronounced, both at rest and during reflex ocular movements.

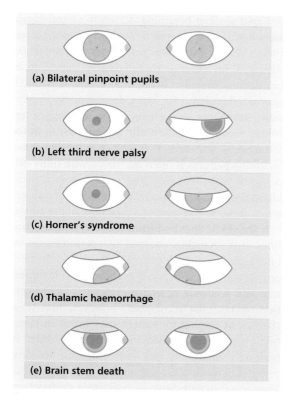

(a) Bilateral pinpoint pupils

(b) Left third nerve palsy

(c) Horner's syndrome

(d) Thalamic haemorrhage

(e) Brain stem death

Fig. 13.2 Pupillary anomalies. (a) Bilateral pinpoint pupils occur with brain stem lesions, opiate and other drug intoxications and with pontine infarction. (b) Left third nerve palsy. There is ptosis, dilatation of the pupil with absence of the light reaction, and slight lateral deviation of the eye. (c) Horner's syndrome. There is ptosis and a small, reactive pupil. (d) In thalamic haemorrhage the eyes tend to 'look towards the tip of the nose', and the pupils are small; later they become large and unreactive as upper brainstem involvement develops. (e) When brain stem death occurs the mid-brain disturbance is manifest by mid-position, fixed (unreactive) pupils, with eye closure.

Doll's head movements

If the patient is too drowsy or stuporose to test voluntary or following eye movements, '*doll's head*' movements should be tested. If possible the patient should be placed supine, although the test can be carried out in any position. The examiner grasps the patient's head with both hands, using the thumbs to hold the eyelids open gently, and firmly rocks the patient's head from side to side through about 70 degrees, and then from passive neck flexion to passive neck extension. The patient's eyes tend to remain in the straight ahead position despite these passive movements of the head, a phenomenon like that found in some children's dolls, i.e. the patient's eyes tend to deviate in the opposite direction to the induced head movement. This movement depends on intact vestibular reflex mechanisms, and is thus a test of the peripheral sense organs involved, the labyrinths and otoliths, and their central connections in the brainstem, including the vestibular nuclei, the medial longitudinal fasciculi and the efferent pathway through oculomotor, trochlear and abducent nerves and their nuclei. Sometimes lesions in these structures can be recognized during the doll's head test by the presence of disturbances in ocular movements consistent, for example, with an abducent or oculomotor nerve palsy. Absence of the reflex on one side indicates an ipsilateral pontine lesion, but complete absence of doll's head movements may be found both in extensive structural lesions in the brainstem and in deep metabolic coma. *In most patients with drug-induced coma, however, doll's head ocular movements are intact.*

Caloric reflexes

Brainstem function can also be assessed by testing caloric reflexes. In the comatose patient, irrigation of the external auditory meatus on one side with at least 20 ml of ice-cold water induces slow conjugate deviation of the eyes towards the irrigated side after a few seconds' delay. In the awake or drowsy patient this slow tonic deviation is masked by a fast, coarse nystagmus towards the opposite side. Normal caloric nystagmus is characteristically also found in cases of psychogenic coma. After a few minutes' delay the opposite ear should also be tested. It is important to inspect the tympanic membrane on each side *before* irrigating the external auditory meatus since it is unwise to perform this test in the presence of a large perforation, or if there is an active otitis media.

Spontaneous ocular movements

Occasionally in patients with infarction or other structural lesions in the posterior fossa *spontaneous ocular movements* may be observed. These may be accompanied by marked ocular divergence, sometimes with elevation of one eye and depression of the other. Rarely there may be a spontaneous 'see-saw' nystagmus in which one eye rotates up and the other down, the movements alternating at a very slow rate. *Rapid ocular oscillations* may occur especially after poisoning with tricyclic antidepressant drugs, and a slow, once or twice a second, conjugate downward *bobbing* movement is sometimes a sign of cerebellar haemorrhage or tumour. In *thalamic haemorrhage* the pupils are pinpoint, and the eyes seem to be looking downwards as if at the patient's own nose. *Rapid conjugate lateral movement*, at a rhythm and rate reminiscent of cerebellar nystagmus, occurring in an unconscious patient should suggest focal motor seizures originating in the contralateral frontal lobe. Such seizures are often accompanied by deviation of the head and eyes in the direction of the 'nystagmoid movement', but not necessarily by a fully developed focal seizure involving face and limbs on the same side. Nystagmus itself cannot occur in the comatose patient because it requires ocular fixation to develop the fast, corrective phase.

PATTERN OF BREATHING

Alterations in the rhythm and pattern of breathing are an important aspect of the assessment of the unconscious patient.

Cheyne–Stokes (periodic) respiration

In Cheyne–Stokes respiration, breathing varies in regular cycles. A phase of gradually deepening respiration is followed, after a period of very deep rapid breaths, by a phase of slowly decreasing respiratory excursion and rate. Respiration gradually becomes quieter and may cease for several seconds before the cycle is repeated. Depressed, but regular breathing at a normal rate occurs in most drug-induced comas, but *Cheyne–Stokes respiration* can occur in coma of any cause, especially if there is coincidental chronic pulmonary disease. Cheyne–Stokes breathing in a comatose patient is a sign of a large unilateral space-occupying lesion with brainstem distortion, e.g. subdural haematoma, or of bilateral lesions from other causes, e.g. cerebral infarction or meningitis.

Kussmaul breathing

Deep sighing, rapid breathing at a regular rate should immediately suggest metabolic acidosis. Metabolic ketoacidosis or uraemia is the commonest cause of this acidotic (Kussmaul) breathing pattern, but a similar pattern may occur in some patients with respiratory failure, and in deep metabolic coma, especially hepatic coma.

Central pontine hyperventilation

Deep, regular breathing may also occur with rostral brainstem damage, whether due to reticular pontine infarction or to central brainstem dysfunction secondary to transtentorial herniation associated with an intra- or extracerebral space-occupying lesion. This breathing pattern is called *central neurogenic (pontine) hyperventilation*. Interspersed deep sighs or yawns may precede the development of this respiratory pattern.

Rapid shallow breathing occurs if central brainstem dysfunction extends more caudally to the lower pons. When medullary respiratory neurones are damaged, for example by progressive transtentorial herniation, irregular breathing (*ataxic respiration*) may develop. Irregular, slow, deep, gasping respirations, sometimes associated with hiccups, suggest terminal medullary failure. In patients with raised intracranial pressure, this sequence of abnormal breathing patterns is often associated with other evidence of brainstem dysfunction, including a rising blood pressure, a slow pulse, flaccid limbs, absence of reflex ocular movements and dilatation of the pupils.

It should be apparent from the foregoing descriptions that changing patterns of respiration in an unconscious patient, particularly the development of central neurogenic hyperventilation, provide important and relatively objective evidence of deterioration. It must be recognized, however, that these changes in respiratory pattern may occur in structural lesions with raised intracranial pressure, in brainstem infarction and less commonly in some varieties of metabolic coma, especially hepatic coma. They are thus indicative of brainstem dysfunction, but not of its causation (Box 13.7).

MOTOR RESPONSES

It is often difficult to elicit signs of focal cerebral disease in the unconscious patient. The presence of focal neurological signs implies localized dysfunction in the central nervous system, and is important in considering the causes of altered consciousness (Box 13.8). If progressive brainstem dysfunction

BOX 13.7 Coma with hyperventilation (and low $Paco_2$).

- Metabolic acidosis
- Diabetic ketoacidosis
- Brainstem lesion, e.g. stroke
- Rising intracranial pressure
- Bacterial meningitis
- Renal failure
- Liver failure
- Pneumonia complicating brain lesion

from raised intracranial pressure with transtentorial herniation has occurred, focal signs indicative of the causative lesion may no longer be recognizable. However, papilloedema is usually present in such cases. In the drowsy or stuporose patient it may be possible to recognize a hemianopia by testing the response to visual menace or, sometimes, by testing for optokinetic nystagmus (page 296). Visual threat, or menace, consists of threatening the patient's face, in first the left, and then the right field. Normally this threat induces rapid eye closure or a flinch. It is necessary to obtain the patient's attention transiently to assess any meaningful response and the test is, unfortunately, only rarely useful. Hemiplegia may be evident either from abnormal flaccidity of the arm and leg on the affected side or, in the stuporose or lightly comatose patient, by absence of spontaneous movements on that side. Noxious stimuli, for example pinching the skin of the forearms and thighs, deep rubbing pressure with a hard object applied to the sternum or, often most effective, lightly pricking the skin and mucous membranes near the nasal orifices on both sides will fail to induce movement of the paralysed limbs. Sometimes in a patient with a dense hemiplegia the cheek blows flaccidly in and out with each breath on the side of hemiplegia. The tendon reflexes may be asymmetrical, but in most comatose patients both plantar responses are extensor (see page 310). It should be noted that *asymmetry* of these motor responses is the important feature to assess.

BOX 13.8 Causes of coma with focal neurological signs.

- Epilepsy (post-ictal state)
- Stroke
- Encephalitis
- Subarachnoid haemorrhage
- Cerebral abscess
- Bacterial meningitis with cortical infarction
- Cerebral venous sinus thrombosis

In both structural lesions and metabolic disorders coma may be accompanied in its terminal stages by *decorticate* or *decerebrate postures*. These may occur asymmetrically and may be apparent, at first, only when induced by noxious external stimuli, such as deep sternal pressure or pinching the skin or Achilles tendon. Decorticate and decerebrate postures are features of severe upper brainstem dysfunction and are thus usually found in association with pupillary abnormalities, absence of doll's head and caloric reflexes and a disturbed breathing pattern. Decerebrate and decorticate postures are found much more commonly with structural coma than with metabolic coma, and thus do not usually occur in patients with drug-induced coma unless there has been additional hypoxic or ischaemic brian injury.

Persistent vegetative state

PERSISTENT STATES OF ALTERED CONSCIOUSNESS

Patients with extensive or diffuse injury to the brain do not always die. In some, partial recovery from coma occurs to a *persistent vegetative state* (see Box 13.9). This term is used to describe patients who appear to be in a state of wakeful unresponsiveness, rather than in a state of unresponsive coma. Despite their apparent wakefulness, patients in a persistent vegetative state make no meaningful response to environmental stimuli.

The patient is immobile, with decerebrate posturing, but appears to be awake, with eyes open, but without purposeful or meaningful response to noxious stimulation. Apparently normal sleep/wake cycles occur through the day and, when awake, the patient's eyes may move slowly and randomly, with preserved spontaneous blinking. Reflex swallowing in response to fluid placed in the mouth, and to salivary

BOX 13.9 Persistent vegetative state (PVS).

- No evidence of awareness of self or environment
- All responses are reflex in nature
- No meaningful or voluntary response to stimulation
- No evidence of language comprehension or expression
- An intermittent sleep/wake pattern
- Preserved cranial nerve responses
- Sufficiently intact hypothalamic (brainstem) autonomic function to allow prolonged survival with nursing and medical care
- Present for more than 1 month

secretion, usually occurs and there may be spontaneous chewing movements. The gag reflex is present, and the patient breathes normally. Relatives often find it difficult to accept that the patient, clearly awake, is not aware. The patient is mute. In patients in a persistent vegetative state for longer than 6 months there is no prospect of recovery.

In *akinetic mutism*, the patient appears awake, as in a persistent vegetative state. The patient shows no awareness of self or environment, but may follow the examiner or a moving object with their eyes. Communication can sometimes be established, even partially, by sign language or by a code based on eye-blinking, and fragmented voluntary movements of the limbs may be possible. If the akinetic mutism is due to a localized lesion or a tumour in the third ventricular region recovery may occur and such patients may have excellent recall of events during the period of illness. It is wise, therefore, to remember that the apparently comatose patient may be able to hear and understand, and may later recall conversations that took place or comments made at the bedside during a phase of apparent coma.

PSYCHOLOGICAL COMA

Psychologically disturbed patients sometimes feign coma. The eyes are actually closed and the patient is usually lying in a resting position, or supine with the arms and legs extended. The eyelids resist attempts to open them and, on forced eye opening, the eyes point upwards exposing the white conjunctiva (Bell's phenomenon) as part of the patient's attempt to maintain eyelid closure. The eyelids close rapidly when released. The slow roving eye movements of organic coma cannot be simulated. Painful stimuli to the limbs may be ignored, but pin prick to the nasal mucosa or to the lips usually elicits volitional grimacing. The pupillary light responses are normal. Cold caloric testing induces nystagmus with the fast phase away from the stimulated side, rather than deviation of the eyes toward the stimulus as would occur in true coma. Examination, especially invasive tests as above, may induce return of co-operation and consciousness, or uncover a disturbed mental state.

INVESTIGATIONS

The investigation of the comatose patient is a component of the clinical management of this problem. The immediate steps to be taken are outlined in Box 13.2. Immediately treatable structural or metabolic disorders require ascertainment and management.

BOX 13.10 Investigations that determine management of the comatose patient.

- Cervical spine X-ray
- CT head scan
- Chest X-ray
- X-ray of suspected fractures/bruised limbs
- Blood for cross-matching
- Check haemoglobin, haematocrit, WBC count
- Drug screen
- Electrolytes and liver function tests
- Blood gases and pH

Investigations are part of this process (Box 13.10). Several, for example blood gas determinations, electrolytes and haemoglobin, require repeated measurement during management. Others, e.g. X-rays of suspected fractured limbs, form part of the initial assessment.

Diagnosis of brain death

With the advent of improved methods of intensive care, and especially of positive pressure ventilation in patients in whom spontaneous respirations have ceased, it has become important to develop new criteria for the diagnosis of death. This has become important not only because of general recognition that brain death may have occurred in certain patients whose respiration has been maintained with a ventilator, although both the body temperature and the systemic circulation continue to be maintained spontaneously, but also because it is important to recognize the value of organ transplantation, for example the kidney, from such patients to others. In both these situations the diagnosis of brain death must be certain before any decision is made to cease attempts to keep the patient alive. A conference of the Royal Colleges and Faculties of the United Kingdom considered this problem in 1976 in the light of previous attempts to define brain death, the changing needs of medical practice, and public concern about the issue, and agreed the following guidelines, which have since been validated in many clinical studies, and are accepted worldwide.

A. Conditions in which the diagnosis of brain death should be considered

- The patient is deeply comatose, being incapable of response to any stimulus, other than reflex responses.

a There should be no suspicion that this state is due to depressant drugs. No such drugs should have been administered in the previous 24 hours.

b Primary hypothermia as a cause of coma should have been excluded.

c Metabolic and endocrine disturbances that can be responsible for or can contribute to coma should have been excluded.

- The patient is being maintained on a ventilator because spontaneous respiration had previously become inadequate or had ceased altogether.

  a Muscle relaxants and other drugs should have been excluded as a cause of respiratory failure.

- There should be no doubt that the patient's condition is due to irremediable structural brain damage. The *diagnosis of a disorder that can lead to brain death* should have been fully established.

B. Diagnostic tests for confirmation of brain death
All brain stem reflexes are absent

- The pupils are fixed in diameter and do not respond to sharp changes in the intensity of incident light.
- There is no corneal reflex.
- The vestibulo-ocular reflexes are absent.
- No motor responses within the cranial nerve distribution can be elicited by adequate stimulation of a somatic area.
- There is no gag reflex response to bronchial stimulation by a suction catheter passed down the trachea.
- No respiratory movements occur when the patient is disconnected from the mechanical ventilator for long enough to ensure that the arterial carbon dioxide tension rises above the threshold for stimulation of respiration. In practice this is best achieved by ventilating the patient with 5% CO_2 in oxygen for 5 minutes before disconnection. This ensures a $PaCO_2$ of 8.0 kPa (60 mmHg). A period of 10 minutes' observation for respiratory movement should then be carried out.

C. Other considerations

- Repetition of testing.
  The interval between tests must depend upon the primary pathology and the clinical course of the disease. In some conditions the outcome is not so clearcut, and in these cases it is recommended that the tests should be repeated. The interval between tests depends upon the progress of the patient and might be as long as 24 hours.

- Integrity of spinal reflexes.
  It is well established that spinal cord function can persist after insults that irretrievably destroy brainstem functions.
- Confirmatory investigation
  Electroencephalography is not necessary for the diagnosis of brain death. Other investigations such as cerebral angiography or cerebral blood-flow measurements are also not required for the diagnosis of brain death.
- Body temperature.
  The body temperature should not be less than 35°C before the diagnostic tests are carried out.
- Specialist opinion and the status of the doctors concerned.
  Only when the primary diagnosis is in doubt is it necessary to consult with a neurologist or neurosurgeon.
- A decision to withdraw artificial support should be made after all the criteria presented above have been fulfilled and can be made by any of the following combination of doctors:

  a a consultant who is in charge of the case and one other doctor;

  b in the absence of a consultant, a deputy, who should have been registered for 5 years or more and who should have had adequate experience in the care of such cases, and one other doctor.

  [modified from *Lancet* (1976) 2: 1069–1070]

These recommendations fall into three groups, parts A, B, and C. The patient must be deeply comatose and on a ventilator, and it must be clearly established that the patient's coma is due to *irremedial structural brain damage* (part A). Drug-induced coma, hypothermia and metabolic causes of coma and relaxant drugs must have been clearly excluded as a cause of ventilatory failure. If these conditions are fulfilled brain death may be diagnosed if no brainstem reflexes can be demonstrated (part B). Repeated tests are necessary but the interval between such tests depends on the pathology and the course of the disease. Purely spinal reflexes can persist after total brainstem destruction but it must always be remembered that decorticate and decerebrate postures are far from necessarily irreversible phenomena and therefore that their presence does not inevitably indicate that brain death has occurred. Indeed some authorities would doubt a diagnosis of brain death if such reflexes persisted. All these tests should be carried out at a body temperature not less than 35°C (part C).

Electroencephalographic and other studies, such as angiography, are not necessary for diagnosis of brain death but absence of brain electrical activity in an electroencephalogram, recorded for not less than 20 minutes at an amplification of 5 μV/cm provides very strong confirmatory evidence of cerebral death, provided that depressant drugs have not been given.

In the past, it has been recommended that such an isoelectric electroencephalogram should be recorded twice not less than 6 hours apart before brain death is diagnosed, but this is no longer regarded as necessary in the UK. It is recommended that at least two doctors, one registered for not less than 5 years, should be consulted *independently* in the diagnosis of brain death before a decision to withdraw ventilatory and other support is made.

CHAPTER 14

The examination of women

General points

When a history is taken and an examination performed tact, discretion, consideration and the maintenance of proper confidentiality are fundamental, as some of the most intimate details of a woman's life are being elicited. All patients have complex expectations of their doctors, and it is reasonable to conform to these insofar as they allow the process of medical diagnosis to proceed smoothly. A genuine interest in the problem presented, combined with a gentleness of manner, allows both doctor and patient to feel at ease while the process of assessment continues. Adequate time should be allowed for the history and examination, but a sense of direction is essential as it can become difficult to separate the important from the trivial.

Presenting problems and gynaecological history

General open-ended questions, such as 'What made you think there was something wrong?' or 'What happened then?' are better than more specific ones in the early stages of history-taking. It is especially important to avoid questions which imply criticism, for example, when assessing a request for termination of pregnancy: 'How could you have forgotten to take your pill?' Such a question will probably ruin the basis for continuing a constructive interview. Later it is acceptable to ask specifically, 'Which pill were you using?' or 'Did you have any episodes of vomiting or diarrhoea about the time you conceived?' Once the interview is progressing satisfactorily, an opportunity must be made to ask about *menstrual upset*, *post-coital bleeding* and *dyspareunia* (pain or difficulty with intercourse), as these symptoms, if present, will need further investigation. Sometimes a woman may be too apprehensive to discuss her problems freely, particularly if the doctor is both young and male. This should be acknowledged as soon as it is recognized; open discussion will often resolve this anxiety. If necessary, the help of a female medical or nursing colleague should be sought.

Psychosexual problems can be especially difficult to elicit and may need several sessions or the help of others who have particular skills in that specialty.

Menstruation—the cyclical loss of sanguineous fluid from the uterus in mature women—is recorded as the days of menstrual loss and the duration of the interval from the first day of one period to the onset of the next. An additional note is useful, e.g. the character of the loss and the daily variation throughout the period. Specific labels like *menor-rhagia*, *metrorrhagia* or *polymenorrhoea* should only be used if the pattern conforms exactly to that definition. Where the problem is infertility, specific questions should be asked about the timing and frequency of intercourse, and if dyspareunia or other sexual difficulties have occurred. Women with these problems will not be embarrassed by such questions as they will be expecting them. If *prolapse* has developed (where a woman has noticed a bulge at the introitus), other associated symptoms of bladder or pelvic floor disturbance and backache should be sought.

History of current and previous pregnancies

If a woman presents with pregnancy, ascertain as gently as possible if it is welcomed or not. Remember that although relatively few pregnancies are planned, by the time of birth most babies are genuinely wanted. In particular, ask the date of the *last menstrual period* (*LMP*) with a note as to its likely accuracy. Also record the previous menstrual pattern before conception and whether these were natural cycles or due to the use of the contraceptive pill. The *expected date of delivery* (*EDD*) of the child can be calculated providing a natural 28-day cycle has been present for some months prior to the conception cycle. The EDD is then 9 months and 7 days from the onset of the last menstrual period (i.e. 280 days or 10 lunar months; the date of delivery is 266 days from the date of conception when this is known). Clearly this is only an approximation as calendar months are not of a standard length, and *term* is regarded as a time stretching from 37 to 42 weeks from the last menstrual period. This degree of variation should be explained to the pregnant woman from the outset, since some correction may be required to the estimate of the EDD as information about the pregnancy accumulates.

These data should be assembled chronologically in 3-monthly periods (*the trimesters*) and should be related to those events which would be expected to occur at an equivalent stage of a healthy pregnancy. The estimated duration of the pregnancy from the last menstrual period to the time of the examination is called the *gestation*. The course and outcome of previous pregnancies must be explored, as these are essential guides to the progress of the current pregnancy. However, the woman's age will have changed and the circumstances may also be quite different,

e.g. change of partner. Where early loss of pregnancy has occurred previously it must be established whether this was by *spontaneous abortion* ('miscarriage') or *therapeutic termination of pregnancy* ('abortion') and on how many occasions it occurred. The gestation, onset of symptoms leading to miscarriage or the method of termination, complications and any treatment must be noted. Valuable additional information includes the time taken for the woman to return to a normal menstrual pattern after the event. The outcome of previous pregnancies is recorded as a *live birth*, a *neonatal death* or a *stillbirth*.

The birth of a child showing any signs of independent life is recorded as a *live birth*. This now usually occurs beyond 24 weeks' gestation (or 500 g weight), but with improved neonatal care, viability of a fetus may soon be obtained from an even earlier stage. If such a child dies, that event in the UK requires a death certificate. In the UK, since the Human Fertilization and Embryology Act (1990), if the child is born dead after 24 completed weeks, it is recorded as a *stillbirth* and requires a stillbirth certificate, and burial. If the child is born dead at an earlier gestation it is regarded as an *abortion* and neither stillbirth certificate nor formal burial is necessary.

The foregoing statements relate to the legal requirements, but it is important to remember that all parents who lose children under any of these circumstances will need compassionate consideration and emotional support as well as professional counselling (e.g. from SANDS, the Stillbirth and Neonatal Death Society, or similar organization). When a child has been born its gestation weight (to see if this was appropriate for gestational age), and condition at birth should be ascertained. Any complications of pregnancy, delivery or the puerperium should be enumerated, as should the developmental 'milestones' of the child. Where events are uncertain, making enquiries at the hospital where the delivery occurred can be vital.

A woman's *gravidity* is described by the notation *para x + y*, where *x* is the number of babies delivered, whether live births or stillbirths, and *y* is the number of pregnancies the woman has had. The latter should include any ectopic pregnancies and abortions prior to 24 weeks' gestation, whether the fetus was born dead, or born alive but too premature to survive, including both spontaneous abortions and terminations of pregnancy. *Parity* is defined as the number of babies delivered older than 24 weeks gestation, i.e. when a baby is considered to be viable.

Past medical history

Besides its general value this should be explored with particular reference to the problems under investigation, e.g. gangrenous appendix related to infertility, a previous blood transfusion producing antibodies related to subsequent loss of pregnancy, etc. It is essential to know of any present or previous medical disorders, e.g. diabetes mellitus, especially when pregnancy, further medical therapy, or operative treatment is being considered.

Medication or treatment history

Any medication taken regularly, or even occasionally, must be recorded. The effects of alcohol and tobacco are often aggravated by a poor diet, and when drug abuse exists (associated with an increased risk of hepatitis and HIV infection), it must also be recognized. Allergic reactions should be recorded and clearly displayed, as this information may be required in a hurry when the patient is unable to respond.

General and associated system assessment

Remember that changes in appetite and weight, responses to normal exercise and variations in sleep patterns are all relevant to a wide variety of obstetric and gynaecological problems. An estimate of the *frequency* and *volume* of urine passed, with a specific note about *nocturia* or *dysuria*, should be recorded. The presence of *urgency*, an overwhelming desire to micturate, which may or may not result in incontinence; or *stress incontinence*, the involuntary leakage of urine from the full bladder when the intra-abdominal pressure is raised, should be assessed. The latter is very common in a minor degree, particularly after childbirth or in the menopause.

Family, marital and social history

The woman's employment, her spouse's employment, their home conditions and the length of their relationship are of great importance when assessing prospects for recovery from illness or the support of the child. The ethnic origins of the family will sometimes give a clue to underlying disease, such as the presence of tuberculosis or a haemoglobinopathy. An actual or supposed history of cancer is one of the underlying anxieties most frequently confessed at interviews.

When a congenital abnormality is suspected in the offspring of relatives, a detailed family history is important, and in some disorders antenatal diagnosis is possible, e.g. in haemophilia and thalassaemia.

Examination

General

This process will have started at the very beginning of the history-taking by observing appearance, gait, demeanour and responsiveness, and by the general assessment of intelligence and educational level. Any aggressiveness or abnormality of affect should be noted and should provoke the question 'Why?' in the doctor. The presence of a chaperone for the physical examination is important for a male doctor, but such a person may inhibit the process of history-taking and so should only be used when the patient needs to undress for the specific needs of the physical examination. Once this has been done, measurements of height and weight and their ratio are made, as they can be particularly difficult to assess if the patient is first seen when in bed. Note too the secondary sexual development, and hair distribution.

The first physical contact with the woman should already have been achieved at the time of greeting with a handshake, and it is important that this non-threatening process should be continued by following a sequence which is predictable, such as the following.

- Hands (to assess the pulse)
- Arms (blood pressure)
- Eyes (conjunctivae)
- Head, chest (heart)
- Breasts
- Abdomen
- Legs.

Breast examination

See page 21.

Abdominal examination

The system of examination described in Chapter 5 should be followed, but in addition, the possibility of pregnancy must be considered in the age range 12-55 years, or even later with newly developed fertility techniques. When an abdominopelvic mass is present its characteristics and size, either in centimetres measured from the symphysis pubis upwards, or estimated as weeks gestation of an equivalent size pregnancy are recorded. If ascites is suspected check the supraclavicular and inguinal lymph nodes and look for an associated hydrothorax.

ABDOMINAL EXAMINATION IN PREGNANCY

Before inspecting the abdomen, make sure the light is good, the room comfortably warm, and that there is maximum exposure (Box 14.1). Particular note

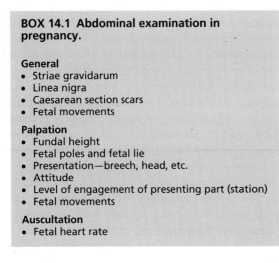

> **BOX 14.1 Abdominal examination in pregnancy.**
>
> **General**
> * Striae gravidarum
> * Linea nigra
> * Caesarean section scars
> * Fetal movements
>
> **Palpation**
> * Fundal height
> * Fetal poles and fetal lie
> * Presentation—breech, head, etc.
> * Attitude
> * Level of engagement of presenting part (station)
> * Fetal movements
>
> **Auscultation**
> * Fetal heart rate

should be made of *striae gravidarum, linea nigra*, previous *Caesarean section scars* and any visible *fetal or other movements*. Ideally the patient is examined flat, but she may be more comfortable semi-recumbent. Ask about any tender areas before palpating the abdomen, so that, initially at least, these can be avoided. Comfort and gentleness can be enhanced by using the flat of the hand as well as the examining fingers; this assists the process of relaxation and allows the outline of a mass or pregnant uterus to be defined more readily. If there is a particular need to undertake an uncomfortable examination, this should be explained to the patient and left to the very end. Remember too, that palpation may produce uterine contractions which can obscure the details of the uterine contents.

The size of the uterus is traditionally estimated from *fundal height*, even though this is only one dimension of a globular mass which is subject to a variety of displacements. Under normal circumstances the fundal height is just above the symphysis pubis at 12 weeks' gestation, at the umbilicus at 22 weeks and at the xiphisternum at 36 weeks. When

the fundus is equidistant from the symphysis pubis and the umbilicus, the gestation is 16 weeks and when equidistant from the xiphisternum and umbilicus it is about 30 weeks. From 36 weeks the fundal height is also dependent on the level of the *presenting part*, and it will reduce as the presenting part descends into the pelvis (Fig. 14.1). Comparative assessments can be made by measuring either the symphysis–fundal height or the minimal girth measured at the level of the umbilicus, as each of these measurements has a correlation with gestation.

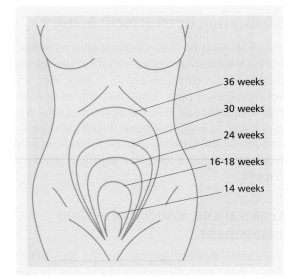

Fig. 14.1 Approximate fundal height with changing gestation.

Next, determination of the number of *fetal poles* will allow the assessment of the fetal axis and in consequence the *fetal lie* (Fig. 14.2). This is the relationship of the long axis of the fetus to the long axis of the uterus. To confirm the lie, the location of the fetal limbs and back should be identified.

The *presentation*, e.g. whether cephalic, breech, or otherwise, must be assessed. At term, over 95% of babies present by the head, but at 30 weeks only 70% do so because of the greater mobility of the fetus and the relatively larger volume of amniotic fluid. The *breech* can usually be distinguished by its size, texture and ability to change shape. However, an ultrasonic examination may be necessary to confirm the clinical diagnosis.

If the baby presents by the head, the smallest diameters which are presented to the pelvis occur when the head is well-flexed, i.e. a vertex presentation. Flexion of the head is termed the *attitude*, and decreasing amounts of flexion lead to brow or face presentations which may cause difficulty in labour, often requiring delivery by Caesarean section. For a breech presentation an equivalent assessment is made to determine if the breech is *extended* (frank breech), *flexed* (complete), or *footling* (incomplete) breech. Once the presenting part has a relationship to the pelvis, that relationship can be vertical, the *level* (Fig. 14.3), or rotational, the *position*. When the flexed head presents, the fetal occiput is termed the *denominator*. When the face presents, the denominator is the mentum (chin) and when the breech presents it is the sacrum. Thus the position with a vertex presentation can now be defined as left occipito-lateral (LOL) or right occipitolateral (ROL), etc. The common positions of the head before the onset of labour are LOL 50%, ROL 25%. This relationship changes during the course of labour because of internal rotation and at the end of labour the common presenting positions are left occipito-anterior (LOA) 60% and right occipito-anterior (ROA) 30%.

The level of the presenting part can be assessed by abdominal or vaginal examination. *Engagement* of the presenting part occurs when the largest diameters have passed through the pelvic brim. The number of fifths of the head palpated through the abdominal wall indicates its level (Fig. 14.4). Thus, if there are three or more fifths palpable, the baby's head will be unengaged. If less than three-fifths are palpable, then the baby's head is probably engaged in the pelvis, but this does depend on the overall size of the fetal head and of the pelvis. Sometimes it is difficult to be sure whether the presenting part is engaged, and it must be remembered that the pelvic brim has an angle of approximately 45 degrees to the horizontal when the mother is lying flat. However, if the abdominal wall is reasonably thin the unengaged head can be palpated by the examiner's fingers passing round the maximum diameter and beginning to meet above the pelvic brim. When this does not occur, the widest diameter must be below the

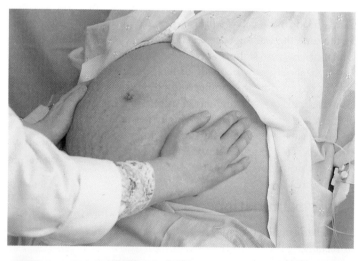

Fig. 14.2 Method of abdominal palpation to determine fetal lie and location of back.

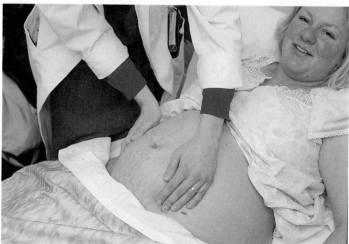

Fig. 14.3 Method of abdominal palpation to determine presenting part.

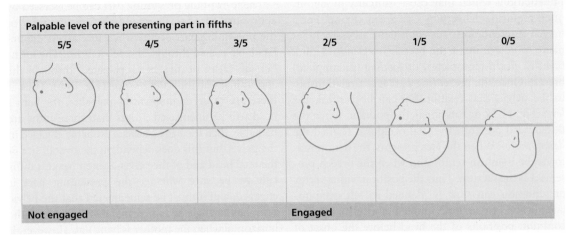

Palpable level of the presenting part in fifths					
5/5	4/5	3/5	2/5	1/5	0/5

Not engaged   Engaged

Fig. 14.4   The vertical relationship of the presenting part to the pelvic inlet (the level).

examining fingers. Fixity of the presenting part in the pelvis is also a guide to engagement.

The level of the presenting part on pelvic examination is termed the *station*. Engagement of the baby's head in the pelvis will usually have occurred by the time the leading edge reaches the level of the ischial spines (zero station).

A note should now be made of fetal movements, both as recorded by the mother and observed by the examiner during the examination. A record is made of the *fetal heart rate* (*FHR*), normally between 120 and 160 beats/min, and finally the *volume of liquor* is estimated. This requires considerable practice as it changes through pregnancy (Fig. 14.5).

Pelvic examination

The pelvic examination may be undertaken vaginally or rectally.

VAGINAL EXAMINATION

As the examination proceeds it is most important to explain every step to the patient. Begin by inspecting the perineum in the dorsal or left lateral position (Box 14.2). A good light is required and an assistant is necessary. Women who use tampons or who have borne children should be able to tolerate a gentle vaginal examination. For those who cannot use tampons or whose hymen is intact, pelvic examination

BOX 14.2 Vaginal examination.

Inspection

Digital palpation
- Locate cervix
- Bimanual palpation
- Assessment of uterus
- Pelvic masses or tenderness
- Ovaries and fallopian tubes

Speculum examination

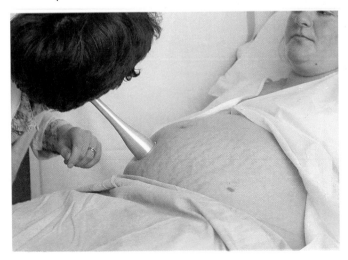

Fig. 14.5   Listening over the fetal back to the fetal heart with a Pinard stethoscope.

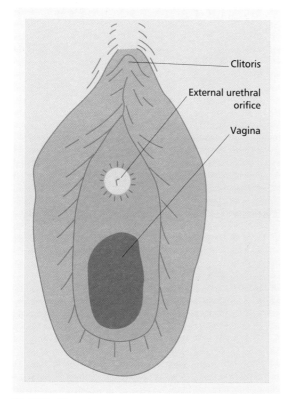

Fig. 14.6 The vulva.

may be undertaken per rectum. Any inflammation, swelling, soreness, ulceration or neoplasia of the vulva, perineum or anus is noted (Fig. 14.6). Small warts (condylomata acuminata) appearing as papillary growths may be seen scattered over the vulva; these are due to the *human papilloma virus*. The clitoris and urethra, which may be difficult to see, are inspected, and the patient is asked to strain and then to cough to demonstrate uterovaginal prolapse or stress incontinence (Fig. 14.7). If the latter is a presenting problem it is important that the bladder is reasonably full and that more than one substantial cough is taken, as the first frequently fails to demonstrate leakage of urine.

For a digital vaginal examination, thin disposable polythene gloves are used on each hand and the examining fingers are lightly lubricated with a water-based jelly. With the patient in the supine position and with her knees drawn up and separated, the labia are gently parted with the index finger and thumb of the left hand while the index finger of the right hand is inserted into the vagina, avoiding the urethral meatus and exerting a sustained pressure on the *perineal body* until relaxation of the perineal musculature occurs. The full length of the finger is then introduced, assessing the vaginal walls in transit

until the cervix is located. At this stage a second finger can be inserted to improve the sensitivity of the digital examination or alternatively a speculum can be used if a cervical smear is required. The examination is continued with the left hand placed on the abdomen above the symphysis pubis and below the umbilicus (Fig. 14.8).

The hand provides gentle directional pressure to bring the pelvic viscera towards the examiner's fingers in the vagina and serves to assess the size, mobility and regularity of abdominopelvic masses in a bimanual manner. The *cervix* is then identified; it is approximately 3 cm in diameter with a variably sized and shaped dimple in the middle, the *cervical os*. The os is normally directed posteriorly when the uterus is anteflexed and anteverted. The consistency of the cervix is firm and its shape is irregular when scarred. Increased hardness of the cervix may be caused by fibrosis or carcinoma. A soft cervix usually indicates the possibility of pregnancy; even greater caution and gentleness is then necessary. The mobility of the cervix is usually 1–2 cm in all directions and testing this movement should produce only mild discomfort. When attempts are made to move the cervix in the presence of pelvic inflammation, particularly in association with ectopic pregnancy, extreme pain (*cervical excitation*) occurs.

Next the size, shape, position, consistency and regularity of the *uterus* and the relationship of the fundus of the uterus to the cervix is estimated. Bimanual examination also enables palpation of the *ovaries* and *fallopian tubes*, although these can be difficult to feel when healthy. The pouch of Douglas is then explored through the posterior fornix via the arch formed by the insertion of the uterosacral ligaments into the cervix. Skill increases with practice.

SPECULUM EXAMINATION

This is an essential part of gynaecological examinations and if it is omitted for any reason then the examination must be regarded as incomplete. Several vaginal specula are available. These include the *bivalve* type, e.g. Cusco's, used for displaying the cervix (Fig. 14.9), the single or double-ended *Sims' (duckbill) speculum*, used to retract the vaginal walls, and *Ferguson's speculum*, a tube used to allow the inspection of the cervix when vaginal prolapse is so severe that a bivalve speculum fails to provide a sufficient view. Speculum examination of the vagina can be undertaken in the dorsal or left lateral position, but the examination for prolapse is always

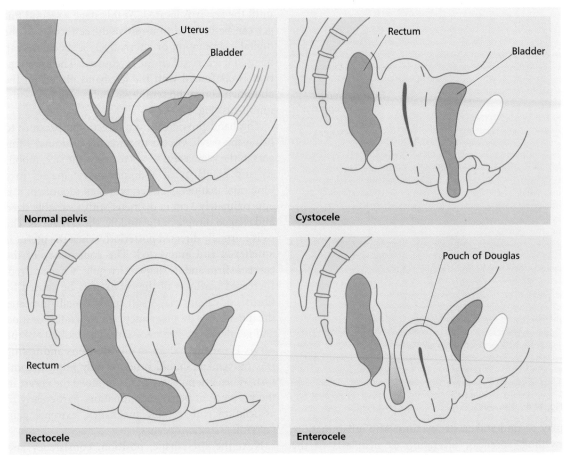

Fig. 14.7   In cystocele there is downward prolapse of the anterior part of the pelvic floor, straightening the angulation of the bladder neck and leading to urinary incontinence. In rectocele the posterior part of the pelvic floor is mostly affected, sometimes with associated faecal incontinence. In some patients the whole pelvic floor is weak with double incontinence, or with prolapse of the uterus. In enterocele there is a prolapse of viscera in the pouch of Douglas as part of severe pelvic floor weakness

undertaken in the left lateral position. The speculum should be warmed to body temperature and lubricated with water or a water-based jelly. All the necessary equipment, e.g. spatulae, slides, forceps, culture swabs, etc. should be prepared before the examination begins (Fig. 14.10).

Technique for speculum insertion and for cervical (Papanicolaou) smear examination
The procedure is explained to the patient and then she is asked to lie on her back. The labia are separated with the left hand as for the bimanual examination. Then, holding the lightly lubricated bivalve speculum in the right hand and using the index finger and thumb of the left hand to separate the introitus, the speculum is inserted with the handle directly upwards, which allows it to be accommodated by the vagina (which is H-shaped in cross-section). When it has been inserted to its full

length, the blades of the speculum are opened and manoeuvred so that the cervix is fully visualized. The screw adjuster or ratchet on the handle is then locked so that the speculum is maintained in place. The presence of discharge and the condition of the cervical epithelium, its colour, any ulceration, scars and retention cysts (*Nabothian follicles*) are all recorded.

In order to detect the presence of cervical precancer, an Ayre's or similar spatula is used so that the tip is an appropriate shape. The tip of this instrument is placed firmly against the cervical os, so as to allow the removal of surface cells from the whole of the *squamocolumnar junction* when the spatula is rotated through 360 degrees. An alternative is the brush which more effectively samples the endocervix. A smear of the vaginal walls can then be taken with the other end of the spatula in order to obtain cells for hormonal assessment. These materi-

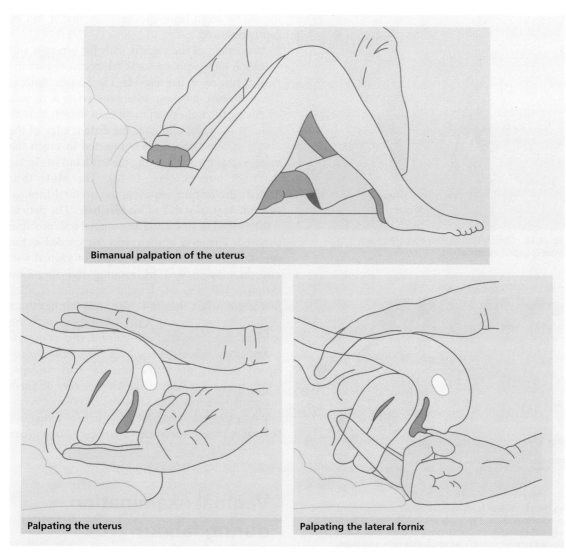

Bimanual palpation of the uterus

Palpating the uterus

Palpating the lateral fornix

Fig. 14.8 Bimanual examination of the pelvis.

als are spread thinly on to microscope slides and immediately placed in a fixative. An example of a stained slide is shown in Fig. 14.11. At the same time a wet slide for the assessment of *monilia* (*Candida albicans*) or *Trichomonas vaginalis* can be prepared and a culture swab taken from the endocervix or vaginal vault and placed in a bacteriological transport medium. In addition a Gram-stained smear can be prepared for the detection of *Neisseria gonorrhoeae* as Gram-negative intracellular diplococci. An aqueous solution of iodine and potassium iodide can be applied to the cervix: the normal mucous membrane, which contains glycogen, stains dark brown. Those areas of abnormality which fail to take up the stain can then be identified (*Schiller's test*). The screw of the speculum is then released and

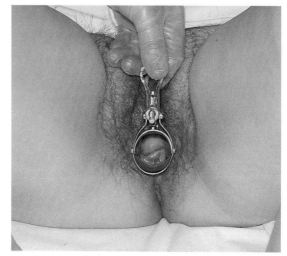

Fig. 14.9 Cusco's speculum used to display the cervix.

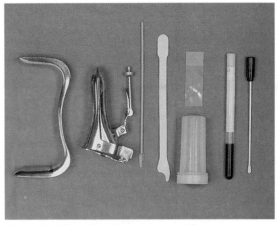

Fig. 14.10 Clinical instruments prepared for a gynaecological examination.

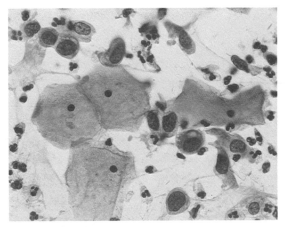

Fig. 14.11 Smear from uterine cervix. Cells scraped from the uterine cervix. There are several abnormal squamous cells indicating *in situ* carcinoma of the cervix. Large pink-stained normal superficial squamous cells and many inflammatory cells are also included. (Papanicolaou stain, ×160.)

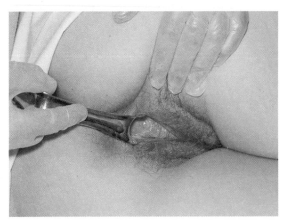

Fig. 14.12 Sims's speculum used to display the anterior vaginal wall.

the blades freed from the cervix so that it can be gently removed.

Assessment of the vaginal walls for prolapse and fistulae is done with a duckbilled speculum with the patient turned on her left side. The best exposure is given by Sims' position, where the pelvis is rotated by flexing the right thigh more than the left, and by hanging the right arm over the distant edge of the couch. A Sims' speculum is inserted in much the same way as formerly, using the left hand to elevate the right buttock (Fig. 14.12). The blade then deflects the rectum, exposing the urethral meatus, anterior vaginal wall and bladder base. The patient is then asked to strain and any vaginal wall prolapse is noted. The level of the cervix is recorded as the speculum is withdrawn. The posterior vaginal wall can then be viewed by rotating the speculum through 180 degrees. Uterine prolapse is called *first-degree* when the cervix descends but lies short of the introitus, *second-degree* when it passes to the level of the introitus, and *third-degree (complete procidentia)*, when the whole of the uterus is prolapsed outside the vulva. Vaginal wall prolapse which may occur with, or be independent of, uterine prolapse consists of *urethrocele, cystocele, rectocele* or *enterocele* (prolapse of pouch of Douglas). Several of these anatomical variations usually occur together.

Vaginal examination during labour

During labour a digital vaginal examination must be made to determine:
- dilatation and effacement of the cervix;
- the presence or absence of amniotic membranes and the state of the liquor;
- the level of the presenting part;
- absence of pulsating umbilical cord, especially if the membranes are ruptured;
- the degree of moulding of the fetal head, or the presence of caput succedaneum; and
- the size and shape of the maternal bony pelvis.

For this examination, because of the possibility of ascending infection, the vulva is swabbed clean with an antiseptic such as chlorhexidine in water and sterile surgical gloves must be worn. Initially an assessment is made of the vagina, which should normally be warm and moist. If it is dry and hot, infection should be suspected. Next the extent of *cervical dilatation* is estimated in centimetres (10 cm is equivalent to full dilatation) and the thinness and elasticity of the cervix, which increases with dilatation, is also assessed. The *level* of the presenting part is measured in centimetres from the ischial spines and noted by a minus sign if above, and a plus sign if below that level. If caput succedaneum occurs, there may be difficulty in estimating both the exact level, and also the position of the presenting part because of the masking of the fontanelles. In these circumstances the *position* can then be assessed by the location and direction of a fetal ear.

The method of estimating maternal pelvic dimensions is described in textbooks of obstetrics. These measurements must be adequate if a vaginal delivery is to be achieved safely.

Rectal examination

(see also pages 102–103)

This is a valuable gynaecological procedure, but it may be perceived by the patient as the most uncomfortable part of the whole examination. When vaginal examination is not possible or not acceptable, rectal examination permits bimanual assessment of the pelvic viscera and is particularly valuable in assessing problems which are located in the pouch of Douglas, the uterosacral ligaments, or the rectovaginal septum. Sometimes disease arising in the rectum, e.g. diverticular disease, can masquerade as a gynaecological problem.

Investigations

A number of investigations are commonly used in gynaecology and obstetrics.

Pregnancy testing

URINE
The most readily available pregnancy tests depend on the demonstration of *human chorionic gonadotrophin* (*HCG*) in the urine. The sensitivity of these tests varies, but some tests detect as little as 50 mUl HCG. As the developing placental tissue produces increasing amounts from about 10 days post-fertilization, very early diagnosis of pregnancy is now possible.

BLOOD
Even earlier detection of pregnancy is possible by radioimmunoassay of the beta-subunit of HCG in blood—a highly specific test.

Bacteriological and virus tests

Bacteriological and virus tests used in gynaecology and obstetrics include the following.
- Swabs from the endocervix, vagina, uretha and rectum may be needed for sexually transmitted diseases.
- Bacteriological midstream urinalysis (MSU) is important in both obstetrics (for suspected bacteriuria) and gynaecology (for example, for suspected urge incontinence).
- Tests for toxoplasma, rubella, cytomegalovirus and herpes simplex (TORCH) cover those viruses most likely to be damaging to a pregnancy.

Endometrial biopsy (Fig. 14.13)

The commonest investigation undertaken in gynaecology is sampling of the endometrium. This is performed by a dilatation of the cervix and curettage to obtain histological material from the cavity of the uterus. Dilatation of the cervix is painful and thus an anaesthetic is needed. The biopsy is not always representative and may fail to make a diagnosis in up to one-third of cases. Other methods of cell sampling have been developed, including surface cytology from uterine scrapings, or from larger quantities of aspirated materials which do not require anaesthesia.

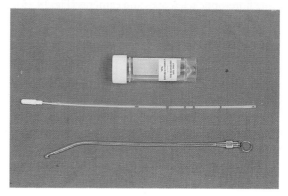

Fig. 14.13 An endometrial biopsy curette, a pipette cell sampler and fixing medium.

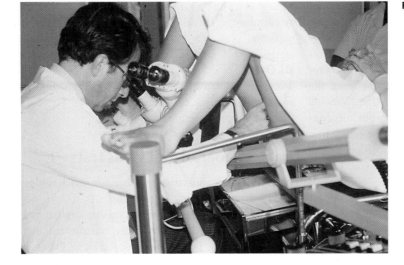

Fig. 14.14   Colposcopy.

Colposcopy

Colposcopy is a technique to visualize the cervix or vaginal vault with a low-power binocular microscope to detect precancerous abnormalities of the cervical epithelium (Fig. 14.14). Usually an abnormal cervical smear will have alerted the doctor to the need for further investigation. This can be undertaken on an out-patient basis, by exposing the cervix, treating it with acetic acid and viewing it through the colposcope to identify the degree, site and extent of the cervical pathology which has produced the abnormal smear. Once this has been done, biopsy and appropriate treatment, e.g. laser destruction or surgical excision, by knife or large loop electrodiathermy, can be undertaken.

Hysteroscopy

This is a method of viewing the cavity of the uterus using fibre-optic telescopes and cameras (Fig. 14.15).

Ultrasound

Ultrasound generated from a piezoelectric crystal transducer is propagated through tissues at variable velocity depending on the tissue density. The echo time can give an estimate of the size and consistency of the object scanned. This technique appears safe; more than 75 million people have been exposed to ultrasound *in utero* without apparent deleterious effect.

Clearly the assessment of gestational age, the presence of fetal abnormality, multiple pregnancy, the

site of the placenta, and monitoring of these factors as pregnancy progresses are important in obstetric care. Ultrasound is also useful in gynaecology in determining the size and relationships of pelvic masses to the viscera.

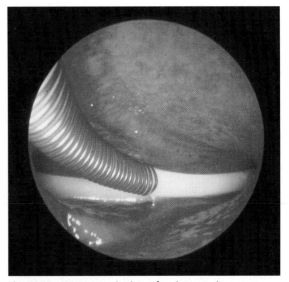

Fig. 14.15   Hysteroscopic view of an intrauterine contraceptive device *in situ*.

Radiological investigations

HYSTEROSALPINGOGRAPHY

This is used to image the uterine cavity and fallopian tubes after a radiopaque medium has been installed into the uterus but is now used less than before if hysteroscopy and falloposcopy are available (Fig. 14.16).

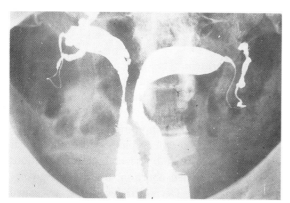

Fig. 14.16   An abnormal hysterosalpingogram: uterus didelphys (double uterus).

LATERAL X-RAY PELVIMETRY

This is used to assess the diameters of the pelvic inlet when cephalopelvic disproportion could exist. It is indicated if there is to be a breech birth, so that the aftercoming head can be certain to pass through the pelvis without obstruction when an emergency arises or when facilities for CT pelvimetry do not exist.

CT SCANNING AND MRI

CT scanning has proved less useful in gynaecology than was originally anticipated. MRI, however, offers an alternative to ultrasound and to X-ray for imaging during pregnancy; it uses no ionizing radiation and no harmful biological effects have been detected at magnetic field strengths (0.2–2.0 tesla) in current usage. Good images are obtained with excellent differentiation of maternal and fetal tissues. Unlike ultrasound, no artefacts from bone or bowel gas occur. Echo planar imaging is useful to reduce fetal movement artefact and increases potential for the study of fetal physiology and pathology.

Laparoscopy/pelvicoscopy

Visualization of the pelvic and abdominal viscera is valuable if it can be done without a major injury to the abdominal wall (Fig. 14.17). This can be achieved by using a fibre-optic telescope illuminated by a light source kept remote from the patient. It is then possible to inflate the abdomen with carbon dioxide under general or local anaesthesia, so that the anterior abdominal wall is lifted away from the viscera, allowing inspection of the abdominal and pelvic contents. The main uses of laparoscopy are diagnostic, e.g. in the investigation of pelvic pain or infertility, and therapeutic, e.g. in sterilization proce-

dures or in the treatment of a rapidly increasing number of pelvic lesions. Modern laparoscopy utilizes multiple puncture techniques with high-quality television monitors and video recorders.

Tests of fetal well-being

Besides those tests made to ensure the good general health of the mother, e.g. haemoglobin, Veneral Disease Research Laboratories test and bacteriuria screen, a number of other investigations of variable complexity can be utilized to check the fetus *in utero*. It is reasonable to use some of these tests in every pregnancy as in about 10% of mothers the outcome of apparently uncomplicated pregnancy is unpredictable. In addition, anonymous testing for asymptomatic HIV in inner London shows a small number of positive results. HIV testing is *not* carried out, however, in the ordinary clinical management of pregnancy.

BIOLOGICAL TESTS

Before using these tests it is important to explore the woman's attitude to the possible results. For example, would she want intervention if an abnormality was discovered? Detailed counselling by a trained professional is essential.

Chorion biopsy (chorionic villus sampling)

This is a method of obtaining chorionic material at 8–10 weeks of pregnancy, either through the cervix or directly through the abdomen so that the genetic

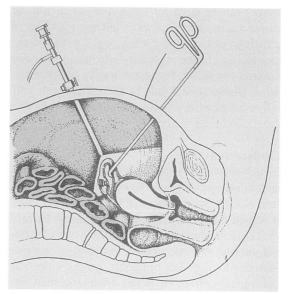

Fig. 14.17   Diagram of a laparoscopy.

constitution or biochemical function of fetal cellular material can be determined. It is useful for the diagnosis of Down's syndrome, of thalassaemia, and in a number of other hereditary conditions. Early diagnosis allows the therapeutic termination of abnormal pregnancy, increasing the safety and acceptability of that procedure. There is still an increased risk of spontaneous abortion after the chorion biopsy and this technique is used only in specialized centres.

Amniocentesis

Samples of amniotic fluid can be used for:

Chromosome analysis. This is undertaken at 12–18 weeks of pregnancy and is currently much safer than chorion biopsy. The amount of desquamated fetal cells obtained is much smaller in quantity than from chorion biopsy and cell culture is necessary (which takes about 3 weeks) before a chromosomal diagnosis is made. This test is mostly used for prenatal diagnosis of Down's syndrome, in which abnormalities on chromosome 21 are characteristic, and when other chromosome abnormalities are suspected.

Bilirubin concentration. This is sometimes measured in amniotic fluid during the latter part of pregnancy in order to assess the health of a baby affected by maternal rhesus isoimmunization.

DNA analysis. Fetal cells obtained by amniocentesis, chorionic villus sampling or cordocentesis (see below) can be used for DNA analysis of nuclear chromatin in order to directly test for a number of genetically-determined diseases, e.g. Tay-Sach's disease and Duchenne muscular dystrophy, in families known to be at risk. Both DNA testing and chromosomal studies should only be carried out with fully informed parental consent, and with the help of a genetic counselling service.

Cordocentesis

In this procedure a needle is inserted through the abdominal wall and into the amniotic sac to obtain fetal blood from the placental insertion of the cord. It is used when chromosomal abnormality, haemophilia, haemoglobinopathies, inborn errors of metabolism, fetal viral infections or fetal anaemia are suspected. Although the procedure carries more risk than amniocentesis, it is less traumatic than fetoscopy while permitting rapid diagnosis.

BIOCHEMICAL TESTS

Early pregnancy

Alpha fetoprotein. This is a normal fetal protein which passes from the fetus into the amniotic fluid and maternal serum. The maternal concentration of this protein varies in a predictable way with gestation. At 16 weeks' gestation increased levels suggest fetal spina bifida or anencephaly. However, similar levels can be caused by several other conditions including threatened abortion, multiple pregnancy and exomphalos. Decreased levels are associated with the presence of an infant with Down's syndrome. A computed risk of Down's syndrome can be produced from maternal weight, gestation, parity and race, measured against alpha fetoprotein, HCG and unconjugated oestriol.

Late pregnancy

Human placental lactogen (HPL). This hormone can be measured in maternal serum and is of some predictive value as to the state of the fetus in later pregnancy: low levels correlate with a low placental mass and a poor fetal prognosis, but lack of precision means the test is now little used.

Labour

Fetal health in labour can be assessed by checking the liquor for the presence of meconium, by checking the responsiveness of the fetal heart rate, and by monitoring fetal movements. In addition to these simple clinical tests, *fetal pH* assessed on a scalp blood sample can be used to detect acidosis. This is particularly useful if labour is prolonged, complicated or known to be high-risk, e.g. in diabetic mothers. The fetal scalp is displayed using an amnioscope and a small sample of capillary blood is obtained. If the pH of the sample is below 7.2 then delivery is an urgent priority.

BIOPHYSICAL TESTS

Fetal movements

In some cases of placental insufficiency fetal movements decrease or stop 12–48 hours before the fetal heart ceases to beat. In a healthy pregnancy fetal movements increase from the 32nd week of pregnancy to term, but the 12-hour daily fetal movement count falls below 10 in only 2.5% of normal pregnancies. Thus a variety of counting systems which are used by mothers for correlating fetal movement and fetal welfare have been devised.

Fig. 14.18 Cardiotocography equipment.

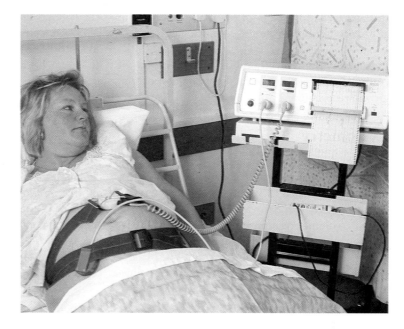

These can alert the mother that more sophisticated forms of surveillance are required.

Ultrasound

Visualization by real time. Sequential ultrasonic scanning to detect the presence of symmetrical or asymmetrical growth retardation or changes in fetal activity, breathing, movements, etc. can be used to assess placental function. If it becomes clear that fetal growth has halted or the child's survival *in utero* is in doubt, then delivery should be planned.

Cardiotocography (CTG). Assessment of the fetal heart rate and its variation with fetal and uterine activity can be recorded antenatally with ultrasound using the Doppler principle (Fig. 14.18). A pressure transducer is attached to the abdominal wall so that variations in uterine activity can be superimposed on the ultrasound recordings. The production of an accurate recording requires patience and considerable interpretive skills.

When the membranes rupture during labour, a more accurate recording of the fetal heart rate can be produced by an electrode attached to the fetal scalp (Figs 14.19 and 14.20).

Doppler blood flow. Studies of the circulatory changes in the umbilical, aortic and cerebral fetal circulation as well as the maternal arteries can give

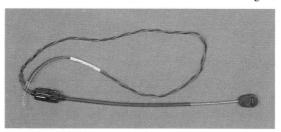

Fig. 14.19 Fetal scalp electrode.

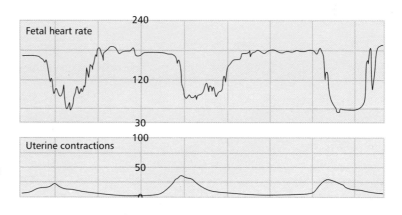

Fig. 14.20 An abnormal cardiotocograph showing late variable decelerations, during uterine contraction, with fetal tachycardia.

further clues to the state of the fetus, especially in already compromised clinical circumstances.

Placental volume. Ultrasound measurements of placental volume also help in the prediction of fetal growth retardation.

Cystometry

Voiding difficulties are initially investigated by checking for urinary tract infection. Assessment of postmicturition bladder volume or coincident pelvic masses by pelvic ultrasound is a useful next step. The pressure/volume relationships of bladder filling, detrusor and sphincter activity and urethral flow rate can be assessed with a cystometrogram. The bladder is catheterized and filled slowly with sterile saline. The volume and pressure at which bladder filling is perceived, and at which a desire to micturate is felt are noted. The urinary flow rate can be measured. In developments of this test electromyographic (EMG) activity in the external urethral sphincter can be measured, and the urethral pressure profile established, the latter visualized by X-ray video recording. This is being replaced by real-time ultrasound assessment of bladder neck activity and descent. In *stress incontinence* urinary flow commences at low bladder pressure because of sphincter incompetence; in *urge incontinence* urinary flow develops at low bladder volumes because of uninhibited detrusor activity. Reflux and overflow also show as urethral leakage. Incontinence can also result from a defect in the anatomical integrity of the urinary tract, e.g. a congenital abnormality or fistula.

CHAPTER 15

The examination of children

Introduction

'If a child cries when you examine it, then it's probably your fault.' This rather sweeping statement was made by the late John Apley, an eminent paediatrician in Bristol. The basic philosophy is right. The examiner cannot avoid some discomfort in some parts of the physical examination, but during most of the examination the child should be contented. This is the essence of the art of examining children. A child who struggles and screams is afraid, and the examiner must spend time trying to gain their confidence. The consulting room must have a range of toys suitable for all ages, and the child should be allowed to play with whatever takes their fancy. If old enough the child should be allowed to explore the room, although dissuaded from playing with expensive or potentially dangerous equipment. Younger children will be sitting on their parent's lap,

and for some of the time regarding you with suspicion. Do not be afraid to stop what you are doing to pull a face or offer a toy that seems to have caught the child's attention.

As the family enter the room, they should be greeted in a friendly way. If you can cause laughter in the first few minutes, you will see a young child responding and relaxing. White clinical coats have little part to play in paediatric practice; they frighten and intimidate most children, and it is best not to wear one.

While talking to the mother, an essential part of the examination is to watch the child. Does the child look unwell? Is he or she interested in the surroundings and exploring them, or apathetic? Watch the child running around: Are there any obvious abnormalities in the gait? Is the face normal, or are there features of abnormal development? Are there any obvious physical abnormalities? Is breathing unusually noisy? Does the child seem well-nourished, or wasted?

History

The history (Box 15.1) will normally be taken from the mother, but when you are seeing an older child, involve him or her by asking relevant points such as the site of a pain etc. Always take notice of what the mother is saying, and listen to her complaints. Do not be tempted to interrupt a mother in full flow to try and ask what you think is a clever question. The mother will know what is worrying her about her child, and any interruptions should be to guide her rather than try and impose your diagnosis on her. Most of all, do not keep looking at your watch or the pile of notes in front of you. A mother and child must be made to feel that they have your whole attention, and that you have all the time in the world for them. Other relatives tend not to be such good historians as the parents, and if well-meaning relatives try to give you the history, make it very clear that it is the parent's view you need, even if this involves the use of an interpreter. Older children are quite capable of giving a history of their current problems and should be encouraged to do so. All the time you are talking to the parents, keep watching everything that the child is doing and their reactions.

BOX 15.1 History-taking in children: categories to include.

- Birth
- Milestones
- Mental and physical development
- School
- Specific illnesses, accidents, etc.
- Immunizations
- Contacts and travel
- Family history
- Social history
- Consanguinity and genetic risk

The structure of the history is no different from that of an adult, consisting of presenting complaint, history of the present illness, and history of any previous illness. In children, enquire particularly as to the nature and severity of *previous illnesses*, the age at which they occurred, e.g. infectious diseases, seizures, bowel disturbances, upper respiratory tract infections, discharging ears and cough. In the case of a cough, always ask when it is worse (for example, asthma sufferers tend to cough at night and when running around), and if vomiting or a 'whoop' is present. Has the child been taking any drugs? Has he or she ever been in hospital, and if so, what was wrong? Have there been any accidents, physical injuries, burns or poisoning incidents?

Next the examiner should pay more specific attention to the *pregnancy, newborn period and developmental progress*. The following questions may be useful.
- Was the mother well during her pregnancy?
- Did she have any particular illnesses, or was she taking any drugs, including alcohol?
- Was the baby born at term?
- What were the birth weight and type of delivery?
- Were there any problems in the newborn period? There should be particular enquiry about jaundice, breathing and fits or feeding difficulties.
- How was the baby fed?
- If bottle-fed, which milk was used?
- When were solid foods introduced?
- Were vitamin drops given and, if so, how many?
- Was the weight gain satisfactory?

At this point it is worth asking if the parents have kept any record of child health clinic attendance, such as a 'baby book', containing dates of attendance at hospital or clinic, weights, immunizations, etc.

It is important to ask about the '*milestones of development*': When did the child first sit up, smile, crawl, walk and talk? Fuller details will be found below (page 377).

General questions should include the following.
- What are the child's present habits with regard to eating, sleeping, bowels and micturition?
- What sort of child is he or she?
- Is he or she robust or moody?
- Does he or she cry a lot?
- How does the child compare with siblings or friends of the same age?
- If of school age, what school does the child go to, and how is he or she getting on?
- Does the child miss much time from school and, if so, why? Ask the child if they like school, and one or two questions about it, such as who is their best friend, and the name of their teacher.

Ask about *routine immunizations*, and if they have all been given.

The *family history* is next:
- How old are the parents?
- How many children are there in the family?
- What are their ages and sex?
- Have there been any stillbirths, miscarriages or other childhood deaths in the family?
- Are there any illnesses in the siblings, parents or any near relatives?

The *social history* must be approached with a

degree of diplomacy, and sometimes it is more prudent to leave deeper probing to a subsequent occasion. It is important to know about living conditions, and whether either or both parents are employed. If the mother is working, there is some daily separation from the child. Ask if the child has ever been separated from her for any time in the past, as this may be the basis of a variety of behavioural difficulties. Find out if the child's parents live together and whether there is any difficulty in the relationship. Is there a supportive family structure involving other relatives, e.g. grandparents. If the family are immigrants, it is important to know how long they have been in their new country. The depth of enquiry in a paediatric social history must always be judged on an individual basis. If the family think that you are prying too much, you may lose the rapport that you have been building up.

Now may be the time to consider talking either to the child or to the parents without the other party being present. This may be particularly valuable in the case of adolescent children, who are often rather resentful of their parents telling you all their problems, and this is the opportunity for them to relax with you. Ask them about the illness, and also a little about themselves and their interests. Parents may also welcome an opportunity to talk in private with you, and it is often during such discussion that the real reason for the consultation emerges. This can be accomplished most easily while the child is undressing or dressing.

By this time you should already have formed an impression of the child, the family, and their relationship, and you are now ready to proceed with the examination. By now, a younger child should have found you such a fascinating person that they will be prepared to co-operate with you in most parts of the physical examination. Alternatively, the child may have become so bored that he or she is asleep. In either case physical examination should present no problems. If the child is crying loudly by now, then you are in for a difficult time, and you should be asking yourself where you went wrong.

Examination

Older children will usually co-operate sufficiently to be examined lying down, and routine physical examination is no different from an adult examination. A younger child should be examined sitting on his or her mother's lap, as any attempt to get them to lay down will result in instant distress. Always talk to children, however young; do not be afraid of looking silly if the result is a co-operative child. Those parts of the examination which are painful or unpleasant should be left until last: if an attempt is made to examine a child's throat at the outset, the immediate response will be a crying child. Offer the child something to play with—even a stethoscope will be a source of amusement to a young infant. Try to follow the scheme set out in Boxes 15.2 and 15.3.

> **BOX 15.2 Assessments to include in the examination of children.**
>
> - Observe
> - Listen
> - Play
> - Palpate
> - Specific clinical tests
> - Other 'background' tests

Start the examination by asking the mother to undress the child. Do not let her hurry. Remember that even very young children may be modest, and prefer to keep their underpants on. Wash your hands while the child is being undressed. Examination should now proceed by the usual method of inspection, palpation, percussion and auscultation; however, no set routine can be followed, and the examination is by regions rather than by systems. Each child will dictate the order of the examination by their reactions to various procedures (Box 15.3).

In general, start with the least threatening manoeuvres. Note again the state of nutrition now that the child is undressed. If there are bruises except on the shins of young children, be suspicious of non-accidental injury. Are there any obvious rashes to be seen? Are there any naevi or other skin anomalies?

> **BOX 15.3 Schema for examination of children.**
>
> - Feet
> - Hands and pulse
> - Face
> - Head
> - Neck
> - Abdomen
> - Chest
> - Neurological
> - Eyes and fundoscopy
> - Genitalia, groins, anus
> - Other invasive clinical tests

The limbs

Often feet are the easiest place to start. There is nothing threatening to the average child about a doctor tickling their feet. This simple trick gives you the first opportunity to touch the child, and will also allow the feet to be checked for a variety of problems such as minor varus deformities, overriding toes, or such minor plantar abnormalities as flat feet. It is then very easy to run your hands over the child's legs at the same time, noting any knee or other bony abnormalities. Note any muscle wasting or tenderness, and the movements of the knee and ankle. At the same time an assessment of the muscle tone should be made, as this seems to the child just an extension of the funny game already being played by this strange but interesting doctor. It is easy to notice at the same time whether the skin is dry or moist, and to feel any skin lesions that you may have noticed. All the time the child's reactions should be watched. Is he or she still your friend? Be prepared to stop what you are doing if the child seems to be getting upset, and spend a few minutes trying to re-establish the rapport that you have just built up.

By now there should be no major objections to the rest of the body being felt. The *arms and shoulders* should be examined next, followed by the *hands*. Do the hands have a single palmar crease, as seen in children with Down's syndrome and in a variety of other syndromes, as well as in a small proportion of normal children? Feel the *wrists* for widening of the epiphyses of the radius and ulna—a sign of rickets. Try to feel the pulse and count it, although this will be difficult in a plump, young infant; the rate is best counted at this age when auscultating the chest.

The head, face and neck

Look at the child's face and ask yourself the following questions .
● Does it look normal?
● If not, what are the abnormal features?
● If the baby looks odd, then do not forget to look at the parents. It may then be obvious that what you regard as abnormal may be nothing more than a family trait. If the appearance is still not too clear, ask who the baby looks like.
● Does the child have a large tongue?
● Are the ears in the normal position, or are they low-set and abnormal in any way? There are many hundreds of syndromes diagnosable by the facial appearance, and the salient features should be carefully noted.

Next note the shape of the *head*. It may be abnormally shaped, owing to premature fusion of the sutures, small if the baby is *microcephalic*, or globular if the baby is *hydrocephalic*, sometimes with dilated veins over the skin surface. It is often asymmetrical (*plagiocephalic*) in normal infants who tend to lie with their heads persistently on one side (Fig. 15.1).

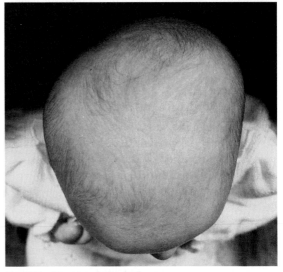

Fig. 15.1 Plagiocephalic skull.

Assuming that you are still friends, there should be no objection to your feeling the child's head now. Leave the measurement of the head circumference to a little later in the examination, as some babies find this a little frightening, and may start crying. Feel the anterior fontanelle. It is normally small at birth, enlarges during the first two months, and then gradually decreases in size until final closure. It is normally closed by 18 months of age, but can close much earlier, and has been reported as staying open in a few normal girls until $4\frac{1}{2}$ years of age. Delayed closure may be seen, however, in *rickets, hypothyroidism* and *hydrocephalus*. An assessment of the tension of the anterior fontanelle is important. In health it pulsates and is in the same plane as the rest of the surrounding skull. A tense, bulging fontanelle indicates *raised intracranial pressure*, but it does also become tense with crying. A sunken fontanelle is a feature of dehydration. The posterior fontanelle is located by passing the finger along the sagittal suture to its junction with the lambdoid sutures. It should normally be closed after 2 months of age. While feeling the head, any ridging of the sutures should be noticed, suggesting premature fusion (*craniostenosis*), or overriding of the sutures if the head is small (*microcephaly*). The sutures tend to be separated in the neonatal period, and there is sometimes a continuous gap from the forehead to the posterior part of the posterior fontanelle. Sutures close rapidly, and are normally ossified by 6 months of age.

Having assessed the skull, the *neck* can be checked, paying particular attention to the presence of lymph nodes. It is common in childhood to feel small lymph nodes in the anterior and posterior triangles of the neck, as they enlarge rapidly in response to local conditions such as tonsillitis. Examination of other lymphatic areas can be carried out at a later stage of the examination—the inguinal nodes when the napkin area is checked, and the axillary nodes when the chest is examined. In young babies the sternomastoid muscles should be checked for the thickened area known as a sternomastoid tumour.

The abdomen

The abdomen can be a little difficult to examine if the baby is crying, but most infants will be quite happy sitting on their mother's lap (Fig. 15.2). If they are crying, it is sometimes possible to quieten them by placing them over their mother's shoulder, and examining them from behind. Small infants can be given a feed to quieten them. Look for any obvious distension or for peristaltic waves suggesting intestinal obstruction. Remember that in children up to the age of 3 years the abdomen is rather protuberant. Note the umbilicus, and whether or not there is a hernia. Palpation should be gentle and light. The liver edge can be felt in normal children up to the age of 4; it can be anything up to 2 cm below the costal margin. When enlarged, the spleen may be felt below the left costal margin,

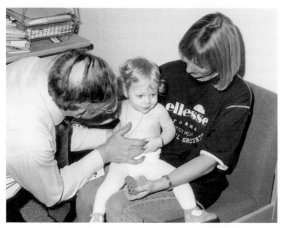

Fig. 15.2   Baby sitting on mother's lap while the abdomen is examined.

and in infancy it is more anterior and superficial than in the older child or adult. Slight enlargement of the spleen is common in children with many infections. Faecal masses can be felt in constipated children, and a full or distended bladder presents as a mass arising from the pelvis. Abdominal tenderness is best detected by watching the child's facial expression during palpation. Deep palpation of the kidneys can be carried out last. Although it would be logical to examine the groin area at this time, it is often better to do this at a slightly later stage. If the child has cried persistently, it is still possible to examine the abdomen by the method of *ballottement*—as the baby breathes in, the abdominal muscles relax, and abdominal viscera and other masses, if present, can then be palpated.

The chest

So far, nothing has been done that should cause the child any concern. Examining the chest, however, introduces the stethoscope, which sometimes worries babies. It helps to have earlier let the baby play with the stethoscope. Check for any asymmetry, and in girls for any breast development. Minor degrees of pes excavatum are a source of great anxiety to many parents, but are not usually of any importance. Indrawing of the lower ribs (*Harrison's sulcus*) may be seen in obstructive airway disease, either from asthma or a blocked nasopharynx from adenoidal hypertrophy. Note any recession when breathing, and count the respiratory rate. In a newborn infant it should be 40 breaths/min, by the second year it has fallen to 30 breaths/min and by 5 years of age to 20 breaths/min. A child with pneumonia will have a grunting respiration, which is due to reversal of the normal respiratory rhythm. The grunting expiration is followed by inspiration, and then a pause. Thickening of the costochondral junction is felt in rickets (*rachitic rosary*). Palpate the anterior chest wall for the cardiac impulse and for thrills. In children under the age of 5 years the apex is normally in the fourth intercostal space just to the left of the midclavicular line. Vocal fremitus is rarely of any clinical value in children. The axillary nodes may now be felt in the same way as in adults.

Percussion of the chest is useful in older children, but in young children and infants it is only rarely of value. Percuss very lightly, and in babies directly, tapping the chest wall with the percussing finger rather than using another finger as a pleximeter. The chest is more resonant in children than in adults.

A stethoscope with a small bell chest piece is suitable for auscultation of the child's chest. Often it is less threatening to examine the back of the chest first, and much more information about the lungs can be learnt in this way. Listen for the breath sounds and adventitious sounds. Because of the thin chest wall, breath sounds are louder in children than in adults, and their character is more like the bronchial breathing of adults (*puerile breathing*). Upper respiratory tract infections in children often give rise to loud, coarse rhonchi, which are conducted down the trachea and main bronchi. All is not lost if the child is crying, as this is associated with deep inspiration, and this is the time to listen for the character of the breath sounds.

When auscultating the front of the chest, the child's immediate instinct is to push the stethoscope away. Some doctors attach a small toy to the tubing to attract attention, while others prefer to distract the child with toys held in the hand (Fig. 15.3). The normal splitting of the first and second sounds is easier to hear in children than in adults. Venous hums and functional systolic flow murmurs are often heard in normal children. Count the heart rate in young children. The normal rates are as follows.

- newborn infant 140 beats/min
- 1-year-old 110 beats/min
- 3-year-old 100 beats/min
- 8-year-old 90 beats/min
- 11-year-old 80 beats/min.

Up to this point in the examination, the baby will have been examined mainly from behind. Take the opportunity to check for spinal abnormalities such as scoliosis or kyphosis, which may otherwise be missed. If there has been no need to stand the baby up at this time, examination of the back can be deferred until the neurological examination, or

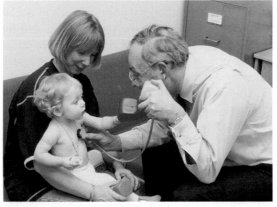

Fig. 15.3 Attracting the attention of a 10-month-old baby whilst examining her heart.

when the baby is moving around when the examination has been completed.

Neurological examination

The neurological examination can usually be carried out in the normal way, as in older children, but in younger children the extent of the neurological examination will depend on the child's age and willingness to co-operate. Already a great deal should have been learnt from initial observations. If the child is walking, the gait should have been observed and muscle tone assessed. Note any abnormal movements.

- Tics or habit spasms are repetitive but purposeful movements, such as shrugging of the shoulders or facial grimacing.
- Choreiform movements are involuntary, purposeless jerks which follow no particular pattern.
- Athetoid movements are writhing and more pronounced distally.

Co-ordination can best be checked by watching a child at play. It is useful to have toys available which require a degree of co-ordination, such as a toy farm or garage. Otherwise, a modification of the finger–nose test using a toy held in the hand can be used. If the child is old enough, watching them dressing or doing up shoelaces are good ways to assess co-ordination.

Check *muscle tone* if this has not already been carried out. Pick the child up if there is still a friendly relationship. This gives a good idea of the feel of a child and of the muscle tone. If the child is hypotonic, it will feel as though he or she is slipping through your hands. Muscle power is difficult to check in young children except by watching playing habits, and assessing power by ability at a variety of lifting games. Always remember to check for neck stiffness. It is detected more readily by resistance to passive flexion of the neck than by testing for Kernig's sign.

Testing of *sensation* is difficult in young children, and is probably best omitted unless there is a strong suspicion of neurological disease.

Testing the *cranial nerves* takes a little ingenuity. Eye movements are relatively easy using a toy moved in different directions in front of the baby's face; many young infants like poking out their tongue, which will check the 12th cranial nerve. If the child can be made to smile, and even if crying, any asymmetry of facial movements can be seen.

Getting a child's limbs into the correct position to

test *tendon reflexes* may take some time. Often they can be elicited by using a finger rather than a patellar hammer. Tendon reflexes in young infants tend to be brisk, and the plantar responses are extensor up to 18 months of age. The persistence of an extensor response beyond the age of 2 years indicates an upper motor neurone lesion. Primitive responses should have disappeared by 3–4 months of age; their persistence indicates significant neurodevelopmental dysfunction. The primitive reflexes will be considered further in the section on examination of the newborn (see page 381).

The eyes

The eyes should now be checked. Inspect them for conjunctivitis, cataracts or congenital defects such as colobomata. It is very important to check for *squints*, as immediate ophthalmological referral is necessary, however young the infant. Squints are checked for by shining a light in the eyes from in front of the face; the light reflex should be at the same position in each cornea. A *cover test* should then be used (see Chapter 12), employing a doll or some other appropriate toy on which a child can focus their gaze. Pupillary accommodation and light reactions can be noted at the same time. Examination of the *fundus* is particularly difficult in infants, and forcible attempts to keep the eyes open will only make the procedure more difficult. Older children will focus on toys or distant people. In younger children only fleeting glimpses of the fundus are likely. It should be possible to see the red reflex, and sufficient of the disc to detect papilloedema.

The testing of vision, hearing, and certain motor functions in young children is included in the section on developmental screening examination (see page 377).

With the possible exception of the eye examination, nothing so far should have upset a baby unduly. The following examinations should be carried out at the end of the consultation, as they are more likely to upset the child.

The genitalia, groins and anus

The nappy and underpants can now be removed if it is necessary to examine the groin or anus. In boys, notice the penis. This is often a source of worry to many parents, especially the lack of retraction of the foreskin. Old wives' tales abound, and few parents

realize that the foreskin will only rarely retract under the age of 5 years, they should be informed that forcibly attempting retraction is not only painful but can also result in *balanitis*. Check the hernial orifices, and see if the testes have descended. To feel the testis, make sure that your hand is warm, and place a finger in the line of the inguinal canal; advance the finger towards the scrotum. This will prevent the cremasteric reflex causing the testis to disappear into the inguinal canal, which tends to happen if the scrotum is approached from below. Having located the testes in the correct place, it is important to demonstrate the normality of the boy to his parents. It is not unusual to find a testis in the inguinal canal in young babies, but it can usually be pushed into the scrotum without too much difficulty. Nothing needs to be done other than to review the boy after a few months, as the testis can be expected to descend into its normal position with increasing maturity.

In girls, check the vulva for soreness or discharge, and for abnormalities such as polyps. Fusion of the labia is not uncommon, so check that they separate normally. Enlargement of the clitoris suggests endocrine disorder.

Check for inguinal lymph nodes at this time, and palpate the femoral artery. If the femoral artery cannot be palpated, this suggests coarctation of the aorta, which requires cardiological assessment.

Examination of the anal margin can best be carried out by gently separating the buttocks with one hand on either side; the anal orifice can then be seen easily, and inspected for fissures, which are not uncommon. Rectal examination is rarely necessary in children, and if carried out should be done with the little finger, which should be advanced very slowly. A little while spent talking and waiting will help.

The nose, ears, mouth and throat

The worst parts of the examination as far as the child is concerned are the nose, ears, mouth and throat.

The *nose* need only be examined superficially, looking for nasal patency, any deviation of the septum, or the presence of polyps. Older children are quite good at sniffing, and this will give some idea of nasal patency.

A co-operative child will allow you to look into his or her *ears* but, if not, the child should be held by the mother, as shown in Fig. 15.4. Held in such a way, the child can be kept still long enough for the eardrums to be inspected.

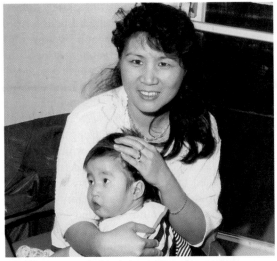

Fig. 15.4 How to hold a baby to allow the ears to be examined. The mother faces the baby to one side, and holds him firmly with one arm around the head, and the other around the upper arm and shoulder.

The *mouth* and *throat* can be examined by encouraging a co-operative child to 'show me your teeth'; an open mouth will then allow a clear view of the mouth and fauces. If uncooperative, the child will need to be held as shown in Fig. 15.5. Sometimes it is not too disastrous if the child cries at this point, as this will give a very clear view of the teeth, the tonsils, and sometimes even the epiglottis. A spatula is a terrifying instrument to the average child, causing most children to clamp their teeth shut. If this happens, the spatula should be forced on to the back of the tongue to induce a gag reflex. Whatever means are used to

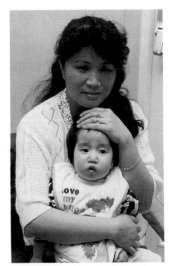

Fig. 15.5 How to hold a baby to allow the mouth and throat to be examined. The baby faces the examiner, with the mother holding him firmly with one hand on the forehead, and the other holding both arms.

open the mouth, the state of the teeth and mucous membranes should be noticed, as well as the tonsils and fauces. Note especially the white patches of *Candida* infections, and Koplik's spots seen in measles.

The child should now be allowed to move freely about the room, allowing a further assessment of gait, and of any marked skeletal abnormalities.

Examination of the hips must *always* be carried out in younger children and infants (see page 384).

The general physical examination of the child, with the exception of the special examinations described in the following sections, has now been completed. It is to be hoped that you have retained the friendship of the child. Once the child is dressed, the examiner should sit quietly with the parents and explain what has been found. It is always best to have finished dressing the child before talking to the parents; they are then more likely to consider what you have to say if they are not worrying about buttons or shoelaces. Always involve an older child in the discussion—he or she has every right to know what is wrong. Even young children can be told that they will be all right. Never under any circumstances deceive a child. If they find you out they will never believe you again.

Special examinations

The following examinations are important.

Height and weight

Measurements of height and weight are essential in the examination of children. Height can be measured in children over the age of 2 years against a wall-mounted gauge. Younger children can be measured lying down on special measuring boards. All measurements should be made under standard conditions, and children should be weighed unclothed. If the child keeps any clothes on, this should be noted against the weight, so that subsequent weights can be taken with the child wearing the same quantity of clothing. Childhood is a period of growth, the pattern of which may be adversely affected by many disturbances of health, as well as social deprivation. Heights and weights should be compared with those of healthy children of similar sex, age and build, and for this purpose percentile charts are essential. It is

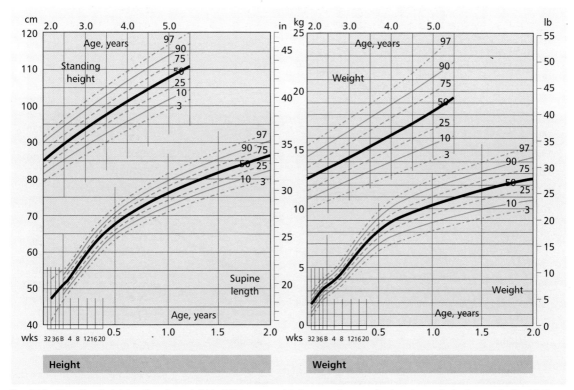

Fig. 15.6 Standing height and nude weight in UK boys aged 0–5 years. Age on abscissa: in weeks before and after birth (B) and in years as relevant. The curves show the percentiles as indicated, the black curve shows the 50th percentile.

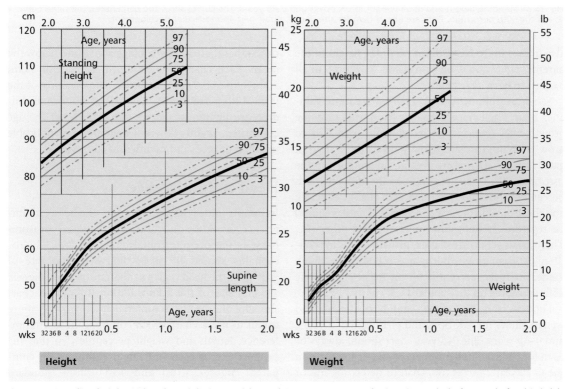

Fig. 15.7 Standing height and nude weight in UK girls aged 0–5 years. Age on abscissa: in weeks before and after birth (B) and in years as relevant. The curves show the percentiles as indicated, the black curve shows the 50th percentile.

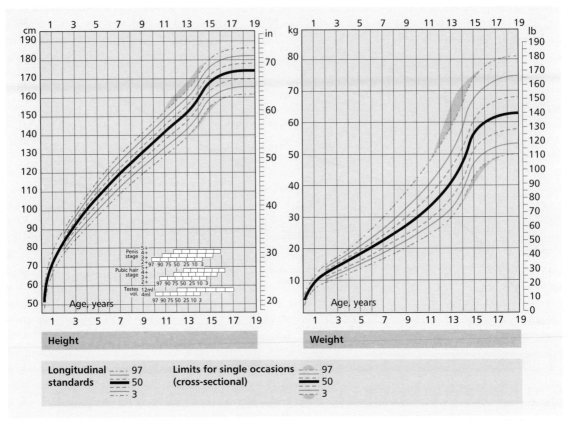

Fig. 15.8 Standing height and nude weight in UK boys aged 0–19 years. The curves show the percentiles, the black curve shows the 50th percentile. Data are also shown for the penile, pubic hair and testicular development.

also important to have some idea of the height of the parents, as it would be unrealistic to expect small parents to have large children.

Serial measurements over a period are more valuable than single measurements, and will give the growth rate—*growth velocity*. A child who fails to grow at an appropriate velocity needs to be investigated further. However, a child presenting for the first time outside the area between the 10th and 90th percentiles should be regarded with slight suspicion, and those outside the 3rd and 97th percentiles should be regarded as unhealthy unless proved otherwise. There are as yet no satisfactory growth charts for children of Asian origin born in the UK. As a rough guide, the mean percentile for an Asian child is the 25th percentile on the standard UK charts.

Figures 15.6–15.9 show standard height and weight charts for UK boys and girls aged 0–5 years, and 0–19 years. The 0–5 year chart should always be used for children under 5 years of age, as the scale on the 0–19 year chart is too small to detect the minor weight changes which can be important in indicating disease at this age. It will be seen from the percentile

charts that there is a wide range above and below the mean. Each chart shows the 3rd, 10th, 25th, 50th, 75th, 90th and 97th percentiles. The meaning of the term '10th percentile' is that 10% of all normal children are lighter or shorter, respectively, at the age concerned. Slightly different standards are applicable in different races and in different countries.

Head circumference

In infants under the age of 2 years, the head circumference should be measured. The standard measurement is the occipitofrontal circumference. Hydrocephalus should be suspected when the rate of growth of the head is greater than normal for the sex, age and size of the infant. Rather than use a chart showing the head circumference alone, it is more useful to use a chart which combines head circumference, length and weight percentiles, so that the proportions of each individual child can be compared. Figures 15.10 and 15.11 show standard height, weight and head circumference charts for boys and girls. An additional advantage of these

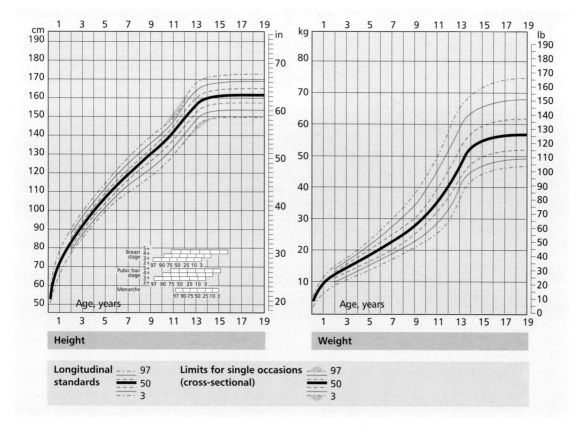

Fig. 15.9 Standing height and nude weight in UK girls aged 0–19 years. The curves show the percentiles, the black curve shows the 50th percentile. Data are also shown for the breast and pubic hair development and for the onset of menstruation.

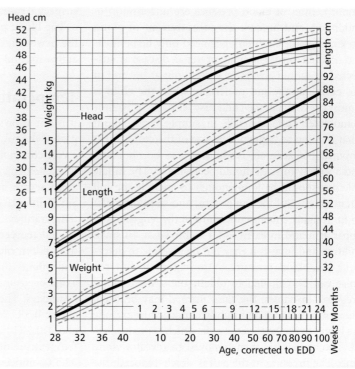

Fig. 15.10 Standard height, weight and head circumference in UK boys aged between 0–2 years. On the abscissa, the lefthand scale refers to development prior to 40 weeks, i.e. before birth, and the scale on the right to the postnatal age in weeks and months. EDD, expected delivery date.

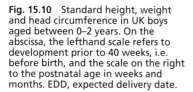

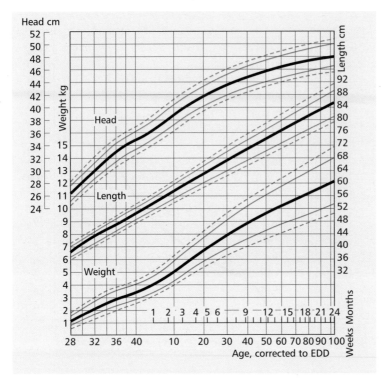

Fig. 15.11 Standard height, weight and head circumference in UK girls aged 0–2 years. On the abscissa, the lefthand scale refers to development prior to 40 weeks, i.e. before birth, and the scale on the right to the postnatal age in weeks and months. EDD, expected delivery date.

charts is that they allow for prematurity, and so separate charts for pre-term babies are not necessary.

Blood pressure

Abnormalities of blood pressure are uncommon in childhood, and because the measurement of blood pressure can be frightening it need only be be measured when cardiovascular or renal disease is suspected. It should always be carried out at the end of the examination, and preferably when the child is almost dressed. Let the child play with the sphygmomanometer cuff, and talk in simple terms about what is going to happen. The size of the cuff is most important if accurate readings are to be obtained, and a variety of sizes should be available. The inflatable bag should be long enough to encircle the full circumference of the upper arm, and should be of a width roughly equal to one-third of the length of the upper arm and forearm as far as the wrist. In small children and infants it may not be possible to determine the blood pressure by auscultation, but the pulse can be palpated to obtain the systolic blood pressure. In babies, the *flush method* may be used. The arm is held up and tightly bandaged to exclude the blood to the level of the cuff, which is then inflated. The bandage is then removed to reveal a white limb. The pressure in the cuff is slowly reduced; the point at which the skin flushes is an approximate indication of the systolic blood pressure. Doppler techniques more accurately measure blood pressure in children, but these are not always available. The blood pressure in the legs must be measured in all suspected cases of coarctation of the aorta.

The blood pressure in the arms is about 65/45 in the newborn, 75/50 at 1 year, 85/60 at 4 years, 95/65 at 8 years, and 100/70 mmHg at 10 years of age.

Temperature

It is not always necessary to take the temperature as part of the routine examination of children. Fever is a very common finding in children, and may be due to excitement, exercise and minor infections, as well as to severe infections and other serious illnesses. Small infants often respond to infection with low temperatures.

Oral temperature measurements should be used in children older than 5 years. In smaller children and infants the thermometer can be placed in the axilla or groin. Rectal temperatures are rarely taken nowadays. The temperature in the axilla or groin is about 0.5°C lower, and the rectal temperature is about 0.5°C higher than the oral temperature. The temperature of normal children is between 36.5 and 37.5°C, and is about 1°C higher in infants than in older children. Rapid rises of temperature to 39.5 or 40°C are not uncommon in children under 5 years of age, and may be associated with a convulsion.

Stools

Never be afraid to see a dirty nappy, or stool. This is part of the examination of a baby, and it is important to know the normal stool appearances in childhood. The stools of a breast-fed infant may be loose and green or pasty and yellow. They have a characteristic odour. Infants fed on cows' milk preparations pass stools of a paler yellow colour and of a much firmer consistency. Babies fed on the newer, modified cows' milk preparations have clay-coloured or greenish stools. The character of the stool in older children is more variable than in adults. Some healthy children pass frequent, loose stools containing undigested vegetable matter, 'toddler's diarrhoea'. The stools of children with coeliac disease and cystic fibrosis are bulky, odiferous and quite characteristic.

Urine

Collection of urine specimens in infants is difficult, and special techniques are required. It is not uncommon for a baby to pass urine while being examined. If you are lucky, and happen to have a sterile container available, a 'clean catch' specimen can be obtained. Alternatively, specially made sterile plastic containers with an adhesive opening can be applied to the washed genitalia. Faecal contamination can be a problem with specimens collected in this way, and it may be necessary to resort to suprapubic aspiration of bladder urine, a procedure which is not difficult in infants.

Developmental screening examination

Development is the normal process of maturation of function which takes place in the early years of life. It may be modified by emotional difficulties, environment, and physical defects and illnesses. Lack of intellectual stimulation, and of the normal experiences of childhood, may result in apparent retardation of development.

All infants should have a simple developmental screening examination at regular intervals. Table

15.1 lists the important milestones, and as part of the history-taking and physical examination it should be a routine to carry out a brief developmental screening examination.

It is usual to consider development under four main headings:

1 Movement and posture
2 Vision and manipulation
3 Hearing and speech
4 Social behaviour.

Screening for developmental delay involves testing the child's performance of a few skills in each of the four fields of development, and comparing the results with the average for children of the same age. The range of normal developmental progress is wide, and the milestones shown in Table 15.1 are those of an average normal baby. Delay in all fields of development is more significant than delay in one only, and severe delay is more meaningful than slight delay. There are considerable individual variations, and lateness in one particular area should not be taken as evidence of mental handicap or cerebral palsy without other corroborating features.

Allowance must always be made for those infants who were born prematurely, at least until the age of 2 years, by which time they should have caught up.

Techniques used

The same rules apply to techniques used in developmental screening as to those of general physical examination. Time has to be spent gaining the friendship of the child. This time can be profitably utilized by offering, for example, a 10-month-old baby a small toy to see how the child grasps it and reacts to it. Let the baby play with the toys and bricks while sitting on his or her mother's lap, and if the child remains suspicious, get the mother to offer the various objects. As with all parts of the examination, much more is learnt by simply watching a child play and his or her reactions to the surroundings.

In the UK, developmental screening is usually carried out by questionnaire administered by the health visitor at 8, 18 and 24 months. The health visitor is trained in developmental skills and will refer on to a doctor babies about whom there is any suspicion.

Testing vision

Much will be learnt about a child's vision by observation. Notice whether the child is looking around

Age	Movement and posture	Vision and manipulation	Hearing and speech	Social behaviour
6 weeks	When pulled from sitting to supine, head lag is not quite complete (Fig. 15.13) When held prone, head is held in line with body When prone on couch, lifts chin off couch Primitive responses persist	Looks at toy held in mid-line Follows a moving person	Vocalizes with gurgles	Smiles briefly when talked to by mother
4 months	Holds head up in sitting position, and is steady Pulls to sitting with only minimal head lag (Fig. 15.14) When prone, with head and chest off couch, makes swimming movements Rolls from prone to supine Primitive responses gone	Watches his or her hands Pulls at his or her clothes Tries to grasp objects	Turns head to sound Vocalizes apparently appropriately Laughs	Recognizes mother Becomes excited by toys
7 months	Sits unsupported Rolls from supine to prone Can support weight when held, and bounces with pleasure When prone, bears weight on hands	Transfers objects from hand to hand Bangs toys on table Watches small moving objects	Says 'Da', 'Ba', 'Ka'	Tries to feed him- or herself Puts objects in mouth Plays with paper
10 months	Crawls Gets to sitting position without help Can pull up to standing Lifts one foot when standing	Reaches for objects with index finger Has developed a finger–thumb grasp Will place objects in the examiner's hands, but not release them	Says one word with meaning	Plays 'peep-bo' and 'pat-a-cake' Waves 'bye-bye' Deliberately drops objects so that they can be picked up Puts objects in and out of boxes
13 months	Walks unsupported May shuffle on buttocks and hands	Can hold two cubes in one hand Makes marks with pen	Says two or three words with meaning	Understands simple questions such as 'Where is your shoe?' May kiss on request Tends to be shy
15 months	Can get into standing position without support Climbs upstairs Walks with broad-based gait	Builds a tower of two cubes Takes off shoes	Will say around 12 words, but mostly gobbledegook	Asks for things by pointing Kisses pictures of animals Can use a cup
18 months	Climbs stairs unaided, holding rail Runs and jumps Can climb on to a chair and sit down	Builds tower of three cubes Turns pages of a book two or three at a time Scribbles Takes off gloves and socks Unzips fasteners	Is beginning to join two words together	Recognizes animals and cars in a book Points to nose, ear, etc. on request Clean and dry but with occasional accidents Carries out simple orders

Table 15.1 Normal developmental milestones.

the room and at particular toys, or staring at nothing in particular, especially if there are random or nystagmoid eye movements; the latter suggests that the child is unable to see. When he or she picks toys up, is accommodation normal? The routine examination of the eye has been dealt with in the first part of this chapter.

Checks of *visual acuity* are not easy in young babies. By 6 weeks of age, infants should be following their mother with their eyes and by 6 months of age they should be able to follow a rolling ball at 3 metres. This is the basis of one method of visual testing at this age. The ability of the child to follow rolling balls of differing diameters gives an accurate assessment of visual acuity. From the age of approximately $2\frac{1}{2}$ years, the *Sheridan–Gardiner test* is used. This is a simple comparison test, with the examiner indicating letters or familiar toys on a board, and asking the child to indicate a similar object on a board held by the mother. The acuity is the ability of the child to pick out the smallest objects (Chapter 10).

Testing hearing

Hearing is normally checked for the first time between 6 and 8 months of age. There are special techniques (e.g. brainstem auditory evoked potential studies) for testing the hearing of newborn babies but these are indicated only in those babies at greatest risk of impaired hearing, e.g. when there is a family history of deafness, and in babies who have received ototoxic antibiotics such as aminoglycosides.

Although distraction testing, as explained below, is still carried out in some centres, this test has a large observer error and many children shown subsequently to be deaf pass the distraction test! It is more usual now to use a questionnaire, concentrating in particular on high-risk factors (see Box 15.4), and specifically on the parent's perception of the child's hearing.

To carry out the distraction test, the baby sits on his or her mother's lap, facing outwards. It helps if an assistant can sit facing them to distract the child with toys etc. (but not funny noises). The examiner then makes a series of soft noises to one side or the other but behind mother and child and out of the child's line of vision (Fig. 15.12). The sounds used are a special high-frequency rattle, a bell, a spoon in a cup, and the rustle of tissue paper or a whisper. At 6 months of age a baby should turn to the source of the sound when it is about 45 cm from their ear. By 9 months a baby reacts more quickly, and localizes the

---

BOX 15.4 Hearing questionnaire for 8-month-old babies.

CHILD'S NAME: ....

DATE OF BIRTH: ....

A HIGH RISK FACTORS FOR DEAFNESS

1. **FAMILY HISTORY** of deafness which required special education or hearing aid fitting in childhood or an inherited condition known to be associated with childhood deafness, even though there is no known deafness in the family. YES | NO

2. **CONGENITAL MALFORMATIONS** either of chromosomal, syndromic or unknown aetiology including craniofacial, branchial arch and cervical spine dysmorphologies; cleft palates; and pinna malformations even if unilateral but excluding isolated ear pits and tags. YES | NO

3. **CONGENITAL INFECTION** to include clinically apparent rubella, cytomegalovirus, toxoplasmosis, herpes and syphilis and also any maternal history of possible infection in pregnancy even in the absence of neonatal stigmata. YES | NO

4. **PERINATAL ILLNESS** requiring admission to the Special Care Baby Unit but only to include those babies with:
   i) Gestation of less than 32 weeks
   ii) Birth weight of 1.25 kg or less
   iii) An Apgar score of 3 or less at 5 minutes
   iv) Cerebral illness, e.g. intraventricular haemorrhage, convulsions, meningitis
   v) Apnoea requiring ventilation for 4 hours or more
   vi) Jaundice where exchange transfusion has been considered or undertaken
   vii) Administration of aminoglycosides at potentially toxic levels. YES | NO

5. **POSTNATAL ILLNESS** of bacterial meningitis, head injury with loss of consciousness or neurological disease. YES | NO

B HEARING RESPONSES

Go through parents' 'hearing' information leaflet with parents. Try to elicit from them clear examples of the baby's responses to loud and quiet sounds.
Having done this

1. Do the parents have any concerns about the baby's hearing? YES | NO

2. Do you have any concerns about the baby's hearing? YES | NO

BOX 15.4 (continued)

C VOICE AND SPEECH DEVELOPMENT

The baby should enjoy using his or her voice freely with variation in pitch and tone.

The baby should have started making repetitive consonant/vowel sequences—'baba', 'mum-mum', i.e. babbling.

1. Do the parents have any concerns about the baby's speech development? | YES | NO |

2. Do you have any concerns about the baby's speech development? | YES | NO |

D MIDDLE EAR PROBLEMS

1. Has the baby had recurrent ear infections requiring treatment? | YES | NO |

2. Has the baby had recurrent upper respiratory tract infections thought to be associated with hearing loss? | YES | NO |

If YES to any of the above, refer the baby to the Secondary Audiology Clinic (or to the Tertiary Clinic if suspected of having a severe loss).

E Is there parental consanguinity?
| YES | NO | UNCERTAIN |

Do not make a referral on this factor alone but, if present, take particular care at this and subsequent interviews.

ACTION

F Has a referral been completed? | YES | NO |

If yes, to whom?

Signature of Interviewer ....

Name (Please Print) ....

Date of Interview ....

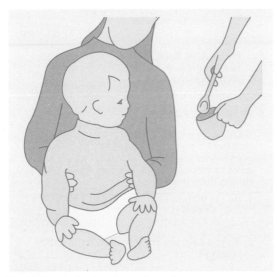

Fig. 15.12   Testing hearing at 6 months.

sound at a distance of 90 cm. If the child fails the test on the first occasion, it does not automatically mean that he or she is deaf, but the test should be repeated after a further month. If the child still fails, he or she should be referred for audiological testing.

Head control

By 4 months babies can normally keep their head in line with the trunk when pulled from supine to sitting, and when held in the sitting position will keep their head upright. Before this age the head lags behind the trunk (Figs 15.13 and 15.14).

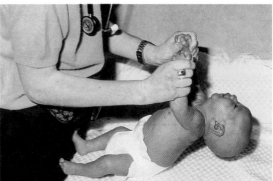

Fig. 15.13   Head control at 6 weeks of age.

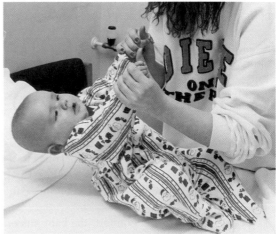

Fig. 15.14   Head control at 4 months of age.

Table 15.1 shows the normal developmental milestones up to the age of 18 months, by which time obvious deviations from normal development will be apparent. Beyond this age developmental testing is more specialized, and is not the concern of this chapter. A baby who appears to have delayed development on screening will need further specialized assessment to establish causation and treatment.

Examination of the newborn

The routine examination of the newborn infant (Box 15.5) is designed to assess the general state of health and to detect congenital abnormalities. It is recommended that all babies should be examined within the first 24 hours of life, and again before the end of the first week. Many parts of the examination of the newborn infant are similar to the techniques described above for older babies and children.

BOX 15.5 Checklist for examination of the newborn.

- Apgar score 5 min after birth
- Weight, length, head circumference
- Passage of urine and meconium
- Alertness and wakefulness
- Skin colour: cyanosis, jaundice
- Birthmarks
- Sacral development: Down's syndrome etc.
- Skull and fontanelles
- Eyes
- Mouth and tongue
- Neck: branchial cysts
- Limbs: digits and palmar creases, talipes
- Chest
- Abdomen and umbilicus
- Perineum and genitalia
- Neurological assessment: movements and tone, reflexes, the cry

---

The neurological status at birth has implications for the future development of the child, and has been used as an indicator of brain damage sustained during or shortly after birth. The *Apgar score* (Box 15.6) is in general use as part of this assessment. An Apgar score of 6 or less at 5 minutes after birth is associated with neurological deficit in about 10% of cases, but a low score 1 minute after birth is less predictive of brain damage. A high Apgar score at 5

BOX 15.7 The Apgar score.

In each of the five categories a score of 0, 1 or 2 is awarded, giving a maximum score of 10. A score of 7–10 is *good*, 3–6 *moderate CNS depression*, and 0–2 *severe CNS depression*.

- Heart rate
- Respiratory effort
- Muscle tone
- Reflex irritability
- Colour

---

minutes, on the other hand, may not recognize focal brain injury or infarction.

Weight, length and head circumference (occipito-frontal) will usually have been measured by the midwife. Note the time of passage of the first urine and meconium, which is the dark green, sticky stool of the newborn baby in the first few days of life.

Always examine a newborn baby in front of his or her mother, and involve her at all stages by explaining what you are doing. Have the baby undressed, and in a warm place. Always have warm hands, and treat the baby gently, leaving the most unpleasant parts of the examination until last. Talk or even sing to the baby—he or she is as aware of what is going on as an older child, and should be afforded the same courtesy.

Much of the time can be spent just watching the baby noting the state of awareness. If the baby is awake, seemingly looking around and not crying, examination of the nervous system will yield much information.

The skin

Note the colour of the skin. *Peripheral cyanosis* is a common finding in the normal newborn, but *central cyanosis* indicates cardiac or respiratory disease. So-called '*traumatic cyanosis*' affects the head and neck, and is produced by confluent petechial haemorrhages; it is most often seen after prolonged or obstructed labour. Jaundice is common *after* 48 hours in most pre-term and some term babies, and is considered physiological. However, jaundice *within* 48 hours of birth has to be considered pathological; the commonest cause is haemolytic disease of the newborn, but any baby jaundiced before 48 hours or after 7 days of age needs to be investigated.

Look for birthmarks, which are either pigmented lesions or haemangiomata. Most babies have a collection of dilated capillaries on the upper eyelids and nape of the neck (sometimes called '*stork bites*'), which fade after a few weeks. Some babies develop a crop of small papules on the trunk during the first week (*erythema toxicum* or *urticaria neonatorum*). They are of uncertain cause, of no significance and usually fade after a few days. Superficial peeling of the skin, especially over the periphery, is common, and is most apparent in post-term and some small-for-gestational-age babies. *Milia* are whitish, pinhead spots concentrated mainly around the nose. They are sebaceous retention cysts, and can be felt with the finger. They usually disappear within a month. *Lanugo hair* may cover the body, especially in pre-term babies and some dark-haired babies. It usually disappears over the first 2 or 3 weeks. Colour of hair at birth is no guide to subsequent hair colour. *Mongolian blue spot* is the name given to the normal dark blue areas of pigmentation commonly seen over the sacrum and buttocks or back of the legs in black or Asian babies.

The face

Look at the face for obvious abnormalities such as Down's syndrome and other indications of craniofacial maldevelopment. Check the position of the ears, and whether they are normal and symmetrical. Accessory auricles are small, pedunculated skin tags, usually just in front of the ears, and can be dealt with by tying them off at the base. Make sure that the upper lip is intact.

Once superficial examination has been completed, more formal examination takes place; again, it should be regional rather than by systems, starting with the head and working down.

The head

Inspect and palpate the head. The bones of the cranial vault, being relatively soft and connected only by fibrous tissue, alter in shape readily in response to external pressure. Moulding of the skull takes place during birth, with overriding of the sutures. It usually disappears after a few days. The *caput succedaneum* is an area of oedema of the scalp over the presenting part of the head during labour. It pits on pressure and is not fluctuant. A *cephalhaematoma* is a subperiosteal haematoma which appears a few days after birth as a large, cystic swelling limited to the area of one of the skull bones. It tends to resolve relatively slowly over a few months, and may leave a calcified edge. The anterior fontanelle varies considerably at birth, but should be checked, as described above (page 368).

The eyes

The eyes can best be examined when the baby has his or her eyes open spontaneously. Alternatively the eyelids can be held open by an assistant, although this tends to make the baby cry. Sometimes a baby will open the eyes if given a feed. The iris gives no indication of its future colour, and is usually greyish-blue in Caucasian infants. A bluish tinge to the sclera

is usual. Tears before 3–4 weeks are unusual. Even though newborn infants can see, eye movements tend to be random, often giving the impression of a transient squint. Subconjunctival haemorrhages show as a dark red patch covering the sclera, sometimes ringing the cornea. They commonly follow normal deliveries, and despite their alarming appearance are of no consequence and disappear after a few weeks. Look for evidence of conjunctivitis and check for other abnormalities as described above (page 371).

The mouth and tongue

Look inside the mouth; this is easy if the baby is crying, and a spatula will not be needed. If the baby is quiet and content, this part of the examination may be left until later. Make sure that there is no cleft of the palate, and note particularly whether the uvula is normal. A bifid uvula indicates a submucous cleft of the palate which requires surgery. Rounded, thickened areas are often seen on the lips, more especially on the lower lips and are known as *suckling blisters.* This is a misnomer, as despite their name, they do not contain fluid. *Epithelial pearls* are small, white areas, best seen on the hard palate. Occasionally teeth are present at birth. They are usually incisors, and can be green in colour. If loose, they are best removed. *Macroglossia* is seen in babies with Down's syndrome, congenital hypothyroidism, Beckwith's syndrome and in some normal children.

The neck

The neck of a newborn baby seems rather short, and may be considered abnormal by the inexperienced. Rarely, cystic swellings are seen; *dermoid cysts* and *thyroglossal cysts* in the midline, or *branchial* cysts just in front of the upper third of the sternomastoid muscle.

The limbs

Examine the limbs for abnormalities. Extra digits on the hand are not uncommon, but are rarer on the feet. Look for a single transverse palmar crease, which is classically seen in babies with Down's syndrome, but in addition is found in a variety of dysmorphic syndromes, as well as in some normal infants. Common foot abnormalities to look for are syndactyly or talipes equinovarus; the latter requires immediate orthopaedic referral.

The chest

The general appearance and shape of the chest should be noticed. Breast enlargement with exudation of a milky fluid from the nipples is sometimes seen in newborn infants of either sex. This is due to transferred maternal hormones, and disappears in a few days without causing problems. Resist the temptation to squeeze the breasts, as this may result in infection (*mastitis*). Make sure that the clavicles are intact. Note the symmetry of the chest wall, the pattern of respiration, and whether there is any indrawing on inspiration. The remainder of the chest examination is as described earlier in this chapter for older children (page 369), percussion of the chest is of even less value at this age. Transient systolic murmurs are extremely common in the first few days, and may reflect the closing ductus arteriosus, or non-specific flow murmurs, as discussed earlier.

The abdomen

The abdomen of a newborn baby usually seems a little distended, and it moves with respiration. Slight divarication of the rectus muscles may occur, and this exaggerates this abdominal bulging. The liver edge is palpable 2–4 cm below the costal margin, and the lower poles of both kidneys can be felt easily. The bladder should not be palpable if the baby has just passed urine. Check the umbilical stump. It should contain two arteries and one vein. A single umbilical artery is associated with an increased incidence of congenital abnormalities, especially of the renal tract. The umbilical cord should become dry, and then separate between the 6th and 10th day. Some moistness of the stump then remains for a further few days. Sometimes excess granulation tissue accumulates, to form a small granuloma; this can be treated by local application of a silver nitrate stick.

The perineum and genitalia

Examine the perineum for hypospadias, hydroceles, hernias or undescended testicles. Look for patency of the anus; an imperforate anus is easily overlooked unless it is specifically checked for. While looking at the buttocks and anus, see if there is a sacral dimple, which is usually a blind-ending pit and of no significance. Make sure that the back is straight and that there are no gross spinal lesions, especially spina bifida. Check female external genitalia for clitoral enlargement or labial fusion. It is not unusual for girls to have a mucous vaginal discharge, and sometimes bleeding. This is the result of transferred maternal hormones, and is usually transient. Make sure that the femoral pulses are palpable.

Neurological assessment

Combine a formal neurological examination with observation of the baby's behaviour. No two babies react in the same way, but there is a broad, general pattern which applies to most. Spontaneous movement normally takes place when the baby is awake, consisting of alternating flexion and extension. Any marked difference between the two sides is abnormal. The fingers are more fully flexed than later in childhood, but spontaneous opening and closing of the hands takes place. The thumb may be tucked under the fingers.

The normal position of a newborn baby is that of flexion. When lying prone, the baby's legs are usually drawn up under the abdomen. If the baby is crying, look for any weakness or paralysis in the face suggesting injury to the facial nerve, or any deficiency of arm movements suggesting injury to the brachial plexus. Note the limb tone and, although tendon jerks are difficult to elicit at this age, they should be checked, using a finger rather than a tendon hammer.

PRIMITIVE REFLEXES

Primitive responses are present in the normal newborn infant, and disappear at variable times up to the fourth month of age. They are responses to specific stimuli, and depend to some extent on the infant's state of wakefulness. The absence of one or more of these reflexes in the newborn infant may indicate some abnormality of the brain, a local abnormality in the affected limb, or a neuromuscular abnormality. Persistence of primitive reflexes beyond the fourth month of life should alert you to the possibility of developmental delay. These reflex responses are as follows:

Rooting reflexes

In response to a touch on the cheek, a baby will turn his or her head towards the stimulus. Stimulation of the upper lip causes opening of the mouth, pouting of the lips, and tongue movements. Sucking itself is a reflex, and failure of the sucking response beyond the 36th week of gestation suggests significant neurological impairment.

Palmar and plantar grasp

A finger placed across the palm will cause a flexion and grasping of the finger. A similar response is seen if a finger is placed on the plantar surface of the foot, but the grasp is not as strong.

Stepping reflex

The baby is held upright, and the feet placed on a firm surface. As the foot presses down on the surface, the other leg flexes at the hip and knee in a stepping movement. As this response is alternated from one leg to the other, the baby makes a walking movement.

The Moro reflex

This is the best known of the primitive reflexes, but it must not be forgotten that because it is a 'startle' reaction it will make the baby cry. It should therefore be left to the end of the examination. Always be gentle in carrying out the test, and make sure that the baby is well-supported. The baby's body is supported with one arm and hand, and the head with the other hand. The hand holding the head is then lowered a few centimetres, allowing the baby's head to drop back (Fig 15.15). In a positive response the baby abducts and extends the arms, and then flexes them. A clearly unilateral response suggests some local abnormality, such as a fracture or brachial plexus injury in the arm on the side that does not respond.

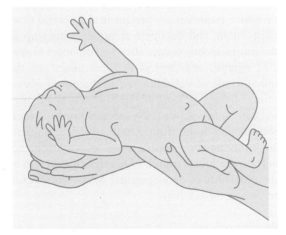

Fig. 15.15 Eliciting the Moro reflex.

Assessment of gestation

Although a full assessment of gestation is beyond the scope of this chapter, a rough approximation of the baby's gestational age should always be made, espe-cially if the baby is small. This can be made from a combination of maternal menstrual data, and size and appearance of the baby. The flexed position of the baby at term has already been mentioned, and the more immature the baby, the less flexed he or she will be. Certain physical criteria are the basis of more formal assessments. Among these are the shape and form of the ears: Is the pinna flat against the skull and unfolded, or is it folded over with a good development of cartilage? The degree of breast formation, the degree of ossification of the skull, and opacification of the skull to transillumination with a bright light are important specific features.

A neurological assessment, especially of muscle tone and movement, and the development of certain reflexes will also give a guide to gestation. For example, by 32 weeks the baby will turn his or her head towards a diffuse light; by 34–36 weeks sucking and neck-righting reflexes will have developed.

At the end of the examination of the newborn infant, a comment should always be made of the estimated gestation.

Examination of the hips

The examination of the hips is essential but should be left to the end of the assessment because it is very uncomfortable for the baby. It is illustrated in Figs 15.16 and 15.17. It is usual to differentiate between a tendinous 'click' and the typical 'clunk' of a hip moving in and out of its socket. The latter is more a feeling than an actual noise. Skin creases on the upper posterior thigh may be asymmetrical, but this is not a reliable sign of dislocation; similarly, limita-

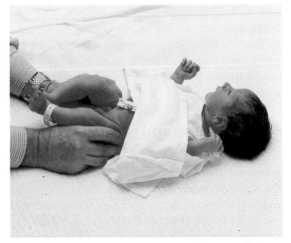

Fig. 15.16 Stage 1 of the examination of the hips: the hips are flexed, medially rotated, and pushed posteriorly. This will dislocate dislocatable hips.

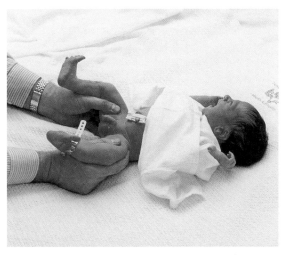

Fig. 15.17 Stage 2 of the examination of the hips: the hips are abducted, and a 'click' or a 'clunk' is felt for (see text). Note the position of the examiner's hands, with the thumbs on the medial aspect of the thigh, and the fingers over the lateral trochanters.

tion of abduction is not absolutely reliable. If there is any doubt about the hip, ultrasound examination should be carried out. Routine ultrasound examination of the hips of all newborn babies is now being carried out in some centres to screen for congenital dislocation. If any doubt still remains, orthopaedic referral is essential.

Screening for genetic disorders

There are a number of disorders for which screening is available by urine testing at birth, and others which may be tested for by measurement of white blood cell enzymes, e.g. gangliosidosis and other lipid storage disorders. In most of these, tests are not carried out routinely except in genetically isolated populations, or in families known to be at risk. In the UK all newborn infants are screened for phenylketonuria, by a simple urine test. If positive, dietary management is offered to prevent the mental and development retardation that would otherwise develop. Increasingly, direct DNA analysis for genetic disorders is becoming available for many inherited disorders.

Having now completed the examination, the newborn baby should be dressed and, as in every examination of children, your findings must be conveyed to the parents.

Conclusions

Throughout this chapter, emphasis has been placed on getting to know the child, and treating him or her as gently as possible. Time has to be spent getting the child's confidence and indeed building up your own confidence in handling him or her. This can only be acquired by examining children at each and every opportunity. One of the most rewarding parts of paediatrics is when a child sits on your lap and plays happily with you. If you can achieve this, you know how to examine children.

CHAPTER 16

The examination of elderly people

Introduction

It is appropriate to think of elderly people in three distinct groups: the young old (65–74), the old old (75–84), and the oldest old (85+). The social and biological characteristics of people in each of these groups is sufficiently distinct to make these categories meaningful. The emphasis in the training of health care workers, and medical students in particular, is upon disease because the detection, investigation, treatment and prevention of disease is the justification for medicine, its one specific function. However, even when detected and treated disease often leaves disabilities. The majority of elderly, frail and disabled people, including those with severe functional impairments, live in private households. Many depend to a greater or lesser extent upon those who contribute to their social networks, whether informally or formally.

Social networks

The informal network of support consists of kin, i.e. nuclear and extended family, and of friends and neighbours (Box 16.1). This network is usually small in size and has a long history of contact with the old person whether rewarding, hostile or mixed. Though

> **BOX 16.1 Social networks.**
>
> **Informal**
> • Family, friends and neighbours: available, concerned and committed, familiar, flexible
>
> **Formal**
> • Financial entitlements: pension and other income
> • Statutory services: health care and social services
> • Voluntary services: church and charity

less skilled than a formal network it has the great advantage of availability at all times, of being able to deal with unexpected events and emergencies and of being flexible, familiar and continuous.

The formal network of support consists first of any basic financial entitlements, e.g. retirement and supplementary pensions, etc. The statutory agencies themselves carry out Governmental economic and social policies and actually provide a service; for example, in the UK these include the National Health Service including the general practitioner, district nurse, health visitor, and the local authority Social Services Department, e.g. social worker, home help, meals-on-wheels, day centre. Finally, there are the voluntary organizations, such as charities, and the local church.

No assessment of an older person, with even slight disability, is complete without a description of those people available to help.

Presentation of disease

Two major factors influence the recognition of disease processes in elderly people:

• acceptance of ill-health with a subsequent delay in seeking help
• atypical presentation of disease processes.

Acceptance of ill-health and disease as 'ageing', with its resultant disabilities, means that many elderly people *expect* to be frail and rarely complain or seek help early. Dramatic complaints, e.g. severe pain, or vomiting blood, may elicit an appropriate call for help but less life-threatening episodes are often accepted as part of the ageing process. Coming to terms with some disability or change is necessary at all ages and acceptance is part of survival. However, the tacit acceptance of deterioration in, for example, eyesight, hearing, teeth and feet may lead to treatable conditions being ignored and consequent loss of independence.

The fact of atypical presentation in old age is one of the most essential elements for the student and practitioner to comprehend. The term 'geriatric giants' (Box 16.2) refers to a set of symptoms and signs that occur in old age that may have as their cause *any* disease process. Diseases as diverse in aetiology as pneumonia, myocardial infarction or drug toxicity may present *classically* or as one of the geriatric giants.

> **BOX 16.2 'Geriatric giants': major clinical syndromes that may result from any disease process.**
>
> • Immobility
> • Falls
> • Incontinence
> • Pressure sores
> • Confusion

A useful analogy is a seizure occurring in a child. This is a symptom not a diagnosis. The latter could be, for example, a febrile illness, epilepsy, meningitis or head injury. In the same way that a fit is not a normal childhood event, falls or incontinence should not be treated as part of the normal ageing process.

There are two other important aspects concerning the unique presentation of disease in old age. One is the concept of *multiple pathology* being present and the other is the recognition of the *social presentation* of disease, and the response that can subsequently occur. Multiple pathologies may be causally linked, although more typically they are not. The art of diagnosis and management is in identifying and treating the most important clinical problems, and utilizing a multidisciplinary approach that compensates for as many of the other associated deficits as possible.

This holistic approach to care of the elderly recognizes that geriatric medicine has a lot to do with social problems. 'Social admission' is a pejorative term in a hospital setting. It usually indicates a lack of history-taking and examination that should have uncovered a disease process resulting in a social response (e.g. relatives leaving a person in the Accident & Emergency Department or neighbours calling a social worker or the police 'to do something'). Recognition of this social presentation of disease allows multiple problems to be identified and treated more easily.

History

To provide adequate assessment of elderly people several aspects of the history are crucial (Box 16.3).

> **BOX 16.3 History-taking: points to note.**
>
> • The introduction
> • Timing, interest
> • Position and comfort
> • Vision, hearing, cognition
> • Environment
> • Use of multiple sources of information
> • Interview versus interrogation

The introduction is extremely important (Box 16.4). It should be straightforward, relatively formal and should respect the dignity of the person. Eye contact, a greeting, an outstretched hand (expecting a returned handshake), your name and the purpose of the meeting are all that are required to begin with.

> **BOX 16.4 Observations during the introduction.**
>
> • Can the patient see and hear you?
> • Is behaviour normal?
> • Is language normal?
> • Does the patient understand your role as a doctor?
> • Is the patient at ease, or in pain?
> • Is there evidence of support from family or friends?

These relatively simple gestures can provide a wealth of information in the first few minutes. Can the person see you? Do they smile in response to your smile? Depressed and very anxious patients may avoid eye contact. The hand contact is useful. Some patients with dementia may not respond—not recognizing the meaning of the social gesture. Frightened elderly patients may continue to clutch one's hand. An unwillingness to let go may also indicate a positive grasp reflex, a primitive reflex usually indicating frontal lobe damage and found in advanced dementia. Giving your name and purpose puts people at ease and can also be used later to assess short-term memory. Ask the person 'What is your name?'; be alert for hearing impairment. The reply indicates how a person wishes to be addressed; alternatively a person may be specifically asked.

Make sure that both the patient and yourself are comfortable. The patient should be asked specifically and asked if they need to use the lavatory. Sit at the same height. Ask whether the patient usually wears glasses and ensure they are put on; the same applies to hearing aids and false teeth. Deafness is such a common problem that any situation where elderly people are seen regularly should have a communication aid (from ear trumpet to electronic aid). If the person is deaf note the presence of a hearing aid, sit at the same height with your face well lit (to help lip reading) and *do not shout*.

Talking at the bedside in a busy environment is accepted practice. This is not privacy and is the wrong place to discuss sensitive issues such as incontinence, to test for cognitive impairment or to explore depressive symptoms. A quiet room is necessary to do the job properly.

Although medical students are taught to start with the presenting complaint and history of the presenting complaint the patients are not! Let the elderly patient tell the story, but help with the time sequence. Inevitably some patients will start with 'It all started when I was injured in the War'. They are really making a statement about personal self-worth and respect and politeness dictates that you should listen to a little of the story. You may use it to collect information that you were planning to ask about later.

Try to avoid interrupting a patient's story. Some patients give a rapid account of things, others are much slower. Try to adjust your pace to that of the patient, a long lifespan means a lot more potential information. However, you may need to interrupt and re-direct the conversation and everyone develops their own technique to avoid losing rapport. Do not behave as a 'busy person', but relax and show you have time to listen. The task is to talk with the patient and the skill is to make the patient feel they have your complete and undivided attention. History-taking with an elderly person can be a time-consuming but ultimately rewarding process. If you are unavoidably called away during the interview, apologize and explain what is happening. Try to avoid telephone interruptions, the person you are with is almost always more important.

Activities of daily living (ADL)

In young patients a brief systems enquiry concerning all the major bodily systems (see Chapter 1) can be used to rule out significant serious or life-threatening problems. In older patients this approach may not be appropriate; a systems enquiry can be time-consuming, producing spurious symptoms, many of which are not immediately relevant. Some sort of sifting procedure is needed. An enquiry about activities of daily living (ADL) provides a useful screen (see Table 16.1).

In general, patients who can dress, get about outdoors, are continent, can do their own housework and cooking, and manage their own pension do not require much immediate enquiry other than about their presenting problem. Among the old old and the oldest old, such patients are the exception. If a daily living task cannot be carried out then it is necessary to make a detailed enquiry focusing on the reason for this.

It is useful to obtain a 'pre-morbid' ADL enabling you to describe what the patient was usually able to do before they became ill. This provides a rough goal for the outcome of treatment. A patient who was unable to get in and out of the bath, who could not dress unaided and who was incontinent prior to suffering a stroke or heart attack is not likely to recover to a trouble-free life. One cannot make the assumption that a person was free from disability before the onset of an acute illness.

Drug history

The elderly are prescribed more medication than any other age group. A treatment history checklist is useful when enquiring about current and past medications (Box 16.5).

Many patients do not take all or any of their prescribed medication. Checking dates on bottles and a

Item	Categories
Bowels	0=incontinent (or needs to be given an enema)
	1=occasional accident (once per week)
	2=continent
Bladder	0=incontinent/catheterized, unable to manage
	1=occasional accident (max once every 24 h)
	2=continent (for over 7 days)
Grooming	0=needs help with personal care
	1=independent face/hair/teeth/shaving (implements provided)
Toilet use	0=dependent
	1=needs some help but can do something alone
	2=independent (on and off, dressing, wiping
Feeding	0=unable
	1=needs help cutting, spreading butter, etc.
	2=independent (food provided in reach)
Transfer	0=unable—no sitting balance
	1=major help (one or two people, physical), can sit
	2=minor help (verbal or physical)
	3=independent
Mobility	0=immobile
	1=wheelchair independent (includes corners)
	2=walks with help of one (verbal/physical)
	3=independent (may use any aid, e.g. stick)
Dressing	0=dependent
	1=needs help, does about half unaided
	2=independent, includes buttons, zips, shoes
Stairs	0=unable
	1=needs help, (verbal, physical), carrying aid
	2=independent
Bathing	0=dependent
	1=independent (may use shower)

Table 16.1 The Barthel ADL Index (total score 20).

The Barthel Index should be used as a record of what a patient does, not as a record of what he could do. The main aim is to establish the degree of independence from any help, physical or verbal, however minor and for whatever reason. The need for supervision means the patient is not independent. Performance over the preceding 24–48 h is important but longer periods are relevant. A patient's performance should be established using the best available evidence. Ask the patient or carer but also observe what the patient can do. Direct testing is not needed. Unconscious patients score '0' throughout. Middle categories imply that the patient supplies over 50% effort. Use of aids to be independent is allowed.

tablet count can act as a rough guide to compliance. Medicine cabinets often contain old medication kept for use in the event of future problems and many elderly people will change a new medication for an older, tested remedy without telling the doctor. Traditional treatments are also often used.

It is often necessary to be critical of the history and check key points. Indeed most students are familiar with that sinking feeling when the consultant, having heard the student's history-taking, asks two or three questions of the patient that appear to totally contradict the main thrust of the history just elicited. The simplest method of corroboration is to go over the key symptoms with the patient a few hours after the initial interview. However, it is essential to get whatever help you can from collateral sources of information. Obtain all old case notes.

Most important of all talk to a close relative or friend whenever possible. The telephone can be a vital piece of equipment for history-taking with elderly patients.

A comprehensive history in an elderly person requires appropriate time and effort devoted to the process.

BOX 16.5 Areas to cover in a treatment history.

- Current medication
- Previous hospital and family doctor medication
- Treatment from 'alternative' practitioners
- Self-medication
- Past bad experiences with medicines
- Other non-drug treatments
- Medicines kept in the home

Examination

General

Always praise a patient for their co-operation and performance. Do not complete the examination in silence—your patient may think that you have found something sinister. Explain what you are doing as you go and comment reassuringly on what you find. It can take time to undress elderly patients but it is useful to use that time to observe your patient's abilities.

Ask patients to remove their clothes themselves. Consider whether the patient can reach their feet and manage their buttons. Is the balance mechanism good? Can the patient get on to the examination couch unaided? These points may help in making a diagnosis; any difficulty with undressing may need to be assessed by an occupational therapist with a view to determining any special needs at home.

Once undressed keep the patient comfortable and use a blanket to protect their dignity. If the patient is agitated, or if you are intending a vaginal or rectal examination a nurse should be present to assist. In the elderly the *temperature* is not always high even with obvious infection. If the temperature is low it must be measured with a low-reading rectal thermometer. Weigh the patient, record the result and *always* test the urine.

Special considerations

Skin

Wrinkles are mainly due to past exposure to ultraviolet light and hence are not usually seen in covered areas. Elderly skin can bruise easily (*senile purpura*) and some people have skin like transparent tissue paper, especially on the backs of the hands and forearms (Figs 16.1 and 16.2). The skin around the eyes may show yellow plaques—*Dubreuilh's elastoma.* Some solar-induced changes to be aware of include keratoacanthoma, basal cell carcinoma, squamous cell carcinoma and malignant melanoma. The most common skin lesion noted is the small red Campbell de Morgan spot, a benign lesion seen most often on the trunk and abdomen.

Leg ulcers are extremely common in old age. Approximately 50% of leg ulcers are due to venous

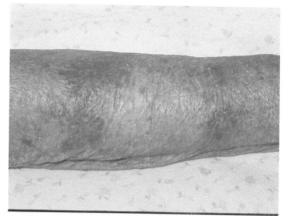

Fig. 16.1   Transparent skin and senile purpura.

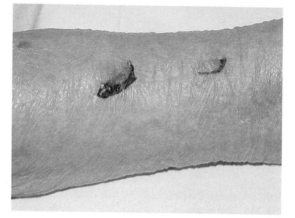

Fig. 16.2   Transparent skin.

stasis (Fig. 16.3), 10% to arterial disease and 30–40% are mixed. Examination should include palpating the peripheral pulses and measurement of ankle blood pressure using a Doppler meter to determine whether the arterial circulation is adequate. The Doppler is used instead of a stethoscope in the lower limb. The resting pressure index (RPI) is calculated using the formula:

$$RPI = \frac{\text{Brachial systolic pressure}}{\text{Pedal systolic pressure}}.$$

An RPI of 1.0 is normal; an RPI below 1.0 may indicate arterial disease, when the blood pressure at the ankle is less than that at the elbow.

Check cutaneous pressure areas, especially heels, hips and sacrum for signs of skin breakdown (*pressure sores*).

Cardiovascular system

Age-related structural and functional changes in the cardiovascular system account for a slight increase in

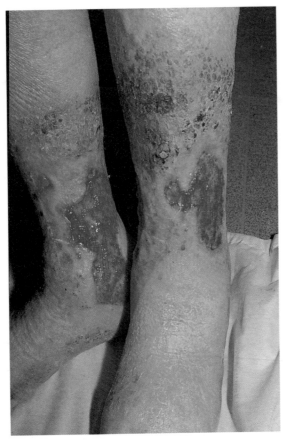

Fig. 16.3 Leg ulcers.

mean blood pressure with increasing age. Heart valves, especially the aortic valve, can become less mobile, exacerbated by atheromatous disease and calcification. This causes an ejection systolic murmur, heard best in the aortic area, and common in the elderly. Degeneration and calcification of the mitral valve can result in either apical ejection murmurs or the more common pansystolic mitral regurgitant murmur (see Chapter 8). Heart rate increase in response to stress, e.g. exercise, illness or pyrexia, is less effective in advanced old age.

A lying and standing (or sitting) blood pressure is mandatory in the examination of all elderly patients. A drop in systolic blood pressure on standing of more than 30 mmHg is defined as postural hypotension, a considerable cause of morbidity in the elderly. As in younger patients, the character of the carotid pulse should be noted. All peripheral pulses should be examined and their presence or absence noted. Peripheral vascular disease is common in the elderly, and palpation of vascular pulsation can be difficult due to atheroma or oedema. In the lower limbs Doppler measurement (see above) can be used to assess the peripheral circulation. The clinical signs of cardiac disease, e.g. valve lesions or congestive heart failure, do not alter in old age. Assessment of retinal vessels for signs of disease, such as hypertension and diabetes, can prove difficult due to the frequent presence of cataracts in old people.

Respiratory system

With ageing the elasticity of the lungs declines, so that the lungs become more distensible. The lung fields on a chest X-ray may therefore appear overinflated. Kyphosis, due to intervertebral disc degeneration and osteoporosis, and calcification of the costal cartilages makes the chest wall more rigid. Chest expansion measurements are thus reduced. Counting the respiratory rate is one of the most useful screening examinations for elderly people. At rest the normal rate will be around 15 breaths per minute. Anxiety may push this up to 20 per minute. With respiratory distress caused, for example, by heart failure or pneumonia the respiratory rate increases in order to maintain gas transfer and avoid hypoxia. It is not until rates increase to 35–40 per minute that a person looks obviously short of breath, so it is necessary to count the rate over at least half a minute. The physical signs of respiratory system disease, for example, cyanosis, lip pursing and tachypnoea, are the same as in younger patients.

Coarse basal crackles caused by air-trapping due to the loss of elasticity can make interpretation of breath sounds difficult. In a sick elderly person a chest X-ray is essential, regardless of the presence or absence of signs and symptoms of pulmonary disease. Previous films, if available, help in interpretation. A major problem for ill elderly people is the position required for a good-quality posteroanterior film. A sympathetic and experienced radiographer is essential. Common changes on the X-ray include calcification from old tuberculosis, calcification in chondral cartilages and major blood vessels, pleural calcification from past pneumonia and old rib fractures.

Vision and the eyes

Visual acuity should be assessed and any loss of vision noted, together with a history of the development of the visual disorder. Acute and chronic causes of loss of vision should be considered during the examination (Box 16.6).

The eyes may be sunken due to loss of periorbital fat; this may be severe enough to cause drooping of

BOX 16.6 Common causes of acute and chronic loss of vision.

Acute
- Retinal detachment
- Vascular (central retinal artery/vein thrombosis)
- Angle-closure glaucoma

Chronic
- Cataract
- Macular degeneration
- Open-angle glaucoma
- Diabetic retinopathy

the upper lid (*ptosis*) and redundant skin at the lateral borders, but may be a feature of normal ageing.

The loss of fat can also cause the lower eyelid to curl in (*entropion*) and irritate the cornea, causing redness and watering (*epiphora*). The laxity also enables the eyelid to fall outwards slightly (*ectropion*) with the same results. A whitish rim around the iris (*arcus senilis*) is a zone of lipid deposition around the periphery of the cornea.

Hearing

If deafness is suspected the external ear must be inspected for wax. However, deafness is most often due to presbyacusis, an age-related degeneration of the cochlear hair cells. If a hearing aid is being worn make sure it is switched on. Communication is aided by raising your voice (but *not* by shouting), obtaining attention, sitting face to face, reducing background noise and speaking slowly and clearly.

Nervous system

Consideration of higher cortical function (language, perception and memory) is too often omitted from routine testing. It is essential that the mental state be assessed early in the interview and the results recorded in the notes (see below). It is important to recognize difficulties with communication, and to consider this possibility if the history proves difficult to elicit or understand. Communication is a two-way process that involves understanding and comprehension, as well as the production of appropriate speech. Communication problems can be considered in terms of:
- disorders of language (*dysphasia*);
- disorders of articulation (*dyspraxia, dysarthria*); and
- disorders of voice (*dysphonia*) or of fluency (*dysfluency*).

Dysphasia is the difficulty in encoding and decoding language and hence can be *receptive*, in which the comprehension of incoming speech is lost, or *expressive*, when speech formation is impaired. Usually both these problems coexist. Dysphasia is usually associated with a left hemisphere lesion. Dyspraxia is difficulty initiating and carrying out voluntary movements, for example of the tongue, and hence can affect speech. It results from damage to the parietal lobe. Dysarthria (see page 282) is a term used to describe impaired articulation, the effects being on the rate and clarity of speech. Causes include stroke, Parkinson's disease, motor neurone disease and multiple sclerosis. Dysphonia, an abnormality of the voice, e.g. hoarseness, can be due to anxiety, vocal abuse, disease such as carcinoma of the larynx or hypothyroidism, and can follow surgery to the throat or even a general anaesthetic with intubation. Dysfluency (stammer) is found in people of all ages, but can develop after brain trauma.

Pencil and paper tests can be invaluable in providing a global measure of mental competence. One test is to present a circle of about 10–15 cm diameter and ask the patient to fill in the numbers of a clock face (Fig. 16.4). This test will be abnormal in patients who have visual impairments, who have difficulty carrying out purposeful actions (*apraxia*), who have perceptual problems especially involving the right parietal lobe, or who are cognitively impaired.

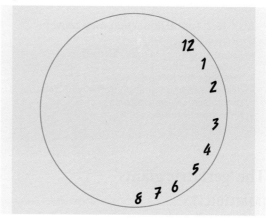

Fig. 16.4   Clock face drawing.

In addition to the formal assessment of the peripheral nervous system by examining muscle bulk and tone, power, sensation and tendon reflexes, it is essential to observe the *walking* or gait pattern in every patient. The tendon reflexes do not change necessarily in the elderly, although it is common for the ankle jerks to be diminished or hard to elicit in very old people.

Examination of the gait may reveal subtle evidence of hemiparesis, poor balance (see Box 16.8), or the furniture-clutching gait of the patient with long-standing mobility problems. This assessment also provides an objective check of at least one activity of daily living. Occasionally patients report that they are capable of carrying out activities when in reality they cannot. Always check the toenails for chiropody problems (e.g. onychogryphosis) where a 'painful' gait is seen.

Gastrointestinal

The majority of elderly people are edentulous. If dentures are used they should be worn during the examination so that problems with fit, e.g. poor speech or eating difficulties, can be corrected early. Leucoplakia appears as small white patches on the oral mucosa. It is associated with repeated mucosal trauma and may become malignant. Varicosities on the underside of the tongue are seen in about 40% of elderly people; their significance is unknown though vitamin C deficiency has been implicated.

Rectal examination is required as part of a full examination and especially if there are symptoms implying lower gastrointestinal, pelvic or prostatic disease. Constipation severe enough to cause faecal impaction is not uncommon and can have serious consequences (Box 16.7).

BOX 16.7 Faecal impaction may cause:

- Faecal incontinence (ball valve effect with spurious diarrhoea)
- Intestinal obstruction
- Restlessness and agitation in the confused (but *never itself causes confusion*)
- Retention of urine
- Rectal bleeding

The 'geriatric giants'

IMMOBILITY

The immobile elderly patient is one of the most common clinical presentations in geriatric practice. Every case requires careful history-taking to discover the underlying problem or problems. The patient should be asked specifically what happened. In assessing this question and the answer given always try to separate cause from effect. Frequently the patient has several problems of which immobil-

ity is but one. The prognosis for recovery, however, is largely determined by the underlying cause of the patient's immobility. The crucial part of the history is the time frame. Sudden immobility should be straightforward to diagnose, yet stroke and impact-ed subcapital fracture can be missed. A steady deterioration in mobility over several years implies a chronic process, e.g. Parkinson's disease and osteoarthrosis. A stepwise decline indicates a disease that has periods of exacerbation and remission, e.g. multiple sclerosis, recurrent minor strokes or rheumatoid arthritis. Repeated rapid swings between full mobility and total immobility over a few days indicates recurrent medical problems, e.g. heart failure and urinary tract infection. The most difficult patients are those in whom the disease process caused immobility a long time ago and the picture is now clouded by the complications of immobility.

Within the bounds of common sense the patient should be asked or helped to stand up and a few steps attempted. This may reveal that a patient can walk but is immobile because he or she is unable to get out of a chair or bed unaided. Alternatively a confused patient may not have mentioned pain on standing, effectively preventing attempts to move. A chair-shaped patient indicates a duration of immobility longer than a few days. If the patient has no concept of walking *apraxia*, an inability to carry out a purposeful sequence of activity despite normal power and sensation, should be suspected. This is usually due to stroke, dementia or to a confusional state. Tentative steps with clutching of helpers may indicate loss of confidence following a fall. A dramatic staggering to the nearest bed, chair or nurse followed by an award-winning collapse suggests that a behavioural cause is possible.

Sometimes a diagnostic gait pattern is found. The broad-based, unsteady gait of *ataxia*; the *apraxic* gait with rapid small steps like a slipping clutch or with feet apparently glued to the floor; the *Parkinsonian* gait with loss of postural reflexes, festination, a fixed posture, tremor, rigidity, hypokinesia of face and limbs, excess salivation and seborrhoea; the gait of *stroke* with dragging of one leg; and the *myopathic* waddling gait due to weak proximal muscles, e.g. from osteomalacia, are typical examples. Gait abnormality is a common problem, of course, in the presence of *osteoarthrosis* of joints, and of local problems with the feet, especially when there is *local pain*. Always remember that immobility in elderly patients is almost always a multifactorial problem.

FALLS

Falls are common in old age and are more common amongst women than men. The incidence of falls over a period of a year in an elderly population is approximately 30%, ranging from trivial tripping-over to major life-threatening events. The aim of history-taking and examination of an elderly person seen because of falls is to diagnose the underlying *pathological* process or processes (Box 16.8). The physiological changes of ageing may well be super-imposed, making it a difficult task to sort out the underlying cause.

It is obvious that even a single fall should lead to a detailed history and examination. Witnesses should always be questioned too. In a patient who was previously well, a search must be made for new acute illness. If none is present the fall may be 'accidental' and due to ageing, or to environmental factors. Information about the pattern of any previous falls can be helpful; in particular their frequency, relationship with posture or time of day, any residual symptoms following the fall and any avoiding steps taken by the patient should be ascertained. Falls that occur on changing posture, particularly on standing from lying, suggest postural hypotension. A trip may occur simply as a result of poor postural reflexes associated with ageing, but may be aggravated by poor vision. Sometimes bifocal glasses can give a distorted view, leading to accidental falls. The absence of any warning implies a sudden event usually of a neurological or circulatory nature. The most useful investigation of elderly fallers is to watch them walking.

INCONTINENCE

Incontinence is an involuntary loss of urine or faeces in an inappropriate place. A full clinical history with careful attention to the history of bladder and bowel function prior to the present illness (from both patient and relatives) will help to differentiate between loss of ability to control excretion and failure to identify or get to an acceptable place. Clinical examination, including a rectal and a vaginal examination, and culture of a mid-stream specimen of urine are all essential (and will often give a good indication as to the cause of the problem). An incontinence chart kept for a few days may suggest a recognizable pattern of urinary and/or faecal incontinence. The specialist help of a continence adviser may be needed. Causes of urinary incontinence include infection, stress incontinence, detrusor instability, overflow, prostatism, neurogenic bladder, uterine prolapse, cystocele and atrophic vaginitis.

Box 16.8 The causes of falls in elderly people.

Premonitory
- Forerunner of acute, usually infectious illness

Medication
- Multiple drug therapy
- Psychotropic drugs
- L-Dopa
- Antihypertensives

Postural hypotension
- Drugs
- Alcohol
- Cardiac disease

Neurological disease
- Multiple strokes
- Transient ischaemic attack
- Parkinson's disease
- Cerebellar disease
- Epilepsy
- Age-related loss of postural reflexes
- Spastic paraparesis (usually due to cervical spondylosis)
- Peripheral neuropathy with sensory loss

Circulatory system disease
- Silent myocardial infarction
- Vasovagal attack
- Cardiac dysrhythmias especially Stokes–Adams disease and atrial fibrillation
- Postural

Musculoskeletal disease
- General muscle weakness (e.g. due to systemic malignancy)
- Muscular wasting due to arthritis
- Unstable knee joint
- Myopathy, e.g. osteomalacia

Miscellaneous
- Drop attacks
- Hypoglycaemia
- Cervical spondylosis
- Alcohol
- Elder abuse (e.g. physical mistreatment)
- Poor vision
- Multisensory deprivation:
  —deafness
  —poor vision
  —labyrinthine disorder
  —peripheral neuropathy

Causes of faecal incontinence include bowel disease such as carcinoma of the rectum, diverticular disease and laxative abuse. Faecal overloading and impaction and neurogenic bowel may also present with faecal incontinence.

PRESSURE SORES

Necrosis of skin, adipose tissue and muscle caused by pressure occurs rapidly in acutely and chronically ill elderly people. The mean capillary pressure in the skin of healthy medical students is approximately

25 mmHg. No measurements are available for normal elderly people let alone those who are ill. External pressures on the skin greater than 25 mmHg lead to occlusion of cutaneous blood vessels; the surrounding tissues, including the skin, then become hypoxic. A bedridden patient easily generates pressures in excess of 100 mmHg especially over the sacrum, heels and greater trochanters (96% of pressure sores occur below the level of the waist).

About 80% of pressure sores are superficial (Fig. 16.5). They occur mainly in dehydrated and incontinent patients exposed to sustained pressure, especially developing postoperatively. The majority of these sores are preventable. Any sore will deepen if the pressure is not relieved. Deep sores (Fig. 16.6) are formed when localized high pressure applied to the skin cuts off a wedge-shaped area of tissue, usually adjacent to a bony prominence.

All at-risk patients should have anti-pressure protection started immediately a new illness or injury occurs, whether at home or in hospital. Clinical scales to determine the kind of risk, such as the Norton scale (Table 16.2) are often used in nursing management. These scales allocate a numerical score to at-risk features, e.g. incontinence, immobility, sensory loss, body weight and nutrition, conscious level. All pressure area sites must be inspected at the first clinical assessment and again at regular intervals during the illness. Many patients need active management of their pressure areas. A most effective medium-priced prevention and treatment is an alternating pressure air mattress (APAM). The horizontal cells (Fig. 16.7) inflate and deflate over a short cycle, constantly supporting the patient but providing periods of low pressure at all sites.

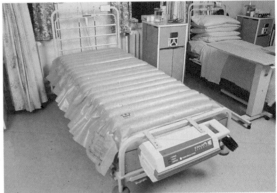

Fig. 16.7   An alternating pressure air mattress (APAM).

CONFUSION

The term confusional state describes an abnormal mental state in which the patient is disoriented in time, place and person, often in the context of other, global disturbances of mental function. *Delirium* (see Chapters 2 and 12) is an acute confusional state with global mental impairment and altered consciousness. *Dementia* is a chronic confusional state with global mental impairment in an alert patient. Delirium with increasing confusion can occur in a patient with dementia.

Acute confusional state (delirium) is one of the most common forms of organic brain syndrome. In most such patients there are physical and mental abnormalities that need urgent assessment. Failure to recognize it and hence to diagnose and treat the underlying condition can have fatal consequences for the patient. Failure to assess a person's level of cognitive functioning on admission and to monitor it periodically during hospitalization can also result in a missed diagnosis of acute confusional state. Multiple coexisting causative factors are common. The differential diagnosis includes acute or chronic confusion, e.g. mild underlying dementia with an

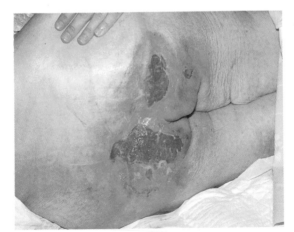

Fig. 16.5   Superficial pressure sores.

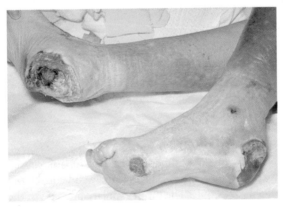

Fig. 16.6   Deep pressure sores.

Physical	Neural	Activity	Mobility	Incontinence
4 Good	4 Alert	4 Ambulant	4 Full	4 None
3 Fair	3 Apathetic	3 Walks with help	3 Slightly limited	3 Occasional
2 Poor	2 Confused	2 Not bound	2 Very limited	2 Usually
1 Very poor	1 Stupor	1 Bedfast	1 Immobile	1 Double

Table 16.2 Norton scale for pressure sores. Low scores carry a high risk.

additional acute problem, and acute functional psychosis (*pseudodelirium*).

Chronic confusional states must have been present for at least three months to be labelled as such. There is usually loss of function in multiple areas (e.g. intellectual function, memory, language). There are, however, reversible causes even of such long-lasting confusion, e.g. drugs, depression and endocrine abnormalities, and appropriate diagnosis and treatment may produce improvement. Chronic confusional states become increasingly common in old age (10% above age 65 years, 20% above age 80 years) but are not a component of normal ageing. Regardless of age a search for the cause is warranted. The differential diagnoses include benign senescent forgetfulness, amnestic syndromes and depression (*pseudodementia*).

The two most common causes of dementia are Alzheimer's disease (AD) and multi-infarct dementia. AD is a clinical diagnosis made on the history, and by excluding other disorders. Clinical criteria for multi-infarct dementia include the presence of dementia with the history of a stepwise deteriorating course, a patchy or uneven distribution of cognitive deficits and focal neurological signs. Other characteristic features (*the Hachinski score*), include the presence of hypertension, signs of atherosclerotic disease elsewhere, emotional lability, pseudobulbar palsy, dysarthria and transient depression. Investigations in chronic confusional states are aimed at identifying potentially reversible causes. At the same time vulnerable frail patients should not be expected to undergo unpleasant tests and scarce resources should be used appropriately.

The confused elderly patient

'Patient confused, no history available' speaks volumes about the training and attitudes of the medical profession. Confused patients deserve better. It is crucial to establish early on whether the patient is orientated in place, time and person. One must also decide whether the patient is alert. It is important to use a standard test of mental function (Box 16.9). Explain to the patient that you wish to test their memory. With experience, it is possible to check most of the items in the mental test score by working them into your introductory talk with the patient. Deafness and speech impairments (such as nominal dysphasia) can make people appear very cognitively impaired. Depressed patients tend to do poorly on mental test scores. If a problem is detected with a simple test it is best to proceed to a more in-depth assessment using the Mini-mental State Examination (page 46). Assessments of mental state are most valuable when used and recorded on the same patient over a period of time.

BOX 16.9 Abbreviated mental test (AMT): total score 10 (one point for each item).

- Age
- Time (to nearest hour)
- Address for recall
- Year
- Where do you live (town or road)?
- Recognition of two persons
- Date of birth (day and month)
- Year of start of First World War
- Name of present Monarch/Prime Minister
- Count backwards 20-1

Envoi

Finally, always remember to treat an elderly patient, as any other patient, as a whole person.

Other issues

Ethnic elders

Many countries have people from a wide range of ethnic groups, all of whom contribute to its social and economic productivity. Ethnic populations are usually derived from migrations of relatively young people, and these people age. Services, particularly social services, provided for ethnic elders are generally inadequate. This is partly because of a desire among the host population for assimilation and acculturation to occur, partly because of an assumption that the extended family will cope with the majority of problems and partly because of lack of understanding and awareness of the problems. In the UK the health issues experienced by ethnic elders (with the exception of tuberculosis) are similar to those of the indigenous population: heart attacks, strokes, diabetes and cataracts. Health services would be more sensitive to the needs of ethnic minorities if emphasis were placed on the following: employment of staff from ethnic minorities; more widespread use of trained interpreters; better signposting; and provision of health education material in appropriate languages.

Elder abuse/inadequate care

There are many types of abuse (physical, psychological, financial, sexual, etc.) but all can be described as representing the effects of inadequate care and of unmet needs. The victim is typically an elderly woman, functionally impaired and living at home with an adult son, daughter or husband, but any elderly person may be at risk. The abusers tend to be sons, and psychological or emotional abuse predominates. Abusers are usually dependent on their victims for finances, lead stressful lives and themselves have health and financial problems, especially alcohol and psychological difficulties.

Risk factors include progressive disabling illnesses, breakdown of communication and isolated or substandard living conditions. Factors in identification include frequent visits to doctors by carers preoccupied with their own problems, marked changes in a carer's lifestyle inducing extra stress, and poor perception of the dependency of the older person by the carer. Recognition of elder abuse is made difficult by the physiological and pathological changes that occur with ageing, e.g. senile purpura. The presence of some of the usual manifestations of inadequate care, especially abrasions, pressure sores and malnutrition, should raise the *possibility* of elder abuse. Assessment includes not only a physical examination but also a sensitive and full social history including a sympathetic questioning of the carer's role. The client's mental state must be assessed and recorded. A diagnosis of suspected abuse or of inadequate care must not be made hastily, and expert help from a social worker, psychiatrist, or clinical psychologist may be necessary in recognition and management. Elder abuse is itself redolent with guilt.

CHAPTER 17

The genitalia and sexually transmitted diseases

Introduction

There is still unwarranted stigma and shame attached to sexually transmitted diseases. Two aspects of sexually transmitted diseases are ever-present. First, an infected patient indicates that at least one other person is also infected. Thus treating a patient in isolation will not control the spread of these diseases. Second, a patient may harbour more than one sexually transmitted disease (Box 17.1). Remember that babies, innocent partners and victims of rape and sexual abuse can also be affected.

The interview and examination must be carried out in privacy and with confidentiality. The staff should be sympathetic, without a disapproving or moralistic attitude. As with other clinical problems, diagnosis is achieved by history (Box 17.2), examination and relevant laboratory tests. Following diagnosis, effective treatment and contact tracing/partner

---

BOX 17.1 Sexually transmitted agents (diseases).

Bacteria
Treponema pallidum (Syphilis)
Neisseria gonorrhoeae (Gonorrhoea)
Chlamydia trachomatis of D-K serovars (50% of 'non-specific' genital infection)
Chlamydia trachomatis of LGV 1-3 serovars (Lymphogranuloma venereum)
Haemophilus ducreyi (Chancroid)
Calymmatobacterium granulomatis (Granuloma inguinale/Donovanosis)
Gardnerella vaginalis, anaerobes (Bacterial vaginosis)
Shigella species (Shigellosis)
Salmonella species (Salmonellosis)
Ureaplasma, mycoplasma (Some cases of 'non-specific' genital infection)

Viruses
Herpes simplex virus types 1 and 2 (Genital herpes)
Human papilloma virus (Genital warts)
Molluscum contagiosum virus (Molluscum contagiosum)

Human immunodeficiency virus (AIDS and related diseases)
Hepatitis A, B, C and Delta viruses
Cytomegalovirus

Fungal
Candida albicans (Thrush/moniliasis/candidiasis/candidosis)

Ectoparasites
Phthirus pubis (Pediculosis pubis)
Sarcoptes scabiei (Scabies)

Protozoa
Trichomonas vaginalis (Trichomoniasis)
Entamoeba histolytica (Amoebiasis)
Giardia lamblia (Giardiasis)

Nematode
Enterobius vermicularis (Enterobiasis)

BOX 17.2 History in sexually transmitted disease.

- Urethral discharge
- Dysuria
- Urinary frequency
- Vaginal discharge
- Dyspareunia
- Genital ulcer
- Painful scrotal swelling
- Pubic/genital itch
- Genital rash
- Anorectal symptoms

---

notification should be instituted promptly. Sexually transmitted diseases in children should alert one to the possibility of sexual abuse although non-sexual transmission can occur.

History

Presenting symptoms

URETHRAL DISCHARGE

This is nearly always a complaint of men. Ensure that the discharge is from the urethra and not from under the foreskin. Ascertain the colour, amount and duration of the discharge. A purulent discharge suggests gonorrhoea while 'non-specific' urethritis and *Trichomonas vaginalis* are more likely to give rise to scanty mucoid or mucopurulent discharge. Sometimes the patient only notices the discharge in the morning or by the staining of his underwear.

DYSURIA

Urethral pain on passing urine may be described as burning or stinging. False dysuria may occur if urine comes into contact with inflamed areas on the prepuce or vulva (*vulvitis*).

URINARY FREQUENCY

Frequent passage of urine, usually in small quantity, suggests bladder infection or involvement of the trigone of the bladder from ascending urethritis. It can also indicate anxiety.

VAGINAL DISCHARGE

Ask if it is itchy or offensive. An itchy vaginal discharge is suggestive of thrush or, occasionally, trichomoniasis. Smelly discharges are usually due to trichomoniasis, bacterial vaginosis, or retained foreign bodies such as tampons. Physiological discharge can occur after sexual stimulation or during pregnancy but is not itchy or offensive. Vaginal discharge may also arise from gonococcal or chlamydial cervicitis.

DYSPAREUNIA

This is pain on sexual intercourse (see Chapter 14). In women, superficial dyspareunia is pain deep in the vagina and can be due to vulvitis. Deep dyspareunia is pain deep in the vagina and may result from pelvic inflammatory disease, endometritis and other gynaecological diseases, particularly endometriosis.

GENITAL ULCER

This is described as a 'sore'. Ask if it is painful or recurrent. *Painful ulcers* are usually due to herpes, chancroid, Stevens–Johnson syndrome, Behçet's disease or trauma, whereas a *painless ulcer* may be due to syphilis or lymphogranuloma venereum. However, a painful ulcer does not exclude syphilis. The evolution of the ulcer is important. Genital herpes may start with local irritation followed by erythema, a group of papules, then blisters which ulcerate and crust before healing. If the infection was acquired in a tropical country, chancroid and granuloma inguinale should also be considered. Ask whether the patient has applied any medicament which may interfere with microbiological tests.

PAINFUL SCROTAL SWELLING

This may indicate acute epididymo-orchitis which may complicate a sexually transmitted disease, or acute surgical emergencies such as torsion of the testis and strangulated inguinal hernia. It is important to remember that neoplasm of the testis may sometimes present as a painful swelling. Acute epididymo-orchitis in sexually active men below the age of 35 is likely to result from gonococcal or chlamydial infection, and above the age of 40 from bacterial urinary tract infection such as that due to *Escherichia coli*.

PUBIC AND GENITAL ITCH

This usually due to pediculosis pubis, scabies or other inflammatory genital conditions such as allergic dermatitis, but may be psychological. Ask if sexual or household contacts also complain of itch. In pediculosis pubis, patients may notice 'crabs' and nits on the hair shaft. Itching at night is suggestive of scabies and is likely to be generalized except for the face.

GENITAL RASH

Itchy rash on the glans penis and prepuce is seen in thrush, scabies and inflammatory dermatological conditions such as lichen planus.

ANORECTAL SYMPTOMS

Anal soreness or pain, itch, rectal discharge, pain on defecation, feeling of incomplete defecation (*tenesmus*) and constipation may occur in infective proctitis. Anal itch (*pruritus ani*) may be secondary to rectal discharge or due to thrush, anal warts, dermatitis and poor anal hygiene. If the itch is worse at night, threadworms in particular should be considered. Pruritus ani is also commonly psychological in origin. Sexually transmitted enteric infections in homosexual and bisexual men may present with diarrhoea.

Other aspects of the history

A *past history* of genitourinary problems, sexually transmitted diseases, gynaecological diseases and obstetric problems is important. In women, the *gynaecological history*, e.g. dyspareunia, pelvic inflammatory disease and cervical dysplasia, and the *obstetric history*, e.g. stillbirths, miscarriages or babies with ophthalmia, may be significant. The *menstrual history* is vital. A delayed menstrual period with unilateral lower abdominal pain may be due to ectopic pregnancy rather than salpingitis. A change in the menstrual cycle may be due to pelvic inflammatory disease. Intrauterine *contraceptive devices* predispose to pelvic inflammatory disease, while the use of condoms may prevent infection. Oral contraceptives can predispose to thrush. Ask whether the patient has taken any *drugs*, especially antibiotics, in recent months. Allergy to antimicrobials, particularly to penicillin, must be noted. Where appropriate, drug abuse should be asked about.

Sexual history

The patient's confidence should first be obtained by enquiring into non-threatening aspects of the medical history, then moving into more personal details such as contraception and, in the case of women, the menstrual history, before proceeding to the sexual history. Details of the sexual history should be obtained by simple questions. Ascertain the date of exposure (When did you last have intercourse/'sex'?), particulars of contacts over recent months (if married, When did you last have intercourse/'sex' with your wife/husband? followed by When did you last have intercourse/'sex' with someone else?), and whether with regular partners, casual contacts or prostitutes. Are sexual partners traceable, e.g. place of intercourse (which town, whether abroad)? If there are several contacts, it is useful to identify them by first names. The possibility of homosexual or bisexual contact should be ascertained (Do you have intercourse/'sex' with men, women or both?).

The incubation period of infection may be assessed from the date of exposure to the onset of symptoms, and hence the probable cause. Tropical sexually transmitted diseases should also be considered in patients presenting with genital problems acquired in the tropics. A history of intercourse with homosexual or bisexual men, injecting drug users or with persons in or from an area of high *human immunodeficiency virus* (*HIV*) endemicity may suggest acquired immune deficiency syndrome (AIDS) as the cause of multisystemic symptoms and signs in a patient.

The *type of sexual practice* will dictate the sites from which to take tests. It is also helpful to understand some of the common or unfamiliar terms which may be used in relation to sexual practices. 'Straight sex' indicates heterosexual (peno-vaginal) intercourse. Ask whether the person also practises insertive or receptive oro-penile intercourse (Do you have 'oral sex'?).

Certain practices in homosexual or bisexual men ('gay sex') may predispose to particular infections; for example, if there is oro-anal contact, the possibility of intestinal pathogens should be considered. Hepatitis B and HIV infection are more common in those practising receptive peno-anal intercourse. Ask whether he practises insertive ('*active*') or receptive ('*passive*') peno-anal intercourse (When did you last have 'anal sex'? or simply, Are you 'active', 'passive' or both?). Some homosexual patients practise oro-anal intercourse ('rimming'), insertive or receptive brachio-anal intercourse ('fisting'), and, rarely, urinating on to each other ('watersports') or using faeces during intercourse ('scat').

Some heterosexual couples also practise peno-anal intercourse. This should be enquired for if rectal infection is found in women, although this commonly occurs without having 'anal sex' in association with infection at other genital sites. Sex 'toys' or 'dildoes' (artificial penises) are objects inserted into the rectum or vagina. 'Fisting' and 'toys' may cause injury presenting as an acute abdomen. 'Bondage', in which the person is tied up during sex, may be associated with masochism (sexual gratification through the infliction of pain on another). This should be suspected if injury marks without an obvious cause are present on the body.

The use of condoms should be enquired into irrespective of whether the patient is using other methods of contraception. Condom usage should be advised if the person is at risk of acquiring or transmitting sexually transmitted diseases including AIDS. It is important to remember that many infections which may initially be acquired through non-sexual means, for example, hepatitis B and HIV infection amongst injecting drug users and haemophiliacs, may then be transmitted through sexual intercourse. Advice on non-penetrative 'safer sex' practices such as body rubbing, dry kissing and masturbating each other, can be given to infected individuals who do not wish to practise penetrative intercourse.

Genital examination

The patient is examined in a well-lit room. Other non-infective genital diseases should be looked for. Gloves should be worn if genital infection is suspected.

Male genitalia

THE PENIS

Note the appearance and size of the penis, the presence or absence of the prepuce, and the position of the external urethral orifice. Examine the penile shaft for warts, ulcers, burrows and excoriated papules of scabies and rashes. In the uncircumcised, establish that the prepuce can readily be retracted by gently withdrawing it over the glans penis. This allows inspection of the undersurface of the prepuce, the glans penis, the coronal sulcus and the external urethral orifice (meatus) for warts, inflammation, ulcers and other rash. Always remember to draw the prepuce forwards after examination, otherwise *paraphimosis*, painful oedema of the glans due to constriction by a retracted prepuce, may ensue.

Phimosis is narrowing of the preputial orifice, thereby preventing retraction of the foreskin. This predisposes to recurrent episodes of infection of the glans penis (*balanitis*), the prepuce (*posthitis*), or both (*balanoposthitis*). *Circinate balanitis* of Reiter's

disease appears as erythematous eroded lesions which coalesce with a slightly raised and polycyclic edge. Multiple small yellow or white submucous material known as *Fordyce's spots* may be seen on the inner prepuce. These are ectopic sebaceous glands and do not require treatment. In unhygienic patients, *smegma*, which is greyish-white cheesy material arising from Tyson's glands, may accumulate under the prepuce.

Hypospadias is a congenital abnormality in which the external urethral orifice is not at the tip of the glans penis but opens at its ventral surface in the midline, anywhere from the glans to the shaft or even in the perineum. *Epispadias*, a similar opening situated on the dorsal surface of the penis, is rare.

Tiny regular papules arranged in rows around the coronal sulcus are *coronal papillae* and may be mistaken for warts. The coronal sulcus is the commonest site for a chancre. The classical Hunterian chancre, described as a single, painless, indurated ulcer with a clean base, is present in only about 40% of cases of primary syphilis. The meatus is examined for inflammation, urethral discharge, narrowing (stricture) and warts. Retract the lips of the meatus to examine for the presence of meatal chancre and intrameatal warts.

Look at the scrotal skin for any redness, swelling or ulcer. Lift the scrotum to inspect its posterior surface. Tiny dark red papules of *angiokeratoma* or round, firm, whitish nodules of *sebaceous cysts* can sometimes be seen. *Scabies* causes erythematous nodular lesions on the scrotum and glans penis. If intrascrotal swelling is present observe whether it appears to extend into the groin and note whether both testes are in the scrotum. *Ulceration* can result from a gumma, or from fungation of an underlying tumour of the testis.

THE TESTES

Now place the right hand below the scrotum and palpate both testes. Arrange the hands and fingers as shown in Fig. 17.1; this 'fixes' the testis so that it cannot slip away from the examining fingers. The posterior aspect of the testis is supported by the middle, ring and little fingers of each hand, the right hand being inferior. This leaves the index finger and thumb free to palpate. Gently move the index finger and thumb over the anterior surface of the body of the testis and feel the lateral border with the index finger and the medial border with the pulp of each thumb. Note the size and consistency of the testis and any nodules or other irregularities. Now very

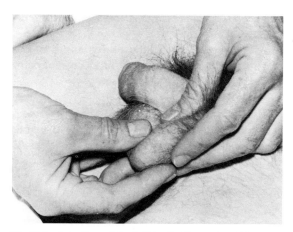

Fig. 17.1 Palpation of the left testis. Gloves should be worn if genital infection is suspected.

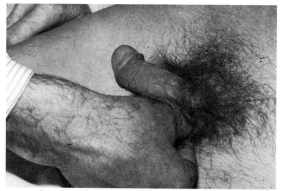

Fig. 17.2 Palpation of the left spermatic cord. Gloves should be worn if genital infection is suspected.

gently approximate the fingers and thumb of the left hand (the effect of this is to move the testis inferiorly, which is easily and painlessly done because of its great mobility inside the tunica vaginalis). In this way the upper pole of the testis can be readily felt between the approximated index finger and thumb of the left hand. Next move the testis upwards by reversing the movements of the hands and gently approximating the index finger and thumb of the right hand, so enabling the lower pole to be palpated. The normal testes are equal in size, varying between 3.5 and 4 cm in length. A unilaterally enlarged testis must be considered malignant, particularly if painless. In old age, testes may become atrophic. In younger men testicular atrophy often indicates chronic liver disease, usually alcoholic in aetiology.

THE EPIDIDYMIS

Now palpate the epididymis. The head is found at the upper pole of the testis on its posterior aspect and is felt between the left thumb anteriorly and the index and middle fingers posteriorly. It is a soft nodular structure about 1 cm in length. The tail lies on the posterolateral aspect of the inferior pole of the testis and is felt between the thumb and fingers of the right hand. The tail is also soft but, unlike the head, its coiled tubular structure can usually be made out. Occasionally the epididymis is situated anterior to the testis.

THE SPERMATIC CORD

Finally palpate the spermatic cord (Fig. 17.2) with the left hand. Then exert gentle downward traction on the testis, place the fingers of the right hand behind the neck of the scrotum, and with the thumb placed anteriorly press forward with fingers of the

right hand. The spermatic cord will be felt between the fingers and thumb; it is about 1 cm in width. The only structure that can be positively identified within it is the *vas deferens*, which feels like a thick piece of string.

Repeat the examination on the other side. In the scrotum, hydrocele of the tunica vaginalis or a cyst of the epididymis are common causes of painless swelling; neoplasm of the testis is less common but must be missed. Acute epididymo-orchitis, torsion of the testis, strangulated inguinal hernia and some cases of testicular neoplasm cause a painful swelling. Hydrocele can be demonstrated by transillumination, using a bright light source held in contact with the large testicle, preferably in a darkened room. In swellings of uncertain origin ultrasound is useful.

Remember that the patient should also be examined standing up to look for *varicocele*—dilated tortuous veins in the scrotum like a bag of worms.

ANORECTAL EXAMINATION

In both homosexual and bisexual men, the anorectal region should be examined. Ask the patient to lie in the standard left lateral position with the knees drawn up, or in the knee–elbow position. Examine the anal and perianal skin for *inflammation, ulceration, fissure* and *tags*. Primary syphilis can mimic an anal fissure. Anal tags should not be confused with anal warts (*condylomata acuminata*), which are sessile or pedunculated papillomata. Anal warts in turn should not be confused with the flat warty lesions of *condylomata lata*, which are the highly infectious lesions of secondary syphilis.

Gently insert a proctoscope lubricated with KY Jelly or liquid paraffin and examine the rectal mucosa for pus, inflammation, warts and threadworms. Take rectal tests. If anal warts are present, proctoscopy should be delayed until the warts are treated to prevent introducing the infection into the rectum. In patients who practise frequent peno-anal intercourse the anus will be lax.

Female genitalia

Women are best examined in the lithotomy position. Examine the perineum, vulva, and labia majora and minora for discharge, redness, swelling, excoriation, ulcers, warts and other lesions. In rape and sexual abuse cases, look for evidence of trauma. Redness and swelling of the vulva with excoriations may be seen in thrush and trichomoniasis. Separate the labia and palpate Bartholin's glands; normally they are not felt. Wipe away any contaminating vaginal discharge from the vulva and urethral meatus and insert a bivalve Cusco speculum (Chapter 14) without lubrication. Note any inflammation of the vaginal wall (*vaginitis*) and the colour, consistency and odour of any vaginal discharge. Curdy or cheesy, white discharge suggests *thrush*, frothy greenish-yellow discharge, *trichomoniasis* and off-white discharge, *bacterial vaginosis*. The last two conditions also have a fishy odour. Tests are taken from the posterior fornix of the vagina.

Wipe the cervix with a swab and examine it for *discharge* from the external cervical os, for *ectopy* or 'erosion' (ectopic columnar epithelium), and for *cervicitis*, *warts* and *ulcers*. Warts on the cervix appear as either flat or papilliferous lesions. Take tests, including a smear for *cervical cytology*, to detect dysplasia and cancer of the cervix. This is particularly important because of the association of cervical cancer with genital warts. Then remove the speculum.

Next the urethral orifice is examined for discharge, inflammation and warts. If no obvious discharge is present, milk the urethra gently forward before taking specimens (see page 407).

Examine the anal region for lesions, as in homosexual men. Insert a lubricated proctoscope and examine the rectal mucosa for discharge or inflammation, and take tests.

BIMANUAL EXAMINATION

A bimanual examination is performed to detect pelvic inflammatory disease and abnormalities of the upper genital tract.

COLPOSCOPY

In some cases, the cervix should be examined under magnification using a colposcope. It may show chlamydial follicular cervicitis. In patients with genital warts, white areas after application of 5% acetic acid suggest cervical wart virus infection which can be confirmed by biopsy. Dysplastic change may also be observed and confirmed by biopsy.

PUBIC REGIONS AND GROINS

Examine for *pediculosis pubis* ('crabs') and nits. *Molluscum contagiosum* lesions appear as pearly or pinkish umbilicated papules. Look at the groins for *tinea cruris*, *thrush* and *erythrasma*. Tinea cruris and erythrasma give rise to a rash with a well-defined border, while in thrush the border is less well-defined and erythematous papules outside the borders known as satellite lesions, are present. Erythrasma lesions show a coral-red fluorescence under Wood's light.

Groin swelling is usually due to hernia or lymphadenopathy. Genital ulceration with tender inguinal lymph nodes (*buboes*) will suggest chancroid lymphogranuloma venereum or herpes; in the first two conditions abscesses may form. In lymphogranuloma venereum, the ulcer may be transient and the buboes may have a grooved appearance resulting from lymphadenopathy above and below the inguinal ligament—'sign of the groove'. Primary syphilis gives rise to painless, mobile and rubbery lymph nodes but they can be painful if the chancre is secondarily infected. Inguinal lymphadenopathy may be part of a generalized involvement as in lymphoma, secondary syphilis or viral infections, e.g. infectious mononucleosis and that due to HIV infection. Granuloma inguinale may give rise to pseudobuboes which are inguinal subcutaneous granulomata.

Human immunodeficiency virus infections

The number of people worldwide with HIV infection has reached pandemic proportions. It is estimated that as many as 13 million people are infected, half of whom live in Africa. North America, South America and Asia each have at least 1 million infected people. There are fewer HIV-positive people in Europe, but the number in Eastern Europe and in the Russian republics is not known. About 300 000 people in the USA alone have, or have died of, AIDS. In Africa the numbers are much larger. HIV-related illnesses have therefore become increasingly important in clinical practice.

The Center for Disease Control in the USA has introduced a widely accepted classification (Box 17.3) of these disorders that is based on the clinical evolution of the immunodeficiency state that leads to the development of the acquired immune deficiency syndrome (AIDS), on average some 8–15 years after infection. AIDS develops more rapidly in infants infected *in utero*, and in the elderly, but less rapidly in people infected by transmission from infected blood products, as in transfusion-related infections.

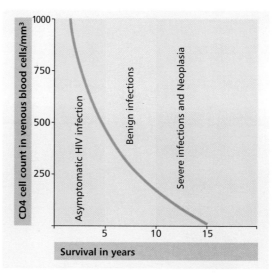

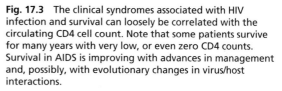

Fig. 17.3 The clinical syndromes associated with HIV infection and survival can loosely be correlated with the circulating CD4 cell count. Note that some patients survive for many years with very low, or even zero CD4 counts. Survival in AIDS is improving with advances in management and, possibly, with evolutionary changes in virus/host interactions.

BOX 17.3 Center for Disease Control (CDC) classification of HIV infection.

Group I: Acute infection
Group II: Asymptomatic stage
Group III: Persistent generalized lymphadenopathy
Group IV: Other diseases
   A: Constitutional disease
   B: Neurological disease
   C: Secondary infectious disease
      C-1: Infectious diseases occurring in AIDS
      C-2: Other infectious diseases
   D: Secondary cancers
   E: Other conditions

HIV infection can also be considered from a more descriptive standpoint as tending to pass through several clinical stages, in which the clinical syndromes are relatively distinctive. The first phase of the illness is the acute seroconversion illness, in which fever, malaise, lymphadenopathy, muscle pain, diarrhoea and sore throat occur, often with erythematous, maculo-papular skin eruption and headache. Oral candidiasis and aphthous ulceration also occur.

The four clinical stages of HIV infection are as follows.

Stage 1. The patient may be asymptomatic, or there may be persistent lymphadenopathy. During this phase of illness the CD4 lymphocyte count (Fig. 17.3) gradually falls, antibodies to the HIV virus appear in the blood, and the HIV antigen may also be detected.

Stage 2. Weight loss, cutaneous and nail-bed fungal infections, with recurrent oral ulceration develop. There is a propensity to frequent upper respiratory tract infections, including sinusitis, and herpes zoster infection has usually occurred.

Stage 3. Weight loss is more marked, with chronic diarrhoea, persistent fever, oral candidiasis, and

oral hairy leucoplakia, a lesion which, unlike candidiasis, cannot be wiped off the mucosa. Bleeding from the mouth and gastrointestinal tract is frequent. Pulmonary tuberculosis is common, and severe bacterial infections occur, especially in the respiratory tract (Fig. 17.4).

Stage 4. A number of life-threatening complications occur in the fully developed stage of the AIDS syndrome. These include severe wasting, anaemia, viral infections of the CNS, including encephalitis and progressive multifocal encephalopathy. In addition, cytomegalovirus disease may involve the lung or other organs, especially the brain, and systemic bacterial and fungal infections, and neoplasms, especially Kaposi's sarcoma (Fig. 17.5) and non-Hodgkin's lymphoma, occur. Atypical mycobacterial infections are also common. Muscular weakness occurs because of the development of polymyositis, neuropathy or spinal cord degeneration.

Assessment of the patient with HIV infection therefore requires a careful history, and a complete examination of the body systems, in order to detect the extent of the disease and its complications. Immunological assessment must include analysis of lymphocyte subtypes, especially CD4 and CD8 counts; selective reduction in numbers of circulating CD4 cells is characteristic of the disturbed immune state.

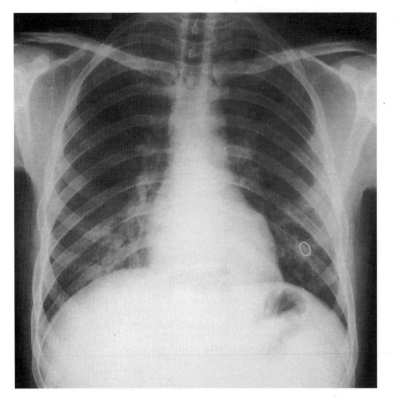

Fig. 17.4 *Pneumocystis carinii* infection in an HIV-positive patient (stage 2–3). Note the ring in the left nipple.

Other retrovirus infections, especially with HTLV-1 virus, also cause disease in humans. HTLV-1 infection is probably also acquired by sexual contact. It is associated with the later development of T cell lymphoma and leukaemia, often with hypercalcaemia, and with a slowly progressive neurological syndrome characterized by a progressive spastic paraparesis (*tropical spastic paraparesis*). These syndromes occur in people in regions where the infection is endemic, such as central Africa, the Caribbean, and parts of Asia.

Systemic examination

Particular attention should be paid to the skin, mouth, eyes, joints and, in late syphilis, the cardiovascular and nervous systems.

The skin

The generalized rash of secondary syphilis is usually non-itchy and commonly involves the palms and soles. Generalized rash can also be seen in acute viral infections such as HIV-seroconversion illness, acute hepatitis B, acute cytomegalovirus infection and infectious mononucleosis. Gummata of the skin may be present in late syphilis. Pustular lesions of disseminated gonococcal infection are seen mainly on the limbs, particularly near joints. Excoriated papules and bur-

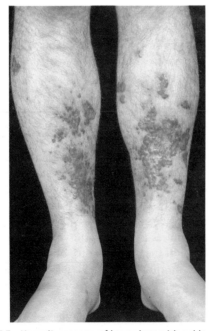

Fig. 17.5 Kaposi's sarcoma of lower legs with ankle oedema in a patient with AIDS.

rows are features of scabies. Purplish nodules or plaques on the skin may indicate Kaposi's sarcoma. A psoriasis-like rash and keratodermatitis of the feet may be present in Reiter's disease. Behçet's disease causes recurrent painful oro-genital ulcers. Stevens–Johnson syndrome can also present with painful oro-genital ulceration and target lesions on the skin.

The mouth

The mouth is a common site for extragenital chancres. Mucous patches and snailtrack ulcers occur in secondary syphilis, and leucoplakia and chronic superficial glossitis in late syphilis. In congenital syphilis, linear scars radiating from the mouth known as *rhagades*, and Hutchinson's incisors—dome-shaped incisor teeth with a central notch—may be present. Genital herpes can spread to the mouth and vice versa if the patient practises orogenital intercourse. In HIV infection, hairy leucoplakia, consisting of persistent white hairy patches on the side of the tongue, oral thrush, consisting of curdy white patches which can be removed leaving behind a raw surface, and gingivitis may be seen. The mouth is also a common site for Kaposi's sarcoma lesions.

The eyes

Conjunctivitis can be due to direct infection by *Chlamydia*, gonococcus or herpes, or can arise indirectly, as in Reiter's disease. Iritis can be seen in Reiter's disease, secondary and late syphilis and in Behçet's disease. Congenital syphilis can present with interstitial keratitis, iritis and choroidoretinitis. *Argyll Robertson pupils* are small irregular pupils seen in neurosyphilis, particularly tabes dorsalis. They are non-reactive to light but the *accommodation reflex* is present.

The joints

Painful joint swelling may be present in Reiter's disease or disseminated gonococcal infection. Charcot's joints in tabes dorsalis are generally painless, deformed and hypermobile; Clutton's joints in congenital syphilis are painless bilateral joint effusions.

Gonococcal and chlamydial infection can cause lower abdominal pain and tenderness if endometritis or salpingitis supervene and right hypochondrial pain and tenderness if perihepatitis (*FitzHugh–Curtis syndrome*) is present.

Special investigations

Urethral discharge

Both gonococcal and non-gonococcal urethritis may be asymptomatic and only discovered by genital tests, or when extragenital complications develop.

The urethral meatus is cleansed with a swab. If there is no visible discharge, the urethra is gently milked forward from the bulb and any discharge noted. A platinum or plastic bacteriological loop is inserted 1–2 cm into the urethra proximal to the fossa navicularis and the urethral material obtained is spread thinly on a glass slide for Gram-staining. Endo-urethral material for gonococcal culture is plated directly on to a suitable culture plate or sent to the laboratory in modified Stuart's transport medium. Positive cultures are tested for antimicrobial sensitivities and beta-lactamase production.

GRAM-STAINING (Box 17.4)
The presence of Gram-negative intracellular diplococci, which appear as opposing bean-shaped cocci within polymorphonuclear leucocytes under the microscope (Fig. 17.6), suggests a diagnosis of gonococcal urethritis. The presence of 10 or more polymorphonuclear leucocytes per high power field ($\times 1000$ magnification) with a negative test for gonococci indicates non-gonococcal urethritis, the causes of which are given in Box 17.5. Exclusion of specific causes of non-gonococcal urethritis such as *Chlamydia trachomatis*, trichomoniasis and non-sexually transmitted disease like bacterial urinary tract infection leads to a diagnosis of 'non-specific' urethritis. However, in the absence of adequate diagnostic facilities, urethritis due to *C. trachomatis* is often included under 'non-specific' urethritis. If a patient has passed urine just before the test, the urethral smear

---

BOX 17.4 Procedure for Gram-staining.

1 Fix the smear on the slide by passing it through a flame twice.
2 Stain with 2% crystal violet for 30 s, then wash with tap water.
3 Stain with Gram's iodine for a further 30 s and wash with water.
4 Decolorize with acetone for a few seconds.
5 Wash with water and counterstain with 1% safranin for 10 s.
6 After a final wash with water, dry by pressing between filter paper.

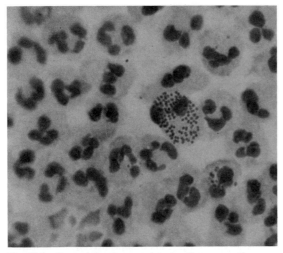

Fig. 17.6 Gram-stained smear showing Gram-negative intracellular diplococci typical of *Neisseria gonorrhoea*.

BOX 17.5 Causes of non-gonococcal urethritis.

Sexually transmitted diseases
Chlamydia trachomatis D-K serotypes
Unknown/Mycoplasma?
Trichomonas vaginalis
Herpes simplex virus
Candida albicans
Intra-meatal warts
Meatal chancre

Non-sexually transmitted diseases
Bacterial urinary tract infection
Tuberculosis
Urethral stricture
Stevens–Johnson syndrome
Benign mucous membrane pemphigoid
Chemical
Trauma
Others

---

may show no polymorphonuclear leucocytes because the urine will have washed out the accumulated urethral material. In such cases the patient should be asked to re-attend for an overnight or late afternoon urethral smear after holding urine for 8 or more hours.

A *wet preparation* is made by mixing urethral material obtained by scraping the urethra using a loop with a drop of normal saline on a slide. This is examined by ordinary or dark ground illumination for *Trichomonas* which appear as ovoid protozoa with beating flagellae and in jerky motion.

If facilities are available for chlamydial culture, epithelial cells obtained with a cotton-tipped wire swab and transported in 2-sucrose phosphate transport medium are used for cell culture to demon-strate chlamydial inclusions. Alternatively, fluorescent staining for chlamydial elementary bodies using monoclonal antibodies or an enzyme-linked immunoabsorbent assay (ELISA) test for chlamydial antigen from genital material can be performed. When such tests can be carried out, about 50% of so-called 'non-specific' urethritis can be due to *C. trachomatis*.

TWO-GLASS TEST

In the two-glass test the patient passes urine into two glasses (or clear plastic cups), approximately 100 ml in the first glass and the rest in the second. The presence of several specks or threads which sink to the bottom in the first glass, with a clear second glass indicates *anterior urethritis*; if there are threads in both glasses, *posterior urethritis* is indicated. Hazy urine in both glasses is commonly due to phosphaturia and this clears with the addition of acetic acid. If the urine still remains hazy and there is pus in the urethral smear, this suggests either sexually transmitted 'non-specific' urethritis with ascending infection in the bladder, or bacterial urinary tract infection with descending non-sexual infection to the urethra. To obtain a presumptive diagnosis, the second glass of urine is centrifuged and the deposit Gram-stained. In 'non-specific' urethritis with ascending infection, there will be polymorphonuclear leucocytes only, whereas in bacterial urinary tract infection the smear will also show bacteria. The latter can be identified by a mid-stream urine culture. Rarely, renal tuberculosis may present with urethritis and hazy urine, which is abacterial on Gram-staining as in 'non-specific' infection. The urine must be checked for sugar, protein, blood and other abnormalities as indicated (Chapter 6).

The presence of urethritis a week or more after successful treatment for gonorrhoea indicates that the patient has *post-gonococcal urethritis*, a non-gonococcal urethritis unmasked following treatment for gonorrhoea.

Vaginal discharge

A smear of the discharge can be Gram-stained to look for the spores and pseudomycelia of thrush and for 'clue cells' indicative of bacterial vaginosis. 'Clue cells' are vaginal epithelial cells covered with *Gardnerella vaginalis*, which are Gram-variable but mainly Gram-negative coccobacilli. If after adding 10% potassium hydroxide to two drops of the discharge a fishy ammoniacal odour is produced, this constitutes a positive *amine test*. This, together with a vaginal pH > 5.0, is suggestive of bacterial vaginosis. A wet-film preparation is examined for *Trichomonas*. Cultures for *Candida* and *Trichomonas* are also performed.

Gram-stained smear and culture of cervical secretion for gonorrhoea are performed routinely. If facilities are available, a cervical test for *Chlamydia trachomatis* should also be performed. If genital herpes is suspected, a cervical specimen for herpes culture should be collected.

Urethral and rectal specimens for Gram-staining and cultures for gonorrhoea should be performed routinely in new patients. A chlamydial culture from the rectum may also be indicated.

In those who practise peno-oral intercourse, a pharyngeal swab should be taken for culture for gonorrhoea and chlamydia. A Gram-stained smear from the throat for gonorrhoea is useless because of the presence of other *Neisseria*.

Genital ulcer

To investigate the cause of a genital ulcer, the base of the ulcer is first thoroughly cleansed with normal saline, then gently squeezed until a drop of serum exudates. A coverslip is applied to the drop which will adhere to it. This is put on to a glass slide and pressed down firmly between filter paper. The slide is examined under the *dark-field microscope* for the characteristic morphology and movements of *Treponema pallidum* (Fig. 17.7)—bending itself at an angle, rotating forward on its long axis or alternating between contraction and expansion of its coils. Dark-field examination should be repeated for several days if syphilis is suspected.

Sometimes dark-field microscopy may be negative from suspected syphilitic ulcers, particularly if the

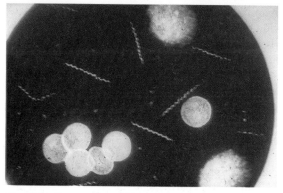

Fig. 17.7 *Treponema pallidum* seen under the dark-field microscope. The thread-like treponema can be seen, together with pus cells from a urethral discharge.

patient has used a topical antiseptic or antibiotic cream. If regional lymph nodes are enlarged, a *lymph node aspiration* can be performed. After infiltration of the skin with 1% lignocaine, 0.2 ml of normal saline is injected into the node, the needle moved around in the node and then aspirated. A drop is placed between a glass slide and coverslip, pressed between filter paper and examined under the dark-field microscope. In oral chancres, commensal treponemes may be confused with *Treponema pallidum*: because of this, immunofluorescent staining for pathogenic treponemes of serum from the ulcer, air-dried on a slide, is advisable.

If herpes is suspected, the base of the blister or ulcer is swabbed and the swab placed in a viral transport medium for herpes culture. Diagnosis of granuloma inguinale is based upon the demonstration of *Donovan bodies*, which stain in bipolar fashion giving a 'safety pin' appearance within the cytoplasm of mononuclear cells in a Giesma-stained tissue smear. Tissue is obtained by infiltrating the edge of the ulcer with 1% lignocaine, and removing a small piece from the edge which is then smeared onto a glass slide or crushed between two glass slides. If chancroid or lymphogranuloma venereum is suspected, culture for *Haemophilus ducreyi* and *Chlamydia trachomatis* of the lymphogranuloma venereum serovars respectively, may be indicated using material obtained from the ulcer or bubo.

Serological tests for syphilis

There are two groups of serological tests for syphilis: the non-specific tests for antilipoidal antibody such as Venereal Disease Research Laboratories (VDRL), Kahn and Wassermann tests, and the specific antitreponemal antibody tests such as *T. pallidum* haemagglutination (TPHA), fluorescent treponemal antibody absorption (FTA-Abs) and *T. pallidum* immobilization (TPI) tests. The VDRL test has superseded most of the other non-specific tests. Although non-specific, it is useful for following-up patients, particularly those who have been treated for primary or secondary syphilis, when the test should become negative within 6 months. After successful treatment of latent or late syphilis, the specific tests usually remain positive while the VDRL test may slowly revert to negative but commonly remains positive in lower titre. A greater than twofold dilution or fourfold increase in antibody titre following treatment indicates recrudescence or reinfection.

The presence of a positive VDRL test on two occasions with negative specific tests and the absence of any evidence of treponemal disease indicates a *biological false-positive* reaction. Acute false-positive reactions may be due to acute febrile infections such as pneumonia, malaria and infective endocarditis, pregnancy and vaccination; they last less than 6 months. Chronic false-positive reactions may indicate autoimmune diseases such as systemic lupus erythematosus, but can also occur in intravenous drug abusers, lepromatous leprosy and old age.

All patients should be screened for syphilis with serological tests such as the VDRL and TPHA. These tests should be repeated after 3 months if initial tests are negative. If primary syphilis is suspected, the FTA-Abs test is also performed as this is usually the first serological test to be positive. In babies with suspected congenital syphilis, the FTA-Abs tests using an IgM conjugate should be requested because of passive transfer of maternal IgG antibodies across the placenta. When treponemes cannot be demonstrated, positive results must be confirmed by a second set of tests before treatment is started.

Endemic treponematoses such as yaws, bejel and pinta may result in positive serological tests for syphilis. It is not possible to differentiate the treponematoses by serological tests.

Investigations in homosexual and bisexual men

Gram-stained smears from the rectum and cultures from the rectum and throat of homosexual and bisexual men should also be obtained to exclude gonorrhoea, in addition to routine tests as for heterosexual men. In cases of proctitis, cultures for herpes and *Chlamydia* may be indicated.

All homosexual and bisexual men should also be screened for hepatitis B surface antigen (HBsAg) and antibody (anti-HBs). The presence of HBsAg indicates that the patient is infectious whereas anti-HBs indicates that the patient is immune. If both tests are negative vaccination against hepatitis B should be offered. If hepatitis is present, other infective causes such as secondary syphilis, hepatitis A and C as well as non-infective causes should be excluded.

Screening for antibody to HIV, the causal agent for AIDS, is advisable for patients at risk of infection because of the possibility of early intervention with anti-HIV agents and preventive treatment against opportunistic infections such as *Pneumocystis carinii* pneumonia. The test may also be indicated to confirm or exclude HIV infection as a cause of problematic medical illness. Consent from the patient for the test to be carried out is desirable. Patients should be counselled as to the medical, social and emotional consequences before performing the test. Facilities for counselling, support and follow-up of patients with positive tests should be available. Patients have lost their jobs, developed psychiatric problems and even committed suicide following the finding of a positive HIV test.

Homosexual and bisexual men with diarrhoea should have their stools examined for *Giardia, Amoeba, Shigella, Salmonella, Cryptosporidium* and cytomegalovirus, the last two being associated with AIDS. Threadworms may also be present.

Ophthalmia neonatorum

Ophthalmia neonatorum is defined as purulent conjunctivitis in the first 3 weeks of life. It should be differentiated from 'sticky eyes' that frequently result from blocked lacrimal ducts.

Ophthalmia neonatorum is commonly due to gonorrhoea, *Chlamydia* or non-sexually transmitted bacteria. A Gram-stained conjunctival smear can be a useful guide. The presence of polymorphonuclear leucocytes with Gram-negative intracellular diplococci is presumptive evidence of gonorrhoea but rarely may indicate *Branhamella catarrhalis* infection; culture must be carried out for full identification. The presence of pus cells with bacteria indicates bacterial ophthalmia, whereas the presence of pus alone suggests chlamydial ophthalmia. A Giemsa-stained conjunctival smear may show chlamydial inclusions in the cytoplasm of epithelial cells. A rapid diagnostic test using monoclonal antibody staining for chlamydial elementary bodies can provide results within 30 minutes. Cultures for gonorrhoea, *Chlamydia* and other bacteria should be performed as mixed infections may occur.

Chest symptoms such as staccato cough and rapid breathing with poor feeding in the absence of fever may indicate chlamydial pneumonia. Auscultation of the chest may be normal but the chest X-ray may show consolidation.

If the ophthalmia is due to gonococcal or chlamydial infection, it is important to check the parents and their sexual partners.

CHAPTER 18

The blood

Introduction

The recognition and analysis of blood disorders begins with the history and physical examination. Knowledge gained from the clinical assessment can then be used to select appropriate haematological investigations and treatment.

History

The history belongs to the patient. Let the patient tell you about their problems simply and without interruption. People vary enormously in their ability to give an accurate and coherent account of their symptoms but they must be given an opportunity to tell their story.

Symptoms in blood disorders are usually due to the effects of too few or too many red cells, white cells or platelets, or the result of too little or too much blood clotting power. This makes it quite easy to organize a group of direct questions after the patient's initial story and to build on the information given.

Because many blood disorders are inherited, the past and family histories assume great importance. The patient in front of you may have few complaints and it may even be better to begin with a full past or family history before moving on to the history of the current problem. Drugs often have profound effects on the blood and a full review of medication taken should never be omitted, while social aspects are of great importance in those with lifelong or life-threatening diseases.

Anaemia

Anaemia is a laboratory diagnosis and is present if the haemoglobin concentration is reduced. There are often no symptoms, especially if anaemia develops slowly, but eventually oxygen delivery to the tissues is affected and the following symptoms may develop.

- *Lassitude* is so common that it is an unreliable guide to anaemia or its severity.
- *Dyspnoea* appears at first only on exertion but, as anaemia progresses, shortness of breath can occur at rest.
- *Palpitations* may simply be the patient's way of describing rapid, vigorous beating of the heart. Irregular palpitations imply some additional disorder and anaemia will exacerbate any vascular insufficiency. This can lead to deterioration of angina pectoris, intermittent claudication or cerebral ischaemic symptoms which are rarely due to anaemia alone.
- *Pallor* is often the complaint of friends and relatives rather than the patients themselves. The degree of pallor is difficult to assess because of variation in the skin pigmentation and thickness.

411

Unfortunately no single symptom leads directly to a diagnosis of anaemia but associated symptoms may be very useful in differential diagnosis.

IRON DEFICIENCY

Iron deficiency usually develops quite slowly and symptoms may not be very prominent, even at low haemoglobin concentrations. *Glossitis* with papillary atrophy and *angular stomatitis* (cheilosis) may result in a sore mouth. In extreme cases this may be associated with *dysphagia* to form the Paterson–Kelly or Plummer–Vinson syndrome. The patient may complain of *brittle nails* which are often spoon-shaped (*koilonychia*).

The history may reveal evidence of dietary lack, particularly in strict vegetarians or of disorders leading to poor absorption of iron, such as a previous history of gastrectomy. Chronic blood loss may be due to menorrhagia, aspirin ingestion, gastrointestinal neoplasm, peptic ulcer, hookworm or haemorrhoids. This means that the diagnosis of iron deficiency is not complete without an indication of its cause and the nature of the investigations carried out will depend on the clinical assessment of each case.

DEFICIENCY OF VITAMIN B$_{12}$

In addition to the symptoms and signs of anaemia, deficiency of vitamin B$_{12}$ may result in mild jaundice and the patients or their relatives may notice a lemon yellow tinge to the skin. The tongue may become red, smooth and sore and the patient may complain of indigestion or diarrhoea. In some cases *subacute combined degeneration of the spinal cord* develops with damage to the corticospinal tracts and dorsal columns and a peripheral neuropathy resulting in an abnormal gait with motor and sensory loss.

The history may reveal a previous gastrectomy or disease of the terminal ileum. A *very* strict vegetarian diet is a cause of B$_{12}$ deficiency in Asian communities in the West.

Pernicious anaemia remains the most common cause of vitamin B$_{12}$ deficiency in the UK and usually presents in later life. It is due to an autoimmune disease of the stomach resulting in loss of intrinsic factor and the classical description is of an elderly, grey-haired, pale person, with lemon yellow skin, a smooth sore tongue and an abnormal gait. In practice many patients are now diagnosed before they become seriously ill due to the frequency of simple screening laboratory investigations. The condition tends to run in families and elderly people with a family history are especially worth screening, as are those with a personal or family history of autoimmune thyroid disease.

DEFICIENCY OF FOLIC ACID

Folic acid deficiency causes the same type of anaemia as vitamin B$_{12}$ deficiency but for different reasons. There is often a history of a poor diet, lacking in green vegetables or there may be evidence of generalized malabsorption as in coeliac disease, often with accompanying diarrhoea. Pregnancy or any condition such as haemolytic anaemia, in which the demand for folic acid increases, may result in deficiency and the effects of folic acid deficiency can be felt quite suddenly, especially when an increased demand for the vitamin is accompanied by infection. Neurological damage is not a feature of this disorder.

HAEMOLYTIC ANAEMIAS

Anaemia due to premature destruction of the red blood cells may be congenital or acquired. The congenital forms have a history of anaemia and usually jaundice dating from early life, often accompanied by a family history. They are usually due to intrinsic abnormalities of the red cell membrane (e.g. congenital spherocytosis), metabolism (e.g. glucose-6-phosphate dehydrogenase deficiency) or haemoglobin structure (e.g. sickle cell disease). Acquired haemolysis is usually of recent onset and results from the cells being exposed to the destructive effects of antibodies, toxic chemicals, poisons or direct injury.

The patient presents with a variable degree of anaemia and jaundice, though in mild cases the latter may be absent. The spleen is often palpable. In severe long-standing haemolysis of congenital origin the increased red cell production tends to limit growth with distortion of the bones of the skull and face due to bone marrow hyperplasia. Typically this results in abnormal facies and radiological thickening of the diploë. There is a tendency for skin ulceration of the lower legs to occur.

When red cell destruction is acute the ability of the body to absorb haemoglobin within the circulation is exceeded and *haemoglobinuria* occurs. Depending on its severity this may impart a 'smoky' appearance to the urine or it may appear frankly bloody or even black (blackwater fever of falciparum malaria). Where haemolysis is extravascular or not so severe as to swamp albumin and haptoglobins then haemoglobin does not appear in the urine but there is an increase in urinary urobilinogen from the enterohepatic circulation and the urine darkens on standing. In haemolytic anaemia no bilirubin appears in the urine because the excess plasma bilirubin is unconjugated.

Some forms of haemolytic anaemia are associated with special symptoms.

Congenital membrane defects

Hereditary spherocytosis is a typical example of a congenital red blood cell membrane defect. It has an autosomal dominant inheritance although the family history is sometimes negative. Anaemia may present at birth and can be severe throughout childhood, being exacerbated by intercurrent illness or surgery. The spleen is enlarged and splenectomy is curative.

Red cell enzyme defects

A breakdown in the mechanism of red cell carbohydrate metabolism may occur either in the pentose phosphate pathway, where deficiency of glucose-6-phosphate dehydrogenase (G6PD) is the more common defect, or in the Emden–Meyerhof glycolytic pathway which is particularly affected by a lack of pyruvate kinase. Both of these important inherited disorders may be associated with haemolytic anaemia.

Pyruvate kinase deficiency gives rise to chronic haemolysis and splenomegaly which is improved by splenectomy. G6PD deficiency is X-linked and occurs particularly in Afro-Caribbean and Mediterranean peoples. Mildly affected subjects (Afro-Caribbean) only develop haemolysis after treatment with drugs such as antimalarials, some analgesics and antibiotics, but the more severely affected Mediterranean people are also sensitive to the fava bean and its pollen (*favism*). Whatever the initial stimulus, brisk intravascular haemolysis with haemoglobinuria may occur. The haemolysis is self-limiting, once the cause is withdrawn and new cells with a higher enzyme content are released into the circulation. It should be noted that female heterozygotes are not immune from haemolysis because each red cell contains the enzyme produced from either the normal or the abnormal X chromosome, but not both.

Haemoglobin disorders

Abnormal haemoglobins may arise as a result of substitution of variants of haemoglobin A, or normal adult haemoglobin formation may be reduced as in the thalassaemia syndromes.

The most important variant haemoglobin is haemoglobin S which, when deoxygenated, becomes insoluble and is liable to crystallize within the red

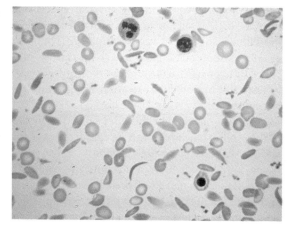

Fig. 18.1 Sickle haemoglobin disease (peripheral blood). In homozygous disease (HbSS), sickle cells and target cells are present together with occasional nucleated red cells. Heterozygotes (HbSA) have a normal peripheral blood.

cells. The resulting membrane damage gives the cell a characteristic sickle shape (Fig. 18.1) which hampers its flow through the blood vessels and results in its destruction. People who are homozygous for the defect (HbSS) have *sickle cell disease*. They are mostly of Afro-Caribbean or Mediterranean origin and have a life-long severe haemolytic anaemia characterized by ill-health, pallor, jaundice and painful crises. These crises affect the bones, abdomen and chest and are due to microvascular obstruction. Symptoms begin at about six months of age as haemoglobin F production declines and crises appear intermittently, often following dehydration or infection. The spleen, which is often enlarged during childhood, later disappears due to infarction causing a liability to bacterial infection which may be life-threatening. Persistent ulceration of the skin, especially on the leg, may occur (Fig. 18.2). The severity of sickle cell disease is

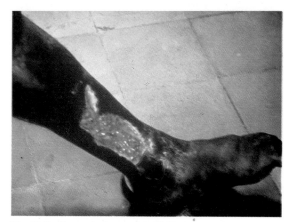

Fig. 18.2 Haemolytic anaemia (sickle haemoglobin disease); leg ulcer.

highly variable both from its physical effects and from the patient's ability to cope with a very distressing illness. The heterozygous condition (HbSA) is usually asymptomatic although crises can be provoked by hypoxia. The heterozygous disorder is easily detectable by a solubility test or haemoglobin electrophoresis.

The *thalassaemias* are due to a failure of globin chain production, which can be found all over the world. However, *beta-thalassaemia* is most commonly found in Mediterranean or Asian peoples. In *beta-thalassaemia major* both beta genes are affected and there is a lifelong haemolytic anaemia in which symptoms of pallor, jaundice and failure to thrive begin at six months of age, the spleen enlarges and facial and cranial bone growth is abnormal (Fig. 18.3). There are no painful crises but premature death occurs due to anaemia unless regular transfusions are given. Even with transfusion, development is not entirely normal and haemolysis together with iron overload results in failure of sexual development, endocrine abnormalities and heart disease. Attempts to correct these abnormalities by splenectomy and iron chelation therapy have been partly successful. By contrast those with *beta-thalassaemia minor*, in whom one beta gene is affected, have only a mild anaemia which closely resembles iron deficiency anaemia, and is asymptomatic. The *alpha thalassaemia syndromes* are more complex because there are two alpha genes per chromosome. The deletion of all four alpha genes is not compatible with life, while the loss of one or two genes is of little clinical importance. The loss of three alpha genes results in a moderate haemolytic anaemia known as *haemoglobin H disease*, owing to the presence of HbH (β_4) in the blood. The majority of patients come from the Far East where two alpha gene deletions on one chromosome is a relatively common occurrence.

Patients with haemoglobin disorders should be offered genetic counselling especially when they are at risk of having children with sickle cell disease or thalassaemia major. A full family history is important so that appropriate support can be provided, based on proper information.

Acquired haemolytic anaemia

Antibiotics, toxic chemicals, poisons, drugs and direct injury can all cause haemolysis and a well-taken history may reveal the exact source of damage.

Autoantibodies of IgG class tend to cause extravascular haemolysis with anaemia, jaundice and splenic enlargement but without haemoglobinuria. IgM class antibodies are usually more active in the cold and fix complement so that increased haemolysis may occur in cold weather and intravascular haemolysis with haemoglobinuria is more likely.

APLASTIC ANAEMIA

Failure of the bone marrow (Fig. 18.4) results in anaemia, leucopenia and thrombocytopenia leading to pallor, increased risk of infection and abnormal bleeding. When a diagnosis of aplasia is made it is important to consider the probable cause, although in up to 50% of cases none is ever determined.

Possible causes are:

- irradiation
- drugs
- chemicals
- infection
- autoimmune disease.

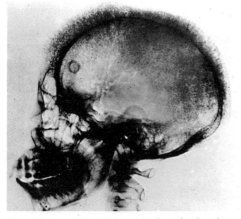

Fig. 18.3 'Hair-on-end' appearance in the calvarium in thalassaemia.

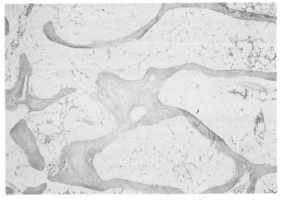

Fig. 18.4 Trephine bone marrow biopsy. The marrow is acellular and there is bone resorption in this patient with aplastic anaemia.

Polycythaemia

Polycythaemia means 'too many red cells in the blood' but by convention the term is also used to indicate an increase in the haemoglobin concentration. There are often no symptoms in the early stages and the condition goes unnoticed by the patient. Relatives may be the first to notice the ruddy complexion or *plethora* of polycythaemia but eventually headache, tinnitus and a feeling of fullness or muzziness in the head develops. As the haematocrit (packed cell volume) rises there is an increasing risk of heart attack, stroke and peripheral ischaemia, all of which are, of course, common without polycythaemia.

Some cases are due to hypoxia secondary to congenital heart disease or chronic lung disease while others arise from renal conditions or rare tumours. These produce pure red cell excess with the symptoms outlined above. They are distinct from *polycythaemia rubra vera* (PRV), a proliferative bone marrow disorder in which the spleen is often enlarged and the white cell and platelet count increased. In PRV patients often complain additionally of itching (*pruritus*), especially when taking a hot bath. Patients with polycythaemia and with high platelet counts are particularly at risk of thrombotic episodes or, paradoxically, of a bleeding tendency.

Leucopenia

The major consequence of leucopenia is infection. In patients with blood disorders this may be severe and persistent. The patient's ability to localize infections is limited so that rapid spread or even septicaemia develops. Fever and pneumonia are common but non-specific.

Mouth ulceration is a frequent presenting symptom and, in the presence of thrombocytopenia, this is often associated with bleeding. Patients with bone marrow disorders often present to their dentists.

Anal ulceration is an unpleasant and dangerous complication of leucopenia. It may be the sole presenting feature but often complicates severe diarrhoea.

Patients often develop opportunistic infections. These are infections with unusual organisms, such as fungi, which rarely cause disease in normal individuals. Common viruses such as herpes zoster (causing chickenpox and shingles) and herpes simplex, cause more serious illness than usual when the white cell count is low.

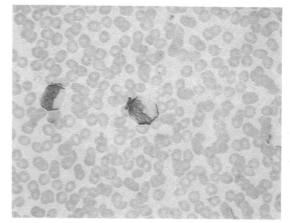

Fig. 18.5 Glandular fever (peripheral blood). Atypical mononuclear cells are visible.

As a general rule a lack of granulocytes (*neutropenia*) is associated with bacterial infection while a lack of lymphocytes (*lymphopenia*) is associated with disease due to viruses or more exotic organisms like *Pneumocystis carinii* and *Toxoplasma*.

Leucocytosis

Leucocytosis may be a normal response to infection or injury and is then associated with the symptoms of the disorder that have led to it. Thus pneumonia will cause fever, cough, sputum and granulocytosis, while patients with infectious mononucleosis (glandular fever, Fig. 18.5) complain of malaise, a sore throat and lymph node enlargement and have a T cell lymphocytosis.

In many haematological malignancies excess white cells accumulate in the peripheral blood (Figs 18.6, 18.7 and 18.8), bone marrow and lymphoreticular

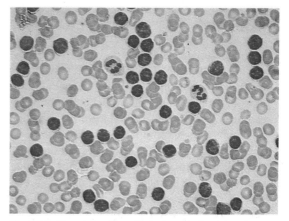

Fig. 18.6 Chronic lymphocytic leukaemia (peripheral blood). The white cell count is increased and most of the white cells are small lymphocytes.

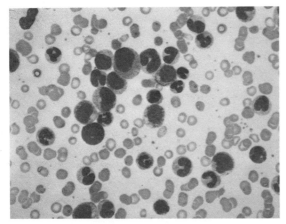

Fig. 18.7 Chronic granulocytic (myeloid) leukaemia (peripheral blood). There is an increased number of granulocytes, most of which are mature neutrophils. A few more primitive cells are also present.

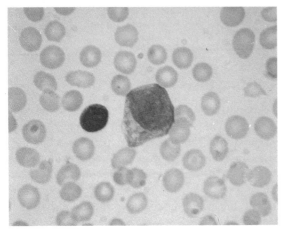

Fig. 18.8 Acute myeloblastic leukaemia (peripheral blood). The myeloblast in the centre of the field contains a cytoplasmic Auer rod.

system and cause symptoms through a variety of effects.

- *Displacement.* If the bone marrow is displaced then anaemia, a lack of effective white cells and thrombocytopenia will develop.
- *Organ infiltration.* Patients may complain of enlargement of lymph nodes or the sensation of dragging or pain in the left hypochondrium which can arise from an enlarged spleen. If the lymph nodes in the mediastinum (Fig. 18.9) become sufficiently large as a result of lymphoma they may cause mediastinal obstruction with venous engorgement of the head and respiratory embarrassment whilst in the abdomen large nodes may cause lymphatic and/or venous obstruction in the lower limbs. Bone pain may be severe where there is marked bony infiltration and pathological frac-

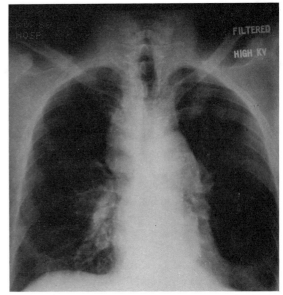

Fig. 18.9 Mediastinal lymph node enlargement in Hodgkin's disease.

tures may occur. When the meninges are invaded symptoms of headache and neck stiffness may be prominent and deposits may damage the spinal cord or the brain resulting in paralysis and sensory loss. Lymphomas may also present with orbital involvement (Fig. 18.10).

- *The white cell count.* When the white cell count is very high this alone causes symptoms, due to failure of the peripheral circulation. Examples include dyspnoea, visual loss, peripheral ischaemia and priapism.

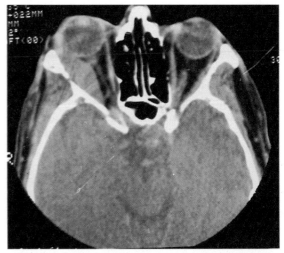

Fig. 18.10 CT scan showing orbital lymphoma. There is a mass in the right orbit arising from the lateral wall and involving the lateral rectus muscle that is causing displacement of the eye forwards and of the optic nerve medially.

- *Systemic effects.* A variety of symptoms are caused by the systemic effects of white cell tumours. These include fever without evidence of infection, weight loss, pruritus, polyneuropathy, myopathy, renal failure, hyperviscosity and haemolytic anaemia.

Myelomatosis

In multiple myelomatosis, osteolytic lesions may be seen in bones, especially the skull (Fig. 18.11). In some patients myeloma presents with a single bony mass, the solitary plasmacytoma.

Bleeding

Bleeding after injury is an everyday experience for healthy people and it can be very difficult to decide whether or not apparently excessive bleeding is due to a blood disorder. Serious congenital conditions, such as severe haemophilia, usually become obvious in early childhood but can be misdiagnosed as non-accidental injury. Milder bleeding disorders (see Fig. 18.12) can remain undetected into old age, especially in men who have not undergone surgery in earlier adult life. Spontaneous easy bruising is a common complaint of normal women and is usually not associated with abnormal bleeding or a demonstrable haemostatic abnormality. It is the frequency and persistence of blood loss together with the minimal severity of injury required to produce it which

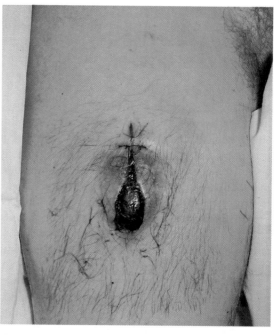

Fig. 18.12   Haematoma following an intramuscular injection in a patient with mild haemophilia.

should alert the physician to the likelihood of a haemostatic defect, while volume of loss is a poor guide.

First it is important to establish whether excessive bleeding has taken place or not. This may be very difficult as 'a little blood goes a long way'. A history often has to be taken from the anxious mother of a child who has bled after dental extraction or tonsillectomy and it is useful to have some objective evidence of excessive haemorrhage from another source, such as the need for blood transfusion.

The next step is to find out whether the bleeding was spontaneous or precipitated by trauma. Typical spontaneous bleeding occurs from the nose (*epistaxis*) or into joints and muscles, although it should be noted that the latter are moving parts subject to minor injury. Bleeding after minor injury may be abnormal if it is persistent from cut surfaces or if bruising results in haematomas with solid centres and marked discoloration of surrounding tissues. Tonsillectomy, dental extraction and severe injury or major surgery are likely to result in significant problems if a haemostatic defect is present.

A history of blood in vomit (*haematemesis*), altered blood in the stools (*melaena*) or blood in the urine (*haematuria*) should be noted but all are fairly common in the population at large, as is bleeding

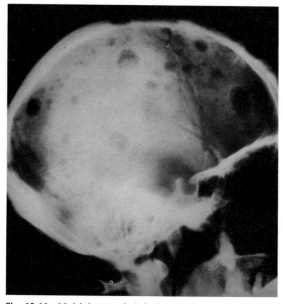

Fig. 18.11   Multiple osteolytic lesions in the skull in myelomatosis.

from the gums and heavy periods. The presence of small blood spots in the skin or mouth (*purpura*) is typical of thrombocytopenia but may have other causes.

It is important to question the patient closely about previous incidents involving excessive bleeding, including events in childhood, and to establish any pattern of inheritance, interviewing relatives if necessary. The drug history begins with questions about aspirin ingestion because aspirin is found in so many proprietary preparations which patients may not regard as 'drugs'. The effect of a single dose of aspirin can last for a week and during this time tests of platelet function will be valueless. It is also important to make sure that the patient is not taking oral anticoagulants.

Finally the patient's social circumstances should be explored. Contact with dangerous chemicals might indicate a cause for thrombocytopenia, while some occupations will not be open to people with significant haemostatic defects.

Haemorrhage due to *vessel wall and platelet defects* tends to be from mucous membranes and into the skin. In patients with *hereditary telangiectasia* (see Fig. 1.1) bleeding occurs from the nose, mouth and gastrointestinal tract and also sometimes from the urinary tract. Patients with *thrombocytopenia* also suffer from nose bleeds and purpura and bleed excessively after surgery. The degree of haemostatic defect depends on the number of circulating platelets. The presence of purpura does not, however, indicate definite thrombocytopenia; patients with *Henoch–Schönlein (anaphylactoid) purpura* (see Fig. 3.11) develop purpura due to immune complex deposition in the skin while the platelet count remains normal.

In patients with *coagulation defects* primary haemostasis, which relies on platelet endothelial interaction may be normal but haemorrhage occurs after surgery or injury, often after a short delay. In severe coagulation defects spontaneous bleeding may occur, especially into joints and muscles, but intra-abdominal and intracranial bleeding are well described. Closed bleeds may develop over a long period of time, causing mass effects and difficulty in diagnosis. Thus bleeding into the ilio-psoas muscle on the right-hand side may mimic appendicitis (Fig. 18.13), and a cerebral tumour may be suspected rather than a cerebral haematoma. In von Willebrand's disease both platelet endothelial interaction and the coagulation mechanism are abnormal and

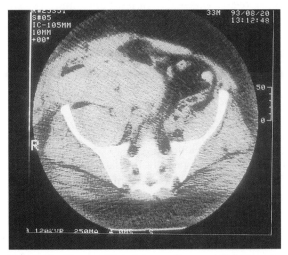

Fig. 18.13 CT scan of the abdomen (haemophilia). There is a large haematoma in the right psoas region causing right-sided abdominal pain and swelling.

there is a mixed clinical picture although the platelet function defect predominates.

Thrombosis

This subject is by no means confined to the blood but haematologists have increasingly come to realize that some congenital and acquired blood disorders can give rise to thrombosis, especially in the venous system.

The approach to the history in a patient with a thrombotic disorder must emphasize the past history and the family history. The nature, severity, site and duration of thrombosis must be established by enquiring about swelling and pain in the calves and thighs, discoloration of the skin of the lower legs and breakdown of the skin of the ankles and feet. Acute venous thrombosis leads to sudden pain and swelling with oedema, usually in the lower limbs but sometimes in the arms, while chronic venous insufficiency leads to long-standing discomfort and an increase in the size of the limb, sometimes with varicose eczema or ulceration. Polycythaemia with thrombocytosis can lead to peripheral ischaemic symptoms of pain and discoloration in the toes, often when there is a good general circulation, and aspirin produces symptomatic relief, in sharp contrast to the clinical features of atheromatous vessel occlusion which is not due to a haematological disorder. Autoimmune disease can also lead to thrombosis and miscarriage, as in systemic lupus erythematosus.

Special blood tests to investigate those with

thrombosis are usually confined to patients aged less than 40 years or who have had recurrent thrombosis or give a positive family history. Despite this limitation a precise cause for such a thrombotic tendency is found in only about 10% of cases studied, illustrating that much has yet to be learned on this topic.

Physical examination

The lymph nodes, liver and spleen are especially important but the skin gives invaluable information about anaemia, infection and bleeding tendencies. A full physical examination must not be neglected as many blood disorders have general effects, and many illnesses in general may affect the blood.

The lymph nodes

Figure 18.14 shows the distribution of the principal lymph node groups which may be felt. These areas should be examined and if lymph nodes are found the following points should be considered.

- How many nodes are palpable?
- What is their approximate diameter in centimetres?
- What is their consistency?
- Are they discrete or confluent?
- Are they mobile or fixed?
- Is the skin in the vicinity of the nodes abnormal?

Tender lymph node enlargement often occurs in the axilla or groin if there is a local infection and chronic, mild or symptomless enlargement of groin nodes due to past infection is a common finding. Glandular fever usually causes tender enlargement of cervical or occipital nodes but the associated symptoms of a sore throat and malaise with fairly rapid resolution should prevent confusion with more serious illnesses. In the lymphomas painless enlargement of the cervical group of nodes is common and more than one node or node group may be affected. The enlarged lymph nodes may be either discrete or matted. The para-aortic nodes can usually only be felt if there is substantial enlargement, as may occur in the more serious lymphomas, and mediastinal nodes can only be detected clinically if they cause superior mediastinal obstruction. If lymph node biopsy is planned it is best to choose a cervical or axillary node rather than one in the groin because the histological appearances of inguinal nodes are frequently distorted by past infection.

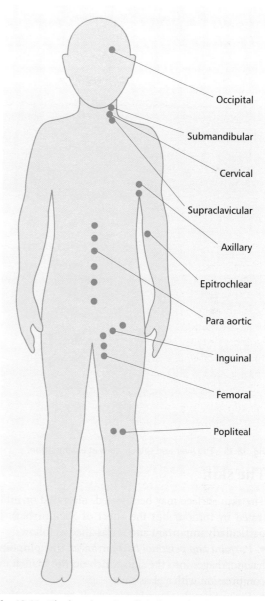

Fig. 18.14 The lymph nodes: clinical examination.

The liver and spleen

Blood disorders often cause marked enlargement of the liver and spleen. The examination should begin in the iliac fossae to avoid missing the edge of an organ which has reached the level of the pelvic inlet. If the liver and spleen are palpable (see pages 91–93) they should be measured in centimetres during natural expiration. A suitable landmark on the costal margin is the midclavicular line and the measurement should be from this point to the furthest extent of the organ (Fig. 18.15).

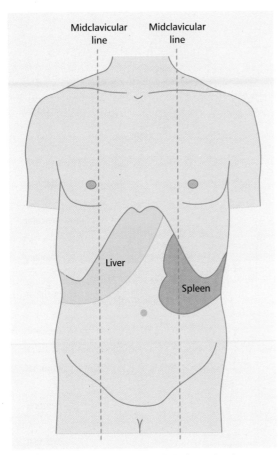

Fig. 18.15 The liver and spleen: clinical examination.

The skin

The skin surface may be infected, ulcerated or infiltrated by tumour but the effect of haemorrhage is particularly important and is classified as follows:

• *Purpura and petechial haemorrhages*: tiny pinpoint haemorrhages into the skin which do not blanch on compression with a glass slide
• *Ecchymoses*: haemorrhages which are larger than petechiae and with more obvious confluence
• *Bruises*: substantial bleeding resulting in confluent deposition of blood, often multicoloured in appearance as the bruise resolves and sometimes associated with an obvious haematoma.

Purpura due to thrombocytopenia is particularly prominent in dependent areas, most commonly on the front of the lower legs, but it may be seen anywhere over the skin surface or in the fundus oculi. Anaphylactoid purpura (Henoch–Schönlein) (see Fig. 3.11), which is due to circulating immune complexes and is unrelated to blood disease, is usually distributed over the backs of the legs and the buttocks. A severe, generalized haemorrhagic rash may follow the use of ampicillin in patients with glandular fever. Bruises often have no haematological significance but if they are extensive with an obvious firm haematoma beneath them then they may indicate a coagulation defect. *Telangiectases* are small dilated blood vessels which may be visible on the skin surface, particularly the lips. They blanch on compression and are sometimes a source of severe haemorrhage when the nose, gastrointestinal tract or bladder is affected.

The conjunctivae should be inspected for pallor or jaundice; the latter is usually mild if it is due to haemolysis.

The skin of the face may be plethoric in polycythaemia while in the dermatitis sometimes associated with lymphomas the whole skin surface may be bright red (*l'homme rouge*). Central cyanosis is best diagnosed by inspection of the lips and tongue and is found in methaemoglobinaemia. Dusky pigmentation, due to a mixture of iron deposition and melanin, is seen in haemochromatosis and haemosiderosis and dark pigmentation is seen in varicose eczema. Patchy depigmentation (*vitiligo*) is a feature of pernicious anaemia but often has no special significance.

The mouth

Cracking of the skin at the corner of the mouth due to iron deficiency is known as *angular cheilosis*. The *white plaques* of thrush or oral candidiasis are commonly seen in patients with blood disorders, and ulceration of the mouth or fauces may be due to leucopenia. These lesions are often associated with cold sores on the lips due to herpes simplex infection. Bleeding in the mouth, especially around the gums, is a familiar feature of thrombocytopenia, and palatal purpura is a well-described sign of glandular fever. The tongue may be smooth or red in various forms of anaemia.

The anus

The anal area is also very vulnerable to infection and ulceration in patients with leucopenia. Where there is also thrombocytopenia the risks of bleeding and haematoma formation combine to create a potentially dangerous combination.

The fundus oculi

Fundal haemorrhages are often visible in disorders of haemostasis, especially thrombocytopenia. When blood viscosity is increased, as in macroglobu-linaemia or chronic granulocytic leukaemia with a high white cell count, there may be engorgement of retinal vessels with papilloedema and retinal haemorrhage.

Talking to patients with serious blood diseases

Patients suffering from leukaemias, lymphomas and haemophilia have serious, painful and unpleasant illnesses which, although treatable, none the less still often result in premature death. It is therefore of the utmost importance to allow adequate time for discussion with patients and their relatives. Frequent counselling interviews will be necessary to explain the nature and progress of the condition. In general, a truthful and accurate discussion of the condition, together with a realistic assessment of the course and prognosis should be given. It is important, however, to reveal only as much information as can be handled at any one interview. This requires sympathy, tact and clinical judgement, and these skills can only be gained by experience. Physicians have to be prepared to cope with the patient's and relatives' responses to bad news; these can be experienced as anger, rejection and denial as well as grief. The help

which nursing staff, social workers and other health workers can provide in supporting patients in these circumstances cannot be overemphasized.

Laboratory examination

The blood is easily sampled and laboratory examination plays a critical role in the analysis of haematological disorders and the choice of appropriate treatment. A venous blood sample is placed in a tube containing dipotassium ethylenediaminetetraacetic acid (EDTA: Sequestrene). A 4.0-ml sample is sufficient for analysis in automatic autoanalyser equipment.

Blood for blood grouping is taken in a plain glass tube and allowed to stand at room temperature for 10 minutes; a clot will form and serum can be separated.

Blood is collected in a heparinized tube for chemical measurements, e.g. plasma iron concentrations.

The red cells and haemoglobin

Estimation of the red cell indices (Tables 18.1 and 18.2) provides invaluable information for the basic

Table 18.1 Normal red cell values.

	Men	Women
Red cell count ($\times 10^{12}$/litre)	4.4–6.1	4.2–5.4
Haemoglobin (g/dl)	13.0–18.0	11.5–16.5
Haematocrit (packed cell volume)	0.40–0.54	0.37–0.47
Mean corpuscular volume (MCV) (fl)	75–99	75–99
Mean corpuscular haemoglobin (MCH) (pg)	27–31	27–31
Mean corpuscular haemoglobin concentration (MCHC) (g/dl)	32–36	32–36

Table 18.2 Typical red cell values in anaemia.

	Iron deficiency	Macrocytic anaemia
Red cell count ($\times 10^{12}$/litre)	4.9	2.7
Haemoglobin (g/dl)	10.4	10.4
Haematocrit (packed cell volume)	0.35	0.32
Mean corpuscular volume (MCV) (fl)	72	119
Mean corpuscular haemoglobin (MCH) (pg)	21	38
Mean corpuscular haemoglobin concentration (MCHC) (g/dl)	29	32

In these two examples there is a similar degree of anaemia (haemoglobin 10.4 g/dl). Note the differences in size (MCV) and haemoglobinization (MCHC) of the red cells in the two types of anaemia. The MCH is increased in the macrocytic anaemia because the red cells are *larger* than normal. In iron deficiency, on the other hand, the MCH is reduced because the red cells are smaller than usual, and also because they are poorly haemoglobinized. Generally, in iron deficiency anaemia the red cell count is well maintained, but in macrocytic anaemia the red cell count is lower.

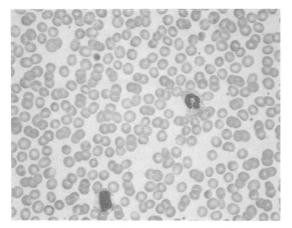

Fig. 18.16   Normal peripheral blood. The red cells show little variation in size or shape. A neutrophil granulocyte and a lymphocyte are visible and platelets are scattered through the film.

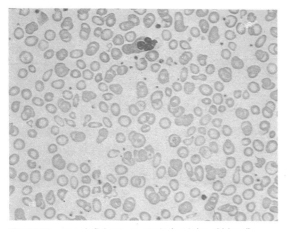

Fig. 18.17   Iron deficiency anaemia (peripheral blood). Hypochromia, microcytosis, anisocytosis and target cells are shown.

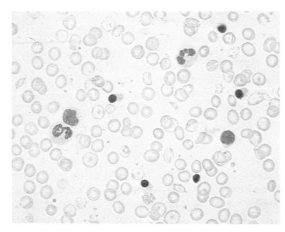

Fig. 18.18   Beta-thalassaemia major (peripheral blood). There is hypochromia, microcytosis and anisocytosis. Target cells and nucleated red cells are numerous. In beta-thalassaemia minor the peripheral blood looks like that of iron deficiency.

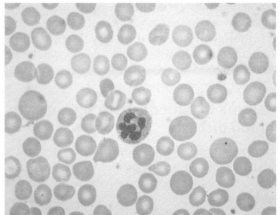

Fig. 18.19   Macrocytic anaemia (peripheral blood). Macrocytosis, anisocytosis, poikilocytosis and a hypersegmented neutrophil granulocyte are shown.

differentiation of the type of anaemia. These indices are calculated from the *haemoglobin concentration*, the *haematocrit* (packed cell volume) and the *red cell count*.

The morphological features of individual red cells (Fig. 18.16), as seen on a peripheral blood film, often provide clues to the nature of the anaemia. *Normocytic red cells* are found in acute blood loss, and in the anaemia of chronic disorders. *Hypochromia and microcytosis* are usually associated with iron deficiency (Fig. 18.17) but also occur in thalassaemia (Fig. 18.18), sideroblastic anaemia and the anaemia of chronic disease. The estimation of plasma iron, total iron binding capacity, serum ferritin and haemoglobin analysis enables them to be distinguished.

Macrocytosis (Fig. 18.19) is typical of vitamin B_{12} and folic acid deficiency and is also seen in any cause of increased erythropoietic activity. The presence of marked variation in red cell size and shape (*anisocytosis* and *poikilocytosis*) together with a reduction in the number of granulocytes, many of which have hypersegmented nuclei, is typical of vitamin B_{12} or folic acid deficiency. Confirmation is by specific assay, and by bone marrow examination; megaloblastic erythroblasts and giant metamyelocytes are seen (Fig. 18.20).

Spherocytosis is typical of red cell damage due to many causes. Important examples are hereditary spherocytosis and autoimmune haemolytic anaemia.

The white cells

The white cell count ranges from 4 to 11×10^9/litre in the normal adult. In health a typical result would be:

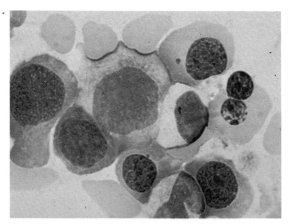

Fig. 18.20 Megaloblastic bone marrow. The majority of cells are megaloblastic erythroblasts showing failure of nuclear development and abnormal nuclear morphology.

- Neutrophils   60%
- Lymphocytes   30%
- Monocytes   6%
- Eosinophils   6%
- Basophils   1%.

Variations of normality are very wide and values are different for infants and young children.

Haemostasis

CLINICAL TESTS

Most tests of haemostasis are performed in the laboratory but the *bleeding time* is a clinical test which assesses platelet endothelial interaction without involving the clotting mechanism. A small wound is made in the forearm under controlled conditions and the time taken for the bleeding to cease is measured. The test should not be performed on patients with thrombocytopenia.

Ivy's method for bleeding time

Place a cuff around the upper arm, inflated to 40 mmHg. After cleaning the forearm make two puncture marks in the forearm skin with a standard lancet, taking care to avoid damaging superficial veins. Remove the blood oozing from the wounds every 15 seconds with filter paper, *without* pressing on the skin, until bleeding ceases. This usually takes less than 9 minutes. Take the average of the two experiments. This test is difficult to standardize, but an abnormal result is a useful indicator of abnormality.

LABORATORY TESTS

A peripheral blood film should always be examined and particular attention paid to platelet numbers and morphology. The standard screening tests are the platelet count and the tests which measure the various parts of the coagulation mechanism (Fig. 18.21).

Platelet count

The normal range of platelet count is 150–400 $\times 10^9$/litre. Platelet numbers can be estimated roughly from the peripheral film and this examination is usually enough for emergencies. Platelets can also be counted visually but automatic machines are usually used.

The platelet count is reduced in bone marrow failure from any cause and in conditions where peripheral destruction of platelets takes place for immunological reasons (e.g. idiopathic thrombocytopenic purpura) or because of trapping and/or destruction by an enlarged spleen (e.g. myelofibrosis). Thrombocytopenia also develops after massive blood transfusion as stored blood does not contain viable platelets. When the platelet count is above 100×10^9/litre no clinical symptoms arise; between 50 and 100×10^9/litre bleeding may occur after major surgery or trauma and between 20 and 50×10^9/litre after minor trauma. Below 20×10^9/litre spontaneous haemorrhage, including haematuria, may occur and purpura is very likely. At very low platelet counts there is a risk of fatal cerebral haemorrhage.

The platelet count is increased in many myeloproliferative diseases and thrombocytosis may occur in Hodgkin's disease or after chronic haemorrhage or splenectomy. Sometimes thrombosis or bleeding may occur as a result.

Many qualitative platelet defects are described. Apart from the effects of aspirin ingestion most of these are very rare.

The prothrombin test and ratio (PTR)

The PTR is the most commonly performed coagulation test and measures the extrinsic coagulation pathway (factors VII, X, V, II and I; Fig. 18.21). Citrate is used as an anticoagulant. Platelet-poor plasma is obtained by centrifugation and is added to an equal volume of brain extract at 37°C (tissue thromboplastin). After recalcification with calcium chloride a clot forms in approximately 15 seconds using normal plasma. The test is compared with that obtained from a pooled normal control and the result is expressed as a ratio of the control sample, i.e. if the test sample takes 30 seconds to clot, the ratio is 2.0. Brain thromboplastin is now

Fig. 18.21 The coagulation and fibrinolytic mechanisms.

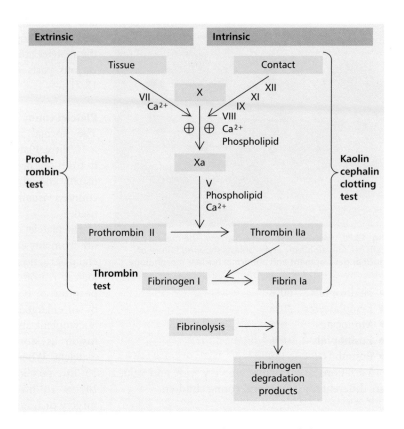

standardized internationally to give an International Normalized Ratio (INR).

Situations in which PTR is abnormal include:
- the use of oral anticoagulants (therapeutic range 2.0–4.0) and heparin
- Hepatic failure
- Haemorrhagic disease of the newborn
- Intravascular coagulation
- Malabsorption of vitamin K.

In practice the test is usually performed to control the dose of oral anticoagulants (e.g. warfarin). These vitamin K antagonists inhibit the formation of the procoagulant factors II, VII, IX, and X as well as the anticoagulant factors proteins C and S. The prothrombin ratio is chosen mainly because it is easy and rapid to perform.

The kaolin cephalin clotting test (KCCT)

The KCCT, also known as the partial thromboplastin test (PTT), again uses citrated platelet-poor plasma and measures the intrinsic coagulation pathway (factors XII, XI, IX, VIII, X, V, II, I; Fig. 18.21). Plasma is added to a mixture of kaolin (surface contact) and cephalin (phospholipid) and is incubated at 37°C. After recalcification with calcium chloride a clot forms in approximately 40 seconds. The result is

not usually expressed as a ratio and the test is more difficult to standardize than the PTR.

Situations in which the KCCT is abnormal include:
- haemophilia (factor VIII or IX deficiency)
- Von Willebrand's disease (factor VIII deficiency with associated factor VIII-related platelet defect)
- contact factor deficiency (factor XII or XI deficiency)
- anticoagulant therapy
- hepatic failure
- intravascular coagulation.

Factor VIII and IX deficiency (haemophilia) make up over 90% of inherited bleeding coagulation defects and the test is used to screen for these conditions. It has also been used for the laboratory control of heparin treatment.

The thrombin test (TT)

An equal volume of thrombin (or a calcium and thrombin mixture) is added to citrated platelet-poor plasma. A clot forms in about 10 seconds. Only the final reaction of fibrin formation from fibrinogen is measured (see Fig. 18.21). The test is abnormal in the presence of hypofibrinogenaemia, dysfibrinogenaemia, heparin or fibrinogen degradation products (FDPs). It is used to monitor heparin therapy and in the diagnosis of intravascular coagulation. Specific tests are performed depending on the clinical findings and the results of the screening tests.

The bone marrow

In the adult, blood production is confined to the skull, spine, pelvis, and upper ends of the long bones. It is often necessary to examine the bone marrow in disorders of the blood and this can be done either by aspiration with a syringe and a specially designed needle or by removing a core of bone marrow tissue (*trephine biopsy*). Aspirates may be taken from the manubrium or body of the sternum or from the anterior or posterior iliac crest, but trephine samples must be obtained from the iliac crest.

Bone marrow aspirates can be spread on slides and stained in the same way as peripheral blood, or they may be examined histologically after formalin fixation. Trephine samples are fixed in formalin and processed before examination.

EXAMINATION

The principles of examination of the bone marrow aspirates are the same as those for the peripheral blood, but the slide must be examined under the low power of the microscope to assess cellularity in the fragments at the ends of the trails and to assess megakaryocyte numbers. Erythropoiesis, granulopoiesis, lymphocytes and plasma cells are examined under the high power of the microscope and a search is made for any evidence of infiltration by cells not usually found in the bone marrow (e.g. carcinoma cells). It is important to stain the aspirate by Perls' ferrocyanide Prussian blue method to assess

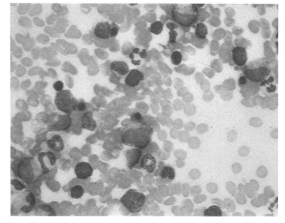

Fig. 18.23   Normal bone marrow aspirate. Nucleated red cells, granulocyte precursors and mature cells are present in this high-power photomicrograph.

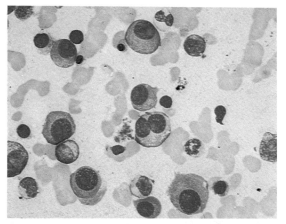

Fig. 18.24   Myelomatosis (bone marrow). The marrow is infiltrated with plasma cells and one binucleate form is present. The red cells show rouleaux formation.

iron (haemosiderin) in fragments and erythroblasts.

Bone marrow appearances are illustrated in Figs 18.4, 18.22, 18.23 and 18.24.

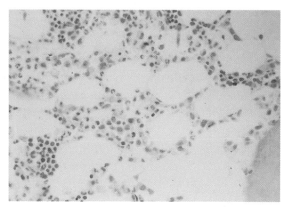

Fig. 18.22   Trephine bone marrow biopsy showing a normally cellular marrow.

CHAPTER 19

Parasites in the blood and faeces

Introduction

Parasitic diseases of humans are a major health problem in tropical countries, especially where clean water is in short supply, and some are also epidemic in the West. It is important to be able to recognize parasitic infestations by microscopy and, when possible, by serological investigations (see Figs 19.1 and 19.2). The more important of these methods are described in this chapter.

Parasites in the blood

The blood forms a habitat for several parasites of major importance. There are three categories: the bacteria, protozoa and helminths or worms (Table 19.1). The main approaches to their diagnosis, often used in combination, are:
- direct diagnosis (finding the parasite);
- indirect diagnosis (finding antibodies to the parasite); and
- circumstantial diagnosis (by identifying the unique pathological changes found in the disease).

The following discussion covers these areas and is focused primarily on the major haemoparasitic diseases. The reader is recommended to consult larger works for information on the other diseases not covered here but listed in Table 19.1.

Malaria

Despite intensive worldwide attempts to contain it, malaria remains the most serious and widespread protozoal infection of humans. Current worldwide statistics estimate a prevalence of some 489 million cases of clinical malaria, of which around 2.3 million are fatal annually. The disease has a wide distribution essentially between 60°N and 40°S of the Equator. Importation of malaria into non-malaria-endemic regions is becoming an increasing problem.

The classical clinical features of malaria infections are paroxysms of fever; most patients present with fever of unknown origin. Since malaria is an emergency in which any delay in diagnosis or treatment may substantially increase morbidity and mortality, it is vital to take a blood sample as soon as possible into EDTA for malaria diagnosis. After blood collection, thin blood films stained with Giemsa should be made immediately and examined microscopically for parasites using ×600 magnification and scanning at least 100 fields before concluding that no parasites are present. Even then, malaria cannot be excluded by a single negative film and a repeat blood sample should be examined several hours later and a thick blood film also made.

A haematology screen using either manual techniques or automated apparatus, such as the Technicon H2, provides useful clues to the presence of malaria. The presence of the disease should be suspected if there is:
- a low white blood cell count ($<4 \times 10^9$/litre);
- thrombocytopenia ($<150 \times 10^9$/litre); or
- increased numbers of atypical lymphocytes ($>4\%$).

Identification of the species of malaria and the percentage of red cells infected are important for subsequent management and treatment. Four species of malaria parasite are involved, each with characteristic morphological and staining properties.

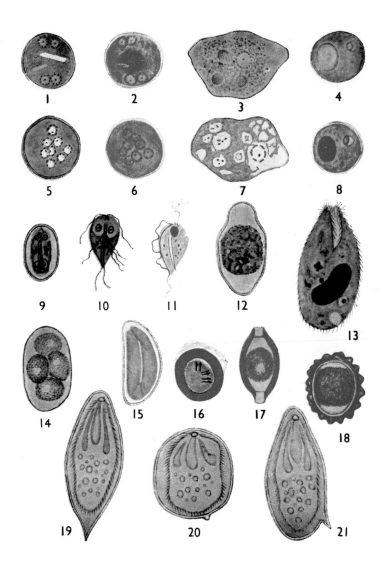

Fig. 19.1 Intestinal parasites.

1 *Entamoeba histolytica.* Fully developed four-nucleated cyst, containing chromatid bodies, as seen in saline preparations. ×1500.

2 *Entamoeba histolytica.* Four-nucleated cyst as seen in iodine preparation. ×1500.

3 *Entamoeba histolytica.* Active form, containing included red blood cells, as seen in saline preparations. ×1500.

4 *Iodamoeba bütschlii.* Cyst, as seen in saline preparations. Note the unstained glycogen vacuole. ×1500.

5 *Entamoeba coli.* Fully developed eight-nucleated cyst, as seen in saline preparations. ×1500.

6 *Entamoeba coli.* Eight-nucleated cyst stained by Lugol's iodine solution. ×1500.

7 *Entamoeba coli.* Active form, as seen in saline preparations. ×1500.

8 *Iodamoeba bütschlii.* Cyst stained by Lugol's iodine solution. ×1500.

9 *Giardia lamblia.* Cyst form, stained by Heidenhain's haematoxylin. ×1500.

10 *Giardia lamblia.* Active form, stained by Heidenhain's haematoxylin. ×1500.

11 *Trichomonas hominis.* Stained by Giemsa's method. ×1500.

12 *Isospora belli (I. hominis).* Undeveloped oocyst as passed in human faeces. ×500.

13 *Balantidium coli.* Active form stained by Heidenhain's haematoxylin. ×350.

14 Ova of *Ankylostoma duodenale* (hookworm). ×500.

15 Ova of *Enterobius vermicularis* (threadworm). ×500.

16 Ova of *Taenia solium* and *T. saginata* (tapeworms). ×500.

17 Ova of *Trichuris trichiura* (whipworm). ×500.

18 Ova of *Ascaris lumbricoides* (roundworm). ×500.

19 Ova of *Schistosoma haematobium.* ×300.

20 Ova of *Schistosoma japonicum.* ×300.

21 Ova of *Schistosoma mansoni.* ×300.

All magnifications approximate.
Drawings by W. Cooper.

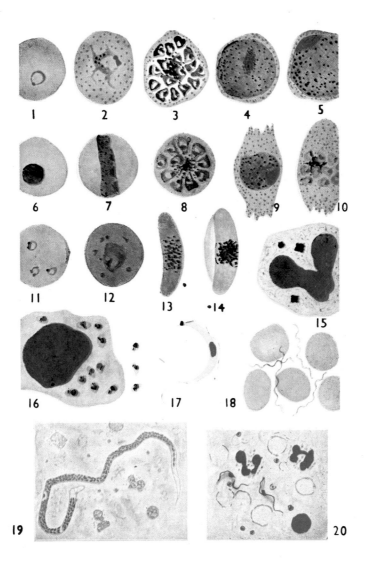

Fig. 19.2 Parasites of the blood.
1 *Plasmodium vivax.* Ring stage. ×2000.
2 *Plasmodium vivax.* Amoeboid form. ×2000.
3 *Plasmodium vivax.* Fully developed schizont. ×2000.
4 *Plasmodium vivax.* Male gametocyte. ×2000.
5 *Plasmodium vivax.* Female gametocyte. ×2000.
6 *Plasmodium malariae.* 'Compact' form. ×2000.
7 *Plasmodium malariae.* 'Band' form. ×2000.
8 *Plasmodium malariae.* Fully developed schizont. ×2000.
9 *Plasmodium ovale.* Female gametocyte. ×2000.
10 *Plasmodium ovale.* Fully developed schizont. ×2000.
11 *Plasmodium falciparum.* Red blood corpuscles containing various types of young ring. ×2000.
12 *Plasmodium falciparum.* 'Old' ring, showing altered staining reaction and Maurer's dots. ×2000.
13 *Plasmodium falciparum.* Male gametocyte or crescent. ×2000.

14 *Plasmodium falciparum.* Female gametocyte or crescent. ×2000.
15 *Plasmodium falciparum.* Pigment in polymorphonuclear leucocyte. ×2000.
16 *Leishmania donovani* from a spleen smear. Some lying free and others within the cytoplasm of an endothelial cell. ×2000.
17 *Trypanosoma cruzi.* Adult form as seen occasionally in the blood of patients suffering from Chagas' disease. ×2000.
18 *Borrelia recurrentis.* ×2000.
19 *Filaria loa.* ×600.
20 *Trypanosoma rhodesiense* as seen in a thick blood film of patients suffering from trypanosomiasis. ×1000.

Drawings by W. Cooper.

	Species	Vector	Reservoir host	Disease
Bacteria				
Spirochaetes	*Borrelia duttoni*	Tick	None	Tick-borne relapsing fever
	Borrelia burgdorferi	Tick	Rodents	Lyme disease
Gram-negative	*Bartonelia bacilliformis*	Sandflies (*Lutzomya*)	None	Oroya fever
Protozoa				
	Plasmodium spp.	Mosquito (*Anopheles* spp.)	None	Malaria
	Trypanosoma spp. (African)	Tsetse flies (*Glossina*)	Game, domestic animals	African trypanosomiasis (Sleeping sickness)
	Trypanosoma cruzi (S American)	Reduviid bugs	Dogs	S American trypanosomiasis (Chagas' disease)
	Leishmania spp.	Sandflies (*Phlebotomus*)	Dogs	Leishmaniasis (visceral and cutaneous)
	Babesia spp.	Ticks	Cattle, rodents	Babesiosis
Helminths				
	Wuchereria bancrofti	Mosquito (*Culex, Aedes*)		Filariasis (Elephantiasis)
	Loa loa	Horsefly (*Chrysops*)		Loaiasis
	Brugia malayi	Mosquito (*Mansonia*)	None	Filariasis (Elephantiasis)
	Mansonella perstans (*Dipetalonema perstans*)	Mosquito (*Cullicoides*)		Filariasis

Table 19.1 The major blood parasites.

PLASMODIUM FALCIPARUM

This species produces falciparum malaria, formerly known as malignant tertian malaria. It is the most widespread and serious form of malaria, accounting for 80% of malaria cases worldwide. The parasite has a high multiplication rate, infecting red cells of all ages, and therefore produces the highest parasitaemias. The incubation period is 8–15 days following the bite of an infected *Anopheles* mosquito, when the classical *ring stages* can be seen in the peripheral blood. The parasite divides by binary fission within erythrocytes, a process known as erythrocytic *schizogony*, to produce infected red blood cells (*schizonts*) containing 8–32 individual *merozoites* which go on to invade new erythrocytes when the schizont ruptures (schizogony). This erythrocytic cycle takes 48 hours to complete.

The ring forms consist of a rim of cytoplasm which stains blue and a small nucleus or chromatin dot which stains purple. *P. falciparum* can be distinguished from other species in that the rings are small and delicate, with multiply invaded cells in severe infections, double chromatin dots and marginal or accole forms (Fig. 19.3a and b). Unlike the situation in other species of *Plasmodium*, the trophozoites and schizonts of *P. falciparum* withdraw from the peripheral circulation and sequester in the internal organs, in particular within capillaries in the brain. Thus, these two stages are never seen in the periph-

eral blood. Characteristic of falciparum infections, usually of long duration (as occurs in semi-immune individuals from malaria-endemic regions), is the presence of a few crescent-shaped male and female *gametocytes*, the sexual stages of the parasite responsible for infection of mosquitoes and transmission of the disease. These gametocytes are easily recognizable (Fig. 19.3b).

In many areas where *P. falciparum* occurs, other malaria species are also transmitted and mixed infections should not be overlooked. It is important that the full number of microscope fields are examined, even when falciparum parasites are viewed in the first few fields.

A heavy parasitaemia indicates a severe infection (although a light parasitaemia does not exclude severe infection) for which the patient requires special management. A falciparum blood film report should therefore always include an estimation of the *parasite density*. A quantitative report also allows a patient's response to treatment to be assessed where parasite resistance to the drugs being used is suspected. Parasite density can be estimated as a percentage of red cells infected or as the number of parasites per microlitre of blood.

Calculation of the percentage of red cells infected. This is performed by counting at least 1000 red cells and expressing the number of parasitized cells as a

Fig. 19.3 (a) *Plasmodium falciparum* taken from *in vitro* culture showing mature erythrocytic schizonts containing individual merozoites (M) (b) Blood film from an African child with *P. falciparum* infection showing the classical sickle-shaped gametocyte. (c) Erythrophagocytosis by a peripheral blood monocyte of a non-parasitized red cell (arrow) in a falciparum infection. (d) *P. vivax* showing the large amoeboid ring (R) and gametocyte (G). The infected red cell is enlarged and the cytoplasm contains Schuffner's dots. (e) Thin blood film from a patient in Thailand showing the rare occurrence of dual invasion of red cells by *P. vivax* and *P. falciparum*. Single invasion of *P. falciparum* is also present as indicated by the small fine rings with double chromatin dots typical of this species (photograph courtesy of M. Guy). (f) Classical 'band' trophozoite of *P. malariae* where the cytoplasm of the parasite lies diagonally across the red cell which does not contain Schuffner's dots. (g) *P. ovale* showing the typical appearance of a trophozoite (T) within an oval-shaped red cell with fimbriated edges and the large rings of this species in a doubly invaded erythrocyte. Like *P. vivax*, the red cells contain Schuffner's dots.

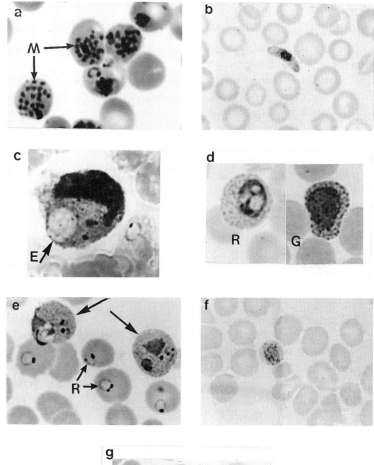

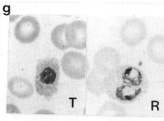

percentage of this number. Most parasitaemias give a value from 1 to 10%. When 10–20% of cells are infected the prognosis is serious; with 20–30% it is grave, and over 30% it is exceptionally grave with the chance of fatality.

Measurement of the number of parasites in 1 μl of blood. Absolute numbers of parasites are estimated by counting parasites against the patient's white blood cell count. Malaria pigment seen within the cytoplasm of monocytes and neutrophils, and occasionally erythrophagocytosis, may be seen in a patient who has recently recovered from an acute attack (Fig. 19.3c).

The World Health Organization (WHO) suggests that the following laboratory indices should be considered as indicative of poor prognosis in falciparum malaria.

- High parasitaemia with > 5% parasitized red cells (250 000 parasites μl/blood)
- Presence of schizonts in peripheral blood films
- Peripheral leucocytosis > 12 000/μl
- High serum tumour necrosis factor alpha (TNFα)
- Haematocrit < 20% (Hb < 7.1 g/dl)
- Blood glucose < 2.2 mmol/litre
- Serum creatinine > 265 μmol/litre
- Raised serum aminotransferases.

Cerebral malaria

Cerebral malaria is the most common clinical presentation of severe falciparum malaria and has an associated 50% fatality rate despite treatment. Sequestration of *P. falciparum* schizonts from the peripheral blood and their attachment to endothelial cells, particularly cells of the post-capillary venules in the brain, causes vessel blockage, cerebral anoxia and associated pathological changes. Clinical examination should be performed urgently in two phases and the patient nursed with intensive care facilities.

First, a brief examination should be carried out to establish the diagnosis (to exclude meningitis and neurotropic viruses) and to detect any parasites, hypoglycaemia, anaemia, renal failure and pulmonary oedema.

Second, a more thorough examination should be performed when treatment is underway. Patients who have had an untreated falciparum infection for several weeks invariably present with severe headache, drowsiness, delirium and convulsions. Examination of the fundus in such a patient is an important part of the physical examination since the presence of retinal haemorrhages in non-comatose patients usually indicates that the person is likely to develop cerebral malaria within hours. Many patients are admitted with unrousable coma and display classical decerebrate rigidity. These features of cerebral malaria can be caused by the associated hypoglycaemia and without blood glucose measurements the two cannot be distinguished. However, only a minority of patients respond to intravenous dextrose. In young African children living in malaria-endemic regions, the neurological signs are those of diffuse encephalopathy with symmetrical upper motor neurone signs and brainstem disturbances, including dysconjugate gaze palsies, stertorous breathing, hypertonicity, absent abdominal reflexes, and retinal haemorrhages.

PLASMODIUM VIVAX

Malaria caused by *Plasmodium vivax* is referred to as vivax malaria, formerly known as benign tertian malaria. It is the main cause of malaria in temperate and subtropical regions and is rarely encountered in West Africa where natural resistance is found. The resistance relates to the lack of Duffy blood group antigens on the red cells of the indigenous population which act as receptors recognized by vivax merozoites for successful invasion into erythrocytes. It is the most common parasite seen in patients from the Indian subcontinent.

P. vivax preferentially invades reticulocytes and therefore only rarely do more than 2% of the red cell population become parasitized. Erythrocyte schizogony occurs every 72 hours within the peripheral blood and trophozoites, schizonts and gametocytes can be viewed in blood films. The young ring form is frequently difficult to differentiate from that of *P. falciparum*. However, the late ring and trophozoites are large and amoeboid. The infected red cell is enlarged and if correctly stained shows well-defined Schuffner's dots (Fig. 19.3d). Mature schizonts contain brown pigment and between 12 and 24 merozoites. Mixed infections do occur and dual parasitization of *single* cells by *P. vivax* and *P. falciparum* has been known (Fig. 19.3e).

P. vivax is a relapsing species with each relapse being initiated by the activation and differentiation of latent *hypnozoite* forms within liver cells. If treatment of vivax malaria does not include concurrent treatment (with primaquine) to kill the hypnozoites, then relapses may occur at intervals of up to 3 years or more after the primary attack.

PLASMODIUM MALARIAE

Malariae malaria, formerly known as quartan malaria, is endemic in the tropics and subtropics where, in Africa, it accounts for up to 25% of *Plasmodium* infections and often accompanies infection with *P. falciparum*. Erythrocytic schizogony is slower than in falciparum malaria, taking 72 hours to complete.

Since parasite numbers are normally low (<1% of red cells are infected), laboratory confirmation requires careful examination of a thick blood film backed by a prolonged search on a thin film for identification of species. The ring forms are large ('bird's eye' rings) and the red cell cytoplasm is devoid of Schuffner's dots (unlike *P. vivax* and *P. ovale*). Trophozoites, schizonts and gametocytes can be seen in the blood film. Two useful features that confirm diagnosis of malariae infection are the presence of band form trophozoites (Fig 19.3f) and the occasional compact 'daisy head' schizont containing 8–12 merozoites.

There is no dormant hypnozoite stage in *P. malariae* and thus no relapses.

PLASMODIUM OVALE

Malaria caused by *P. ovale* is referred to as ovale malaria and was previously known as ovale tertian malaria. Like *P. vivax* it is a relapsing species and mixed infection with *P. falciparum* is common. It has a restricted distribution and low prevalence, mainly in West Africa.

All stages of erythrocyte schizogony are found in the peripheral blood and rarely do more than 2% of red cells become parasitized. The rings are large and obvious and multiple invasion is sometimes seen. The red cell cytoplasm contains Schuffner's dots and 20–30% of infected cells take on an oval shape with fimbriated (ragged) ends, especially those containing late trophozoites and schizonts (Fig. 19.3g).

NEW TECHNIQUES TO ASSIST CLINICAL DIAGNOSIS

During the last decade several new techniques have been developed to improve the speed and sensitivity of standard microscopy, although most have limitations in developing countries for technical and financial reasons.

Species-specific *DNA probes*, are available for the detection of *P. falciparum* and *P. vivax*. Probes containing repetitive sequences of *P. falciparum* DNA, are able to detect a parasitaemia of 0.001%. This is less sensitive than standard microscopy, which in the hands of a trained microscopist detects a parasitaemia of 0.0004%. The introduction of the polymerase chain reaction (PCR) technique has increased the sensitivity of molecular probes, which are most suited for mass screening of bloods in epidemiological studies and in blood banks.

Ribosomal RNA (rRNA) probes, developed because rRNA is the most abundant cellular macromolecule and therefore an obvious target, have proved to be more sensitive. Using the *P. falciparum* probe, it has been possible to detect as little as 13 fg of target, representing a parasitaemia of 0.00001%.

A newly developed, commercially available diagnostic test is now available which relies on the staining of parasite DNA and RNA by a *fluorescent probe*. The QBC (quantitative buffy coat) combines concentration of infected red cells by centrifugation (they have a greater density than uninfected cells) with staining of parasites with acridine orange. The manufacturers have designed simple instrumentation and tubes for the use of QBC in rural and tropical environments and claim a sensitivity greater than that of a thick film. Detection of one parasitized cell in the presence of 100 million uninfected cells is claimed.

African trypanosomiasis

Two organisms cause African trypanosomiasis or sleeping sickness:

- *Trypanosoma brucei gambiense* produces *gambiense sleeping sickness*, a chronic debilitating disease found in Central and West Africa, and
- *T. b. rhodesiense* produces *rhodesiense sleeping sickness*, a more acute disease found in Central and East Africa.

Another subspecies, *T. b. brucei* with a similar East African geographical distribution infects only animals. The different subspecies are morphologically identical and can be distinguished with certainty only by biochemical techniques, such as electrophoretic typing of their isoenzymes. The parasite is transmitted by the bite of the tsetse fly (*Glossina* spp.), a genus only found on the African continent.

Although sleeping sickness claims relatively few lives today, the risk of severe epidemics requires that surveillance and active control measures are maintained in endemic regions. This involves the application of specific and reliable diagnostic techniques.

Demonstration of the organism itself is obviously the best diagnostic procedure. Trypanosomes are elongated flagellate protozoa some 14–30 μm long and 1–3 μm broad (Fig. 19.4). The flagellum arises from an organelle called the kinetoplast, which contains double-stranded DNA, and this feature has been exploited for the development of molecular probes (see below). The circulating forms are termed *trypnomastigotes* and these multiply by binary fission within the blood and subsequently invade a wide variety of tissues including the brain during the late stages of the disease.

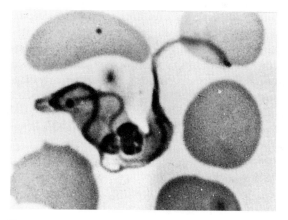

Fig. 19.4 Trypomastigote of *Trypanosoma brucei brucei* dividing by binary fission. It has two flagella, nuclei and kinetoplasts.

DIAGNOSIS

Confirmation of the clinical diagnosis (hepatosplenomegaly, lymphadenopathy, anaemia, thrombocytopenia, wasting and altered mental state) is as follows.

Examination of blood for trypnomastigotes. During early infection actively mobile parasites may be seen in wet blood preparations and Giemsa-stained blood films, although this is often unsuccessful as a result of the small number of parasites present, and to the daily fluctuations in detectable parasite numbers (*T. b. rhodesiense* is easier to find than *T. b. gambiense*). Trypanosomes must not be confused with microfilariae (see below) which may be present in the blood of the same donor.

Miniature Anion Exchange Column concentration (MAEC). The Sephadex anion 'minicolumn' permits the detection of very small numbers of trypanosomes in specimens of blood or cerebral spinal fluid (CSF). It is an invaluable diagnostic aid in individual patients and has also been used in field studies.

Whole blood from the patient is added to the column and washed through with an appropriate buffer. The red cells adhere to the column but the less strongly charged trypanosomes pass through in the eluate and can be concentrated by centrifugation. Full details of this technique and availability of MAEC kits can be obtained from the WHO.

Examination of lymph node aspirates. Cervical lymphadenopathy, especially in the posterior triangle of the neck ('*Winterbottom's sign*'), is an important clinical diagnostic feature of gambiense sleeping sickness which calls for gland puncture. The trypanosomes are easily identified in the wet preparation and their identity confirmed by staining. This is a valuable and simple means of providing early diagnosis.

Examination of cerebral spinal fluid (CSF). After several months (*T. b. rhodesiense*) or years (*T. b. gambiense*) trypanosomes invade the central nervous system, resulting in a meningoencephalitis. A lumbar puncture should, therefore, be performed in patients with confused mental state. In such instances and in contrast with viral meningitis, tuberculous meningitis and neurosyphilis, the CSF will reveal a lymphocyte pleocytosis and an increased protein content, of which IgM represents >10%. Trypanosomes may also be seen in stained films of a centrifuge deposit or by using CSF applied to the minicolumn described above.

Testing for anti-trypanosome antibodies. Tests used in the serological diagnosis of trypanosomiasis include an indirect fluorescent antibody test (IFA) and an enzyme-linked immunosorbent assay (ELISA) using commercially available antigens. The card agglutination test (CATT) is a recent addition to the commercial market and is widely used (particularly for field surveys) to assist in the diagnosis and control of gambiense trypanosomiasis. Anti-trypanosomal IgM can be detected using this simple test which agglutinates freeze-dried trypanosomes fixed to the card.

DNA probes. DNA probes have yet to be completely evaluated. Analysis of trypanosome DNA reveals that in *T. b. brucei*, for example, highly repetitive sequences represent 12% of total nuclear DNA, making species-specific DNA probes a reality for diagnosis. In addition, kinetoplast DNA (kDNA) minicircles are present at approximately 5000–10 000 per genome and thus represent good candidates for use in a sensitive DNA hybridization assay.

ADDITIONAL FEATURES OF AFRICAN TRYPANOSOMIASIS

Analysis of blood and serum from a trypanosomiasis patient will reveal an anaemia, thrombocytopenia, raised erythrocyte sedimentation rate (ESR) and autoagglutination and rouleaux formation of red cells. The two latter features result from the exceptionally high serum IgM (7–10 times the local mean).

South American trypanosomiasis

Trypanosoma cruzi causes South American trypanosomiasis or *Chagas' disease*. As the name implies, it occurs only in the Americas, especially in tropical and subtropical Latin American countries. It is estimated that around 16–18 million people are infected and 65 million at risk of infection. Chagas' disease is the main cause of chronic heart disease in these parts, where some 20–30% of all infected will develop Chagasic cardiomyopathy.

T. cruzi is naturally transmitted through contact with the faeces of an infected haemophagus bug of the family Reduviidae—the cone-nose or kissing bugs. The faeces contain the infective *trypomastigotes* which are deposited on mucous membranes, particularly around the eye, as the bugs feed. The parasites enter through the bite wound or penetrate the membrane. Once in the bloodstream trypomastig-otes invade reticuloendothelial and other tissue cells, especially those of the heart muscle, nerves, skeletal muscle, and smooth muscle of the gastrointestinal tract. Once within the cell they lose the flagellum and become *amastigotes*, multiplying by binary fission. Parasites in the heart cause severe myocarditis, especially in the early stages of infection. The severity of the acute myocarditis seems to seal the eventual fate of the sufferer from chronic cardiac changes which include dysrhythmias of various types, cardiomegaly and complete heart block resulting in sudden death. Muscular degeneration and denervation of segments of the alimentary tract cause mega-oesophagus, megastomach and megacolon (*megasyndrome*) which can be detected radiologically.

Chronic Chagas' disease is incurable, although there are two drugs (Nifurtimox and Benznidazole) used for very early infection (early diagnosis is difficult).

DIAGNOSIS

Several techniques are available for diagnosis as follows.

Detection of trypanosomes in the blood. Try-panosomiasis may be detected in peripheral blood films in early acute infections. As is the case with African trypanosomiasis, only very few trypomastig-otes are present. They are characteristically U- or C-shaped.

Xenodiagnosis. This is an alternative technique often used in chronic cases. Uninfected, susceptible, laboratory-reared bugs are fed on the patient's blood. If trypanosomes are ingested they will multiply and around 25 days later trypomastigotes will be found in the faeces or rectum of the bug.

Serology. The incidence of transfusion-acquired Chagas' disease is very high in some Latin American countries, and serological techniques for the detection of anti-*T. cruzi* antibodies have been developed for the screening of blood donors. The main tests are haemagglutination and immunofluorescence. DNA probes are currently being evaluated.

Visceral leishmaniasis

The leishmaniases comprise several diseases caused by different species of the intracellular protozoan parasite *Leishmania*, of which ten infect humans. The leishmaniases are grouped together under three headings: *cutaneous leishmaniasis*, *mucocutaneous leishmaniasis* and *visceral leishmaniasis*. This section will only deal with the life-threatening visceral disease where the parasite takes up residence intracellularly within reticuloendothelial cells. The disease is spread by the bite of an infected sandfly (*Phleboto-mus*). Visceral leishmaniasis, or kala-azar, in the Old World is caused by *L. donovani* subspecies (*L. d. donovani* and *L. d. infantum*). It is widely distributed, not being confined to the tropics, and can be found in the Mediterranean basin, the Atlantic coast of Portugal, tropical Africa, parts of South America and Central and East Asia.

When an infected sandfly bites a human, flagellate forms of the parasites (*promastigotes*) enter the blood and invade reticuloendothelial cells, notably those of the spleen and liver, where they differentiate into non-flagellate *amastigotes*. These are round oval bodies from 2 to 5 μm in diameter, containing a large nucleus and rod-shaped kinetoplast (Fig. 19.5a) referred to as Leishman–Donovan bodies (*LD bodies*). Amastigotes multiply rapidly inside the

(a)   **(b)**

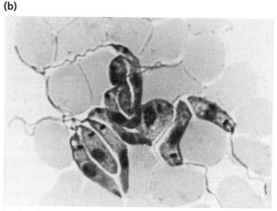

Fig. 19.5 *Leishmania donovani infantum* (a) amastigotes or LD bodies (arrowed) within macrophages in a bone marrow aspirate from a patient with leishmaniasis, and (b) culture of the same bone marrow and differentiation of amastigotes to flagellate promastigotes.

macrophages, eventually leading to rupture of the parasitized cells and dissemination throughout the body, where they are taken up by other phagocytic cells. The incubation period is very variable but is usually between 3 and 18 months.

DIAGNOSIS

Clinically the patient presents with a high temperature and a marked hepatosplenomegaly, lymphadenopathy and characteristic blood changes (see below). If left untreated the infection is invariably fatal, commonly from secondary infections. Severe immunosuppression can make asymptomatic leishmaniasis clinically apparent. Kala-azar should therefore be suspected if the above symptoms are present in an *HIV-positive* patient. Visceral leishmaniasis is often difficult to diagnose and frequently has resulted in incorrect diagnosis such as aplastic anaemia or lymphoma. Only direct diagnosis, that is the demonstration of parasites, is capable of producing true-positive results.

Demonstration of parasites in biopsy specimens. In the human host only intracellular amastigotes can be demonstrated. Biopsy material may be taken from the bone marrow, lymph nodes or, preferably, the spleen. The spleen houses the greatest number of parasitized cells and will frequently give positive results when the bone marrow appears negative. However, splenic puncture is only safe if the organ is large and firm, the patient's platelet count is $>50 \times 10^9$/litre and the prothrombin time normal in order to minimize the risk of bleeding. A film is made of the biopsied material and visualized with a Romanowsky stain. Using oil immersion microscopy, the amastigotes can be seen in groups within mononuclear phagocytic cells. Because the macrophage membrane becomes fragile following parasitization of the cell, it is common for the cell to rupture when the film is being made. Thus amastigotes are frequently found lying free between cells rather than contained within them (Fig. 19.5a). Structurally, amastigotes of *Leishmania* species are similar and differentiation cannot be made on morphological grounds. Occasionally amastigotes can be found in peripheral blood monocytes, especially in Indian and Kenyan visceral leishmaniasis. The blood is centrifuged, the buffy coat removed, stained and examined for amastigotes.

Culture of biopsied material. If amastigotes cannot be seen on the film of the biopsied material, it is important to confirm the presence or absence of *Leishmania* by culturing the aspirated material (which must be maintained in a sterile condition) in insect culture medium at room temperature (24°C) for 3–14 days. The principle is to mimic conditions within the vector gut, so encouraging any amastigotes present to differentiate and emerge from the macrophages as flagellate promastigotes (Fig. 19.5b).

Diagnosis by animal inoculation. If culture facilities are unavailable, biopsied material may be injected intraperitoneally into hamsters which are highly susceptible to infection. After 4–6 weeks, amastigotes are usually found in large numbers in impression smears of the liver and spleen. The one disadvantage of this technique is the long period of time for the disease to reach patency.

Serology for anti-leishmanial antibodies. There are many methods available for use, some commercially available, including IFA and ELISA employing *L. d. donovani* promastigotes as antigen which, because of serological cross-reaction, can additionally be used to diagnose *L. d. infantum.* Unfortunately, cross-reactions also occur with sera from a variety of other infections, including malaria, toxoplasmosis and disseminated tuberculosis, so limiting specificity of the tests.

Molecular probes. Because early identification of leishmaniasis is difficult, even in a well-equipped hospital, improved methods have been much in demand. Present DNA techniques use kinetoplast DNA (kDNA) probes for hybridization to parasites in tissue aspirates. The large DNA differences between different geographical isolates of *Leishmania* has resulted in the development of several thousand recombinant DNA probes which are relatively simple and cheap to prepare. Their more widespread use will open the way for earlier specific treatment and greatly assist epidemiologists concerned with more effective control interventions and the link between variation of clinical disease and geographical isolate.

Characteristic blood changes. Anaemia and thrombocytopenia are typical, but not specific, features of visceral leishmaniasis. One distinctive feature is a marked granulocytopenia, sometimes amounting to an agranulocytosis, another is a gammaglobulinaemia often exceeding 4–5 g/dl.

Filariasis

Filarial worms are nematodes that derive their name from their long hair-like appearance. The adult worms (according to species) live in the lymphatics, connective and other tissues, whereas the larvae, or *microfilariae*, live in the blood. The larvae show what is termed *periodicity*, i.e. they are released periodically into the peripheral blood from lung blood and are therefore found in greater numbers during certain hours. Different species have characteristic periodicities. This is thought to be an adaptation by the parasite to the biting habits of their insect vectors. Being aware of the periodicity of each species is important when taking blood samples for diagnosis of the disease. Greatest numbers of microfilariae may be present during night hours (nocturnal periodicity, e.g. *Wuchereria bancrofti* and *Brugia* spp.) or day hours (diurnal periodicity, e.g. *Loa loa*), although many patients with symptomatic infections have no demonstrable microfilariae in their blood at any time.

The most commonly encountered filarial blood infections are *Wuchereria bancrofti*, *Brugia* spp., *Loa loa* and *Mansonella perstans*.

WUCHERERIA BANCROFTI

This is the most widely distributed of the filarial worms. The most seriously affected areas are India, South-East Asia, China, the east coast of Africa and the Pacific Islands where the parasite causes the disease *Bancroftian filariasis*. The number of infected people is estimated at 81 million worldwide. Infection occurs when larvae are deposited on the skin from an infected mosquito taking a blood meal. The larvae enter the bite wound and make their way to the lymphatics, mature into adults and begin producing more microfilariae which then enter the blood. Adults may live for up to 15 years within the same host. Diagnosis of the disease is made by detection of microfilariae in the blood (which must be collected between 22.00 and 04.00 hours). Microfilariae of *W. bancrofti* are sheathed and large (300 × 10 μm) compared with other species (Fig. 19.6) and can be identified in wet and stained blood films.

Accompanying *W. bancrofti*—indeed, any filarial infection—is a pronounced blood eosinophilia and raised serum IgE. The adults within the lymphatics cause obstruction, especially in the leg, progressing in chronic cases to enormously enlarged limbs called 'elephantiasis'. This may also arise in the arm, breast or scrotum. By this stage microfilariae are rarely

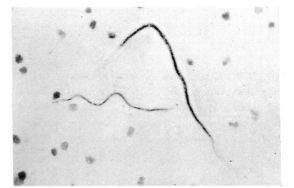

Fig. 19.6 Microfilariae in a blood film. Two species are present—the unsheathed smaller *Mansonella perstans* is readily distinguished from the larger sheathed *Loa loa*.

found in blood films. The dilated lymph vessels occasionally rupture and discharge chyle into the urinary tract, thus producing the milky appearance known as *chyluria*.

BRUGIA

Brugia malayi and *B. timori* cause *lymphatic filariasis* (*Malayan filariasis*) and are endemic in parts of South-East Asia, India, the Philippines, Vietnam and China. The life cycle of the parasite is similar to that of *W. bancrofti*, but frequently gives rise to a symptomless infection. Diagnosis is as for bancroftian filariasis.

LOA LOA

Loa loa (the 'eye worm') causes *loiasis*, also known as subcutaneous filariasis or *Calabar swelling*. The latter are recurrent large swellings seen in the hand, wrists and forearm which last about 3 days and indicate the tracks of the migrating adult worms in the connective tissue. A marked eosinophilia (60–90%) accompanies this phase of the infection. Sometimes the worms can be seen migrating under the conjunctiva causing considerable irritation and congestion. The adult can be extracted with fine forceps after anaesthetizing the conjunctiva.

The disease is endemic in many parts where *W. bancrofti* exists. The diurnal microfilariae can be detected in peripheral blood taken between 10.00 and 15.00 hours. As with the other filarial infections, high numbers of microfilariae should always be reported because serious complications can arise when treating heavily infected persons.

MANSONELLA PERSTANS

Formerly called *Dipetalonema perstans*, this is a very common non-pathogenic species found in tropical

Africa and parts of South America. The microfilariae are much smaller ($190 \times 4 \mu m$) than those of the other species.

Since there is considerable geographical overlap in the distribution of species, it is important to distinguish between the different microfilariae. This is usually made on differences in size, shape, presence or absence of a sheath, nuclei within the tail, and the periodicity.

Parasites in faeces

The major reason for the examination (both macroscopically and microscopically) of a faecal sample is to detect cysts and eggs, and in a minority of cases adult parasites themselves. Because the release of helminth eggs and protozoan cysts is irregular, three, and in some instances, six samples should be examined on separate (preferably alternate) days. In some instances (e.g. when searching for *Entamoeba histolytica* trophozoites—see below), the sample should be examined as soon as possible (preferably <1 hour) after collection in the *fresh* state. Although 'formed' stool samples can be stored at 4°C overnight, examination should, when at all possible, be carried out on the same day. Samples that cannot be delivered to the laboratory promptly can be posted after emulsification in a preservative fluid (e.g. Bayer's solution or methiolate–iodine–formalin) in order to maintain parasites in a recognizable state and to allow a concentration and staining technique to be applied later.

A record of the macroscopical state of the faecal sample should always be kept, especially its composition and colour, and the presence of adult parasites must be recorded.

Microscopic examination involves direct visualization of cysts, ova and parasites, and use of a concentration technique. About 2 mg of faeces should be emulsified in a single drop (less if the sample is fluid) of warm (37°C) saline using a wooden applicator; a coverslip is then applied. When blood and/or mucus is present it should be examined separately, for it is especially likely to contain *E. histolytica* trophozoites. The presence of undigested food, bacteria, yeasts, crystals or fat globules should also be noted. The value of applying a concentration technique (to a 'formed' specimen) is that it significantly increases the likelihood of detecting ova, cysts or lar-

vae, especially when the load of infection is light. Sedimentation (e.g. modified formol–ether sedimentation) or zinc sulphate centrifugal flotation techniques can also be used; in the former, parasites are deposited at the bottom of the tube, and in the latter they float towards the surface of a liquid of high specific gravity, most debris remaining at the bottom. Although they do allow subsequent application of a staining method, concentration techniques destroy trophozoites and distort the cellular exudates.

Protozoa

In clinical practice, the most important protozoan parasite of the gastrointestinal tract, that is, the colorectum, is *Entamoeba histolytica*. Figure 19.7 summarizes methods used for its identification. Table 19.2 summarizes some classical differences between *E. histolytica* and *Entamoeba coli* (and other nonpathogenic amoebae); trophozoites of *E. histolytica* are invasive (and contain ingested host-erythrocytes) only if they belong to an appropriate zymodeme. In amoebic dysentery, direct microscopy of a fresh faecal sample (at 37°C) reveals motile trophozoites and cellular exudate. Presence of cysts of *E. histolytica* in the absence of trophozoites is defined as the *cyst carrier state*. A cellular exudate may coexist with both this and *Balantidium coli*, and also with *Shigella* sp. and *Campylobacter* sp. infection.

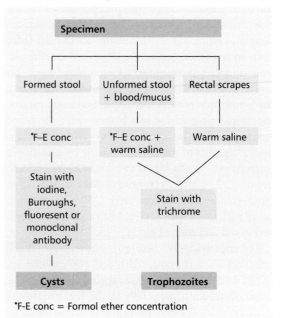

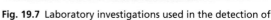

*F-E conc = Formol ether concentration

Fig. 19.7 Laboratory investigations used in the detection of *Entamoeba histolytica* in a faecal sample.

	Invasive *E. histolytica*	*Entamoeba coli*	Other
Trophozoite:			
Occurrence	Present at high cncentration in dysenteric stool	Never at high concentration	Variable
Size	10–60 μm	20–40 μm (often larger than *E. histolytica*)	Usually smaller, but *Balantidium coli* 50–200 μm
Mobility	Active: large pseudopodia	Sluggish, small pseudopodia	Variable
Cytoplasm	Ingested erythrocytes	Never contains erythrocytes	Variable
Cyst:			
Size	9–14.5 μm (usually nearer 10 μm)	14–30 μm (usually nearer 20 μm)	Usually smaller; but *Balantidium coli* 5–60 μm
Nucleus (fewer in young)	4 when mature	8 when mature	1–4
Cytoplasm (chromatoidal bars diminish as cyst matures)	Chromatoid bars present in fresh specimen. Diffuse glycogen	Chromatoid bars rarely seen	*Iodamoeba* sp. has a compact glycogen vacuole
Cyst wall	Thin	Thicker than *E. histolytica*	Variable

Table 19.2 Some differentiating features between *Entamoeba histolytica*, *Entamoeba coli* and other non-pathogenic amoebae.

The presence of polymorphonuclear neutrophils, macrophages, erythrocytes and epithelial cells should be noted. Pus cells and macrophages are present in greater numbers in *Shigella* sp. compared with *E. histolytica* dysentery, whereas the pH of a faecal sample is usually more acid in *E. histolytica* compared with *Shigella* sp. infection. Table 19.3 summarizes other protozoan parasites which may be detected in a faecal sample, together with their site of origin. Some of these are depicted in Fig. 19.1.

Giardia lamblia is a small intestinal protozoan parasite that can cause small intestinal malabsorption, resulting in a faecal sample with a high fat content. While the cyst form is often detectable, albeit intermittently, in a faecal sample, jejunal fluid or biopsy reveals the flagellated trophozoite.

Cryptosporidium sp. and *Isospora belli* (and possibly *Sarcocystis hominis*) can also be associated with

malabsorption and are opportunistic in AIDS. Oocysts are easily recognizable in a faecal sample, jejunal fluid or biopsy.

DIAGNOSIS

There are several useful staining techniques for protozoa. Temporary stains include Lugol's iodine, Burrough's stain, acridine orange and eosin/saline. Permanent stains include Giemsa, a modified rapid Field's stain, and a trichrome method, consisting of a modified Gomori technique. When *Cryptosporidium* sp. and *I. belli* oocysts are being sought, it is essential to use an acid-fast technique, e.g. a modified Ziehl–Neilsen or the phenol-auramine method, since routine stains do not allow easy identification.

Rectal scrapes often give a higher yield of positive results when an *E. histolytica* infection is suspected. Exudate should be obtained proctoscopically and

Usual anatomical site	Amoebae	Flagellate	Ciliate	Coccidia
Small intestine		*Giardia lamblia**		*Cryptosporidium* sp.* *Isospora belli** *Sarcocystis hominis** *Blastocystis hominis**†
Colo-rectum	*Entamoeba histolytica** *Entamoeba coli* *Entamoeba hartmanni* *Iodamoeba butschlei* *Endolimax nana* *Dientamoeba fragilis*	*Chilomastix mesnili* *Trichomonas hominis* *Enteromonas* sp. *Retortamonas* sp.	*Balantidium coli**	

* Pathogenic organism.
† Classification remains undetermined.

Table 19.3 Faecal protozoa.

immediately examined microscopically. Active trophozoites, not necessarily visualized in a fresh faecal sample, may be demonstrable.

Helminths

Worms are the commonest of all intestinal parasites.

NEMATODES (ROUNDWORMS)

Nematodes are all cylindrical, pointed at both ends, and unsegmented. The male is usually smaller than the female. They contain a tough, smooth, outer cuticle and a body cavity containing a well-developed intestinal tract. The mouth may contain rudimentary teeth or cutting plates for attachment to the mucosal surface. The largest nematode parasitic in humans, *Ascaris lumbricoides* (male 15 cm; female 25 cm), may be detected either in a faecal sample or in vomit. Differentiation from the earthworm, which is not infrequently delivered to the laboratory by an anxious patient after it has been noticed in a lavatory, is usually straightforward, the earthworm being browner in colour. The hookworms (*Ankylostoma duodenale* and *Necator americanus*) are much smaller (female approximately 8 mm) and contain two hook-like teeth at the top and two triangular cutting plates at the bottom. These are very important causes of iron-deficient microcytic anaemia in most tropical countries. Both *A. lumbricoides* and hookworm are extremely common in most tropical countries, infecting a very high proportion of the indigenous population.

Enterobius vermicularis (threadworm)

An extremely prevalent nematode (arguably the most common intestinal helminth to afflict the human species), the threadworm is worldwide in distribution. The female is 8–12 mm and the male 2–4 mm in length; the latter dies rapidly after fertilizing the female. The major clinical manifestation is pruritus ani. Both adult worms and eggs can be recovered from perianal skin. Several methods are available. A saline-moistened swab can be gently rubbed around the perianal area and afterwards agitated in a small tube of normal saline to dislodge the eggs. After centrifugation, the supernatant is decanted and the deposit examined microscopically. Alternatively, a sellotape strip can be placed across the anus in the early morning; after removal this is applied (sticky side down) on to a microscope slide.

Trichuris trichiura (the whipworm) is a faecal nematode which causes symptoms only in children when present at high concentration. Eggs are readily detectable in a faecal sample.

Strongyloides stercoralis

This is the most difficult nematode to detect. Ova are not usually detectable in a faecal sample since the eggs hatch to produce larvae before they reach the anus. The larvae (200–250 μm in length) may, however, be demonstrable; a culture technique often allows identification of these even when they are too scanty for detection by a concentration technique.

CESTODES (TAPEWORMS)

Although a number of different species can parasitize humans, the two most common (and important) are *Taenia solium* and *T. saginata*. The importance of *T. solium* (the pork tapeworm) is that its larva is the causative agent in neurocysticercosis. Human infection is acquired by ingestion of *T. solium* eggs. Adult worms can reach a length of 4–8 m. Flat white segments of these worms are easily recognizable. After successful chemotherapy the entire worm (complete with head, neck and strobila) should be passed in the stool. Identification of the head (*T. solium* 1 mm and *T. saginata* 1–2 mm) is important, although it is difficult after praziquantel or niclosamide chemotherapy, both of which tend to dissolve this structure. For identification, a purged stool can be poured through a sieve of fine mesh and examined for the scolex (often broken off from the rest of the body with about 0.5 cm of the neck remaining). When detected it can be squashed in a drop of saline under a coverslip and identified microscopically. It possesses four suckers and a rostellum (a double row of alternating hooks). Various techniques can be used for fixation and staining of adult helminths (these can be found in specialized manuals of parasitology). They are particularly useful for establishing a permanent record.

The fish tapeworm, *Diphyllobothrium latum* (present in Finland and Sweden), may reach a length of 3–10 m in the human bowel. A rare clinical manifestation is macrocytic (B_{12}-deficient) anaemia.

EGGS

Methods used for the concentration of nematode, cestode or trematode eggs are the same as those used for cysts. Eggs of *Schistosoma mansoni*, *S. intercalatum*, *S. matthei*, *S. japonicum* and *S. mekongi* can usually be detected in a faecal sample or rectal biopsy specimen; *S. haematobium* can also occasionally be found in the latter, but causes urinary tract disease.

Figure 19.1 shows diagrams of eggs of human helminths as seen in a faecal sample; once detected, identification of these should be straightforward. All tropical laboratories should possess a collection of examples for use as a reference collection.

Potential difficulties in identification of cysts, eggs and larvae

The greatest problem lies in pronouncing a faecal sample 'negative'. Once evidence of a parasitosis has been established, identification is relatively straightforward. However, misidentification of some non-pathogenic objects as parasites is a major problem; some of the difficulties are as follows.

- Protozoan cysts can be confused with air bubbles, fat globules or yeasts; if iodine is added to the wet preparation the internal structure of the cyst(s) can be visualized.
- Trophozoites of pathogenic strains of *Entamoeba histolytica* must be differentiated from those of non-pathogenic amoebic trophozoites and macrophages.
- Eggs of some helminths, especially those of *Trichuris trichiura* and *Taenia* sp., can be confused with pollen grains.

- *Ascaris lumbricoides* and *Fasciola hepatica* (the liver fluke) eggs can be mistaken for vegetable cells.
- *Strongyloides stercoralis* and hookworm larvae can be confused with hairs or vegetable fibres; the latter are usually tapered at one end, whereas the former are blunt and there is no internal structure.
- Eggs of insects and mites can occasionally be found in a faecal sample—examples of a 'spurious' infection.

Some other potential pitfalls in diagnosis are as follows.

- Charcot–Leyden crystals (breakdown products of eosinophils) are sometimes found when an immune response to a foreign substance has been initiated.
- Undigested starch granules contain concentric rings, and stain blue with iodine; when partly digested they stain red with iodine.
- A cellular exudate and/or erythrocytes may be present in, for example, invasive *E. histolytica* infection.
- Macrophages, which possess a large nucleus compared with *E. histolytica* trophozoites, may be present in colonic amoebiasis.
- Polymorphonuclear leucocytes are present in bacillary dysentery; these are scanty in *E. histolytica* dysentery.
- Epithelial cells can sometimes be visualized in a faecal sample and frequently in material obtained at sigmoidoscopy.

CHAPTER 20

Using the laboratory

Introduction

Co-operation with laboratories requires mutual understanding between clinicians and laboratory workers. Pathology now embraces a series of specialized subjects and clinicians cannot be expected to be familiar with the detailed performance of all tests that they request. However, they should know:
- what investigation to request in given circumstances;
- the *discomfort* and possible *risk* to the patient of an investigation;
- what *information* the pathologist requires about the patient;
- what *specimens* are required and how they should be obtained and transmitted to the laboratory;
- the approximate *cost* in time and money of an investigation;
- the possible *risk* of a specimen to the laboratory worker (infected material or Australia antigen-positive sera);
- how to make the *best use* of the results received from the laboratory. In the case of complicated

investigations, the clinician and the pathologist should agree a programme of investigation and discuss the results.

What investigation to request

The result of any laboratory investigation is only one part of the information required to make a diagnosis. It may have as much or as little significance as any other physical finding. The plan of investigation has to be decided from the facts elicited by history-taking and physical examination. However, the widespread use of automation in haematology and biochemistry means that tests are often performed in a 'package'. It is necessary to know what is offered in each package and to choose the appropriate one, rather than the single test. The availability of these routines should not lead to the abandonment of the eclectic approach that adds to the patient's comfort, the speed of diagnosis and the continued education of the doctor.

Certain investigations are often necessary to monitor the natural history of a disease and its treatment. For example, the white blood cell count has to be followed serially in cases of leukaemia and the sedimentation rate in rheumatoid arthritis. There should therefore be a planned series of repeat tests as is often necessary when following the resolution of a metabolic disorder. Tests should not be repeated without good reason and, if repeated, the interval between them should be decided logically.

What information to send

A source of serious error can be failure to identify correctly the source of a specimen from a given patient. Therefore, laboratories design their request forms with care and it is essential that all details required are filled in accurately and legibly. Usually it is necessary to record the patient's surname and first name, address (or ward and bed number), the hospital serial number and the sex and date of birth of the patient. These details are all the more necessary in parts of the world where many family names are very similar.

Requests must also indicate the exact nature of the material sent, its source and the precise nature of the investigations required. The date on which the specimen is collected must be recorded. For many biochemical tests it is necessary to record the exact time at which the specimen is collected.

It is desirable that the patient's tentative diagnosis should be recorded together with any relevant clinical comment. A note of current antibiotic therapy is necessary with all requests for bacteriological examinations. Similarly, any therapy that might influence biochemical investigations should be recorded.

Collection of specimens

It is essential that specimens reach the laboratory fresh and in the correct kind of container. Specimens are best taken by hand to the laboratory as soon as they are obtained, but they can, if necessary, be sent by post, provided they are suitably packed and labelled 'fragile, with care' and 'pathological specimen'. Such specimens must be placed in a sealed inner container and then packed in a secure carton containing sufficient absorbent material to soak up all the liquid contents if the inner container is broken. Local and international regulations about the transmission of pathological material must be adhered to strictly.

Suitable containers are best obtained from the laboratory that is going to make the investigations. All containers must be perfectly clean and preferably sterile. This is of course essential for bacteriological specimens. Containers for blood should be completely dry. All containers must have properly fitting lids or caps. It is usually essential that the correct container should be used for each investigation (e.g. particular anticoagulants are necessary for different chemical or other blood tests). It is also desirable that the amount of material specified for a particular container should be placed in that container, and not more than the amount specified.

All syringes and needles must be sterile and should either be of the disposable type or be properly sterilized in a laboratory.

Venepuncture

A piece of rubber tubing is used as a tourniquet and applied round the upper arm over the middle of the biceps so as to impede the venous but not the arterial flow. The skin at the bend of the elbow is 'painted' with 0.5% chlorhexidine in 70% alcohol or simply 70% spirit (iodine is expensive and can give rise to severe skin reactions). The skin is rendered tense by the operator's left hand; the syringe with the needle attached is held in the right hand and almost parallel with the patient's arm; the patient is asked to 'make a fist' and then the needle with the bevel upwards is inserted into a prominent vein—the median basilic is usually convenient—and the needle is pointed in the direction of the blood flow. The required amount of blood is then drawn up into the syringe and the tourniquet is removed before the needle is withdrawn, as otherwise a haematoma may form. For some purposes it is necessary to remove the tourniquet as soon as the needle enters the vein, so that free-flowing blood is withdrawn. As soon as the needle is withdrawn a swab is placed on the puncture site and the patient is asked to hold their forearm firmly flexed against their arm for a minute or so. Occasionally a vein in the forearm or wrist may prove more convenient than one at the elbow, but the procedure is then usually more painful. A vein which can be *felt* is generally easier to enter than one which can only be *seen*.

Blood obtained by venepuncture should be placed

immediately in the appropriate container for the test requested. The needle should first be removed from the syringe, since forcing the blood through the needle may cause haemolysis. Appropriate containers for particular investigations should be obtained from the laboratory.

Heparin and sequestrene (EDTA) are the most generally useful anticoagulants. Sequestrene can be used for most haematological investigations and heparin for most simple chemical tests, with the exception of blood glucose, for which bottles containing sodium fluoride are necessary.

For blood group and serological investigations blood should be taken into a dry sterile bottle or tube. If the specimen has to be sent to the laboratory by post, it is best to wait till the blood has clotted. Some serum should then be removed with a sterile needle and syringe, and this serum is sent separately, together with the blood clot.

Other specimens

Urine, faeces, peritoneal fluid, pleural fluid, gastric and pancreatic juice, bile, arterial blood samples, semen, nasal secretions, cerebrospinal fluid, fluid aspirated from cysts, epididymal cysts, cutaneous cysts, etc. and pus may also be collected and sent to the laboratory for examination. Methods appropriate for the collection of these samples are discussed elsewhere in this book.

Making the best use of results

It is merely stating the obvious to say that the interpretation of any laboratory test will depend on the relevance of the test to the presumptive diagnosis and the interpreter's knowledge of pathology, biochemistry and physiology. The task of a clinical laboratory is to put these disciplines to work in the solution of a diagnostic problem.

All tests are subject to errors of performance. Fortunately these are rare, but the clinician will help the pathologist if any 'rogue' result that does not accord with other data is reported back to the laboratory. All results will depend on the precision of the method used and the variability of the quality measured amongst a healthy population.

In non-quantitative tests, as in cytology, there may be false-positives and false-negatives. The laboratory should be able to say with what frequency these may occur. For instance, in cases of bronchial carcinoma, malignant cells are often to be detected in the sputum; however, in a very small proportion of examinations, apparently malignant cells in the sputum will be reported when there is no bronchial carcinoma. The clinician can give some weight to such findings by considering the patient. If the patient is a middle-aged man who smokes heavily, the report of malignant cells would be likely to be a true-positive as bronchial carcinoma is prevalent is such patients. Conversely, if the patient is a non-smoking young girl, the positive sputum report would be likely to be false, and should be reassessed.

For quantitative tests, as in biochemistry and much of haematology, the precision of a test can be determined statistically and its performance monitored within the laboratory and by co-operation with other laboratories.

Precision is the measure of the repeatability of a determination. If the method is very precise the spread of results around the 'true' value will be small and vice versa. The precision of measurement has to be linked to the variations of the 'true' value as found in a population of, say, 1000 healthy people. The results of the measurement performed on this group of normals can be plotted as a Gaussian curve on either side of the mean value. It is conventional to express this normal range as the mean value plus or minus two standard deviations. Although 95% of all normal results will fall within this range, it has to be remembered that 1 in 20 of all normal results will fall just outside the normal range. Therefore a value just outside the range of normal does not necessarily indicate abnormality. It should also be remembered that normal ranges have to be established for the sex and age of the groups studied and also for the method as performed in each laboratory.

Microbiological investigations

Special care is necessary both in the collection and in the transport of specimens for microbiological examination to the laboratory because:
• successful culture depends on the viability of the organisms;
• overgrowth of the normal flora present in the

specimen can hinder detection of the pathogen, which is often present only in small numbers;
• careless collection techniques can lead to cross-contamination with organisms present on the patient's or operator's skin, or in the environment.

Specimens can be taken either to detect the organism directly, or to detect an antibody response to the infecting organism. Direct detection of the organism can be achieved by direct visualization, usually with the aid of a light or electron microscope. Success is dependent on the presence of a relatively large number of organisms in the specimen, for example in pus. If fewer organisms are present a more sensitive technique is necessary. Traditionally this has been achieved by culture techniques, that is, by allowing the organism to multiply.

More modern methods have been developed which detect genes or gene products specific to the organism, allowing direct detection even when only small numbers of the organism are present. The earliest of these methods used immunological principles to detect antigens by complement fixing antibodies. The most recent use the *polymerase chain reaction (PCR)* to detect organism-specific proteins. Although these newer techniques are very sensitive, unless meticulous care is taken both during collection of the specimen and during performance of the test, contamination with other antigens or proteins is a problem that reduces the specificity of the result. In addition, specificity may not be as great as expected when antigens are shared by the organism and by the patient's tissues.

Serological response to infection

Traditionally, antibodies have been detected and assayed in serum. Techniques are now also available to detect an antibody response in other fluids, including CSF and saliva. The total antibody response or the specific IgG and IgM response can be assessed. The total antibody response and the IgG response are useful in measuring the incidence of disease in a community. To identify active current infection it is necessary, in general, either to demonstrate the presence of IgM, or a fourfold increase in titre of total antibody, during the course of the illness.

Tissue discharges, pus, CSF and other fluids

It is important always to send a sufficient quantity of the material to the laboratory. Generally, about 10–15 g of tissue or discharge and up to 25 ml of fluid are necessary. These are substantial amounts of material. If only very small amounts of material are available, e.g. less than an apple pip in size, the material should be sent in a sterile container containing isotonic saline (*never* in formol saline). The best results will be obtained when only small amounts of material are available by asking the laboratory personnel to come to the patient's bedside to make the cultures there (Figs 20.1–20.3).

If it is not possible to submit material for culture in sufficient bulk then a swab may be taken. Ensure

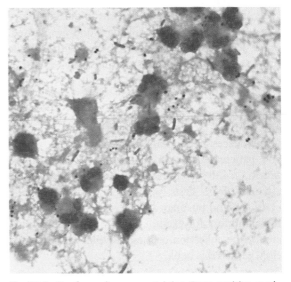

Fig. 20.1 Pus from abscess, containing Gram-positive cocci and Gram-negative rods.

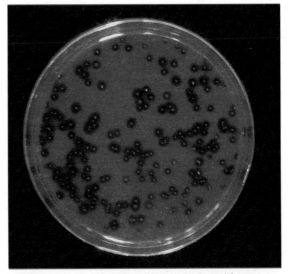

Fig. 20.2 Beta-haemolytic streptococci cultured from a throat swab on a blood agar medium.

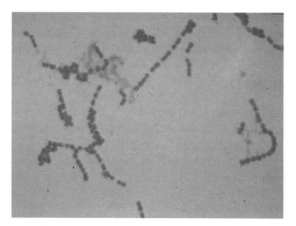

Fig. 20.3 Gram smear of culture of pus showing a growth of streptococci.

that the correct swab, supplied by the laboratory, is used. Swabs will vary according to which pathogen is sought (Box 20.1).

Blood culture

Blood cultures may be set up for bacteria or viruses.

BACTERIAL PATHOGENS

Blood culture for bacterial pathogens is useful in the investigation of almost all infections, although it is necessary for diagnosis in only a few clinical situations. Bacteria are often present in blood in only very low concentrations, and their viability and growth potential may be inhibited by antibiotic treatment. Since so many different infections may be accompanied by septicaemia it is important to inoculate bottles containing a variety of different culture media. The media used should be suitable for aerobic pathogens, anaerobic pathogens, and for fastidious species such as *Brucella* spp., *Mycobacteria* spp., *Leptospira* spp., and for non-bacterial pathogens such as fungi. Antibacterial substances present in the patient's blood can be inactivated by dilution (at least 1:10), by the addition of specific enzymes, e.g. penicillinase, or by absorption by resins.

Before withdrawing blood the patient's skin and the bottle cap should be cleaned with 70% alcohol or alcohol chlorhexidine, and allowed to dry. At least three sets of blood cultures should be taken, preferably before antibiotic therapy is begun. Occasionally, particularly if endocarditis is suspected, it may be necessary to take up to six sets of cultures before a negative result can be accepted.

VIRAL PATHOGENS

Sterile heparinized blood should be sent to the virus laboratory.

SEROLOGY

Clotted blood in a sterile container without additives is required.

Urine culture

Urine specimens (Box 20.2) should be transferred to the laboratory within 1 hour of voiding, unless specific precautions are taken to prevent bacterial multiplication before cultures are set up. Urine specimens may be stored overnight at 4°C. If this is not possible then a commercial kit for culture of the specimen at

---

BOX 20.1 Swabs.

• Plain swab *without* transport medium: Used for hardy microorganisms only; rarely the swab of choice
• Plain swab *with* transport medium: For general bacteriology
• Swab *with* charcoal (black) transport: For *Neisseria gonorrhoeae*, and other delicate bacteria
• Plain swab *with* virus transport medium: Essential to gently squeeze swab in transport medium. Virus transport medium contains antibiotics and is *not* suitable for bacterial culture
• Chlamydial swab *with* transport medium: For detection of *Chlamydia trachomatis* antigen by immunoassay. Designed for use with urogenital and ophthalmic specimens only
• Wire swab *with* transport medium: For isolation of nasal pertussis infection

---

BOX 20.2 Urine collections for microbiological examination.

Catheter specimen of urine (CSU)
Aspirate the urine, via a 21 gauge needle and syringe, from the rubberized part of the tubing connecting the catheter to the collection bag. *Do not collect urine from the tap outlet to the bag.*

Early morning urine (EMU)
Send the entire first-voided specimen, usually about 250 ml, to the laboratory in the large sterile container provided. Three consecutive morning specimens should be taken.

Mid-stream urine (MSU)
A urine specimen is taken during mid-micturition by the patient, after instruction, or with the assistance of a nurse, after the labia or penile orifice have been cleaned with chlorhexidine.

the bedside should be used. Several commercial 'chemical' kits are available, but experience in their sensitivity and specificity is limited at present.

Mid-stream (MSU) or suprapubic aspiration techniques are suitable for general bacterial and viral culture of urine, but are unsuitable for typhoid or tuberculosis. In the diagnosis of the latter infection three early morning urine (EMU) specimens should be submitted to the laboratory. For the diagnosis of schistosomiasis the terminal 5 ml of a freshly voided specimen is required.

Examination of faeces

BACTERIAL PATHOGENS

Human faeces contain approximately 10^{11} organisms/g wet weight as normal flora, whereas gut bacterial pathogens rarely exceed 10^5 organisms/g. Because of the relative scarcity of pathogens in faecal specimens examination of a Gram-stained smear of faeces is not usually performed. However, occasionally in infections caused by *Campylobacter* spp. the typical seagull-shaped Gram-negative bacteria are present in sufficient numbers to be identifiable in a directly stained smear of a faecal specimen.

The mainstay of diagnosis of bacterial infections of the gut is by culture. Correct collection and transportation of the specimen to the laboratory is particularly important, since incorrect technique can lead to the death of the pathogen or to overgrowth by normal gut flora.

Collection of the specimen

Approximately 20 ml of stool should be collected on three separate occasions as early as possible in the illness and placed in three separate, sterile containers. For immediate transfer to the laboratory dry sterile containers are suitable but, if there is a delay in transportation to the laboratory, the faecal specimen should be placed in a suitable preservative, for example in 0.0033 M phosphate buffer mixed with an equal volume of glycerol, at pH 7.0. If possible, include any mucus or blood in the faeces in the specimen submitted.

As there are a large number of bacterial species that can cause diarrhoea, the laboratory will use many different selective culture media in order to increase the isolation rate. It is essential to note on the accompanying request form any relevant clinical details to enable the laboratory staff to seek the most likely pathogens. Important informa-

tion includes a history of travel to potentially endemic areas, prior antibiotic therapy, any known outbreak of sporadic disease, possible contamination of food, and any associated immunosuppressive disease.

VIRAL PATHOGENS

Many of the viruses which cause diarrhoea cannot be cultured. Diagnosis is therefore often made by immunological techniques, or by electron microscopic identification of the virus.

Collection of specimens

In contrast to the techniques used for collection when viral pathogens are suspected, chemical preservatives should not be used. Specimens should be taken into a dry sterile container and sent to the laboratory promptly, or frozen at $-20°C$ ($-70°C$ is optimal but rarely available). For direct detection of viral particles by electron microcopy many particles must be present. Electron microscopy is a specific but not very sensitive technique.

PARASITIC INFECTIONS

This topic is discussed in Chapter 19. For detection of *Entamoeba histolytica* infestation the faecal specimen must be kept at body temperature until it can be examined. Other cysts and ova can be detected by examination of stool sent in a plain sterile container.

The respiratory tract

Material may be taken for detection of bacterial or viral infections. Specimens can be taken from the throat, the nasopharynx, sputum or by bronchoalveolar lavage, as appropriate.

THROAT SWABS

Vigorously swab the tonsillar areas, the posterior pharynx, and any areas of visible inflammation, exudation, ulceration or membrane formation. For bacterial cultures, use a plain swab with transport medium. For viral detection, use a plain swab with virus transport medium. The specimen should be sent immediately to the laboratory, or stored at 4°C; it should not be frozen.

NASOPHARYNX

Specimens of nasopharyngeal secretions are used principally for diagnosis of *Pertussis* infection, an uncommon disorder in developed countries, in which immunization programmes have been largely effective in preventing whooping cough.

The specimen is obtained using a wire pernasal swab. The swab is passed gently along the base of the nostril into the nasopharynx, rotated, removed and placed into transport medium. The laboratory may need prior warning of the arrival of the specimen so that appropriate culture media can be prepared.

For detection of viral pathogens from the nasopharynx an aspirated specimen is obtained using a section catheter.

SPUTUM

For best results an early morning freshly expectorated sputum specimen should be collected in a dry, sterile bottle, preferably with the help of a physiotherapist. For isolation of mycobacteria three consecutive morning specimens should be obtained.

BRONCHO-ALVEOLAR LAVAGE

This technique may be helpful when lower respiratory tract infection is suspected, e.g. *Legionella* spp., *Nocardia* spp., *Pneumocystis carinii*, *Mycobacterium* spp. and *Cytomegalovirus* infections.

The genital tract

Different methods are used for particular clinical problems (Box 20.3).

BOX 20.3 Microbiological investigation of the genital tract.

Neisseria gonorrhoeae infection
• Urethral and/or endocervical (not high vagina), rectal or throat swabs
• Use charcoal transport medium
Chlamydia trachomatis
• Endocervical (not high vaginal) or urethral specimen
• Inoculate in transport medium
• Abnormal specimens will contain pus cells
• Specimen can be stored at 2–8°C
Candida spp. and *Trichomonas* spp.
• High vaginal swab in plain transport medium
Herpes simplex virus (HSV)
• Most successful in first 3 days of infection
• Use plain sterile swab to collect vesicular fluid into viral transport medium
• Air-dried smears of scrapings from base of vesicles can be used for direct examination by immunofluorescence
Pelvic inflammatory disease
• Send endocervical swabs of pus in charcoal transport medium

---

The skin

DERMATOPHYTES AND CANDIDA ALBICANS

Keratinized specimens, e.g. hair, skin scrapings or nail cuttings, should be sent enclosed in black paper, for ease of recognition. Do not use sticky tape.

VIRUS DETECTION

See above (page 448).

The eyes

There are methods for detection of bacterial and viral pathogens.

BACTERIAL PATHOGENS

Conjunctival infection

Using a firm action, thoroughly swab the inner surface of the lower and then the upper eyelid, using a separate swab for each eye. Use a plain swab and a transport medium. For gonorrhoeal infection use a charcoal transport medium.

Intraocular infection

Bedside inoculation of tiny quantities of aspirated material can be performed by the ophthalmologist.

VIRAL PATHOGENS

A swab moistened with sterile saline is used to collect secretions from the palpebral conjunctiva; this is inserted into a transport medium.

Scrapings from cornea or conjunctiva can be collected by the ophthalmologist.

CHLAMYDIA INFECTION

Specimens should contain as many epithelial cells as possible, but should not consist of pus. See above for special precautions.

Chemical tests used in urinalysis

The tests described below for urinary protein, sugar, ketones and urobilinogen have been largely replaced by commercial reagent strip tests that incorporate modifications of the reagents used in these tests into convenient standardized procedures. However, the original versions of these chemical urine tests are reliable and use commonly available reagents; they are therefore still useful when reagent strip tests are not available.

Proteinuria

THE SALICYLSULPHONIC ACID TEST
To 5 ml urine in a test tube add 20% salicylsulphonic acid, drop by drop. The presence of protein is indicated by a cloudy precipitate, best seen against a black background, but up to 25 drops may be required before this forms. Continue to add salicylsulphonic acid until no more precipitate is formed. For ordinary purposes it is sufficient to express the amount present as a haze, cloud or granular precipitate, a haze representing about 20 mg protein per 100 ml; a heavier deposit should be allowed to settle (which may take an hour or so) and the quantity expressed as the proportion of the urine volume occupied by the deposit. If this proportion is one-half, the urine contains about 10 g protein/litre. False-positive results may be due to the presence of radiographic contrast medium; they may also occur in patients treated with sulphonamides, tolbutamide, para-aminosalicylic acid or large doses of penicillin, or if the urine contains a lot of uric acid.

THE BOILING TEST
Fill a small test tube two-thirds full of urine. If this is alkaline, add 10% acetic acid, drop by drop, mixing thoroughly after each drop, until pH 5 is reached as shown by pH indicator paper. Boil the top 2 cm over a flame while holding the bottom of the tube and examine against a dark background. A cloudiness indicates the presence of protein, or of phosphates which have precipitated because loss of carbon dioxide on boiling has made the urine more alkaline. If the precipitate disappears on adding more acid it was due to phosphates; if not, it is precipitated protein. If more than a light cloud persists, boil all the urine, acidifying until no more protein is deposited. Allow to settle and express semiquantitatively as described for the salicylsulphonic acid test. The two tests are comparable in sensitivity.

Treatment with tolbutamide or large doses of penicillin, or the presence of radiographic contrast medium, may cause false-positive results.

Urinary sugar

BENEDICT'S TEST
This is not specific for glucose and a positive reaction is given by any reducing substance present in the urine. To 5 ml of Benedict's reagent add 8 drops of urine, boil for 2 minutes and allow to cool. If a reducing substance is present, a precipitate will appear, varying from a light green turbidity to a red precipitate (Table 20.1). If the reduction is due to glucose, the test gives approximately quantitative results.

Precipitate	Sugar (g/dl)
Light green turbidity	0.1-0.5
Green precipitate	0.5-1.0
Yellow precipitate	1.0-2.0
Red precipitate	2.0 or more

Table 20.1 Benedict's test.

Urinary ketones

ROTHERA'S TEST
A volume of 10 ml of urine is saturated with an excess of ammonium sulphate crystals; 3 drops of a strong freshly prepared solution of sodium nitroprusside and 2 ml of strong ammonia solution are then added. A deep permanganate colour is produced by acetone and acetoacetic acid. If Rothera's test is negative, ketones are absent.

GERHARDT'S TEST
Drop by drop 10% ferric chloride solution is added to 5 ml of urine in a test tube. A precipitate of ferric phosphate usually forms, but disappears again when more ferric chloride is added. The solution becomes brownish-red if acetoacetic acid is present.

Aspirin and other salicylates, phenothiazines, phenol and some other drugs give a similar colour with ferric chloride. Boiling the urine for 5 minutes before adding the ferric chloride destroys acetoacetic acid, but the other substances which react with it are unaffected. If, therefore, urine which has been boiled still gives a positive reaction, it may be inferred that this is not due to acetoacetic acid or to other substances.

A positive ferric chloride reaction is obtained only if acetoacetic acid is present in considerable amount. If the urine reacts to Rothera's test but not to ferric chloride, it may be deduced that only a small amount is present. If both are positive, the patient is severely ketotic and requires urgent treatment.

Urobilinogen and porphobilinogen

EHRLICH'S ALDEHYDE TEST

At room temperature 1 ml of fresh urine is mixed with 1 ml of Ehrlich's aldehyde reagent (2 g paradimethylaminobenzaldehyde, dissolved in 100 ml of 5% hydrochloric acid). After 1.5 minutes 2 ml saturated aqueous sodium acetate is added and mixed, followed by 2 ml of a 3:1 (v/v) mixture of amyl alcohol and benzyl alcohol. The test tube is stoppered and its contents are shaken gently for 1 minute. After the phases have separated a red colour in the upper (alcohol) phase indicates that urobilinogen is present, whilst a similar colour in the lower (aqueous) phase denotes porphobilinogen. Chloroform may be used in the test as an alternative to amyl and benzyl alcohols. It separates more quickly, into the *lower* layer, where the red colour due to urobilinogen may be seen. Normal fresh urine contains enough urobilinogen to produce a weakly positive reaction.

Centigrade and Fahrenheit scales

The centigrade (Celsius) scale is preferred. Table 20.2 shows the relationship of the centigrade and Fahrenheit scales, as far as is likely to be required in clinical work.

To convert Fahrenheit to centigrade:

$$X°F - 32 \times \tfrac{5}{9} = Y°C$$

To convert centigrade to Fahrenheit:

$$X°C \times \tfrac{9}{5} + 32 = Y°F$$

SI units

In this book the Système International (SI) d'Unités has been used a far as possible. This system aims to derive all measurements from seven basic units and to express all measurements as decimal fractions or multiples of these. Of the seven basic units the four which appear in this book are:

Physical quantity	Name of SI unit	Symbol
Length	metre	m
Mass	kilogram	kg
Time	second	s
Amount of substance	mole	mol

and the prefixes indicating the decimal fraction and multiples are:

Fraction	Prefix	Symbol
10^{-1}	deci-	d
10^{-2}	centi-	c
10^{-3}	milli-	m
10^{-6}	micro-	μ
10^{-9}	nano-	n
10^{-12}	pico-	p
10^{-15}	femto	f

1 fluid ounce (fl oz)	= 28 ml
1 gallon UK (gal)	= 4.5 l
1 grain (do not abbreviate)	= 65 mg
1 inch (in)	= 25.4 mm
1 foot (ft)	= 0.3 m
1 ounce (oz)	= 28 g
1 pound (lb)	= 0.45 kg
1 calorie (cal)	= 4.2 J
1 kilocalorie (medical calorie, Cal)	= 4.2 kJ

The litre (= 1 dm³) is also recognized as the unit of volume.

It follows that with the adoption of SI, certain familiar terms are no longer used, as is the case with measures of volume. A cubic centimetre (cc, cm³) is replaced by the millilitre (ml) and the cubic

Centigrade	Fahrenheit	Centigrade	Fahrenheit
110	230	36.5	97.7
100	212	36	96.8
95	203	35.5	95.9
90	194	35	95
85	185	34	93.2
80	176	33	91.4
75	167	32	89.6
70	158	31	87.8
65	149	30	86
60	140	25	77
55	131	20	68
50	122	15	59
45	113	10	50
44	111.2	5	41
43	109.4	0	32
42	107.6	−5	23
41	105.8	−10	14
40.5	104.9	−15	5
40	104	−20	−4
39.5	103.1		
39	102.2	0.54	1
38.5	101.3	1	1.8
38	100.4	2	3.6
37.5	99.5	2.5	4.5
37	98.6		

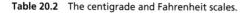

Table 20.2 The centigrade and Fahrenheit scales.

millimetre (cmm, mm³) by the microlitre (μl). In linear measure the micron (μ) should no longer be used; the correct unit is the micrometre (μm). Blood, intra-uterine and intra-ocular pressures are measured in millimetres of mercury (mmHg) and intrathecal pressures in centimetres of cerebrospinal fluid (cm CSF). It is recommended that the medical calorie or kilocalorie should now be converted to the joule (1 kcal = 4186.8 J).

Further information on SI units may be obtained from *The Use of SI Units*, Publication PD 5686 of the

Multiple	Prefix	Symbol
10	deca-	da
10^2	hecto-	h
10^3	kilo-	k
10^6	mega-	M

British Standards Institution, and useful information on the SI units commonly used in medicine and biology is available in *Units, Symbols and Abbreviations: A Guide for Biological and Medical Editors and Authors*, published by the Royal Society of Medicine.

Normal reference values in chemical pathology

These represent only a guide to the range approved in the Royal London Hospital laboratories. Other laboratories may utilize slightly different reference values because of variations in laboratory techniques. In many patients a change in a test result during a period of observation is more important than any single value.

Plasma/serum

Acid phosphatase — Total: up to 11 u/l; prostatic: up to 4 u/l

Albumin — 38-50 g/l dependent on posture

Aldosterone — 100–330 pmol/l after overnight recumbency

Alkaline phosphatase — Adults 25–90 u/l; children up to 250 u/l

Amylase — 30–170 u/l

Anion gap (Na + K) – Cl + HCO₃) — 12–18 mmol/l

Alanine aminotransferase (ALT, GPT) — 7–35 u/l

Ascorbic acid (vitamin C) — Please contact laboratory

Aspartate aminotransferase (AST, GOT) — 7–40 u/l

Bicarbonate — 23–28 mmol/l

Bilirubin — Total: less than 17 μmol/l; direct: less than 6 μmol/l

Calcium — 2.2–2.6 mmol/l

Carotenoids (as β-carotene) — 1.0–5.5 μmol/l

Chloride — 96–108 mmol/l

Cholesterol — See under Serum, below

Cholinesterase (pseudocholinesterase) — 3–8 u/l

Copper — 8–24 μmol/l

Cortisol (marked diurnal variation) — Midnight 20–280 nmol/l; 9.30 a.m. 140–600 nmol/l

Creatinine — Males 62–124 μmol/l; females 53–106 μmol/l

Creatine kinase — Males 25–170 u/l; females 25–150 u/l

Gamma glutamyltransferase (γGT) — Males 6–28 u/l; females 4–18 u/l

Gastrin — 0–200 pg/ml (<40 pmol/l)

Globulins — 18–32 g/l

Glucose, fasting — 3.3–5.3 mmol/l

Haptoglobins — See Haematology list

α-Hydroxybutyrate dehydrogenase (HBD)	Children 92–185 u/l; adults 50–140 u/l
Inorganic phosphate	0.6–1.5 mmol/l
Iron	Males 13–32 μmol/l; females 11–29 μmol/l
Iron binding capacity (TIBC)	44–67 μmol/l
Lactate dehydrogenase (LD)	60–450 u/l
Lead (in whole blood)	Please see later section
Magnesium	0.7–1.0 mmol/l
17 β-Oestradiol	
Follicular	200–400 pmol/l
Mid-cycle	400–1000 pmol/l
Luteal	400–1200 pmol/l
Post-menopausal	<100 pmol/l
Osmolality	282–295 mosmol/kg
Parathormone	See under Serum, below
Potassium	3.5–4.8 mmol/l
Progesterone	
follicular	<3–12 nmol/l
luteal	>33 nmol/l
Prolactin	See under Serum, below
Protein, total	65–80 g/l dependent on posture
Sodium	137–144 nmol/l
Testosterone	Males 9.0–24.0 nmol/l; females 0.5–2.5 nmol/l
Thyroxine, free (free T_4)	8.8–23.1 pmol/l
Thyroid-stimulating hormone (TSH)	Males 0.45–3.8 u/l; females 0.40–4.8 u/l; females >51 years 0.40–5.7 u/l
Transketolase	Please enquire in laboratory
Triglycerides	See under Serum, below
Tri-iodothyronine (total T_3)	1.5–3.1 nmol/l
Urate	Males 240–500 μmol/l; females 170–450 μmol/l;
Urea	2.5–6.6 mmol/l
Vitamin A	0.7–1.5 μmol/l
Vitamin C (ascorbic acid)	Please contact laboratory
25-OH Vitamin D (25-OH cholecalciferol)	>10 ng/ml
Zinc	9–17 umol/l

Blood (whole blood: anticoagulant required: consult laboratory)

Lead	<1.9 μmol/l

Serum (clotted specimen required)

α-Fetoprotein	
Pregnancy: rising values	Consult tables
	Examples: 14 weeks: 32 u/ml
	18 weeks: 110 u/mol
	22 weeks: 184 u/mol
Non-pregnancy	<10 u/ml
Ferritin	Males 16–330 ng/ml (mean 90); females females 4–120 ng/ml (mean 18); Post-menopausal females 12–230 ng/ml (mean 49); iron deficiency <10 ng/ml; iron overload >300 ng/ml

Gonadotrophins
  Follicle-stimulating hormone
    Female
      Follicular   1–10 u/l
      Luteal   6–25 u/l
    Male   1–7 u/l
    Luteinizing hormone
    Female
      Follicular   1–2l u/l
      Mid-cycle   4.5–70 u/l
      Luteal   <1–12.8 u/l
    Male   1–9.7 u/l
Growth hormone   Please enquire in laboratory
β-hCG   Please enquire in laboratory

Lipids
  Cholesterol, total—up to 40 years of age. Higher   Males 3.6–6.7 mmol/l; females 3.5–6.5 mmol/l
    values above 40 years without defined limits
  HDL—cholesterol (fasting)   Males 0.9–1.4 mmol/l; females 1.2–1.7
                                                            mmol/l

  Triglycerides (fasting)   0.8–1.9 mmol
Lipoprotein electrophoresis   Qualitative report
Parathormone (if normal plasma calcium)   Males 0.4–0.9 ng/ml; females up to 0.7
                                                            ng/ml

Placental lactogen (HPL)   Please contact laboratory
Prolactin   60–360 u/l
Protein electrophoresis   Qualitative report

Urine (excretion range per 24 h)

Ascorbic acid (vitamin C)   Saturation test—please contact laboratory
Aldosterone   10–40 nmol
Amylase   100–600 u
Calcium   2.5–7.5 mmol
Catecholamines   Please contact laboratory
Chloride   60–180 mmol
Copper   0.2–0.8 μmol
Creatinine   5.7–17 mmol
HMMA (4-hydroxy-3-methoxymandelic acid)   10–35 μmol
  (VMA) screening test
5-HIAA (5-hydroxindoleacetic acid)   16–75 μmol
Indicans   145–335 μmol
Lead   0–3 μmol
Magnesium   3.3–4.9 mmol
17-Oxosteroids (17-Ketosteroids) ⎫   Oxogenic steroids and related metabolites are
17-Oxogenic steroids (17-ketogenic steroids) ⎬   reported in a urine steroid profile—please
                                              ⎭   contact laboratory

Oestrogens, total, in pregnancy   3–180 μmol/24 h—they show a rising level
                                                            with advancement of pregnancy within
                                                            these limits
                                                          Higher in multiple pregnancies
Oxalate   Males 0.10–0.41 mmol (as oxalic acid);
                                                          females 0.04–0.32 mmol (as oxalic acid)

Porphyrins
   Coproporphyrins
   Uroporphyrins
   Porphobilinogen
Proteins, total
Phosphate
Potassium
Sodium
Urea
Urate, uric acid

150–300 nmol
6–40 nmol
1–10 μmol
10–90 mg
16–48 mmol
50–100 mmol
60–180 mmol
250–500 mmol

Markedly dependent
on dietary intake

Not greater than 3.62 mmol/24 h on a purine-free,
isocaloric diet

Normal reference values in haematology

	Infant	Child	Adult Male	Adult Female
Haemoglobin concentration (g/dl)	13.6–19.6	12	13.5–18.0	11.5–16.0
Red cells ($\times 10^{12}$/l)	4–6	4.5	4.5–6.5	3.9–5.6
Haematocrit (PCV)	0.44–0.64	0.4	0.4–0.54	0.37–0.47
MCV (fl)	106	80	76–96	
MCH (pg)			27–32	
MCHC (g/dl)			32–36	
Reticulocytes (%)			<2	
White cells ($\times 10^{9}$/l)	10–2	5–15	4–11	
Neutrophils		2–6	2–7.5	
Lymphocytes		5.5–8.6	1.5–4.0	
Monocytes		0.7–1.5	0.2–0.8	
Eosinophils		0.3–0.8	Up to 0.4	
Basophils		<0.1	<0.1	
Platelets ($\times 10^{9}$/l)			150–400	
ESR (mm/h)			0–5	0–7

Haemoglobins

	Neonate	Adult
Haemoglobin A (%)	30	97
F (%)	70	1
A_2 (%)	<1	1.5–3.2

Haematinics

	Adult
Plasma iron (μmol/l)	13–32
Total iron binding capacity (TIBC; μmol/l)	47–70
Ferritin (μg/l)	25–400
Vitamin B_{12} (ng/l)	210-920
Serum folate (μg/l)	2–14
Red cell folate (μg/l)	125–600

Haemostasis

	Adult
Platelet count (×10^9/l)	150–400
Bleeding time (template)	Up to 9 min
Prothrombin ratio	1.0–1.3
Partial thromboplastin time (kaolin cephalin clotting time; s)	38–45
Thrombin time (s)	10–12

PCV = packed cell volume; MCV = mean corpuscular volume; MCH = mean corpuscular haemoglobin; MCHC = mean corpuscular haemoglobin concentration; ESR = erythrocyte sedimentation rate.

Appendix

Nomograms

The body surface area is given by the point of intersection with the middle scale of a straight line joining height and weight. Reproduced with permission from Bentley Laboratories.

Adult nomogram

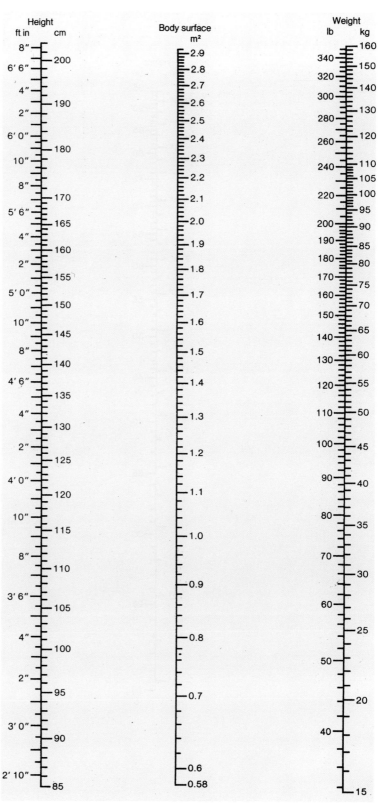

Height		Body surface	Weight	
ft in	cm	m²	lb	kg

Child nomogram

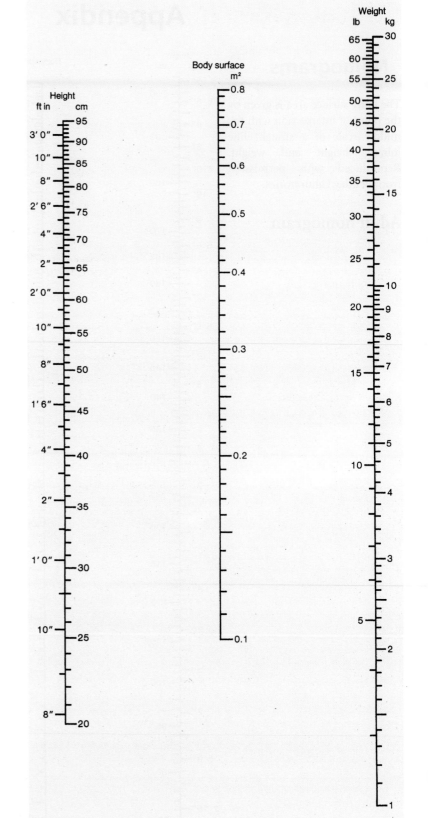

CHAPTER 21

Ethical issues in medicine

Introduction

Successful medical practice requires a relationship of trust between doctor and patient. Although, in family practice this relationship may be built up over several years, in hospital practice and in an emergency it is frequently the case that the patient and the doctor are meeting for the first time. A strict code of behaviour on the part of the doctor is therefore required in order to set the scene for a trusting relationship. It is the function of a code of medical ethics to provide this. Patients will expect a high standard of care when they seek help, and this will include an expectation that they will be consulted about decisions bearing on their treatment, that they be informed about the likely outcome of any treatment offered, and that their right of confidentiality be respected. It is unacceptable for one individual, such as a physician, to attempt to exert unconstrained power over the fate of another individual.

The capacity of a patient to take part in clinical decisions should never be underestimated. Always assume that a patient is able fully to understand the nature of the medical problem, and its implications, whatever their educational level. Remember that the patient will expect to be given the opportunity of a full explanation of the situation. Very often, it will be up to the doctor to introduce this topic at a suitable moment in the consultation. Some patients like to discuss the limits of what they would like to know early in a consultation, and others will define clearly the limits of dissemination of information through their family. These wishes must be respected.

Other issues in considering how and what to tell a patient are often brought to bear. The family may feel that the patient would not be able to take in the information, or that the information would be too terrible a burden for them to bear. The patient may make it clear that they do not wish the family to know about the problem or, sometimes, that they themselves do not wish to know the diagnosis. In all such instances, the needs and rights of the individual patient should be paramount. Should there be any conflict, the patient's interests are, first and foremost, always more important than those of the family. Fortunately such conflicts of interest are very rare, and are often more apparent than real. With discussion they can usually be resolved.

Historical aspects

In ancient Egypt rules of conduct for physicians included adherence to established methods of treatment. Later, the Code of Hammurabi formalized scales of payment for medical services, including penalties for negligence. In ancient Greece the Hippocratic Oath, a code of medical behaviour that underlies all modern clinical practice, required proper instruction of physicians, recognized that the physician's duty was to his patient, a duty that included an injunction to do no harm, and proscribed euthanasia and abortion, together with certain other risky or unacceptable procedures, such as lithotomy or castration. In addition, this Oath recognized the special nature of the doctor–patient relationship, and stressed that this relationship should not be abused. In both the Christian and Muslim worlds the influence of Judaism in medical ethics has been strong, particularly in clarifying the responsibilities of individuals in relation to groups, as in the case of isolation of patients with serious infective conditions. This is an example of a special policy which puts the needs of the group temporarily on a level with those of the individual patient. Similar attitudes prevail in other religious environments.

Autonomy

The fundamental principle underlying the concept of a medical ethic is that of the autonomy of the patient. This means that the patient has the right to decide his or her own medical destiny; the physician may advise, but the patient decides. Upon this notion rests the concept of seeking consent for medical interventions, for research, and for teaching from the patient or, in the case of a minor or a mentally disturbed person, from the patient's lawful parents or guardians. The physician or surgeon, therefore, not only has a duty to advise, but also to explain.

The origin of this medical ethic antedates the Christian era, and is common to Judaism, and to the Muslim world, in addition to all countries whose governance has been influenced by Christianity. It can thus be separated from any apparent religious background, itself an important aspect of the universality of the concept of a medical ethic.

Consent

As a general rule the patient's consent should be sought to any treatment, however minor. In many instances consent is implied, as when a patient presents to a doctor with an injury and asks for treatment. In other circumstances, a minor symptom may lead to the discovery of a serious illness requiring complex investigation and treatment. In this example consent will be required for each stage of the investigation and treatment as part of the unfolding of the diagnosis and the management proposed.

For a patient to give consent sufficient accurate information about the illness must be given to enable the patient to decide whether the proposed treatment is, generally, both acceptable and in their own interests. There are four requirements on the doctor discussing an intervention with a patient.

1 The procedure itself must be described, including the technique and its implications.

2 Information about the risks and complications must be given.

3 Associated risks, e.g. from anaesthesia, or from other drugs that may be necessary, should be described.

4 Alternative medical or surgical investigations or treatments should be discussed, so that the reasons for the specific advice given are clear. In addition the implications of the 'do nothing' option should be discussed.

The procedure

The amount of information divulged will vary according to the context of the discussion, and the needs of the patient as they emerge in the consultation. For example, an operation on the knee of a sportsman has far greater implications than the same operation in the case of a sedentary office worker. It is not appropriate to burden the patient with a textbook approach to medical knowledge. The objective is not to place the patient in the situation of having to decide between conflicting medical data, but to explain why the advice given as to the mode of management recommended is regarded as the best in the circumstances. It may happen, of course, that during discussion other factors come to light that result in the advice being altered. Clearly, this should be accepted as a happy outcome since it implies agreement as to the best course.

Setting the scene

Discussions regarding consent for investigation and treatment are emotionally charged for the patient and often, also, for the doctor. Therefore, try to arrange a suitably quiet and pleasant environment for the discussion, that is free of interruptions, and away from unnecessary observers, such as other patients or unfamiliar nurses or students. Make time for the discussion; *never* appear rushed. Use simple language that the patient can understand. Be patient. If necessary, and with the patient's permission, involve relatives. If there is likely to be a language problem, make sure that an interpreter is available. At the end of the discussion check that the patient has actually understood. If there is any doubt be prepared to have a further discussion; it is often better, in the case of really serious news, to have a discussion about management on several occasions, even once a treatment schedule has commenced.

Implications of consent

In the event that the patient declines the investigation or treatment recommended remember that, not only is this the patient's right, but that the objective of the process of discussion is to allow the patient to understand the management proposed and to come to a decision as to whether or not to proceed with it. Therefore, refusal is *not* a signal for the doctor to disengage from management of the patient but, rather, to continue to provide care to as high a level as is possible and, if necessary, to continue discussion about future management.

If explicit consent is given, the patient and doctor should both sign an appropriate Consent Form. This procedure should be followed for all serious interventions. In hospital this Consent Form will be a standardized form, and a similar form should be used in family or private practice to verify that the discussion took place. The mere act of both parties

signing the form does not constitute proof that consent has been lawfully given. It simply documents that a discussion occurred without describing the context, or giving details of the information described. Generally, however, it will be taken to mean that consent was obtained.

Legal requirements for consent

There are three aspects of consent that are required in law.
1 The patient must be mentally and legally competent to give consent.
2 The patient must have been sufficiently well informed to be able to give consent.
3 Consent must have been given voluntarily, and not under duress.

Competence for consent

Competence is difficult to define. The patient must be able to understand the discussion. If there is doubt as to the patient's competence to give consent, consent should be obtained not only from the patient but, also, from a responsible relative. If necessary, help from senior nursing staff, or even from a psychiatrist should be enlisted.

Special difficulties arise with the unconscious patient. If treatment is necessary in order to save life, treatment can and must be given without waiting for consent. If relatives are available, they should be consulted, but their wishes are not necessarily paramount in the decision to initiate life-saving therapy. In the UK no adult can act as a proxy for another. In some other countries relatives can be given powers of guardianship that allow them to give consent for the other adult person for whom they act as guardian.

Consent for the treatment of children is a matter that must be considered with care. In the UK treatment of a minor, i.e. someone under the age of 16 years, can be given without parental consent, provided that care has been taken to make sure that the child understands the nature of the treatment proposed, and its possible risks, adverse effects and consequences. However, this should be a most exceptional decision. In practice, the parents' consent should almost always be sought. An obvious exception would be in an emergency, for example after a life-threatening head injury. Difficult decisions sometimes arise; for example, when the prescription of contraceptive drugs to a young girl is requested in circumstances where the young person does not wish her parents to know.

Appropriately informed

The point at which a patient can be considered to be appropriately informed is a matter of judgement. Some patients make it clear that they do not wish long and involved discussion, but others are comfortable with the process only when very full explanations have been given. It is often necessary to strike a balance. It is easy to frighten a patient to such an extent by recitation of unwelcome, but rare, possible complications of a procedure that they refuse treatment. This should not be the objective of discussing treatment. If a procedure is so risky that the doctor feels it is not justified, i.e. it is futile, the patient should be advised accordingly rather than being asked to decide for themselves.

Not under duress

This should be self-evident both to the patient and to the doctor. The patient should be given the opportunity to consider the matter after the initial discussion, if necessary. The personal, religious or social beliefs of the doctor must not be allowed to intrude. If this is likely, e.g. in the case of a doctor required to advise on therapeutic abortion, whose religious beliefs forbid this procedure, another doctor should be asked to take over the care of the patient. Remember that duress can arise unexpectedly. A patient may feel that he or she must embark on treatment in order to prevent stress at home. The right course here is to explore the nature of this stressful situation and take steps to alleviate it, in addition to considering medical treatment. Duress may be financial. There must be no financial advantage, constituting bribery or inducement, either to the patient or to the doctor in the management proposed. Political or social duress is an issue that has confronted physicians in many parts of the world in their relations with their patients, and constitutes a particularly difficult problem for an individual to resolve. It is clearly unethical.

Consent for research

Similar rules of conduct apply to the obtaining of consent for research, as for a patient's entry into a clinical trial of a new drug, and for teaching. It should be a condition of all research that the question addressed is relevant, and the protocol is capable of answering the question proposed. These are matters that are the special concern of the clinical investigators, and should have been checked, most thoroughly, by the Research Ethics Committee (see below).

Confidentiality

All aspects of the medical consultation are confidential. This common law duty is recognized by the public and is an essential part of the background to the consultation, since it allows the patient freedom of expression in the knowledge that disclosures made within the confines of the consulting room will not be made available to others. Indeed, in some aspects of medical practice, especially in treating sexually-transmitted diseases, and in much of psychiatric practice, confidentiality is fundamental.

The principle of confidentiality applies also to the medical records. These are held by the doctor, or the practice or, in the case of hospital records, by the hospital itself. Hospital records are not available to those other than the medical and nursing staff treating the patient, and are immune from police powers of search. They are made available, however, with the permission of the patient, and can be used in evidence in court in both civil and criminal cases, once disclosed. The principle of confidentiality of medical information was recognized by Hippocrates, and has been affirmed subsequently, even in modern times, for example, in the Declaration of Geneva of 1968. Although, in the modern hospital, medical information is far more widely available, through a number of different health professionals and administrators, the principle of confidentiality of the record must be strictly followed. In the UK, it is rigorously supported by the General Medical Council and its breach is regarded as a serious matter. In certain other European countries, for example in France, medical confidentiality is protected by the criminal code.

The situations in which confidentiality can be relaxed include:

- when the patient or his legal adviser allows it;
- when it is in the patient's interests;
- if there is an overriding duty to society as a whole;
- in cases of statutory disclosure;
- in certain situations where inspection of medical records is allowed; or
- sometimes after death.

With permission

A common example of relaxation of confidentiality with the patient's permission is when a doctor discusses the patient's problems or takes a history with others present, e.g. medical students or a nurse. The patient should be given the opportunity to ask that others leave.

In the patient's interests

When it is necessary that another family member be informed about the nature of a patient's illness, for example, in order to obtain information essential for effective treatment, it may be judged in the patient's best interests to break confidentiality. Another example might arise if a patient was judged mentally incompetent, and it became necessary to involve the patient's legal adviser to handle the patient's financial and legal affairs during a severe illness. This generally requires permission from a court.

An overriding duty to society

Occasionally confidentiality may be relaxed in the context of a known or possibly pending violent crime. In the case of illness, such as epilepsy or coronary heart disease that might impair the ability to control a vehicle, the responsibility to inform the authorities rests with the patient. In this instance, it is generally thought that it is in the interests of society to encourage voluntary disclosure, thus maintaining the principle of confidentiality between doctor and patient. The clinician does have discretion, however, to break this principle of confidentiality in circumstances entailing serious public risk.

Statutory disclosure

Confidentiality is breached in the case of certain infectious diseases, such as tuberculosis, that are 'notifiable' to the public health authorities. There is also a statutory duty for a doctor to help in the identification of a driver involved in a road traffic accident who, for example, might have attended a surgery or casualty department after the accident. The doctor in the witness box is in a state of privilege, and is protected against any action for breach of confidentiality when instructed by a court to disclose potentially confidential information. Similarly, a court can ask that medical documents be released to it if they are regarded as necessary for the completion of a fair trial of an accused person.

Inspection of medical records

In the UK the case notes themselves belong to the hospital, or the health authority, and not to the patient or to the doctor. Private patient notes belong to the doctor concerned. Patients themselves have a lawful right to inspect their own medical records, and can see any medical reports concerning their own medical condition that have been prepared before they are released to another party. Such medical reports can only be prepared with the permission of the patient, or at the request of a statutory body, as in the context of an order under the Mental Health Act, or in the jurisdiction of a recognized court. Generally, persons other than the patient have no right to inspect the medical records of an individual unless permission is given in writing by the patient, or the records are subject to a subpoena from a recognized court. The inspection of medical records for epidemiological purposes and for medical audit is currently allowed, since these activities are clearly necessary, but there is a need for distinct guidelines to be established relating to these activities in order to protect confidentiality.

This right of access by the patient clearly makes it important to write in the records only statements that can later be justified or defended. Value judgements about a patient are not matters for comment in medical records.

After death

Generally the principle of confidentiality should extend to patients who have died. In the cases of a number of deceased public figures of recent years, e.g. Winston Churchill and John F. Kennedy, this principle was not adhered to on the grounds that there were matters of public interest involved. Whether this was really the case the reader can decide.

Organ donation

When a tissue that can be replaced by the donor's own tissues, such as blood or bone marrow, is given to another patient no special ethical problem arises. When a living donor gives an irreplaceable organ, such as a kidney, difficulties arise. The donor must be of sound mind, not under duress, and must not be placed in a position to gain financially by the gift. In other words, the ordinary principles of consent apply. The sale of organs for transplantation is forbidden in all developed countries, and is rapidly becoming illegal in all countries. Similar considerations apply to the acquisition of donor organs from a minor, a practice about which it is particularly difficult to issue sound guidelines.

Because deceased persons have only limited rights over their organs, statutes have been introduced to regulate the practice of cadaver organ donation. This regulation is still evolving, and varies from country to country. In general, in the UK an organ can be removed from a deceased person if it is known that this was the wish of that person in life, whether for purposes of therapy, research or education, provided that the next of kin agrees. An organ can also be removed with the authorization of the next of kin, without knowledge of the deceased's wishes. However, this requirement has generally not led to the easy acquisition of organs such as kidneys for transplantation in the UK, since the next of kin are often distressed during the crucial and short period when it is possible to use cadaver organs for successful transplantation. In addition, the next of kin are often concerned to follow the supposed wishes of the deceased, or to contact other relatives for a decision and, by the time a decision is made it is too late. In some of the countries of the European Union there is a presumption that a deceased person would have wished to donate organs in the absence of any explicit statement to the contrary. However, this attitude is not general and it seems unlikely that it will become so, since clinicians are unlikely to take organs if they believe that this will cause distress among relatives. Voluntary schemes requiring a decision to consent to organ donation after death are generally preferred in most countries.

Certain religious constraints should be remembered. People of the Muslim faith are forbidden to accept organ donations from animals other than humans, and will not accept porcine products, e.g. pig valve grafts. However, porcine insulin is acceptable, since it consists of a product of the animal and not part of the organs of the animal. Donations of organs from a living patient, e.g. the gift of a kidney from a relative, may be subject to the agreement of two wise men from the community, in addition to the usual ethical procedures required by any hospital in the Western world.

Abortion and the rights of the fetus

The passage of the Abortion Act in the UK in 1967 marked a change in society's attitudes and, broadly, an acceptance by the medical profession of this change, illustrating that concepts of what is ethically acceptable change. None the less, there are still those who for religious or other reasons find the legality of abortion unacceptable. Abortion was forbidden in the Oath of Hippocrates.

Much of the current controversy concerns definition of the age of fetal viability. This has become a particular issue since fetal tissues have begun to be used in the treatment of certain diseases, and even as a source of ova for the management of infertility. Fetal viability is partly determined by medical science, and medical skill in keeping small premature babies alive, and partly by biological factors. If the age of viability becomes a matter for legal definition by statute, it must be recognized that this statute will need to change with advances in medical science. There is a long-standing difficulty in resolving the logical description of the appropriate medical behaviour when the rights of an unborn fetus are seen as in conflict with those of the mother herself.

The issue of viability, therefore, differs from the more philosophical issue of definition of the stage in development at which the fetus becomes a person, imbued with human characteristics, and subject to the same ethical considerations as a child or adult. This issue can be resolved on religious grounds, by defining, as does the Roman Catholic Church, the onset of human life as the moment of conception, or by recognizing the onset of fetal movement, or the external recognition of pregnancy. A simpler definition is that the fetus is invested with human status at the moment that independent existence begins, i.e. after birth. This approach, however, denies the fetus the ordinary ethical considerations of the right to life, or the protection from deliberate or negligent harm, that are accorded to persons, and therefore is likely to be rejected by many thoughtful observers. Because of the dependence of the fetus on its mother, the rights of the fetus are inevitably bound up with those of the pregnant woman.

In recent years there has been an emphasis on the rights of the fetus as a person-in-embryo. It is averred that the fetus has the same rights in common law and in society as a competent adult. In this approach the issue of medical viability becomes of less relevance, since the fetus has rights whether or not it is medically viable.

Resuscitation

Resuscitation is generally available in hospitals in the event that cardiopulmonary arrest occurs unexpectedly. However, this is not always successful, and many patients, recognizing the terminal nature of their illness may request that resuscitation not be attempted. This is an entirely valid request which should be respected once it is clear that the options are clearly understood by the patient.

Not for resuscitation

It sometimes happens that a patient is so seriously ill that there is doubt among medical and nursing attendants that it would be appropriate to resuscitate them in the event that they suffered a cardiac arrest. It should be recognized at the outset that this implies a judgement on the part of those charged with the responsibility of caring for the patient that, in some way, the patient's life is not worth saving. It should be asked whether any physician or surgeon is ever in a position to make such a judgement. Many would think that this is not a matter that one human should decide about another.

However, the question of whether or not resuscitation is to be attempted arises in clinical practice with increasing frequency, as medical technology becomes more complex and more effective, thus prolonging life into situations that would not occur but for the efforts of medical science. The situation most frequently arises when a patient has terminal cancer, and one of the medical or nursing team asks whether the 'crash team' should be called in the event the patient undergoes circulatory or ventilatory collapse. Resuscitation for a few hours or days of further pain and discomfort might be regarded as an unnecessary prolongation of the terminal illness.

The decision to withhold resuscitation is a matter for which it is proper always to seek the patient's full, informed consent. Indeed, the patient's views are paramount, and should be respected whatever the views of the clinicians, nurses or even the relatives. Relatives have no legal rights in a decision about possible resuscitation of another individual. While they may be consulted, and their views noted, they should not be allowed to influence a decision once made by an individual patient, unless it is decided that the patient is not competent by reason of dementia, or some other impairment of judgement, to come to a decision. Overt depression, for example, might be a reason for not accepting a patient's expressed wish not to be resuscitated.

Although it might be thought not helpful to a patient to discuss this issue openly, in fact the reverse is usually the case. Most patients near to death are aware of their situation and welcome the opportunity for full discussion of the issues. Indeed, it may give them the opportunity to discuss matters with their family in a more open manner than would otherwise be possible.

As a general matter of policy it is wise to involve the most senior clinician concerned with the patient's care in discussions about 'not for resuscitation'. Many large hospitals have a Resuscitation Officer, part of whose duties it is to review clinical decisions about resuscitation, since the resuscitation resource needs to be applied uniformly across the hospital, and not be more available to some patients than to others. In many hospitals policies for resuscitation and for withholding resuscitation, in consideration of the issues outlined above, have been agreed by medical and nursing staff. These should be sufficiently flexible to allow change with evolving medical technologies, and with increasing levels of knowledge and involvement of the general public in such issues. It should always be the case, of course, that a patient should be resuscitated when cardiopulmonary collapse is unexpected and the patient's wishes are unknown.

Ethics committees

The Ethics Committee in the UK is concerned with research. It will ascertain that proper arrangements exist for safeguarding the patient's interests at all times, especially with regard to consent and to the recognition of any possible risks associated with a research protocol. Confidentiality must be maintained, and this must include the security of any computer-held records. Research involving human subjects, whether patients or normal subjects, generated by medical staff, medical students, nurses and other paramedical staff is all properly within the remit of the Research Ethics Committee. No research is ethical that is not scientifically valid.

Particular care is required in considering research in the Intensive Care Unit, and in paediatric practice, because of the difficulties of ensuring that consent can adequately be established, and the level of dependence of the patients.

It is the role of the Research Ethics Committee to be impartial and authoritative. Research Ethics Committees in the UK are locally organized, and independent of local hospitals. The Research Ethics Committee functions as an autonomous committee of the health authority (the local component of the Department of Health). It consists of lay members, experienced researchers, and other relevant professionals who understand the wide variety of ethical and legal problems that can arise in research proposals involving human subjects. Research Ethics Committees insist that records related to research should be maintained in a state such that they are available to scrutiny by others for some years after the conclusion of the research, as part of the effort to prevent fraud in research. Adequate safeguards, and agreements for restitution for any harm inadvertently caused to a patient during participation in an approved research protocol, must be in place in the institution concerned. This will often involve an agreement with a sponsoring pharmaceutical company or other responsible organization. There are European and American guidelines and arrangements in force that cover these eventualities that must be adhered to as appropriate for the country concerned.

Review of a research protocol by the established local Research Ethics Committee is a requirement of the process of permission to commence a research protocol in Europe, and is a Federal legal requirement in the USA. Indeed, the results of any research not complying with these requirements is not acceptable to the new products licensing bodies in these two parts of the world. Similar rules pertain in many other countries.

Volunteers in research

Particularly stringent rules relate to the selection of volunteers for research who are not themselves patients. Volunteers, just as the patients and the investigators themselves, should not accept inducements to take part in research. Indeed, such inducements should not in any way form part of a research protocol, except insofar as provision is made to cover incidental expenses and inconvenience. Any financial interest that the investigator or the employing department may have must be clearly acknowl-

edged. Some agreed process of compensation for patients or volunteers in research programmes to whom harm is done, whether inadvertently or as a result of negligence, is a requirement for acceptance by the Research Ethics Committee. This usually involves the need for some form of insurance.

Other ethical problems

There are several other problems that arise in medical practice, several of which are likely to become more important in the coming years.

Medical negligence

Actions against doctors in the courts alleging medical negligence have become more common in many Western countries in recent years. Medical accidents, meaning inadvertent adverse events, are frequent in clinical practice, perhaps occurring in as many as 4% of all medical interventions. Few of these result in any legal action. An accusation of negligence often implies that a doctor–patient relationship has broken down. For the doctor such an action is distressing and sometimes professionally damaging even when shown to be unjustified.

In considering whether there has been negligence it is necessary to establish *causation, harm and breach of professional duty*. Breach of the responsibility of professional duty or care is addressed by asking whether the standard of care afforded the patient fell below that expected. The standard of care expected is that of the ordinary skilled practitioner in the field of expertise in question, practising in the circumstances pertaining. It is not that of the greatest expert in the land. Thus, in assessing possible negligence a court will need to establish what is the ordinary practice, that the doctor did not follow this practice, and that the doctor undertook a course of clinical management that no ordinarily skilled doctor in that specialty would have undertaken if acting with ordinary care.

A mistake in diagnosis is not necessarily negligent, and the test of the standard of care applicable to the ordinary practitioner in the specialty will be applied by the court in considering this. Doctors are expected to keep up to date in their expertise, and this is an aspect that is relevant to this judgement. Doctors in training are expected, by and large, to exercise an appropriate standard of care, and no patient should expect a lower standard of care simply because they are cared for by a junior doctor of less experience. This would clearly be wrong. It is imperative, therefore, that in treating a patient advice and help should be sought at all relevant times from senior colleagues.

Resource allocation

In every country, even the richest, there is a limitation on the availability of medical resources. The distribution of this resource is decided in different ways. In some countries it is decided by the capacity of any individual to pay for private medical care. In others it is made available more generally but to a level decided by the limits of the resource devoted to it by a benevolent, or otherwise, government. The doctor, therefore, is often confronted by a limitation on the capacity to offer a treatment, for one or other of a number of possible reasons.

Since the doctor's responsibility is always first to his or her patient, as an individual, and not to that group of potential patients in the general population that have not yet presented for treatment, this potential limitation of resource is relevant only in the general context of the politics of resource allocation for medicine. The individual patient's rights and the doctor's responsibilities in this matter are clear. The duty to the individual must always take precedence, and every effort must always be made to treat each patient to the best of the doctor's ability and in the best interests of the patient, utilizing such resources that are available from whatever source.

Notwithstanding this duty of care to the individual patient, the doctor does have a duty to society to improve treatments whenever possible, and to make as widely available as possible treatments to those that will benefit from them. Currently, much effort is being expended in trying to establish methods for measurement of benefit in relation to treatments, in order that resource allocation decisions, themselves a problem in medical economics rather than in medical ethics, can more rationally be formulated.

HIV

Testing for HIV requires the consent of the patient or individual. It is usual to counsel the individual before testing, since there are implications for lifestyle, future health, and even employment hinging on the result of the test. Life insurance companies usually require HIV testing only for large insured liabilities.

Genetics

The rapidly evolving availability of relatively accurate genetic testing for susceptibility to inherited diseases, based on the modern understanding of DNA and the genetic code, has raised a number of ethical problems for which most societies are not well prepared. For example:

- Who should have genetic tests done?
- What should be done with the results?
- Who should have access to the information other than the patient, if anyone?
- How should expensive treatments that may be possible for genetically determined disorders be made available?
- Is it socially and economically appropriate to prevent these disorders?

Genetic counselling

Genetic counselling is relatively long-established. The clinical geneticist will usually be asked to assess the risks of genetically determined disease in the context of a known familial occurrence of a disease, e.g. Down's syndrome, Duchenne muscular dystrophy, or cystic fibrosis. There is knowledge about the genetic causation of each of these conditions, and certain tests with probabilities of accuracy are available in assessing the risk for individuals in a family, and for the risk that a planned pregnancy might result in an affected offspring. Major difficulties arise in deciding whether to tell a person, shown by genetic testing to be certain to develop a disease in later life, e.g. Huntington's disease. Such decisions should ideally be made before testing is undertaken at all. Even when offering counselling about the risks for planned pregnancies similar difficulties arise. The social costs in terms of unresolved problems to individuals and their families of offering treatment or prevention for genetic disorders are largely undetermined at this time. Practice in this context will change as knowledge and experience accumulate.

Life insurance and genetic information

There has been concern about the implications of genetic knowledge for life insurance, a problem that is similar to that related to occult HIV infection. The knowledgeable, affected person might obtain insurance knowing of their own risk, thus selecting against the insurance company. Life insurance is a business, and not a form of social security. Clearly it is in the best interests of the insurance company, which has a responsibility toward all its insured clients, to have knowledge of all relevant medical problems affecting a client in order that an appropriate risk can be assigned to an individual policy. However, this concept may need adjustment in the light of the new genetics. It remains the case, of course, that information about an individual should never be divulged to an insurance company, or to any other organization, without the written permission of the individual, and only after the implications have been discussed with the person.

Principles of medical ethics

Several modern attempts have been made to encapsulate the principles of ethical medical behaviour in a series of simple statements. The *Declaration of Geneva* (Box 21.1) represents a modern attempt to restate the Hippocratic Oath in terms acceptable to contemporary students and medical practitioners. *The International Code of Medical Ethics* (Box 21.2)

BOX 21.1 Declaration of Geneva propounded by the World Medical Association, in Sydney (1968).

On admittance to the medical profession:

1 I will solemnly pledge myself to consecrate my life to the service of humanity
2 I will give my teachers the respect and gratitude which is their due
3 I will practise my profession with conscience and dignity
4 The health of my patients will be my first consideration
5 I will respect secrets that have been confided in me, even after the patient has died
6 I will maintain by all the means in my power the honour and noble traditions of the medical profession
7 My colleagues will be my brothers
8 I will not permit considerations of religion, nationality, race, party politics or social standing to intervene between my duty and my patient
9 I will maintain the utmost respect for human life from the time of conception. Even under threat I will not use my medical knowledge contrary to the laws of humanity
10 I make these promises solemnly, freely and upon my honour.

BOX 21.2 International Code of Medical Ethics.

Duties of doctors in general
- To maintain the highest standards of professional conduct
- To practise uninfluenced by motives of profit
- To use caution in divulging discoveries or new techniques of treatment
- To certify or testify only those matters with which the doctor has personal experience
- To ensure that any act or advice that could weaken physical or mental resistance of an individual must be used only in the interest of that individual.

The following are unethical practices
- Any self-advertisement except as expressly authorized in a national code of ethics
- Collaboration in any form of medical service in which the doctor does not have professional independence
- Receipt of any money in connection with services rendered to a patient other than a proper professional fee, even if the patient is aware of it.

Duties of doctors to the sick
- Always remember the obligation of preserving life
- The patient is owed complete loyalty, and all the resources of medical science. Whenever a treatment or examination is beyond the capacity of the doctor, the advice of another doctor should be sought
- A doctor must always preserve absolute secrecy concerning all he knows about a patient, because of the confidence trusted in him
- Emergency care is a humanitarian duty which must be given, unless it is clear that there are others better able to give it.

Duties of doctors to each other
- A doctor must behave to his colleagues as he would have them behave toward him
- A doctor must not entice patients from his colleagues
- A doctor must observe the principles of the Declaration of Geneva.

---

was derived from these principles, and restates them in more direct terms. The *Declaration of Helsinki* (1975) sets out recommendations for the guidance of doctors wishing to undertake biomedical research involving human subjects. The recommendations of the Declaration of Helsinki are generally recognized as relevant to the design of research protocols.

The problems raised by the interaction of modern medical practice with government and with society as a whole are important, and will require much thought and analysis in the future. This chapter cannot pretend to raise all the issues, but should be taken as an introduction to what should be a daily consideration, both in learning about, and in practising medicine.

Index